Frontiers of COVID-19

Sasan Adibi • Paul Griffin
Melvin Sanicas • Maryam Rashidi
Francesco Lanfranchi
Editors

# Frontiers of COVID-19

## Scientific and Clinical Aspects of the Novel Coronavirus 2019

Springer

*Editors*
Sasan Adibi
School of Information Technology
Deakin University
Melbourne, VIC, Australia

Paul Griffin
School of Medicine
University of Queensland
Brisbane, QLD, Australia

Melvin Sanicas
Clinical - Vaccines
Clover Biopharmaceuticals
Zürich, Switzerland

Maryam Rashidi
Inflammation Division
Walter and Eliza Hall Institute of Medical Research
Melbourne, VIC, Australia

Francesco Lanfranchi
Department of Health Sciences (DISSAL)
University of Genoa
Genoa, Italy

ISBN 978-3-031-08044-9 ISBN 978-3-031-08045-6 (eBook)
https://doi.org/10.1007/978-3-031-08045-6



This Springer imprint is published by the registered company Springer Nature Switzerland AG
The registered company address is: Gewerbestrasse 11, 6330 Cham, Switzerland

# Introduction

We are in the midst of a major global pandemic and due to the critical interests, the global scientific community has been desperately seeking out new research and accurate information regarding coronavirus disease 2019 (COVID-19), a contagious viral disease caused by severe acute respiratory syndrome coronavirus 2 (SARS-CoV-2). With the first, second, and in some areas, third waves of the coronavirus pandemic, our knowledge and understanding of this disease have gradually been evolving, which has resulted in revising and oftentimes revising most of our earlier understanding of the dynamics of this virus. Furthermore, we are just at the turning point in the realization of the types of antibodies produced in infected patients and the associated limitations and challenges, which are shaping the global efforts towards the effective development of COVID-19 vaccines. Therefore, we believe the timing is right to have a more comprehensive and highly anticipated book on the recent and ongoing acquired knowledge on COVID-19 and a possible roadmap on how to move forward.

This book aims to present recent clinical manifestations and findings regarding COVID-19 and the roadmap and the prospect of living gracefully alongside COVID-19 along with the existence of this virus in our societies. This work comprises the following four parts:

1. History, Pathogenesis, and Epidemiologic Background of Coronavirus
2. Clinical Observations
3. Interventions and Treatments
4. Current Trends and Future Directions

# Part I: History, Epidemiologic Background and Pathogenesis of Coronavirus

## *Main Topics*

The first part contains introductory chapters presenting the history, pathogenesis, and epidemiology background of COVID-19.

### History of Coronaviruses

Novel Coronavirus (COVID-19) disease is a cascade of a family of contagious diseases, which was discovered in late 2019. The first class of illness was named the Severe Acute Respiratory Syndrome Coronavirus 2 (SARS-CoV-2), which gave rise to a number of related variants, leading to an ongoing pandemic, which has infected over 450 million people worldwide and caused over 6 million fatalities as of March 2022 (https://covid19.who.int/).

### Epidemiology and Demographics of COVID-19

The topic of SARS-CoV-2 genome relates to the importance of key encoded proteins essential for this virus to cause disease, and the diversity of SARS-CoV-2 variants that have so far emerged and their divergence from other coronaviruses.

### Pathogenesis of COVID-19

The mechanism of pathology and the pathogenesis of COVID-19 has now been illustrated by several studies. The SARS-CoV-2 spike protein binds with high affinity to the human angiotensin-converting enzyme 2, or ACE2 receptor, but it can also interact with other receptors and enzymes. Following viral infection, a plethora of subsequent molecular and cellular alterations occur in the host that have been implicated in the progression of the signs and symptoms observed in COVID-19 patients.

## *Chapters Included*

### Chapter 1: Surfaces as a Source for SARS-CoV-2 Transmission

This chapter discusses the role of contaminated surfaces as a potential source for SARS-CoV-2 transmission.

### Chapter 2: Humoral Immune Response in SARS-CoV-2 Infection and Its Therapeutic Relevance

This chapter covers topics such as production of antibodies secondary to SARS-CoV-2 infection, immunological memory to a future reinfection, and the role of antibodies in COVID-19.

### Chapter 3: SARS-CoV-2 Invasion and Pathogenesis of COVID-19: A Perspective of Viral Receptors, Bradykinin and Purinergic System

This chapter covers the role of bradykinin and kallikrein-kinin system in the pathological findings associated with COVID-19, the involvement of purinergic signaling on the modulation of inflammatory process generated by SARS-CoV-2 infection, and possible pharmacological approaches.

### Chapter 4: Genetics and Biological Characteristics of SARS-CoV-2

This chapter covers the SARS-CoV-2 genome and the diversity of SARS-CoV-2 variants and the divergence from other coronaviruses.

### Chapter 5: COVID-19 Impact on Host at Pathophysiological and Cellular Level

This chapter summarizes COVID-19-associated comorbidities, dysregulated inflammation as a key factor to worsening the disease conditions, and the important molecular pathways associated with SARS-CoV-2-associated inflammation.

### Chapter 6: Identification of the COVID-19 Droplet Deposition Path and Its Effects on the Human Respiratory Tract Before and After the Disease: A Scoping Novel Respiratory Mask Design

This chapter describes a well-verified real anatomical model simulating the passage of air in the human upper respiratory system, computed using high-quality Computer Tomography (CT) images, the Fluid-Structure Interaction (FSI) method, and the Discrete Phase Model (DPM) to assess the temporal and spatial motion of the deposition of virus-impregnated droplets in vitro in the upper respiratory system.

### Chapter 7: SARS-CoV-2 Variants: Impact of Spike Mutations on Vaccine and Therapeutic Strategies

This chapter discusses the SARS-CoV-2 variants, their characteristics, and the efficacy of vaccine and therapeutic interventions against these variants. It also summarizes the acquired genetic alterations that have accumulated in these variants and their impact on protein structure and antigenicity.

### Chapter 8: Global Biologic Characteristics of Variants of Concern and Variants of Interest of SARS-CoV-2

This chapter covers the identified variants of concerns (VOCs) and emerging variants of interest (VOIs), their biology, epidemiology, demographics, clinical manifestations, and clinical impact. It also highlights the importance of scale genomic surveillance to strengthen global health.

### Chapter 9: Emergence of COVID-19 Variants and Its Global Impact

This chapter covers the nomenclature of the SARS CoV-2 variants, VOCs and notable variants, reasons for emergence of SARS CoV-2 variants, and the public health impact of viral variants.

# Part II: Clinical Observations

## *Main Topics*

The second part covers clinical observations, including symptoms (respiratory, and gastrointestinal) and complications (neurological and cardiovascular) as well as diagnosis of COVID-19 illness.

### Respiratory Symptoms

COVID-19 is primarily a respiratory disease and is spread by small droplets from coughs and sneezes and reaches the respiratory tract. COVID-19 can affect the upper respiratory system (nose, sinuses, and throat) with flu-like symptoms and the lower respiratory system (airways and lungs) by causing cough with or without mucous or difficulty breathing. Runny nose, headache, fatigue, and sore throat are four fairly common signs in all COVID-19 patients. When infected with the Delta variant, sneezing, persistent cold, and loss of smell and taste are typical. With the Omicron variant, sneezing is common while loss of smell and taste are rare.

### Cardiovascular Complications

COVID-19 can cause a high level of inflammation that can trigger a strong immune response and induce hyperinflammation and blood clots. The blood clots can lead to stroke and heart attacks even in young and healthy people without comorbidities.

### Neurological Complications

Neurological symptoms appear in a significant portion of people hospitalized with COVID-19. These symptoms include loss of taste and smell, headaches, stroke, delirium, and brain inflammation. Evidence suggests that COVID-19 may harm the brain in different ways: attacks specific brain cells directly, reduces blood flow to brain tissue, or triggers production of immune molecules that can harm brain cells.

### Gastrointestinal Symptoms

In COVID-19 patients, gastrointestinal symptoms have been reported with variable onset and severity. Symptoms include anorexia, abdominal pain, diarrhea, nausea, vomiting together with respiratory symptoms. Evidence also shows acute hepatocellular injury, indicated by elevated liver enzymes (i.e., alanine aminotransferase, aspartate aminotransferase, gamma-glutamyl transferase).

### Psychological and Sociological Issues

Early on in the pandemic, COVID-19 patients reported an increase in panic attacks. Now, anxiety in patients is moving from panic to feeling anxious about the future. Increased anxiety caused by COVID-19 has been a factor in increasing eating disorder behaviors. Depression can be triggered when we have to isolate from others. The pandemic has also been reported to make obsessive-compulsive disorder (OCD) responses worse because the threat is no longer an unsubstantiated fear. As families quarantine in close quarters and spend more time together, the chances of marital and family conflicts increase.

## *Chapters Included*

### Chapter 10: Psychological Impacts of the COVID-19 Pandemic

This chapter focuses on the psychological impacts of the COVID-19 pandemic, where it begins with the acute effects of the pandemic in substantially increasing rates of psychological distress and symptoms of psychiatric disorders. At the end, this chapter concludes with the promise of coping and psychological adaptation strategies, drawing from evidence reported during prior pandemics as well as early data reported during the ongoing pandemic.

## Chapter 11: Spatial Epidemiology of COVID-19: Disease Risk, Prognosis, and Complications

This chapter covers the geographic, environmental, behavioral, genetic, and comorbidity differences that have influenced spatial dynamics of COVID-19 transmission and outcomes, regional and country-level hotspots, and factors that create COVID-19 hotspots.

## Chapter 12: Eye Disorders and Neuro-ophthalmic Manifestations

This chapter lists the ocular signs and symptoms among COVID-19 patients, ocular surface clinical presentation, retinal vessel alterations and choroid involvement, ocular motor cranial nerves palsy, and other neuro-ophthalmic manifestations in patients with COVID-19.

## Chapter 13: Evaluation and Management of Dysphagia During the COVID-19 Pandemic

This chapter discusses how a safe and reasonable dysphagia care pathway can be implemented in the context of the COVID-19 pandemic with an understanding of safety precautions, modifications of the investigation setup, and with the application of newer technologies.

## Chapter 14: Gastrointestinal Manifestations of COVID-19 and Inflammatory Bowel Disease in the COVID-19 Era: Clinical Overview and Updated Guidelines

This chapter summarizes the gastrointestinal manifestations associated with COVID-19 including the pathophysiology and molecular pathways, impact on the severity of the disease, and the importance of feco-oral route of infection and viral shedding.

## Chapter 15: Post COVID-19 Conditions: The New Challenge to Mankind

Post COVID-19 conditions have and will continue to have a major impact on the healthcare system in the upcoming years. This chapter covers cardiovascular complications and pulmonary embolism post-COVID and results of the first national survey in Bulgaria.

### Chapter 16: Association of Alpha 1 Antitrypsin Deficiency with COVID-19 Mortality Rate

This chapter summarizes what is known about Alpha 1 antitrypsin (A1AT) (encoded by SERPINA1 gene), an inhibitor of transmembrane protease serine 2 (TMPRSS2), the major host protease that enables entry of the SARS-CoV-2 into host cells by spike (S) protein priming. It outlines the role of A1AT in the prevention of the pathogenesis of COVID-19 and associated complications and its significant potential not only in predicting the susceptibility and prognosis but also in the anti-COVID therapeutic repertoire.

### Chapter 17: Social Cognition Approaches to Understanding and Changing COVID-19 Preventive Behaviors

This chapter provides an overview of the social cognition literature and interventions targeting key psychological constructs as means to adopt and maintain COVID-19 preventive behaviors. It also offers sample materials used in behavior change interventions based on social cognition theory, which could be applied across a broad range of COVID-19 preventive behaviors.

### Chapter 18: Neurological Complications of COVID-19

This chapter covers neurological manifestations and neurological complications of COVID-19 (Neuro-Covid) in order to increase awareness about current and potential emerging complications and to facilitate their early recognition and effective management.

### Chapter 19: The Impact of Covid-19 on Surgical Disease

This chapter summarizes wide ranging implications of COVID-19 for the practice of surgery including COVID-19-induced hypercoagulability that can affect surgical procedures, impact on trauma/acute care surgery and elective surgery, and perioperative effects of COVID-19.

## Part III: Interventions and Treatments

### *Main Topics*

The third part covers interventions and treatments of COVID-19, including oxygen and convalescent plasma therapies, antiviral agents, immune-modulating drugs, treatment of complications, vaccine and psychological interventions.

### Diagnosis of SARS-CoV-2 Infection

Diagnostic tests for SARS-CoV-2 use nucleic acid, antibody (serology), and protein-based detections. Nucleic Acid Amplification Tests (NAATs, such as Reverse Transcription—Polymerase Chain Reaction) and antigen tests are used as diagnostic tests to detect current infection with SARS-CoV-2. Antigen tests generally have similar specificity, but are less sensitive than most NAATs. Correct interpretation of results from antigen tests and confirmatory NAATs, when indicated, is crucial. Antibody tests are used to detect previous infection with SARS-CoV-2 and can aid in the diagnosis of multisystem inflammatory syndrome (MIS) in children (MIS-C) and adults (MIS-A).

### Current Treatments

Several drugs have been approved to treat the different stages of COVID-19, and the living WHO guideline [1] is continuously updated and practice recommendations are offered by the BMJ (https://www.bmj.com/content/370/bmj.m3379).

## *Chapters Included*

### Chapter 20: Pre-hospital Management of COVID-19: Looking for a Future Perspective

This chapter analyzes the most relevant findings confirmed by metanalyses or by randomized clinical trials (RCT), and hypothesizes their reproducibility in a pre-hospital setting. It outlines strategic pre-hospital guidelines for managing COVID-19 patients, including screening procedures and prognostic assessment, multidimensional investigations focused on both negative and positive predictors, treatment criteria, and protocols for adequate ventilation maintenance.

### Chapter 21: Biotechnological Strategies in the Intervention and Treatment of COVID-19

This chapter covers the repurposed known drugs against COVID-19, the first COVID-19 vaccines, natural products, bioactive substances, and vitamins that may have the potential to treat or improve the disease progression in COVID-19 patients.

### Chapter 22: Vitamin D: A Potential Prophylactic and Therapeutic Agent Against COVID-19

A common factor for progressive disease is a low-grade inflammation as seen in those with metabolic syndrome, diabetes, and cardiovascular diseases, to which micronutrient deficiencies such as vitamin D may contribute. This chapter examines the evidence supporting vitamin D's role in prophylaxis and therapeutic administration against SARS-CoV-2 infection and COVID-19.

## Part IV: Current Trends and Future Directions

## *Main Topics*

### Ongoing Clinical Trials for Treatment and Vaccination

"Finding more effective and accessible therapeutics for COVID-19 patients remains a critical need, and WHO is proud to lead this global effort," said Dr. Tedros Adhanom Ghebreyesus, WHO Director-General. The WHO developed the COVID-19 Solidarity Therapeutics Trial (https://www.who.int/emergencies/diseases/novel-coronavirus-2019/global-research-on-novel-coronavirus-2019-ncov/solidarity-clinical-trial-for-covid-19-treatments) to test potential therapies for COVID-19 with the aim of recruiting thousands of patients globally, with standardized data capture, a bigger sample size, and faster and more efficient sharing of study results.

### Future Directions for COVID-19 Management in Clinical Practice and Research

Several groups around the world are conducting research to know more about the post-acute and long-term phases of COVID-19 and to differentiate the direct consequences of SARS-CoV-2 infection from hospitalization and the procedures and treatments required for care of people with severe disease of any etiology.

### Post-COVID-19 or Long COVID

The World Health Organization (WHO) has developed a clinical case definition of post-COVID-19 or Long COVID [2]. It is also known as post-COVID-19 syndrome, post-acute sequelae of COVID-19 (PASC), or chronic COVID syndrome (CCS). According to the authors, post-COVID-19 "occurs in individuals with a history of probable or confirmed SARS CoV-2 infection, usually 3 months from the onset of COVID-19 with symptoms and that last for at least 2 months and cannot be explained by an alternative diagnosis. Common symptoms include fatigue, shortness of breath, cognitive dysfunction but also others and generally have an impact on everyday functioning." Research on post-COVID conditions is ongoing and likely to change rapidly with ongoing research.

## *Chapters Included*

### Chapter 23: Rational Repurposing of Drugs, Clinical Trial Candidates, and Natural Products for SARS-Cov-2 Therapy

This chapter covers the rationale for, and examples of, successful drug repurposing for COVID-19, SARS-CoV-2 molecular targets suitable for repurposing, computational methods for virtual screening, virtual screening results, and implications and promising leads.

### Chapter 24: In Silico Drug Repositioning for COVID-19: Progress and Challenges

This chapter discusses various computational drug repositioning strategies, the challenges to the correct interpretation of existing preclinical and clinical evidence, as well as the generation of new evidence related to drug repurposing.

### Chapter 25: Computationally Repurposed Natural Products Targeting SARS-CoV-2

This chapter summarizes the virtually screened natural products, such as alkaloids, sterols, peptides, polyphenols, and terpenoids, which showed antagonistic potential to host cell recognition, viral attachment and fusion through binding with various receptor-binding regions of SARS-CoV-2 spike protein for ACE2, GRP78, and NRP-1 as well as host cell transmembrane TMPRSS2.

### Chapter 26: Different Platforms, Immune Response Modulators, and Challenges in SARS-CoV-2 Vaccination

This chapter summarizes how the pandemic influenced vaccine development, the implications of the route of immunization and adjuvant's choice for vaccines, and some recommendations to consider for future pandemics.

### Chapter 27: SARS-CoV-2 Vaccine Against Virus: Mission (Im)possible

This chapter outlines the mutations in the viral spike protein and other parts of the virus, the implications for COVID vaccines, and gives suggestions on what the global community can do beyond vaccination, hygiene, and physical distancing.

### Chapter 28: COVID-19 Vaccines Authorized by Stringent Regulatory Authorities and Vaccine

This chapter discusses the different technologies used in vaccine development and the COVID-19 vaccines developed for each modality, the different vaccines that have been approved by any national regulatory authority and the publicly available data for these vaccines, and the knowledge gaps that need to be filled to understand the important questions like durability of protection, the need for a booster, and long-term safety and efficacy against emerging SARS-CoV-2 variants.

### Chapter 29: The Global Evolution of a Pandemic on Clinical Practice

This chapter summarizes the impact of the pandemic on clinical practice including regional variations in rural and urban populations, implications of backlog on hospital system recovery during the pandemic, the impact on providers and patients across many outpatient settings, employee screening protocols, use of personal protective equipment, bed allocation challenges, and reliance upon communication and social media for clinical updates.

### Chapter 30: Anticipated Long-Term Neurobehavioral Outcomes Following COVID-19

This chapter addresses the less familiar encephalopathic, dementia, and behavioral syndromes that will likely be observed as more research is conducted on COVID-19 and provides guidance for clinicians who will undoubtably encounter increased volumes of patients with residual post-COVID-19 neurobehavioral changes.

### Chapter 31: The Road Ahead

This chapter covers the path out of the current pandemic and the road to future directions regarding the next possible phases of COVID-19 and the long-term clinical effects of it for years to come.

## References

1. Agarwal A, Rochwerg B, Lamontagne F, Siemieniuk RA, Agoritsas T, Askie L, Lytvyn L, Leo YS, Macdonald H, Zeng L, Amin W, Barragan F, Bausch FJ, Burhan E, Calfee CS, Cecconi M, Chanda D, Dat VQ, De Sutter A, Du B, et al. A living WHO guideline on drugs for covid-19. BMJ. 2020;370:m3379. https://doi.org/10.1136/bmj.m3379
2. Soriano JB, Murthy S, Marshall JC, Relan P, Diaz JV; WHO Clinical Case Definition Working Group on Post-COVID-19 Condition. A clinical case definition of post-COVID-19 condition by a Delphi consensus. Lancet. 2022;22(4):e102–e107. https://doi.org/10.1016/S1473-3099(21)00703-9

# Contents

# Part I
# History, Epidemiologic Background and Pathogenesis of Coronavirus

# Chapter 1
# Surfaces as a Source for SARS-CoV-2 Transmission

**Günter Kampf**

## Introduction

The role of contaminated surfaces as potential source for SARS-CoV-2 transmission has not been clear at the beginning of the pandemic. In the meantime, however, a lot of research has been performed, resulting in a better understanding of the relevance of surfaces contaminated with SARS-CoV-2.

## Persistence of Infectious SARS-CoV-2 on Surfaces

The persistence of infectious SARS-CoV-2 on inanimate surfaces under laboratory conditions has been described for various materials. In Table 1.1, data are summarized that were obtained at room temperature. On stainless steel, SARS-CoV-2 was mostly below the detection limit after up to 7 days. Similar results were described for plastic, glass, bank notes, paper, Tyvek, nitrile, rubber, polypropylene, metal, and a disposable gown. Persistence was shorter on copper (1 h to >2 days), vinyl (12–24 h), silver (>2 days), and laminate (8 h). In the dark, the virus could not be detected anymore after 4 weeks on different materials.

A higher temperature such as 30 °C or 40 °C and a higher relative air humidity results in a shorter persistence whereas a lower temperature such as 4 °C results in a longer persistence on surfaces [5, 11, 13, 15, 16] although no major differences in persistence were described at 4 °C, 20 °C, and 30 °C in one study [14]. Higher

G. Kampf (✉)
University Medicine Greifswald, Greifswald, Germany
e-mail: guenter.kampf@uni-greifswald.de


S. Adibi et al. (eds.), *Frontiers of COVID-19*,
https://doi.org/10.1007/978-3-031-08045-6_1

**Table 1.1** Persistence of infectious SARS-CoV-2 on different surfaces at room temperature

| Material | SARS-CoV-2 strain | Initial viral load | Below detection limit after | References |
|---|---|---|---|---|
| Stainless steel | Strain USA-WA1/2020 | $10^{4}$ [a] | 12 h | [1] |
| | Strain nCoV-WA1-2020 | $10^{3}$–$10^{4}$ [b] | 2 days | [2] |
| | Strains hCoV-19/Germany/BY-Bochum-1/2020 (B.1.1.70), VOC B.1.1.7 RKI-0026_B.1.1.7 and VOC B.1351 RKI-0029_B.1.351 | $10^{6}$ [b] | >2 days | [3] |
| | SARS-CoV-2 patient strain | $10^{4}$–$10^{5}$ [b] | 3 days | [4] |
| | Strain USA-WA1/2020 | $10^{4}$ [c] | 4 days | [5] |
| | Variant England 02/2020 HCM/V/052, isolate/England/MIG457/2020 (lineage B.1.1.7), isolate/England/H204661641/2020 (lineage B.1.351) | $10^{4}$–$10^{5}$ [a] | 7 days | [6] |
| | Isolate England 02/2020 (EPI_ISL_407073) | $10^{5}$ [a] | 7 days | [7] |
| | Strains hCoV-19/Germany/BY-Bochum-1/2020 (B.1.1.70) and RKI-0026_B.1.1.7 | $10^{6}$ [b] | 7 days | [8] |
| | Strain BetaCoV/Beijing/AMMS01/2020 | $10^{5}$–$10^{6}$ [b] | >7 days | [9] |
| | Strain CoV-19/Canada/ON-VIDO-01/2020 | $10^{6}$ [a] | >14 days | [10] |
| | Strain Australia/SA01/2020 | $10^{6}$ [b] | 28 days [d] | [11] |
| Plastic | Strain nCoV-WA1-2020 | $10^{3}$–$10^{4}$ [b] | 4 days | [2] |
| | SARS-CoV-2 patient strain | $10^{4}$–$10^{5}$ [b] | 5 days | [4] |
| | Isolate SARS-CoV-2/Finland/1/2020 | $10^{4}$–$10^{5}$ [a] | 6 days | [12] |
| | Strain BetaCoV/Beijing/AMMS01/2020 | $10^{5}$–$10^{6}$ [b] | >7 days | [9] |
| | Strain CoV-19/Canada/ON-VIDO-01/2020 | $10^{6}$ [a] | >21 days | [10] |
| Glass | Strain USA-WA1/2020 | $10^{4}$ [c] | 4 days | [5] |
| | SARS-CoV-2 patient strain | $10^{4}$–$10^{5}$ [b] | 5 days | [4] |
| | Strain HKU-001a | $10^{4}$–$10^{5}$ [c] | 5 days | [13] |
| | Strain BetaCoV/Beijing/AMMS01/2020 | $10^{5}$–$10^{6}$ [b] | >7 days | [9] |
| | Strain Australia/SA01/2020 | $10^{6}$ [b] | >28 days[d] | [11] |
| Bank note/paper | Strains hCoV-19/Germany/BY-Bochum-1/2020 (B.1.1.70) and RKI-0026_B.1.1.7 | $10^{6}$ [b] | 3 days | [8] |
| | Isolate England 02/2020 (EPI_ISL_407073) | $10^{5}$ [a] | 5 days | [7] |
| | Strain BetaCoV/Beijing/AMMS01/2020 | $10^{5}$–$10^{6}$ [b] | 5 days | [9] |
| | Strain Australia/SA01/2020 | $10^{6}$ [b] | 28 days [d] | [11] |
| Tyvek | Strain USA-WA1/2020 | $10^{4}$ [c] | 4 days | [5] |
| | Isolate England 02/2020 (EPI_ISL_407073) | $10^{5}$ [a] | 7 days | [7] |
| | Strain CoV-19/Canada/ON-VIDO-01/2020 | $10^{6}$ [a] | >14 days | [10] |

**Table 1.1** (continued)

| Material | SARS-CoV-2 strain | Initial viral load | Below detection limit after | References |
|---|---|---|---|---|
| Copper | Strains hCoV-19/Germany/ BY-Bochum-1/2020 (B.1.1.70) and RKI-0026_B.1.1.7 | $10^{6}$ [b] | 1 h | [8] |
| | Strain USA-WA1/2020 | $10^{4}$ [a] | 4 h | [1] |
| | Strain nCoV-WA1-2020 | $10^{3}$–$10^{4}$ [b] | 1 day | [2] |
| | Strains hCoV-19/Germany/ BY-Bochum-1/2020 (B.1.1.70), VOC B.1.1.7 RKI-0026_B.1.1.7 and VOC B.1351 RKI-0029_B.1.351 | $10^{6}$ [b] | >2 days | [3] |
| Nitrile glove | Strain USA-WA1/2020 | $10^{4}$ [c] | 5 days | [5] |
| | Strain CoV-19/Canada/ON-VIDO-01/2020 | $10^{6}$ [a] | >7 days | [10] |
| Vinyl | Strain USA-WA1/2020 | $10^{4}$ [a] | 12–24 h | [1] |
| | Strain Australia/SA01/2020 | $10^{6}$ [b] | >28 days [d] | [11] |
| Silver | Strains hCoV-19/Germany/ BY-Bochum-1/2020 (B.1.1.70), VOC B.1.1.7 RKI-0026_B.1.1.7 and VOC B.1351 RKI-0029_B.1.351 | $10^{6}$ [b] | >2 days | [3] |
| Laminate | Strain USA-WA1/2020 | $10^{4}$ [a] | 8 h | [1] |
| Ceramics | Strain BetaCoV/Beijing/AMMS01/2020 | $10^{5}$–$10^{6}$ [b] | 7 days | [9] |
| Wood | Strain BetaCoV/Beijing/AMMS01/2020 | $10^{5}$–$10^{6}$ [b] | >7 days | [9] |
| Rubber | Strain USA-WA1/2020 | $10^{4}$ [c] | 4 days | [5] |
| Polypropylene | Strain USA-WA1/2020 | $10^{4}$ [c] | 4 days | [5] |
| Metal | Strain SARS-CoV-2/ München-1.1/2020/929 | $10^{5}$ [b] | 6 days | [14] |
| Disposable gown | Isolate England 02/2020 (EPI_ISL_407073) | $10^{5}$ [a] | 7 days | [7] |

[a]PFU per coupon
[b]$TCID_{50}$ per mL
[c]$TCID_{50}$
[d]In darkness

temperatures have been described to lead to dramatic disruption of viral structural stability, especially when the heat is applied in the dry state [17]. It has been suggested that SARS-CoV-2 may be inactivated by dryness on water absorbent porous materials but sheltered by long-persisting microdroplets of water on waterproof surfaces [18].

The relevance of the rather long persistence on surfaces remains controversial. Viruses from respiratory secretions are embedded in mucus and saliva which probably contain specific antibodies against the virus, high numbers of leukocytes, and intrinsic antiviral activity because of its polyanionic charge which binds to viruses, as well as bacteria and fungi which may influence the environment around the virus

[19]. The applicability of the laboratory findings to real life is in addition doubtful for another reason. In the *in vitro* studies, a high load of infectious virus was typically applied to a small surface. The inoculum is therefore probably a lot higher than those in droplets in real-life situations. As a result, the amount of virus actually deposited on surfaces could be several orders of magnitude smaller [20].

Nevertheless, the findings obtained under laboratory conditions raised the concern that viral shedders in the public may contaminate frequent touch surfaces finally resulting in viral transmission via uncontrolled hand–face contacts. As a result, many public surfaces were subjected to disinfection, for example, in shops, museums, restaurants, public transportation, or sports facilities.

## Detection of Viral RNA on Surfaces

SARS-CoV-2 RNA has been described to be quite stable on surfaces with an average of one $\log_{10}$ reduction in genome copy recovery over 21 days [7]. Laboratory data with SARS-CoV-2 show that $C_t$ (cycle threshold) values of 29.3 (steel surface) or 29.5 (plastic surface) correlate with detection of culturable virus, whereas $C_t$ values of 32.5 (steel surface) or 32.7 (plastic surface) correlate with the detection of nonculturable virus [21].

### *Surrounding of Confirmed COVID-19 Patients in Health-Care Settings*

The presence of SARS-CoV-2 RNA was determined in samples obtained from surfaces in the surrounding of confirmed COVID-19 patients in health-care facilities where it is common practice to clean and disinfect surfaces in the immediate surrounding of patients regularly. That is why the surface treatment prior to sampling may well have influenced the SARS-CoV-2 RNA detection rates. In 32 of the studies, no specific information was available when the last cleaning or disinfection was done prior to sampling [21–51]. In eight studies sampling was done before the next scheduled surface cleaning or disinfection [30, 36, 52–57], and in two studies it was performed prior to cleaning with 1000 ppm sodium hypochlorite [58, 59]. In other studies surface sampling was performed at least 4 h after the last cleaning procedure [60, 61], within 4–7 h after the first daily cleaning [62], 7 h after cleaning and disinfection [63], at least 8 h after any cleaning procedure [64], before and after decontamination [65, 66], or after terminal disinfection [67].

Detection rates were mostly less than 30% (Fig. 1.1). The vast majority of $C_t$-values was at least 30, suggesting a low viral load and the absence of infectious SARS-CoV-2 [22, 23, 27, 30, 33–36, 38–40, 44, 46, 48, 52–54, 57, 63–66, 68].

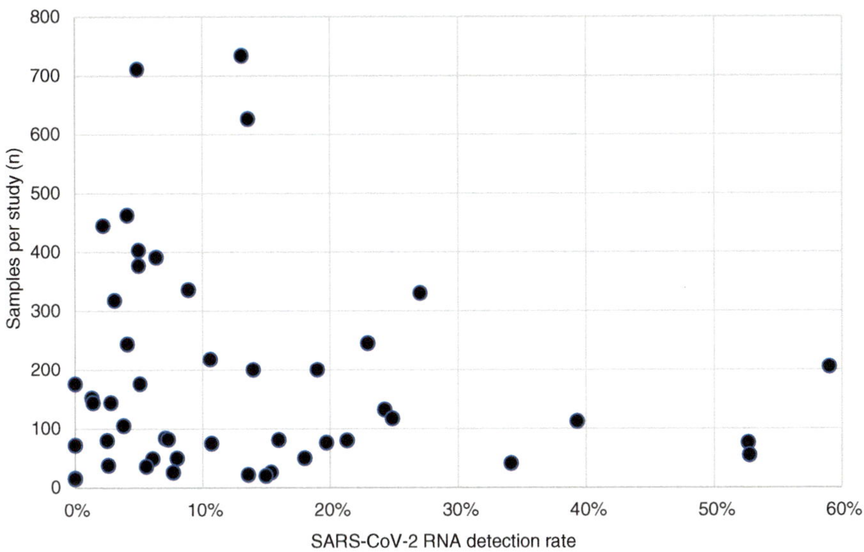


**Fig. 1.1** SARS-CoV-2 RNA detection rates on surfaces in the surrounding of confirmed COVID-19 patients in health care; [21–23, 25, 27, 29–49, 51–69]

## *Surrounding of COVID-19 Patients in Non-Health-Care Settings*

The settings were on a cruise ship during a COVID-19 outbreak [70], in rooms of COVID-19 patients [71], in COVID-19 quarantine hotels [72, 73], in domestic quarantine of COVID-19 cases [74–76], in a clinical microbiology laboratory testing for SARS-CoV-2 [77], in a nursing home during a COVID-19 outbreak [54], in a long-term care facility with 30 asymptomatic COVID-19 cases [54] and on a ferryboat during an ongoing COVID-19 outbreak investigation [54].

Samples were taken in some studies before any cleaning or disinfection procedure was carried out [54, 70, 72, 75]. In one study, however, 50% of the 428 samples were taken before the cleaning and disinfection, the other half was taken after the disinfection procedure [71]. No specific information regarding any prior treatment of surfaces was found in the remaining studies [73, 74, 76, 77].

The detection rate of SARS-CoV-2 RNA on surfaces was mostly between 0 and 20% of all samples (Fig. 1.2) with corresponding $C_t$ values mostly >30 suggesting a low viral load and the absence of infectious SARS-CoV-2 [54, 70, 72–74, 76, 77].

## *Public Surfaces*

Samples were collected from surfaces in various public settings such as public squares, universities, schools, parks, markets, shopping malls, stores, bank notes, water fountains and nozzles, often from high touch surfaces. The epidemiological

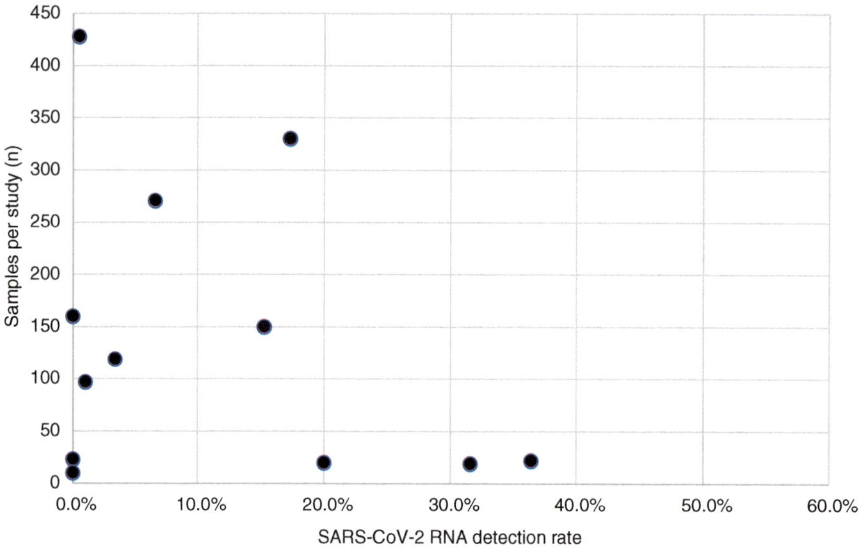


**Fig. 1.2** SARS-CoV-2 RNA detection rates on surfaces in the surrounding of confirmed COVID-19 patients in non-health-care settings [54, 70–77]

situation during the study period was not described in all studies. In Brazil, the study took place in one of the regions with the highest number of notified COVID-19 cases [22]. In the USA, sampling was carried out during a regional COVID-19 outbreak [78]. In Iran, sampling was done during the early stage of a local outbreak [79]. In Italy, surfaces were samples 2–3 months after the national epidemic peak [41] or in supermarkets during a COVID-19 lockdown [80]. In China, a store was chosen for sampling after it was found to be linked to the majority of new cases in the city of Tianjin [81].

The RNA detection rates were low with 0–22.1% (Fig. 1.3), the corresponding $C_t$ values were mostly >30, suggesting a low viral load and the absence of infectious SARS-CoV-2 [22, 78, 80, 81].

## Detection of Infectious SARS-CoV-2 on Surfaces

In some of the studies the investigators tried to detect infectious SARS-CoV-2 by cell culture. In 9 of the 11 studies infectious SARS-CoV-2 could not be detected by cell culture in any sample on surfaces. Only two studies provided evidence that infectious SARS-CoV-2 can be found in the immediate surrounding of COVID-19 patients with 0.7% and 10.5% of the samples being positive (Table 1.2). A major limitation of the results of one study, however, is that seven of eight positive samples were obtained in the surrounding of only one patient with persistent cough and

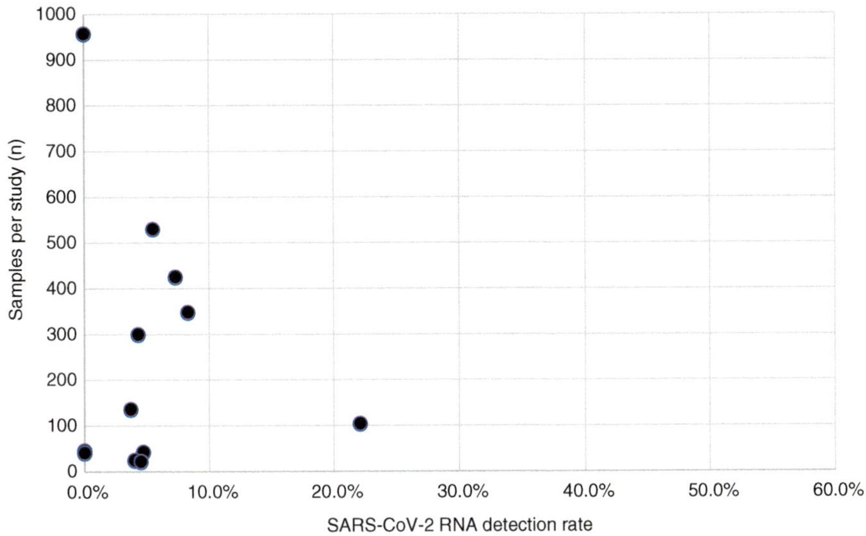


**Fig. 1.3** SARS-CoV-2 RNA detection rates on public surfaces [22, 28, 31, 41, 53, 78–86]

**Table 1.2** Detection rates of infectious SARS-CoV-2 and viral RNA on surfaces in health-care and other settings

| Setting (country) | Types of sampled surfaces (*n*) | Proportion of viral RNA detection (%) | Proportion of infectious SARS-CoV-2 detection (%) | References |
|---|---|---|---|---|
| Diamond princess cruise ship during COVID-19 outbreak (Japan) | Surfaces in cabins of confirmed cases (330) | 17.3 | 0 | [70] |
| | Surfaces of noncase cabins (160) | 0 | 0 | |
| | Surfaces in shared areas (97) | 1.0 | 0 | |
| COVID-19 cases in isolation at home (Germany) | Surfaces in 21 households (119) | 3.4 | 0 | [74] |
| Treatment rooms for COVID-19 patients (England) | High contact surfaces in patient rooms (336) | 8.9 | 0 | [38] |
| Teaching hospital with COVID-19 patients (UK) | Various surfaces in different parts of the hospital (218) | 10.6 | 0 | [21] |
| Households of COVID-19-cases (USA) | Various surfaces (150) | 15.3 | 0.7[a] | [76] |

(continued)

**Table 1.2** (continued)

| Setting (country) | Types of sampled surfaces (*n*) | Proportion of viral RNA detection (%) | Proportion of infectious SARS-CoV-2 detection (%) | References |
|---|---|---|---|---|
| Severe COVID-19-cases in isolation rooms (Republic of Korea) | Surrounding of three patients (76) | 19.7 | 10.5[b] | [68] |
| COVID-19 ICU (Singapore) | Various surfaces in common areas and staff pantry (75) | 10.7 | 0 | [39] |
| COVID-19 isolation unit (Israel) | Various surfaces (55) | 52.7 | 0 | [23] |
| COVID-19 isolation ward (China) | Various surfaces (50) | 8.0 | 0 | [46] |
| COVID-19 isolation ward (Iran) | Various surfaces (50) | 18.0 | 0 | [27] |
| COVID-19 cases in hospitals (Italy) | Various surfaces (26) | 7.7 | 0 | [60] |

[a]Detected on nightstand of index case (corresponding $C_t$-value: 26.4

[b]7 of 8 positive samples obtained in the surrounding of one patient with persistent cough and frequent sputum spitting during sampling

frequent sputum spitting during sampling. It seems therefore likely that swab contamination mostly occurred by cough droplets and sputum.

Similar results were found with other respiratory tract viruses. In hospitals, SARS-CoV-1 RNA could be detected in 5.6% of 85 samples and 27.7% of 94 samples, but cell cultures for infectious SARS-CoV-1 remained all negative [87, 88]. The RNA of H1N1 influenza-A-virus could be found on surfaces of 17.8% from 90 households with confirmed infections in children, but all cell cultures were negative [89]. MERS-CoV RNA was found on surfaces of an isolation ward in 20.3% of the samples, infectious MERS-CoV was isolated in 4.1% of all samples [90]. That is why surfaces were not considered to be a relevant source of SARS-CoV-2 transmission.

The relative decline of viral infectivity on surfaces has been described to be similar with higher and lower initial viral loads. Expected levels of SARS-CoV-2 viable environmental surface contamination would therefore lead to undetectable levels within 2 days [7].

## Probability of Surfaces to Be the Source for SARS-CoV-2 Transmission

A transmission from surfaces may occur via transiently contaminated hands, for example, after contact to a surface contaminated with infectious virus and followed by a hand–nose or hand–mouth contact. Several studies have analyzed the likelihood of fomite transmission for respiratory viruses. One study highlighted the importance of aerosols for rhinovirus transmission, in contrast to a neglectable role for surfaces. In this study, two groups of men played poker, one group was sick with the common cold, the other group was healthy. The healthy group was exposed to infectious virus aerosols simply by being in the same room with the sick group. But they were restrained so that participants could not touch their faces. Cards and chips used in the poker game were transferred to a group of healthy men to play with, and they were instructed to touch their faces frequently. Interestingly, the aerosol-exposed group got sick, while the surfaces-exposed group did not [91]. In another study it was found that only a small fraction of infectious virus is usually found on hands after contact with artificially contaminated surfaces such as 0.1–16% after drying of a high initial viral load of SARS-CoV-2 [8], 1.5% with parainfluenza virus and 0.7% with rhinovirus [92]. In addition, only a small fraction of the viral load can be transferred from contaminated hands to an inanimate surface (0% with human coronaviruses, 0% with parainfluenza virus and 0.9% with rhinovirus) unless the coronavirus is presented in organic load such as feces resulting in 0–16.7% virus transfer [92, 93]. The risk of disease transmission by a hand contact with a contaminated surface followed by a single hand–nose contact is very low and has been described for rhinovirus (0.0486%) and for influenza virus (0.0000000256%) [94]. For SARS-CoV-2 it would need at least 1000 infectious viruses dropped on the mucosa [95] which is very unlikely considering the expectable loss during transfer. House flies have been described to harbor infectious SARS-CoV-2 under laboratory conditions for up to 24 h [96]. Infectious SARS-CoV-2, however, could not be detected on the surrounding surfaces after 4 and 24 h, only SARS-CoV-2 RNA. It is therefore very unlikely that house flies contribute to viral transmission via transiently contaminated surfaces. Seasonality of respiratory tract virus transmission should be considered when interpreting these results. Some factors including humidity can directly influence aerosol stability. Under tropic conditions (warm and humid climates) aerosols or droplets evaporate less water, therefore readily settle on surfaces, which could favor fomite transmission as hypothesized for influenza viruses [97].

Overall, the probability of surfaces to be the source of SARS-CoV-2 transmission is low, especially for public surfaces (Fig. 1.4).

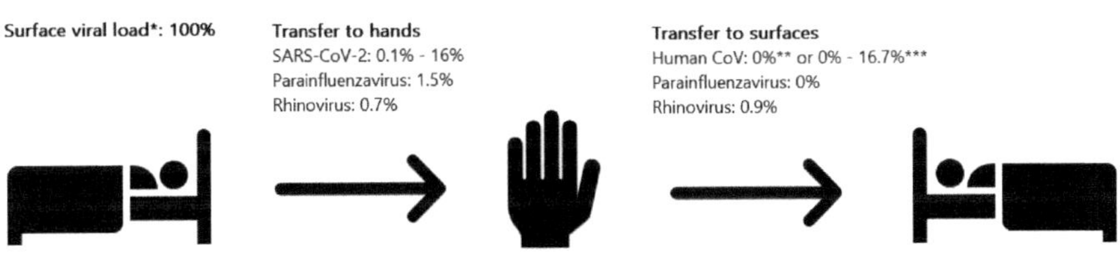


**Fig. 1.4** Transfer probability of infectious respiratory tract viruses including SARS-CoV-2 from surfaces via direct contact (only data available for inanimate surfaces as target for transfer from hands) [8, 92, 93]; *assumed baseline viral load; **no organic load; ***in the presence of organic load (faeces)

## References


1. Ronca SE, Sturdivant RX, Barr KL, Harris D. SARS-CoV-2 viability on 16 common indoor surface finish materials. HERD. 2021;14(3):49–64. https://doi.org/10.1177/1937586721991535.
2. van Doremalen N, Bushmaker T, Morris DH, Holbrook MG, Gamble A, Williamson BN, Tamin A, Harcourt JL, Thornburg NJ, Gerber SI, Lloyd-Smith JO, de Wit E, Munster VJ. Aerosol and surface stability of SARS-CoV-2 as compared with SARS-CoV-1. N Engl J Med. 2020;382(16):1564–7. https://doi.org/10.1056/NEJMc2004973.
3. Meister TL, Fortmann J, Todt D, Heinen N, Ludwig A, Brüggemann Y, Elsner C, Dittmer U, Steinmann J, Pfaender S, Steinmann E. Comparable environmental stability and disinfection profiles of the currently circulating SARS-CoV-2 variants of concern B.1.1.7 and B.1.351. J Infect Dis. 2021;224(3):420–4. https://doi.org/10.1093/infdis/jiab260.
4. Gidari A, Sabbatini S, Bastianelli S, Pierucci S, Busti C, Bartolini D, Stabile AM, Monari C, Galli F, Rende M, Cruciani G, Francisci D. SARS-CoV-2 survival on surfaces and the effect of UV-C light. Viruses. 2021;13(3):408. https://doi.org/10.3390/v13030408.
5. Kwon T, Gaudreault NN, Richt JA. Environmental stability of SARS-CoV-2 on different types of surfaces under indoor and seasonal climate conditions. Pathogens. 2021;10(2):227. https://doi.org/10.3390/pathogens10020227.
6. Pottage T, Garratt I, Onianwa O, Spencer A, Paton S, Dunning J, Bennett A. A comparison of persistence of SARS-CoV-2 variants on stainless steel. J Hosp Infect. 2021;114:163–6. https://doi.org/10.1016/j.jhin.2021.05.015.
7. Paton S, Spencer A, Garratt I, Thompson KA, Dinesh I, Aranega-Bou P, Stevenson D, Clark S, Dunning J, Bennett A, Pottage T. Persistence of SARS-CoV-2 virus and viral RNA in relation to surface type and contamination concentration. Appl Environ Microbiol. 2021;87(14):e0052621. https://doi.org/10.1128/aem.00526-21.
8. Todt D, Meister TL, Tamele B, Howes J, Paulmann D, Becker B, Brill FH, Wind M, Schijven J, Heinen N, Kinast V, Mhlekude B, Goffinet C, Krawczyk A, Steinmann J, Pfaender S, Brüggemann Y, Steinmann E. A realistic transfer method reveals low risk of SARS-CoV-2 transmission via contaminated euro coins and banknotes. iScience. 2021;24(8):102908. https://doi.org/10.1016/j.isci.2021.102908.
9. Liu Y, Li T, Deng Y, Liu S, Zhang D, Li H, Wang X, Jia L, Han J, Bei Z, Li L, Li J. Stability of SARS-CoV-2 on environmental surfaces and in human excreta. J Hosp Infect. 2021;107(1):105–7. https://doi.org/10.1016/j.jhin.2020.10.021.
10. Kasloff SB, Leung A, Strong JE, Funk D, Cutts T. Stability of SARS-CoV-2 on critical personal protective equipment. Sci Rep. 2021;11(1):984. https://doi.org/10.1038/s41598-020-80098-3.
11. Riddell S, Goldie S, Hill A, Eagles D, Drew TW. The effect of temperature on persistence of SARS-CoV-2 on common surfaces. Virol J. 2020;17(1):145. https://doi.org/10.1186/s12985-020-01418-7.
12. Virtanen J, Aaltonen K, Kivistö I, Sironen T. Survival of SARS-CoV-2 on clothing materials. Adv Virol. 2021;2021:6623409. https://doi.org/10.1155/2021/6623409.
13. Chan KH, Sridhar S, Zhang RR, Chu H, Fung AY, Chan G, Chan JF, To KK, Hung IF, Cheng VC, Yuen KY. Factors affecting stability and infectivity of SARS-CoV-2. J Hosp Infect. 2020;106(2):226–31. https://doi.org/10.1016/j.jhin.2020.07.009.
14. Kratzel A, Steiner S, Todt D, V'Kovski P, Brueggemann Y, Steinmann J, Steinmann E, Thiel V, Pfaender S. Temperature-dependent surface stability of SARS-CoV-2. J Infect. 2020;81(3):474–6. https://doi.org/10.1016/j.jinf.2020.05.074.
15. Biryukov J, Boydston JA, Dunning RA, Yeager JJ, Wood S, Reese AL, Ferris A, Miller D, Weaver W, Zeitouni NE, Phillips A, Freeburger D, Hooper I, Ratnesar-Shumate S, Yolitz J, Krause M, Williams G, Dawson DG, Herzog A, Dabisch P, Wahl V, Hevey MC, Altamura LA. Increasing temperature and relative humidity accelerates inactivation of SARS-CoV-2 on surfaces. mSphere. 2020;5(4):00441-20. https://doi.org/10.1128/mSphere.00441-20.
16. Morris DH, Yinda KC, Gamble A, Rossine FW, Huang Q, Bushmaker T, Fischer RJ, Matson MJ, Van Doremalen N, Vikesland PJ, Marr LC, Munster VJ, Lloyd-Smith JO. Mechanistic

theory predicts the effects of temperature and humidity on inactivation of SARS-CoV-2 and other enveloped viruses. Elife. 2021;10:e65902.

17. Sharma A, Preece B, Swann H, Fan X, McKenney RJ, Ori-McKenney KM, Saffarian S, Vershinin MD. Structural stability of SARS-CoV-2 virus like particles degrades with temperature. Biochem Biophys Res Commun. 2021;534:343–6. https://doi.org/10.1016/j.bbrc.2020.11.080.
18. Corpet DE. Why does SARS-CoV-2 survive longer on plastic than on paper? Med Hypotheses. 2021;146:110429. https://doi.org/10.1016/j.mehy.2020.110429.
19. Eccles R. Respiratory mucus and persistence of virus on surfaces. J Hosp Infect. 2020;105(2):350. https://doi.org/10.1016/j.jhin.2020.03.026.
20. Goldman E. Exaggerated risk of transmission of COVID-19 by fomites. Lancet Infect Dis. 2020;20(8):892–3. https://doi.org/10.1016/s1473-3099(20)30561-2.
21. Zhou J, Otter JA, Price JR, Cimpeanu C, Garcia DM, Kinross J, Boshier PR, Mason S, Bolt F, Holmes AH, Barclay WS. Investigating SARS-CoV-2 surface and air contamination in an acute healthcare setting during the peak of the COVID-19 pandemic in London. Clin Infect Dis. 2021;73(7):e1870–7. https://doi.org/10.1093/cid/ciaa905.
22. Abrahão JS, Sacchetto L, Rezende IM, Rodrigues RAL, Crispim APC, Moura C, Mendonça DC, Reis E, Souza F, Oliveira GFG, Domingos I, de Miranda Boratto PV, Silva PHB, Queiroz VF, Machado TB, Andrade LAF, Lourenço KL, Silva T, Oliveira GP, de Souza AV, Alves PA, Kroon EG, de Souza TG, Drumond BP. Detection of SARS-CoV-2 RNA on public surfaces in a densely populated urban area of Brazil: a potential tool for monitoring the circulation of infected patients. Sci Total Environ. 2021;766:142645. https://doi.org/10.1016/j.scitotenv.2020.142645.
23. Ben-Shmuel A, Brosh-Nissimov T, Glinert I, Bar-David E, Sittner A, Poni R, Cohen R, Achdout H, Tamir H, Yahalom-Ronen Y, Politi B, Melamed S, Vitner E, Cherry L, Israeli O, Beth-Din A, Paran N, Israely T, Yitzhaki S, Levy H, Weiss S. Detection and infectivity potential of severe acute respiratory syndrome coronavirus 2 (SARS-CoV-2) environmental contamination in isolation units and quarantine facilities. Clin Microbiol Infect. 2020;26(12):1658–62. https://doi.org/10.1016/j.cmi.2020.09.004.
24. Cheng VCC, Wong SC, Chen JHK, Yip CCY, Chuang VWM, Tsang OTY, Sridhar S, Chan JFW, Ho PL, Yuen KY. Escalating infection control response to the rapidly evolving epidemiology of the coronavirus disease 2019 (COVID-19) due to SARS-CoV-2 in Hong Kong. Infect Control Hosp Epidemiol. 2020;41(5):493–8. https://doi.org/10.1017/ice.2020.58.
25. Chia PY, Coleman KK, Tan YK, Ong SWX, Gum M, Lau SK, Lim XF, Lim AS, Sutjipto S, Lee PH, Son TT, Young BE, Milton DK, Gray GC, Schuster S, Barkham T, De PP, Vasoo S, Chan M, Ang BSP, Tan BH, Leo YS, Ng OT, Wong MSY, Marimuthu K. Detection of air and surface contamination by SARS-CoV-2 in hospital rooms of infected patients. Nat Commun. 2020;11(1):2800. https://doi.org/10.1038/s41467-020-16670-2.
26. Colaneri M, Seminari E, Piralla A, Zuccaro V, Filippo AD, Baldanti F, Bruno R, Mondelli MU. Lack of SARS-CoV-2 RNA environmental contamination in a tertiary referral hospital for infectious diseases in Northern Italy. J Hosp Infect. 2020;105(3):474–6. https://doi.org/10.1016/j.jhin.2020.03.018.
27. Dargahi A, Jeddi F, Vosoughi M, Karami C, Hadisi A, Ahamad Mokhtari S, Ghobadi H, Alighadri M, Haghighi SB, Sadeghi H. Investigation of SARS CoV-2 virus in environmental surface. Environ Res. 2021;195:110765. https://doi.org/10.1016/j.envres.2021.110765.
28. Elbadawy HM, Khattab A, Alalawi A, Dakilallah Aljohani F, Sundogji H, Mahmoud AS, Abouzied M, Eltahir HM, Alahmadey Z, Bahashwan S, Suliman BA. The detection of SARS-CoV-2 in outpatient clinics and public facilities during the COVID-19 pandemic. J Med Virol. 2021;93(5):2955–61. https://doi.org/10.1002/jmv.26819.
29. Escudero D, Boga JA, Fernández J, Forcelledo L, Balboa S, Albillos R, Astola I, García-Prieto E, Álvarez-Argüelles ME, Martín G, Jiménez J, Vázquez F. SARS-CoV-2 analysis on environmental surfaces collected in an intensive care unit: keeping Ernest Shackleton's spirit. Intensive Care Med Exp. 2020;8(1):68. https://doi.org/10.1186/s40635-020-00349-5.

30. Faezeh S, Noorimotlagh Z, Mirzaee SA, Kalantar M, Barati B, Fard ME, Fard NK. The SARS-CoV-2 (COVID-19) pandemic in hospital: an insight into environmental surfaces contamination, disinfectants' efficiency, and estimation of plastic waste production. Environ Res. 2021;202:111809. https://doi.org/10.1016/j.envres.2021.111809.
31. Falahi S, Bastani E, Pakzad I, Rashidi A, Abdoli A, Kenarkoohi A. Environmental surface contamination with SARS-CoV-2: toilets as the most contaminated surfaces in COVID-19 referral hospital. Hosp Top. 2021;2021:1–8. https://doi.org/10.1080/00185868.2021.1969870.
32. Guo ZD, Wang ZY, Zhang SF, Li X, Li L, Li C, Cui Y, Fu RB, Dong YZ, Chi XY, Zhang MY, Liu K, Cao C, Liu B, Zhang K, Gao YW, Lu B, Chen W. Aerosol and surface distribution of severe acute respiratory syndrome coronavirus 2 in hospital wards, Wuhan, China, 2020. Emerg Infect Dis. 2020;26(7):1583–91. https://doi.org/10.3201/eid2607.200885.
33. Hu X, Ni W, Wang Z, Ma G, Pan B, Dong L, Gao R, Jiang F. The distribution of SARS-CoV-2 contamination on the environmental surfaces during incubation period of COVID-19 patients. Ecotoxicol Environ Saf. 2020;208:111438. https://doi.org/10.1016/j.ecoenv.2020.111438.
34. Lee SE, Lee DY, Lee WG, Kang B, Jang YS, Ryu B, Lee S, Bahk H, Lee E. Detection of novel coronavirus on the surface of environmental materials contaminated by COVID-19 patients in the Republic of Korea. Osong Public Health Res Perspect. 2020;11(3):128–32. https://doi.org/10.24171/j.phrp.2020.11.3.03.
35. Lei H, Ye F, Liu X, Huang Z, Ling S, Jiang Z, Cheng J, Huang X, Wu Q, Wu S, Xie Y, Xiao C, Ye D, Yang Z, Li Y, Leung NHL, Cowling BJ, He J, Wong SS, Zanin M. SARS-CoV-2 environmental contamination associated with persistently infected COVID-19 patients. Influenza Other Respir Viruses. 2020;14(6):688–99. https://doi.org/10.1111/irv.12783.
36. Liu W, Li D, Yang C, Chen F, Jia R, Jia L, Xia X, Fan S, Tan Q, Ke Y, Chen Y, Li H, Zhan L, Liu X, You J, Fu X, Li D, Zhang L, Wang C, Han L. Environmental contamination with SARS-CoV-2 in COVID-19 hospitals in Wuhan, China, 2020. Environ Microbiol. 2021;23(12):7373–81. https://doi.org/10.1111/1462-2920.15695.
37. Marotz C, Belda-Ferre P, Ali F, Das P, Huang S, Cantrel K, Jiang L, Martino C, Diner R, Rahman G, McDonald D, Armstrong G, Kodera S, Donato S, Ecklu-Mensah G, Gottel N, Salas Garcia M, Chiang L, Salido RA, Shaffer JP, Bryant M, Sanders K, Humphrey G, Ackermann G, Haiminen N, Beck KL, Kim HC, Carrieri AP, Parida L, Vazquez-Baeza Y, Torriani FJ, Knight R, Gilbert J, Sweeney D, Allard SM. SARS-CoV-2 detection status associates with bacterial community composition in patients and the hospital environment. Microbiome 2021;9(1):132. https://doi.org/10.1186/s40168-021-01083-0.
38. Moore G, Rickard H, Stevenson D, Aranega-Bou P, Pitman J, Crook A, Davies K, Spencer A, Burton C, Easterbrook L, Love HE, Summers S, Welch SR, Wand N, Thompson KA, Pottage T, Richards KS, Dunning J, Bennett A. Detection of SARS-CoV-2 within the healthcare environment: a multi-centre study conducted during the first wave of the COVID-19 outbreak in England. J Hosp Infect. 2021;108:189–96. https://doi.org/10.1016/j.jhin.2020.11.024.
39. Ong SWX, Lee PH, Tan YK, Ling LM, Ho BCH, Ng CG, Wang DL, Tan BH, Leo YS, Ng OT, Wong MSY, Marimuthu K. Environmental contamination in a COVID-19 intensive care unit (ICU)—what is the risk? Infect Control Hosp Epidemiol. 2021;42(6):669–77. https://doi.org/10.1017/ice.2020.1278.
40. Orenes-Piñero E, Baño F, Navas-Carrillo D, Moreno-Docón A, Marín JM, Misiego R, Ramírez P. Evidences of SARS-CoV-2 virus air transmission indoors using several untouched surfaces: a pilot study. Sci Total Environ. 2021;751:142317. https://doi.org/10.1016/j.scitotenv.2020.142317.
41. Piana A, Colucci ME, Valeriani F, Marcolongo A, Sotgiu G, Pasquarella C, Margarucci LM, Petrucca A, Gianfranceschi G, Babudieri S, Vitali P, D'Ermo G, Bizzarro A, De Maio F, Vitali M, Azara A, Romano F, Simmaco M, Romano Spica V. Monitoring COVID-19 transmission risks by quantitative real-time PCR tracing of droplets in hospital and living environments. mSphere. 2021;6(1):e01070. https://doi.org/10.1128/mSphere.01070-20.

42. Ryu BH, Cho Y, Cho OH, Hong SI, Kim S, Lee S. Environmental contamination of SARS-CoV-2 during the COVID-19 outbreak in South Korea. Am J Infect Control. 2020;48(8):875–9. https://doi.org/10.1016/j.ajic.2020.05.027.
43. Somerville CC, Shoaib M, Kuschner CE, Brune Z, Trindade AJ, Benias PC, Becker LB. Prospective analysis of SARS-CoV-2 dissemination to environmental surfaces during endoscopic procedures. Endosc Int Open. 2021;9(5):E701–5. https://doi.org/10.1055/a-1395-6946.
44. Vicente VA, Lustosa BPR, Grisolia ME, Pavini Beato C, Balsanelli E, de Souza Gubert Fruet V, Bordignon Nogueira M, Raboni SM, Carvalho KAT, Flôr IC, Ferreira Voidaleski M, Etchepare RG, Meis JF, Soccol VT, Souza EM. Environmental detection of SARS-CoV-2 virus RNA in health facilities in Brazil and a systematic review on contamination sources. Int J Environ Res Public Health. 2021;18(7):3824. https://doi.org/10.3390/ijerph18073824.
45. Wang H, Mo P, Li G, Chen P, Liu J, Wang H, Wang F, Zhang Y, Zhao Q. Environmental virus surveillance in the isolation ward of COVID-19. J Hosp Infect. 2020;105(2):373–4. https://doi.org/10.1016/j.jhin.2020.04.020.
46. Wang J, Feng H, Zhang S, Ni Z, Ni L, Chen Y, Zhuo L, Zhong Z, Qu T. SARS-CoV-2 RNA detection of hospital isolation wards hygiene monitoring during the Coronavirus Disease 2019 outbreak in a Chinese hospital. Int J Infect Dis. 2020;94:103–6. https://doi.org/10.1016/j.ijid.2020.04.024.
47. Wu S, Wang Y, Jin X, Tian J, Liu J, Mao Y. Environmental contamination by SARS-CoV-2 in a designated hospital for coronavirus disease 2019. Am J Infect Control. 2020;48(8):910–4. https://doi.org/10.1016/j.ajic.2020.05.003.
48. Xu K, Zhang XH, Long XB, Lu X, Liu Z. An environmental study of tracheostomy on eight COVID-19 patients. J Otolaryngol Head Neck Surg. 2021;50(1):3. https://doi.org/10.1186/s40463-021-00494-1.
49. Ye G, Lin H, Chen S, Wang S, Zeng Z, Wang W, Zhang S, Rebmann T, Li Y, Pan Z, Yang Z, Wang Y, Wang F, Qian Z, Wang X. Environmental contamination of SARS-CoV-2 in healthcare premises. J Infect. 2020;81(2):e1–5. https://doi.org/10.1016/j.jinf.2020.04.034.
50. Yung CF, Kam KQ, Wong MSY, Maiwald M, Tan YK, Tan BH, Thoon KC. Environment and personal protective equipment tests for SARS-CoV-2 in the isolation room of an infant with infection. Ann Intern Med. 2020;173(3):240–2. https://doi.org/10.7326/m20-0942.
51. Zhou L, Yao M, Zhang X, Hu B, Li X, Chen H, Zhang L, Liu Y, Du M, Sun B, Jiang Y, Zhou K, Hong J, Yu N, Ding Z, Xu Y, Hu M, Morawska L, Grinshpun SA, Biswas P, Flagan RC, Zhu B, Liu W, Zhang Y. Breath-, air- and surface-borne SARS-CoV-2 in hospitals. J Aerosol Sci. 2020;152:105693. https://doi.org/10.1016/j.jaerosci.2020.105693.
52. Kim UJ, Lee SY, Lee JY, Lee A, Kim SE, Choi OJ, Lee JS, Kee SJ, Jang HC. Air and environmental contamination caused by COVID-19 patients: a multi-center study. J Korean Med Sci. 2020;35(37):e332. https://doi.org/10.3346/jkms.2020.35.e332.
53. Maltezou HC, Tseroni M, Daflos C, Anastassopoulou C, Vasilogiannakopoulos A, Daligarou O, Panagiotou M, Botsa E, Spanakis N, Lourida A, Tsakris A. Environmental testing for SARS-CoV-2 in three tertiary-care hospitals during the peak of the third COVID-19 wave. Am J Infect Control. 2021;49(11):1435–7. https://doi.org/10.1016/j.ajic.2021.08.022.
54. Mouchtouri VA, Koureas M, Kyritsi M, Vontas A, Kourentis L, Sapounas S, Rigakos G, Petinaki E, Tsiodras S, Hadjichristodoulou C. Environmental contamination of SARS-CoV-2 on surfaces, air-conditioner and ventilation systems. Int J Hyg Environ Health. 2020;230:113599. https://doi.org/10.1016/j.ijheh.2020.113599.
55. Shah MR, Jan I, Johns J, Singh K, Kumar P, Belarmino N, Saggiomo KJ, Hayes C, Washington K, Toppmeyer DL, Haffty BG, Libutti SK, Evens AM. SARS-CoV-2 nosocomial infection: real-world results of environmental surface testing from a large tertiary cancer center. Cancer. 2021;127(11):1926–32. https://doi.org/10.1002/cncr.33453.
56. Tan L, Ma B, Lai X, Han L, Cao P, Zhang J, Fu J, Zhou Q, Wei S, Wang Z, Peng W, Yang L, Zhang X. Air and surface contamination by SARS-CoV-2 virus in a tertiary hospital in Wuhan, China. Int J Infect Dis. 2020;99:3–7. https://doi.org/10.1016/j.ijid.2020.07.027.

57. Su WL, Hung PP, Lin CP, Chen LK, Lan CC, Yang MC, Peng MY, Chao YC. Masks and closed-loop ventilators prevent environmental contamination by COVID-19 patients in negative-pressure environments. J Microbiol Immunol Infect. 2020;54(1):81–4. https://doi.org/10.1016/j.jmii.2020.05.002.
58. Cheng VC, Wong SC, Chan VW, So SY, Chen JH, Yip CC, Chan KH, Chu H, Chung TW, Sridhar S, To KK, Chan JF, Hung IF, Ho PL, Yuen KY. Air and environmental sampling for SARS-CoV-2 around hospitalized patients with coronavirus disease 2019 (COVID-19). Infect Control Hosp Epidemiol. 2020;41(11):1258–65. https://doi.org/10.1017/ice.2020.282.
59. Liang En Ian W, Sim XYJ, Conceicao EP, Aung MK, Tan KY, Ko KKK, Wong HM, Wijaya L, Tan BH, Venkatachalam I, Ling ML. Containing COVID-19 outside the isolation ward: the impact of an infection control bundle on environmental contamination and transmission in a cohorted general ward. Am J Infect Control. 2020;48(9):1056–61. https://doi.org/10.1016/j.ajic.2020.06.188.
60. Colaneri M, Seminari E, Novati S, Asperges E, Biscarini S, Piralla A, Percivalle E, Cassaniti I, Baldanti F, Bruno R, Mondelli MU. Severe acute respiratory syndrome coronavirus 2 RNA contamination of inanimate surfaces and virus viability in a health care emergency unit. Clin Microbiol Infect. 2020;26(8):1094.e1091–5. https://doi.org/10.1016/j.cmi.2020.05.009.
61. Jerry J, O'Regan E, O'Sullivan L, Lynch M, Brady D. Do established infection prevention and control measures prevent spread of SARS-CoV-2 to the hospital environment beyond the patient room? J Hosp Infect. 2020;105(4):589–92. https://doi.org/10.1016/j.jhin.2020.06.026.
62. Wei L, Lin J, Duan X, Huang W, Lu X, Zhou J, Zong Z. Asymptomatic COVID-19 patients can contaminate their surroundings: an environment sampling study. mSphere. 2020;5(3):e00442. https://doi.org/10.1128/mSphere.00442-20.
63. D'Accolti M, Soffritti I, Passaro A, Zuliani G, Antonioli P, Mazzacane S, Manfredini R, Caselli E. SARS-CoV-2 RNA contamination on surfaces of a COVID-19 ward in a hospital of northern Italy: what risk of transmission? Eur Rev Med Pharmacol Sci. 2020;24(17):9202–7. https://doi.org/10.26355/eurrev_202009_22872.
64. Lomont A, Boubaya M, Khamis W, Deslandes A, Cordel H, Seytre D, Alloui C, Malaure C, Bonnet N, Carbonnelle E, Cohen Y, Nunes H, Bouchaud O, Zahar JR, Tandjaoui-Lambiotte Y. Environmental contamination related to SARS-CoV-2 in ICU patients. ERJ Open Res. 2020;6(4):00595-2020. https://doi.org/10.1183/23120541.00595-2020.
65. Ong SWX, Tan YK, Chia PY, Lee TH, Ng OT, Wong MSY, Marimuthu K. Air, surface environmental, and personal protective equipment contamination by severe acute respiratory syndrome coronavirus 2 (SARS-CoV-2) from a symptomatic patient. JAMA. 2020;323(16):1610–2. https://doi.org/10.1001/jama.2020.3227.
66. Peyrony O, Ellouze S, Fontaine JP, Thegat-Le Cam M, Salmona M, Feghoul L, Mahjoub N, Mercier-Delarue S, Gabassi A, Delaugerre C, Le Goff J. Surfaces and equipment contamination by severe acute respiratory syndrome coronavirus 2 (SARS-CoV-2) in the emergency department at a university hospital. Int J Hyg Environ Health. 2020;230:113600. https://doi.org/10.1016/j.ijheh.2020.113600.
67. Hofmaenner DA, Wendel Garcia PD, Duvnjak B, Chakrakodi B, Maier JD, Huber M, Huder J, Wolfensberger A, Schreiber PW, Schuepbach RA, Zinkernagel AS, Buehler PK, Brugger SD. Bacterial but no SARS-CoV-2 contamination after terminal disinfection of tertiary care intensive care units treating COVID-19 patients. Antimicrob Resist Infect Control. 2021;10(1):11. https://doi.org/10.1186/s13756-021-00885-z.
68. Ahn JY, An S, Sohn Y, Cho Y, Hyun JH, Baek YJ, Kim MH, Jeong SJ, Kim JH, Ku NS, Yeom JS, Smith DM, Lee H, Yong D, Lee YJ, Kim JW, Kim HR, Hwang J, Choi JY. Environmental contamination in the isolation rooms of COVID-19 patients with severe pneumonia requiring mechanical ventilation or high-flow oxygen therapy. J Hosp Infect. 2020;106(3):570–6. https://doi.org/10.1016/j.jhin.2020.08.014.
69. Barksdale AN, Zeger WG, Santarpia JL, Herrera VL, Ackerman DN, Lowe JJ, Wadman MC. Implementation of a COVID-19 cohort area resulted in no surface or air contamination in

surrounding areas in one academic emergency department. Am J Emerg Med. 2021;47:253–7. https://doi.org/10.1016/j.ajem.2021.04.082.
70. Yamagishi T, Ohnishi M, Matsunaga N, Kakimoto K, Kamiya H, Okamoto K, Suzuki M, Gu Y, Sakaguchi M, Tajima T, Takaya S, Ohmagari N, Takeda M, Matsuyama S, Shirato K, Nao N, Hasegawa H, Kageyama T, Takayama I, Saito S, Wada K, Fujita R, Saito H, Okinaka K, Griffith M, Parry AE, Barnetson B, Leonard J, Wakita T. Environmental sampling for severe acute respiratory syndrome coronavirus 2 during a COVID-19 outbreak on the diamond princess cruise ship. J Infect Dis. 2020;222(7):1098–102. https://doi.org/10.1093/infdis/jiaa437.
71. Wong JCC, Hapuarachchi HC, Arivalan S, Tien WP, Koo C, Mailepessov D, Kong M, Nazeem M, Lim M, Ng LC. Environmental contamination of SARS-CoV-2 in a non-healthcare setting. Int J Environ Res Public Health. 2020;18(1):117. https://doi.org/10.3390/ijerph18010117.
72. Jiang FC, Jiang XL, Wang ZG, Meng ZH, Shao SF, Anderson BD, Ma MJ. Detection of severe acute respiratory syndrome coronavirus 2 RNA on surfaces in quarantine rooms. Emerg Infect Dis. 2020;26(9):2162–4. https://doi.org/10.3201/eid2609.201435.
73. Liu J, Liu J, He Z, Yang Z, Yuan J, Wu H, Zhu P, Fu X, Lin Y, Zhang Y, Zhao Z, He S, Ma X. Duration of SARS-CoV-2 positive in quarantine room environments: a perspective analysis. Int J Infect Dis. 2021;105:68–74. https://doi.org/10.1016/j.ijid.2021.02.025.
74. Döhla M, Schulte B, Wilbring G, Kümmerer BM, Döhla C, Sib E, Richter E, Ottensmeyer PF, Haag A, Engelhart S, Eis-Hübinger AM, Exner M, Mutters NT, Schmithausen RM, Streeck H. SARS-CoV-2 in environmental samples of quarantined households. Viruses 2022;14(5):1075. https://doi.org/10.3390/v14051075.
75. Liu B, Rayment S, Oppenheim FG, Troxler RF. Isolation of human salivary mucin MG2 by a novel method and characterization of its interactions with oral bacteria. Arch Biochem Biophys. 1999;364(2):286–93.
76. Marcenac P, Park GW, Duca LM, Lewis NM, Dietrich EA, Barclay L, Tamin A, Harcourt JL, Thornburg NJ, Rispens J, Matanock A, Kiphibane T, Christensen K, Pawloski LC, Fry AM, Hall AJ, Tate JE, Vinjé J, Kirking HL, Pevzner E. Detection of SARS-CoV-2 on surfaces in households of persons with COVID-19. Int J Environ Res Public Health. 2021;18(15):8184. https://doi.org/10.3390/ijerph18158184.
77. Bloise I, Gómez-Arroyo B, García-Rodríguez J. Detection of SARS-CoV-2 on high-touch surfaces in a clinical microbiology laboratory. J Hosp Infect. 2020;105(4):784–6. https://doi.org/10.1016/j.jhin.2020.05.017.
78. Harvey AP, Fuhrmeister ER, Cantrell M, Pitol AK, Swarthout JM, Powers JE, Nadimpalli ML, Julian TR, Pickering AJ. Longitudinal monitoring of SARS-CoV-2 RNA on high-touch surfaces in a community setting. Environ Sci Technol Lett 2021;8(2):168–75. https://doi.org/10.1021/acs.estlett.0c00875.
79. Gholipour S, Nikaeen M, Mohammadi Manesh R, Aboutalebian S, Shamsizadeh Z, Nasri E, Mirhendi H. Severe acute respiratory syndrome coronavirus 2 (SARS-CoV-2) contamination of high-touch surfaces in field settings. Biomed Environ Sci BES. 2020;33(12):925–9. https://doi.org/10.3967/bes2020.126.
80. Caggiano G, Triggiano F, Apollonio F, Diella G, Lopuzzo M, D'Ambrosio M, Fasano F, Stefanizzi P, Sorrenti GT, Magarelli P, Sorrenti DP, Marcotrigiano V, De Giglio O, Montagna MT. SARS-CoV-2 RNA and supermarket surfaces: a real or presumed threat? Int J Environ Res Public Health. 2021;18(17):9404. https://doi.org/10.3390/ijerph18179404.
81. Liu H, Fei C, Chen Y, Luo S, Yang T, Yang L, Liu J, Ji X, Wu W, Song J. Investigating SARS-CoV-2 persistent contamination in different indoor environments. Environ Res. 2021;202:111763. https://doi.org/10.1016/j.envres.2021.111763.
82. Akter S, Roy PC, Ferdaus A, Ibnat H, Alam A, Nigar S, Jahid IK, Hossain MA. Prevalence and stability of SARS-CoV-2 RNA on Bangladeshi banknotes. Sci Total Environ. 2021;779:146133. https://doi.org/10.1016/j.scitotenv.2021.146133.
83. Gavaldà-Mestre L, Ramírez-Tarruella D, Gutiérrez-Milla C, Guillamet-Roig F, Orriols-Ramos R, Tisner SR, Pàrraga-Niño N. Nondetection of SARS-CoV-2 on high-touch surfaces of public

areas next to COVID-19 hospitalization units. Am J Infect Control. 2021;49(6):840–2. https://doi.org/10.1016/j.ajic.2021.01.007.
84. Karami C, Normohammadi A, Dargahi A, Vosoughi M, Zandian H, Jeddi F, Mokhtari SA, Moradi-Asl E. Investigation of SARS-CoV-2 virus on nozzle surfaces of fuel supply stations in north west of Iran. Sci Total Environ. 2021;780:146641. https://doi.org/10.1016/j.scitotenv.2021.146641.
85. Kozer E, Rinott E, Kozer G, Bar-Haim A, Benveniste-Levkovitz P, Klainer H, Perl S, Youngster I. Presence of SARS-CoV-2 RNA on playground surfaces and water fountains. Epidemiol Infect. 2021;149:e67. https://doi.org/10.1017/s0950268821000546.
86. Singh M, Sadat A, Abdi R, Colaruotolo LA, Francavilla A, Petker K, Nasr P, Moraveji M, Cruz G, Huang Y, Arora A, Chao A, Walker S, Wang X, Rathnayake S, Ragupathy S, Newmaster SG, Hanner RH, Goodridge LD, Corradini MG. Detection of SAR-CoV-2 on surfaces in food retailers in Ontario. Curr Res Food Sci. 2021;4:598–602. https://doi.org/10.1016/j.crfs.2021.08.009.
87. Booth TF, Kournikakis B, Bastien N, Ho J, Kobasa D, Stadnyk L, Li Y, Spence M, Paton S, Henry B, Mederski B, White D, Low DE, McGeer A, Simor A, Vearncombe M, Downey J, Jamieson FB, Tang P, Plummer F. Detection of airborne severe acute respiratory syndrome (SARS) coronavirus and environmental contamination in SARS outbreak units. J Infect Dis. 2005;191(9):1472–7. https://doi.org/10.1086/429634.
88. Dowell SF, Simmerman JM, Erdman DD, Wu JS, Chaovavanich A, Javadi M, Yang JY, Anderson LJ, Tong S, Ho MS. Severe acute respiratory syndrome coronavirus on hospital surfaces. Clin Infect Dis. 2004;39(5):652–7. https://doi.org/10.1086/422652.
89. Simmerman JM, Suntarattiwong P, Levy J, Gibbons RV, Cruz C, Shaman J, Jarman RG, Chotpitayasunondh T. Influenza virus contamination of common household surfaces during the 2009 influenza A (H1N1) pandemic in Bangkok, Thailand: implications for contact transmission. Clin Infect Dis. 2010;51(9):1053–61. https://doi.org/10.1086/656581.
90. Bin SY, Heo JY, Song MS, Lee J, Kim EH, Park SJ, Kwon HI, Kim SM, Kim YI, Si YJ, Lee IW, Baek YH, Choi WS, Min J, Jeong HW, Choi YK. Environmental contamination and viral shedding in MERS patients during MERS-CoV outbreak in South Korea. Clin Infect Dis. 2016;62(6):755–60. https://doi.org/10.1093/cid/civ1020.
91. Dick EC, Jennings LC, Mink KA, Wartgow CD, Inhorn SL. Aerosol transmission of rhinovirus colds. J Infect Dis. 1987;156(3):442–8. https://doi.org/10.1093/infdis/156.3.442.
92. Ansari SA, Springthorpe VS, Sattar SA, Rivard S, Rahman M. Potential role of hands in the spread of respiratory viral infections: studies with human parainfluenza virus 3 and rhinovirus 14. J Clin Microbiol. 1991;29(10):2115–9. https://doi.org/10.1128/jcm.29.10.2115-2119.1991.
93. Dallner M, Harlow J, Nasheri N. Human coronaviruses do not transfer efficiently between surfaces in the absence of organic materials. Viruses. 2021;13(7):1352. https://doi.org/10.3390/v13071352.
94. Wilson AM, Reynolds KA, Sexton JD, Canales RA. Modeling surface disinfection needs to meet microbial risk reduction targets. Appl Environ Microbiol. 2018;84(18):e00709–18. https://doi.org/10.1128/aem.00709-18.
95. Popa A, Genger JW, Nicholson MD, Penz T, Schmid D, Aberle SW, Agerer B, Lercher A, Endler L, Colaço H, Smyth M, Schuster M, Grau ML, Martínez-Jiménez F, Pich O, Borena W, Pawelka E, Keszei Z, Senekowitsch M, Laine J, Aberle JH, Redlberger-Fritz M, Karolyi M, Zoufaly A, Maritschnik S, Borkovec M, Hufnagl P, Nairz M, Weiss G, Wolfinger MT, von Laer D, Superti-Furga G, Lopez-Bigas N, Puchhammer-Stöckl E, Allerberger F, Michor F, Bock C, Bergthaler A. Genomic epidemiology of superspreading events in Austria reveals mutational dynamics and transmission properties of SARS-CoV-2. Sci Transl Med. 2020;12(573):eabe2555. https://doi.org/10.1126/scitranslmed.abe2555.
96. Balaraman V, Drolet BS, Mitzel DN, Wilson WC, Owens J, Gaudreault NN, Meekins DA, Bold D, Trujillo JD, Noronha LE, Richt JA, Nayduch D. Mechanical transmission of SARS-CoV-2 by house flies. Parasit Vectors. 2021;14(1):214. https://doi.org/10.1186/s13071-021-04703-8.
97. Moriyama M, Hugentobler WJ, Iwasaki A. Seasonality of respiratory viral infections. Annu Rev Virol. 2020;7(1):83–101. https://doi.org/10.1146/annurev-virology-012420-022445.

# Chapter 2
# Humoral Immune Response in SARS-CoV-2 Infection and Its Therapeutic Relevance

**Victor Araujo Correa, Amanda Izeli Portilho, Emanuelle Baldo Gaspar, and Elizabeth De Gaspari**

## Introduction

The humoral immune response is an arm of adaptive response, also known as antibody-mediated immune response. It is responsible to protect the extracellular fluids, such as blood and lymph, through the production of effector and memory B cells, which B cells generate antibodies, leading to neutralization, opsonization, complement activation, and modulation of inflammation. Also, it promotes an immunological memory, capable of protecting against future reinfection to the pathogen [1–3]. Upon a reexposure to the pathogen, or, more specifically, to an antigen, the humoral memory response has three typical characteristics: (1) it is more robust and faster than the primary antibody response; (2) it is dominated by high affinity, isotype-switched antibodies; and (3) it is long-lived and self-sustaining, allowing for a rapid complement cascade activation and antibody production [4, 5]. Given all that, antibody production following natural infection or vaccination is essential to combat and prevent infectious diseases.

In 2020, the World Health Organization (WHO) declared COVID-19 as a pandemic disease, which challenged the researchers to understand how the virus stimulates the immune system as soon as possible, in order to discover a way to treat the disease and stop the viral transmission. This chapter intends to discuss the humoral immune response against SARS-CoV-2 infection.

V. A. Correa · A. I. Portilho · E. De Gaspari (✉)
Departamento de Imunologia, Instituto Adolfo Lutz, São Paulo, SP, Brazil

Programa de Pós-Graduação Interunidades em Biotecnologia, Instituto de Ciências Biomédicas, Universidade de São Paulo, São Paulo, SP, Brazil
e-mail: a.izeliportilho@usp.br; elizabeth.gaspari@ial.sp.gov.br

E. B. Gaspar
Embrapa Pecuária Sul, Bagé, RS, Brazil
e-mail: emanuelle.gaspar@embrapa.br


S. Adibi et al. (eds.), *Frontiers of COVID-19*,
https://doi.org/10.1007/978-3-031-08045-6_2

## Pathogens and Antibodies Evolve Together

Antibodies are glycoprotein molecules composed of four chains: two light chains (L) and two heavy chains (H). The domains are linked by disulfide bonds. The intersection of the L and H chains forms the hypervariable region, or complementarity-determining region (CDR). The CDR regions comprise the paratope, which is responsible for the interaction with the antigen's epitope. The analysis of the evolution of CDRs in response to an infection is important: the changes in CDR results from natural selection, aiming to increase the affinity for the target molecule, the epitope, from 1000 to 10,000 times [6–8].

On the other hand, some pathogens present high mutation rates. The exchange of amino acids allows for better adaptation to the environment and improves the performance of the pathogens in front of challenges, like the host's immune response [9].

Given that, through the accumulation of genetic mutations, the host's antibodies and pathogen's antigens coevolve, acting as forces of selection for each other. The coevolution between environment, pathogens, and host was originally proposed by the "Red Queen Theory": it proposes that a successful evolution from one species produces a negative effect on the other species, and vice versa [10, 11].

## Antibody Kinetics After SARS-CoV-2 Infection

SARS-CoV-2 presents two main proteins that are highly immunogenic and able to trigger humoral response: the Spike (S) and the Nucleocapsid (N) proteins. S is divided into S1 and S2 subunits: the first mediates the binding with angiotensin-converting enzyme (ACE)-2 by the receptor binding domain (RBD) and the second mediates the fusion of the virus and the cellular membrane. N is the most abundant viral protein, it binds with the RNA and mediates virion assembly. Membrane (M) and Envelope (E), the other two structural proteins, induce a poor humoral response, probably because of their small molecular size; however, such proteins are studied in cellular response [12, 13].

The immune response to pathogens usually presents initial IgM seroconversion, a result of T-independent humoral response, which is a mark of acute disease that decreases within a few weeks. The following IgG seroconversion, after T cell activation and class switch, is a mark of maturation of immune response and immunologic memory. IgG is the main class of antibody found systemically, and it is often desired for an adequate immune response [2].

Antibody response to acute viral infection is found in patients with COVID-19. As expected, the first antibody detected is IgM, followed by IgG, once the seroconversion rate and antibody levels increase fast during the first 2 weeks following infection. The cumulative seropositive rate reaches 50% on the 11th day and 100% on the 39th day [14]. The IgG titers increase until 2 months after diagnostic, then it reaches a plateau [15]. One study demonstrated that, after 6 months, the positive rate for IgG was maintained, ranging from 92.3% to 95.5%, while the positive IgM rate decreased from 90.4% to 22.7% [16]. Another study demonstrated a durable B cell response, until 8 months after infection [17].

It was demonstrated that 6 months after the infection, the patients continue having an anti-SARS-CoV-2 B cells response, being observed an accumulation of somatic mutations in these cells, and production of antibodies with increased neutralizing breadth and potency [18].

However, subsequent studies described a concomitant IgM/IgG seroconversion. It has also been suggested the value of IgA seroconversion as the first mark of the humoral response against SARS-CoV-2. Thus, the combined serology of IgA/IgG presents higher sensitivity and specificity than IgM/IgG to detect past exposure to the virus [14, 19, 20].

In summary, there are a great number of studies about antibody kinetics after SARS-CoV-2 infection. As expected, not all the results agree with each other, but, in general, it has been proposed that IgA seroconversion happens within 4–6 days post symptoms onset, peaking around 16–20 days and declining after 31–41 days. For IgM, seroconversion starts 4 to 6 days after symptoms onset, the peak happens on days 11 to 15, and then it decreases [20].

## The Role of Antibodies in COVID-19

The description of the immune response in COVID-19 has been an issue and several studies have focused on it. Despite the differences between the investigations conducted, it can be stated that the sole presence of antibodies cannot be used to infer protection against SARS-CoV-2. Studies support that the ideal response is probably a synergetic one, that comprises the innate, humoral, and cellular mechanisms [21].

## Antibody Titers

Studies point that severe infection patients present higher antibody titers than mild infection patients—which could lead one to suggest that antibodies would not bring benefits to the patients. A work demonstrated that this high antibody secretion in severe infection patients could mediate pathogenesis by multiple mechanisms, including tissue damage by activation of inflammatory macrophages [22]. The possible explanation for this is the lack of viral replication control, which induces a persistent viremia and causes an intense or prolonged B cell activation, resulting in a pathogenic B cell production [23].

These high loads of IgG in the alveoli form immune complexes with viral particles, capable of activating the complement system and inducing inflammation in the lungs, a serious issue in COVID-19 [24]. The worry about IgG response was also related to antibody-dependent enhancement (ADE). It happens when antibodies produced by a previous, poor immune response, which are not capable of neutralizing activity or present lower affinity by the pathogen, intensify the current infection, allowing for internalization mediated by the Fcγ receptor, thus favoring the release of pro-inflammatory cytokines and immunopathology. Several studies about SARS-CoV-2 do not corroborate this hypothesis, but it was important to state how the quality of antibodies, rather than the quantity, should be assessed [25].

The expressive presence of anti-N antibodies in severe patients also points to higher viremia, since large amounts of N protein are incorporated into the virion. It is also supported by children showing high anti-S but low anti-N titers: there is a decrease of ACE-2 expression in this age group, which has been related to their reduced risk of suffering from COVID-19; thus, their viremia is expected to be lower when compared with that of adults. Of note, the induction of antibodies through vaccination, training the immune system before the exposure, should not be directly compared with natural infection response [12, 26, 27].

It is still controversial how antibodies and the severity of the disease may affect each other. A study demonstrated that antibody levels were significantly higher in severe than in nonsevere patients, between the second and fifth week after disease onset; but there is no observation for IgG or IgM alone [14]. Another study shows that 3 weeks after the disease, the levels of IgM and IgG to S and N proteins were higher in non-severe and RNA-negative patients than in severe and RNA-positive patients [28]. The same controversial results were observed when the antibody titer is correlated with age and symptoms. In some studies, the age was positively correlated with IgG, IgM, and IgA titers; and especially IgG was correlated with specific COVID-19 symptoms, like fever, sore throat, shortness of breath, and nausea [28, 29]. On the other hand, a study shows that antibody response was independent of patient age, sex, and most preexistent comorbidities [30]. It was demonstrated that male sex, older age, and hospitalization for COVID-19 were associated with increasing antibody response [31].

## Antibodies Functionality

Generally, antibody avidity increases during the infection and remains elevated. The same was observed to SARS-CoV-2: low antibody avidity was reported during early infection, until 3 weeks after symptom onset [32]. However, other studies report that the avidity of naturally induced antibodies did not improve with time [33]. It was also observed that the avidity is higher in hospitalized than in nonhospitalized patients. As an indicator of functionality, anti-spike avidity was correlated with higher neutralizing antibodies (nAbs) titers [34, 35].

It is described that nAbs are needed for virus clearance and it has been considered a key for the protection or treatment of COVID-19. Diverse studies found that nAb levels in asymptomatic or mild cases were lower than moderate or severe cases

[14, 26, 36]. Such results have led previous reports to question the efficacy of nAb-mediated protection in COVID-19 severe cases and have suggested that the enhancement of nAbs is associated with a worst clinical condition [17, 37]. Similarly to antibody titers, which are usually higher in severe cases, the neutralizing activity of the plasma of most symptomatic COVID-19 patients persists up to 6 months [28], whereas in asymptomatic patients, it gradually disappears in 2 months [38]. The interplay between viral load and antibody titers discussed above could also affect the nAb titers.

The study of IgA against SARS-CoV-2 has been encouraged, given the involvement of mucosa in COVID-19 [24]. The seric IgA could reflect the mucosa implication of COVID-19. It was described as the main antibody responsible for early neutralization of SARS-CoV-2, even in less quantity than IgG; thus, it would be capable of penetrating epithelial cells, neutralizing intracellular virus [20, 39]. The secretory-IgA (sIgA), locally produced in the mucosa, was considered as a potential biomarker of SARS-CoV-2 early infection, which could be tested in saliva. With better elucidation of duration and functionality of the immune response, sIgA could also be a correlate of protection, given its ability to control the infection when the virus first enters the host [40]. Moreover, patients with nAbs and anti-spike IgA demonstrated a faster viral control [41].

When the production of antibodies against the structural proteins was analyzed, it was verified that SARS-CoV-2 specific IgM recognition of S and N proteins was transient and disappeared around the 12th week; thus, the IgM response would not contribute to sustained immunity against the virus. Also, there was no correlation between IgM response and the ability of plasma to neutralize the virus in cell culture. Differently, IgG antibodies that recognize the S and N proteins maintain high positive rates for up to 6 months, and particularly RBD-specific IgG were correlated with neutralizing activity, being associated with early virus control [3, 28]. Thus, titers of IgG was not correlated with severe acute respiratory distress syndrome [30].

It was postulated that anti-S or, more specifically, anti-RBD IgG, would be ideal for protection, since it could neutralize the virus by impairing the RBD-ACE-2 binding. Serology studies also suggest that anti-S protein antibodies are maintained over longer periods when compared with anti-N antibodies. Indeed, the S protein or its subunits has been used as vaccine antigens [12, 20, 42, 43].

Because of the lack of drugs capable of inhibiting SARS-CoV-2, convalescent plasma (plasma obtained from recovered patients that present high levels of nAbs) was indicated as a therapeutic option for COVID-19 severe infection patients. The studies that followed this type of intervention varied a lot regarding the number of patients and how the plasma was obtained, which limits the comparisons, but good results were described overall [44].

Serology presents a limited role in diagnosing SARS-CoV-2 infection and assessing the protective status of a person. However, determining the humoral response is an interesting tool for public health, to verify the prevalence of COVID-19 [43]. Despite that, the study of neutralizing activity is useful for immune-based therapy trials [45].

## Antibodies and Reinfection

Until 2020, sporadic cases of reinfection by SARS-CoV-2 were described around the world. In some cases, it was more severe, but in others, an increasing severity was observed. However, with the emergence of variants and as time passed, more cases were documented [46–48]. It was suggested that some people would fail to develop a protective immunity, which would explain the reinfections [17].

However, with the pandemic ongoing, four hypotheses have been developed to explain the cases of more severe reinfection: (1) a very high dose of virus might have led to this second infection and induced more severe disease; (2) the reinfection was caused by another, more virulent, strain; (3) the mechanism of antibody-dependent enhancement might be the cause; and (4) the incomplete avidity maturation after COVID-19 infection did not confer a protective immunity [33, 48–50].

The current knowledge leads to suggest that the most accurate hypothesis is that natural infection is prone to failure in developing an efficient immunologic memory, because of impaired affinity maturation, and high-coverage vaccination is needed to control the pandemic, since it provides a more adequate immune response [33].

## Antibody Production Modulated by Cytokines

As described before, COVID-19 hospitalized patients usually present a stronger IgG avidity and higher nAbs titers than nonhospitalized patients [51]. A study showed that nAb longevity was associated with sustained levels of inflammatory cytokines, up to 180 days after symptoms onset in COVID-19 [52]; furthermore, pro-inflammatory cytokine milieu was correlated with antibody levels against the virus [53].

Some cytokines play an important role in B cell development, as interleukin (IL)-7, which aids in survival and proliferation; IL-4 and IL-6, which influence isotype switching; IL-10, which is important for regulation of the immune response; and Interferon-gamma (INF-γ), IL-12, and IL-17, which participate in B cell development [54–57].

Some studies show that patients with severe COVID-19 exhibit higher levels of IL-2, IL-6, IL-7, IL-10, INF-γ, tumor necrosis factor-alpha (TNF-α), inducible protein (IP)-10, monocyte chemoattractant protein (MCP)-1, macrophage inflammatory protein 1α, and granulocyte-colony stimulating factor than patients with mild and moderate infections. Such cytokine environment stimulates the antibody production and functionality [19, 58, 59].

Even though the cytokine storm induced by SARS-CoV-2 infection contributes to the humoral response, it can also be correlated with increased severity of the disease and favoring uncontrolled inflammation [60]. Considering that, cytokine production becomes a double-edged sword in the case of COVID-19.

## Maternal Antibodies

Maternal antibodies are transferred from mother to child to protect them during their immune system maturation in the first year of life. The majority of maternal antibodies are of IgG isotype, which are preferentially transferred before the birth in utero across placenta; these passively-transferred antibodies enter the bloodstream of offspring and act as a protective shield in the same way as active antibodies [61]. Different from IgG isotype, secretory IgA is transferred to breast milk from mother and protects the gastrointestinal tract against pathogens [62, 63].

It is well described that vaccination of pregnant women can increase neonatal antibodies against influenza, tetanus, diphtheria, and pertussis [64, 65]. Moreover, the WHO reports a 96% reduction of death by neonatal tetanus through the recommendation of certain good practices from 1988 to 2015, including the vaccination of pregnant women [66].

In a study that analyzed the seroconversion of newborns from pregnant women infected with SARS-CoV-2, it was demonstrated that SARS-CoV-2 IgG positive rate among parturients was 80.8%, and half of their infants obtained maternal IgG.

If the mothers were infected earlier and later than 2 weeks before delivery, the IgG rates were, respectively, 18.8% and 81.8% in their infants; after that, they presented a reduction of IgG in the first 2 months of life [67]. In this way, the study demonstrated that the passage of naturally induced maternal antibodies against SARS-CoV-2 is low. On the other side, when prenatal BNT16b2 mRNA vaccination was analyzed, it was observed a robust maternal humoral response, which was effectively transferred to the fetus [68], showing the importance of vaccination against SARS-CoV-2 during pregnancy.

## Conclusion

In this chapter, we have reviewed the humoral response after COVID-19. Our knowledge regarding SARS-CoV-2 has increased dramatically with the pandemic and we still have a long way to go to completely understand the virus and the response it triggers in the human immune system.

It should be noted that the substitution of amino acids in the variable portions of the immunoglobulins brings the advantage of high repertoire variability and greater chances of expression of a highly effective antibody, but this mechanism suffers an important restriction caused by the stability of the resulting protein. The stability of protein folding is constant when analyzing the evolution of proteins [69]; however, the mutations that generate the most specific paratope do not necessarily result in the most stable CDR region—it is a dynamic process. Affinity maturation is one of the easily observable examples of Darwinian evolution: genetic mutations are continuously happening in the coding regions of CDRs and selected immediately, since

B cells which mutations are neutral or beneficial rapidly expand. Emerging pathogens present an excellent opportunity to learn about the coevolution of pathogens and the immune system: evolution is happening right in front of our eyes.

## References


1. Dunkelberger JR, Song WC. Complement and its role in innate and adaptive immune responses. Cell Res. 2010;20:34–50. https://doi.org/10.1038/cr.2009.139.
2. Forthal DN. Functions of antibodies. In: Antibodies for infectious diseases. New York: American Society of Microbiology, Wiley; 2014. p. 25–48.
3. Assadiasl S, Fatahi Y, Zavvar M, Nicknam MH. COVID-19: significance of antibodies. Hum Antibodies. 2020;28:287–97. https://doi.org/10.3233/HAB-200429.
4. Inoue T, Moran I, Shinnakasu R, et al. Generation of memory B cells and their reactivation. Immunol Rev. 2018;283:138–49. https://doi.org/10.1111/imr.12640.
5. Shishido SN, Varahan S, Yuan K, et al. Humoral innate immune response and disease. Clin Immunol. 2012;144:142–58. https://doi.org/10.1016/j.clim.2012.06.002.
6. Eisen HN, Siskind GW. Variations in affinities of antibodies during the immune response. Biochemistry. 1964;3:996–1008. https://doi.org/10.1021/bi00895a027.
7. Berek C, Milstein C. Mutation drift and repertoire shift in the maturation of the immune response. Immunol Rev. 1987;96:23–41. https://doi.org/10.1111/j.1600-065X.1987.tb00507.x.
8. Wang S, Mata-Fink J, Kriegsman B, et al. Manipulating the selection forces during affinity maturation to generate cross-reactive HIV antibodies. Cell. 2015;160:785–97. https://doi.org/10.1016/j.cell.2015.01.027.
9. Van Valen L. Molecular evolution as predicted by natural selection. J Mol Evol. 1974;3:89–101. https://doi.org/10.1007/BF01796554.
10. Liow LH, Van Valen L, Stenseth NC. Red queen: from populations to taxa and communities. Trends Ecol Evol. 2011;26:349–58. https://doi.org/10.1016/j.tree.2011.03.016.
11. Brockhurst MA, Chapman T, King KC, et al. Running with the red queen: the role of biotic conflicts in evolution. Proc R Soc B Biol Sci. 2014;281:20141382. https://doi.org/10.1098/rspb.2014.1382.
12. Dai L, Gao GF. Viral targets for vaccines against COVID-19. Nat Rev Immunol. 2021;21:73–82. https://doi.org/10.1038/s41577-020-00480-0.
13. Paces J, Strizova Z, Smrz D, Cerny J. COVID-19 and the immune system. Physiol Res. 2020;69:379–88. https://doi.org/10.33549/PHYSIOLRES.934492.
14. Zhao J, Yuan Q, Wang H, et al. Antibody responses to SARS-CoV-2 in patients with novel coronavirus disease 2019. Clin Infect Dis. 2020;71:2027–34. https://doi.org/10.1093/cid/ciaa344.
15. Gudbjartsson DF, Norddahl GL, Melsted P, et al. Humoral immune response to SARS-CoV-2 in Iceland. N Engl J Med. 2020;383:1724–34. https://doi.org/10.1056/nejmoa2026116.
16. Liu C, Yu X, Gao C, et al. Characterization of antibody responses to SARS-CoV-2 in convalescent COVID-19 patients. J Med Virol. 2021;93:2227–33. https://doi.org/10.1002/jmv.26646.
17. Dan JM, Mateus J, Kato Y, et al. Immunological memory to SARS-CoV-2 assessed for up to 8 months after infection. Science. 2021;371:eabf4063. https://doi.org/10.1126/science.abf4063.
18. Gaebler C, Wang Z, Lorenzi JCC, et al. Evolution of antibody immunity to SARS-CoV-2. Nature. 2021;591:639–44. https://doi.org/10.1038/s41586-021-03207-w.
19. Huang C, Wang Y, Li X, et al. Clinical features of patients infected with 2019 novel coronavirus in Wuhan, China. Lancet. 2020;395:497–506. https://doi.org/10.1016/S0140-6736(20)30183-5.
20. Ma H, Zeng W, He H, et al. Serum IgA, IgM, and IgG responses in COVID-19. Cell Mol Immunol. 2020;17:773–5. https://doi.org/10.1038/s41423-020-0474-z.

21. Vardhana SA, Wolchok JD. The many faces of the anti-COVID immune response. J Exp Med. 2020;217:1–10. https://doi.org/10.1084/JEM.20200678.
22. Hoepel W, Chen H-J, Geyer CE, et al. High titers and low fucosylation of early human anti-SARS-CoV-2 IgG promote inflammation by alveolar macrophages. Sci Transl Med. 2021;13(596):eabf8654. https://doi.org/10.1126/scitranslmed.abf8654.
23. Woodruff MC, Ramonell RP, Nguyen DC, et al. Extrafollicular B cell responses correlate with neutralizing antibodies and morbidity in COVID-19. Nat Immunol. 2020;21:1506–16. https://doi.org/10.1038/s41590-020-00814-z.
24. Béné MC, de Carvalho BM, Eveillard M, Le Bris Y. Good IgA bad IgG in SARS-CoV-2 infection? Clin Infect Dis. 2020;71:897–8. https://doi.org/10.1093/cid/ciaa426.
25. Halstead SB, Katzelnick L. COVID-19 vaccines: should we fear ADE? J Infect Dis. 2020;222:1946–50. https://doi.org/10.1093/infdis/jiaa518.
26. Atyeo C, Fischinger S, Zohar T, et al. Distinct early serological signatures track with SARS-CoV-2 survival. Immunity. 2020;53:524–532.e4. https://doi.org/10.1016/j.immuni.2020.07.020.
27. Gallo O, Locatello LG, Mazzoni A, et al. The central role of the nasal microenvironment in the transmission, modulation, and clinical progression of SARS-CoV-2 infection. Mucosal Immunol. 2021;14:305–16. https://doi.org/10.1038/s41385-020-00359-2.
28. Wu J, Liang B, Chen C, et al. SARS-CoV-2 infection induces sustained humoral immune responses in convalescent patients following symptomatic COVID-19. Nat Commun. 2021;12:1–9. https://doi.org/10.1038/s41467-021-22034-1.
29. Weisberg SP, Connors TJ, Zhu Y, et al. Distinct antibody responses to SARS-CoV-2 in children and adults across the COVID-19 clinical spectrum. Nat Immunol. 2021;22:25–31. https://doi.org/10.1038/s41590-020-00826-9.
30. Cervia C, Nilsson J, Zurbuchen Y, et al. Systemic and mucosal antibody responses specific to SARS-CoV-2 during mild versus severe COVID-19. J Allergy Clin Immunol. 2021;147:545–557.e9. https://doi.org/10.1016/j.jaci.2020.10.040.
31. Klein SL, Pekosz A, Park HS, et al. Sex, age, and hospitalization drive antibody responses in a COVID-19 convalescent plasma donor population. J Clin Invest. 2020;130:6141–50. https://doi.org/10.1172/JCI142004.
32. Valdivia A, Torres I, Huntley D, et al. Qualitative assessment of SARS-CoV-2-specific antibody avidity by lateral flow immunochromatographic IgG/IgM antibody assay. J Med Virol. 2021;93:1141–4. https://doi.org/10.1002/jmv.26344.
33. Bauer G. The potential significance of high avidity immunoglobulin G (IgG) for protective immunity towards SARS-CoV-2. Int J Infect Dis. 2021;106:61–4. https://doi.org/10.1016/j.ijid.2021.01.061.
34. Benner SE, Patel EU, Laeyendecker O, et al. SARS-CoV-2 antibody avidity responses in COVID-19 patients and convalescent plasma donors. J Infect Dis. 2020;222:1974–84. https://doi.org/10.1093/infdis/jiaa581.
35. Gaspar EB, De Gaspari E. Avidity assay to test functionality of anti-SARS-Cov-2 antibodies. Vaccine. 2021;39:1473–5. https://doi.org/10.1016/j.vaccine.2021.02.003.
36. Zhang B, Zhou X, Zhu C, et al. Immune phenotyping based on the neutrophil-to-lymphocyte ratio and IgG level predicts disease severity and outcome for patients with COVID-19. Front Mol Biosci. 2020;7:157. https://doi.org/10.3389/fmolb.2020.00157.
37. Wang K, Long Q-X, Deng H-J, et al. Longitudinal dynamics of the neutralizing antibody response to severe acute respiratory syndrome coronavirus 2 (SARS-CoV-2) infection. Clin Infect Dis. 2020;73:e531–9. https://doi.org/10.1093/cid/ciaa1143.
38. Lei Q, Li Y, Yan HH, et al. Antibody dynamics to SARS-CoV-2 in asymptomatic COVID-19 infections. Allergy. 2021;76:551–61. https://doi.org/10.1111/all.14622.
39. Sterlin D, Mathian A, Miyara M, et al. IgA dominates the early neutralizing antibody response to SARS-CoV-2. Sci Transl Med. 2021;13(577):eabd2223. https://doi.org/10.1126/scitranslmed.abd2223.

40. Chao YX, Rötzschke O, Tan EK. The role of IgA in COVID-19. Brain Behav Immun. 2020;87:182–3. https://doi.org/10.1016/j.bbi.2020.05.057.
41. Dispinseri S, Secchi M, Pirillo MF, et al. Neutralizing antibody responses to SARS-CoV-2 in symptomatic COVID-19 is persistent and critical for survival. Nat Commun. 2021;12:2670. https://doi.org/10.1038/s41467-021-22958-8.
42. Karthik K, Senthilkumar TMA, Udhayavel S, Raj GD. Role of antibody-dependent enhancement (ADE) in the virulence of SARS-CoV-2 and its mitigation strategies for the development of vaccines and immunotherapies to counter COVID-19. Hum Vaccin Immunother. 2020;16:3055–60. https://doi.org/10.1080/21645515.2020.1796425.
43. West R, Kobokovich A, Connell N, Gronvall GK. COVID-19 antibody tests: a valuable public health tool with limited relevance to individuals. Trends Microbiol. 2021;29:214–23. https://doi.org/10.1016/j.tim.2020.11.002.
44. Lu L, Zhang H, Zhan M, et al. Antibody response and therapy in COVID-19 patients: what can be learned for vaccine development? Sci China Life Sci. 2020;63:1833–49. https://doi.org/10.1007/s11427-020-1859-y.
45. Sewell HF, Agius RM, Kendrick D, Stewart M. Vaccines, convalescent plasma, and monoclonal antibodies for COVID-19. BMJ. 2020;370:m2722. https://doi.org/10.1136/bmj.m2722.
46. To KKW, Hung IF-N, Ip JD, et al. Coronavirus disease 2019 (COVID-19) re-infection by a phylogenetically distinct severe acute respiratory syndrome coronavirus 2 strain confirmed by whole genome sequencing. Clin Infect Dis. 2020;73(9):e2946–51. https://doi.org/10.1093/cid/ciaa1275.
47. Van Elslande J, Vermeersch P, Vandervoort K, et al. Symptomatic severe acute respiratory syndrome coronavirus 2 (SARS-CoV-2) reinfection by a phylogenetically distinct strain. Clin Infect Dis. 2020;73:354–6. https://doi.org/10.1093/cid/ciaa1330.
48. Tillett RL, Sevinsky JR, Hartley PD, et al. Genomic evidence for reinfection with SARS-CoV-2: a case study. Lancet Infect Dis. 2021;21:52–8. https://doi.org/10.1016/S1473-3099(20)30764-7.
49. Guallar MP, Meiriño R, Donat-Vargas C, et al. Inoculum at the time of SARS-CoV-2 exposure and risk of disease severity. Int J Infect Dis. 2020;97:290–2. https://doi.org/10.1016/j.ijid.2020.06.035.
50. Yip MS, Leung NHL, Cheung CY, et al. Antibody-dependent infection of human macrophages by severe acute respiratory syndrome coronavirus. Virol J. 2014;11:1–11. https://doi.org/10.1186/1743-422X-11-82.
51. Moura A, Costa HH, Correa V, et al. S assessment of avidity related to IgG subclasses in SARS-CoV-2 Brazilian infected patients. Sci Rep. 2021;11:17642. https://doi.org/10.1038/s41598-021-95045-z.
52. Chia WN, Zhu F, Ong SWX, et al. Dynamics of SARS-CoV-2 neutralising antibody responses and duration of immunity: a longitudinal study. Lancet Microbe. 2021;6:e240–9. https://doi.org/10.1016/S2666-5247(21)00025-2.
53. Wu F, Liu M, Wang A, et al. Evaluating the Association of Clinical Characteristics with neutralizing antibody levels in patients who have recovered from mild COVID-19 in Shanghai, China. JAMA Intern Med. 2020;180:1356–62. https://doi.org/10.1001/jamainternmed.2020.4616.
54. Abed NS, Chace JH, Fleming AL, Cowdery JS. Interferon-γ regulation of B lymphocyte differentiation: activation of B cells is a prerequisite for IFN-γ-mediated inhibition of B cell differentiation. Cell Immunol. 1994;153:356–66. https://doi.org/10.1006/cimm.1994.1034.
55. Metzger DW. Interleukin-12 as an adjuvant for induction of protective antibody responses. Cytokine. 2010;52:102–7. https://doi.org/10.1016/j.cyto.2010.06.011.
56. Vazquez MI, Catalan-Dibene J, Zlotnik A. B cells responses and cytokine production are regulated by their immune microenvironment. Cytokine. 2015;74:318–26. https://doi.org/10.1016/j.cyto.2015.02.007.
57. Shibui A, Shimura E, Nambu A, et al. Th17 cell-derived IL-17 is dispensable for B cell antibody production. Cytokine. 2012;59:108–14. https://doi.org/10.1016/j.cyto.2012.03.018.
58. Chen G, Wu D, Guo W, et al. Clinical and immunological features of severe and moderate coronavirus disease 2019. J Clin Invest. 2020;130:2620–9. https://doi.org/10.1172/JCI137244.

59. Liu J, Li S, Liu J, et al. Longitudinal characteristics of lymphocyte responses and cytokine profiles in the peripheral blood of SARS-CoV-2 infected patients. EBioMedicine. 2020;55:102763. https://doi.org/10.1016/j.ebiom.2020.102763.
60. Hojyo S, Uchida M, Tanaka K, et al. How COVID-19 induces cytokine storm with high mortality. Inflamm Regen. 2020;40:37. https://doi.org/10.1186/s41232-020-00146-3.
61. Fouda GG, Martinez DR, Swamy GK, Permar SR. The impact of IgG transplacental transfer on early life immunity. Immuno Horizons. 2018;2:14–25. https://doi.org/10.4049/immunohorizons.1700057.
62. Langel SN, Otero CE, Martinez DR, Permar SR. Maternal gatekeepers: how maternal antibody fc characteristics influence passive transfer and infant protection. PLoS Pathog. 2020;16:e1008303. https://doi.org/10.1371/journal.ppat.1008303.
63. Niewiesk S. Maternal antibodies: clinical significance, mechanism of interference with immune responses, and possible vaccination strategies. Front Immunol. 2014;5:446. https://doi.org/10.3389/fimmu.2014.00446.
64. Albrecht M, Pagenkemper M, Wiessner C, et al. Infant immunity against viral infections is advanced by the placenta-dependent vertical transfer of maternal antibodies. Vaccine. 2021;40(11):1563–71. https://doi.org/10.1016/j.vaccine.2020.12.049.
65. Albrecht M, Arck PC. Vertically transferred immunity in neonates: mothers, mechanisms and mediators. Front Immunol. 2020;11:555. https://doi.org/10.3389/fimmu.2020.00555.
66. World Health Organization. Protecting all against tetanus guide to sustaining maternal and neonatal tetanus elimination (MNTE) and broadening tetanus protection for all populations. 2019. https://apps.who.int/iris/bitstream/handle/10665/329882/9789241515610-eng.pdf?sequence=1&isAllowed=y
67. Wang X, Yang P, Zheng J, et al. Dynamic changes of acquired maternal SARS-CoV-2 IgG in infants. Sci Rep. 2021;11:8021. https://doi.org/10.1038/s41598-021-87535-x.
68. Beharier O, Plitman Mayo R, Raz T, et al. Efficient maternal to neonatal transfer of SARS-CoV-2 and BNT162b2 antibodies. J Clin Invest. 2021;131(13):e15031. https://doi.org/10.1172/JCI150319.
69. Lässig M, Mustonen V, Walczak AM. Predicting evolution. Nat Ecol Evol. 2017;1:77. https://doi.org/10.1038/s41559-017-0077.

# Chapter 3
# SARS-CoV-2 Invasion and Pathogenesis of COVID-19: A Perspective of Viral Receptors, Bradykinin, and Purinergic System

**Angélica Regina Cappellari, Julia Brandt de Souza, Daniele Rubert Nogueira-Librelotto, Jéssica Dotto de Lara, Jéssica Carla Martins Couto, Júlia Leão Batista Simões, Margarete Dulce Bagatini, Carlos Fernando Mello, and Micheli Mainardi Pillat**

---

Angélica Regina Cappellari and Julia Brandt de Souza contributed equally with all other contributors.

---

A. R. Cappellari
Laboratory of Molecular Biology, Biovel—Laboratory of Clinical Research and Analysis, Cascavel, PR, Brazil
e-mail: angelica.cappellari@biovel.com.br

J. B. de Souza · J. C. M. Couto · C. F. Mello
Postgraduate Program in Pharmacology, Health Sciences Center, Federal University of Santa Maria, Santa Maria, RS, Brazil
e-mail: julia.brandt@acad.ufsm.br; carlos.mello@ufsm.br

D. R. Nogueira-Librelotto · J. D. de Lara
Postgraduate Program in Pharmaceutical Sciences, Health Sciences Center, Federal University of Santa Maria, Santa Maria, RS, Brazil
e-mail: librelotto.daniele@ufsm.br; jessica.dotto@acad.ufsm.br

J. L. B. Simões · M. D. Bagatini
Graduate Program in Biomedical Sciences, Federal University of Fronteira Sul, Chapecó, SC, Brazil
e-mail: margarete.bagatini@uffs.edu.br

M. M. Pillat (✉)
Postgraduate Program in Pharmacology, Health Sciences Center, Federal University of Santa Maria, Santa Maria, RS, Brazil

Postgraduate Program in Pharmaceutical Sciences, Health Sciences Center, Federal University of Santa Maria, Santa Maria, RS, Brazil

Department of Microbiology and Parasitology, Health Sciences Center, Federal University of Santa Maria, Santa Maria, RS, Brazil
e-mail: micheli.pillat@ufsm.br


S. Adibi et al. (eds.), *Frontiers of COVID-19*,
https://doi.org/10.1007/978-3-031-08045-6_3

## Introduction

The present chapter focuses on the mechanisms of the Severe Acute Respiratory Syndrome Coronavirus-2 (SARS-CoV-2) infection, pathogenesis, and the possible therapeutic strategies targeted to the viral receptors, purinergic and kallikrein–kinin system. SARS-CoV-2 can bind to three main receptors on host cells: angiotensin-converting enzyme 2 (ACE2), CD147 (also known as basigin or EMMPRIN), and CD209. This interaction between spike from virus and receptors on the host cell is the first step for SARS-CoV-2 invasion, intracellular infection cycle, and, later, dissemination of virus among other cells. Recent studies have detailed the mechanism by which cell invasion occurs, evidencing the involvement of several proteins/enzymes and their differential expression on tissues. These routes provide important targets for developing specific and effective anti–COVID-19 drugs, as well as reveal a novel understanding of pathogenesis and tropism of SARS-CoV-2.

Following viral infection, a plethora of subsequent molecular and cellular alterations occurs in the host. These alterations, which include the activation of host defense mechanisms, have been implicated in the genesis of the signs and symptoms observed in COVID-19 patients. In this context, the kallikrein–kinin system has been proposed to play a key role in the pathological findings associated to SARS-CoV-2 infection.

Kinins, such as bradykinin (BK), bind to B1 and B2 receptors (B1R and B2R) and cause several systemic effects. They include increased vasodilation (and consequent hypotension), increased endothelial permeability, driving the edema observed in infected tissue, and bronchoconstriction. Moreover, the activation of the kallikrein–kinin system facilitates inflammation, natriuresis, and blood coagulation. In fact, samples obtained from COVID-19 patients reveal an extreme imbalance in kallikrein–kinin system, increasing BK on a system-wide level (referred to as a "bradykinin storm"). Therefore, we will discuss here the available evidence that indicate a role for the kallikrein–kinin system in the signs and symptoms of COVID-19-infected patients [1, 2].

The inflammatory process is essential for the organism to effectively deal with the SARS-CoV-2 infection. Nevertheless, deleterious excessive and prolonged responses of cytokines and chemokines, such as cytokine storm, can occur. In this chapter, we emphasize the immune responses activated by the extracellular nucleotide adenosine triphosphate (ATP), which is released from several cell types by autocrine secretion or after damage. Current evidence indicates that SARS-CoV-2 infection-induced release of ATP promotes immune cells activation, proliferation, and migration, possibly facilitating inflammation. Therefore, one might reasonably propose decreasing purinergic signalling to attenuate the exacerbated immune response in COVID-19, including the cytokine storm, and reduce inflammation-induced tissue damage.

## Human Cell Invasion by SARS-CoV-2

### *ACE-2 and SARS-CoV-2, The Supposed Main Mechanism*

SARS-CoV-2 is a virus of Coronaviridae family and is the cause of Coronavirus Disease-19 (COVID-19) pandemic since early 2020. SARS-CoV-2, similarly to SARS-CoV and MERS-CoV, enters human host cells by using angiotensin-converting enzyme 2 (ACE-2) as a receptor [3–5]. This is an important and determinant factor of viral infectivity and pathogenesis [6, 7], and understanding these mechanisms may lead to a target for therapeutic treatment [8].

Evolution of COVID-19 infection depends on specific interaction of Spike (S) protein found on the virus surface with ACE-2. SARS-CoV-2 shares 80% of structural similarity with SARS-CoV [9]. Interestingly, Ortega and collaborators (2020) showed that SARS-CoV-2 S protein binds with higher affinity to the human ACE2 receptor (hACE2) than Bat-CoV S protein. Moreover, SARS-CoV-2 receptor binding domain (RBD) has a higher hACE2 binding affinity than SARS-CoV RBD [10]. Such a high affinity for hACE may be the cause of high infectivity and rapid spread of SARS-CoV-2 in humans [10, 11].

First, SARS-CoV-2 recognizes hACE2 as its receptor [7, 8] through binding the S1 subunit (where lies RBD) of the S protein [5]. ACE2 is an enzyme homologous to angiotensin-converting enzyme (ACE) and plays a key role in the renin-angiotensin system (RAS) that maintains blood pressure homeostasis and fluid and salt balance [12–14]. ACE2 is widely expressed in several tissues, including heart, kidneys, blood vessels, gastrointestinal system and pulmonary alveolar epithelia, which are the main targets of SARS-CoV-2 [15]. Viral entry also depends on the transmembrane protease serine protease-2 (TMPRSS-2), which is present in host cells and manages the cleavage of the S1 and S2 subunit of the viral S protein. This protein allows for the fusion of the viral membrane and the host membrane [6, 16, 17]. Finally, SARS-CoV-2 is internalized by endocytosis and viral RNA is released for replication inside of host cells and assembly of new viral particles [18].

SARS-CoV-2 infection downregulates ACE2, increases Ang-II levels and over-activates angiotensin-II type 1 receptor (AT1R) [19]. The Ang-II/AT1R axis has pro-inflammatory, pro-fibrotic, pro-thrombotic, and vasoconstrictor effects, facilitating the occurrence of respiratory diseases, including pneumonia [20, 21]. Metabolic disorders, such as diabetes and hypertension, also downregulate the RAS axis and, for this reason, patients with these comorbidities present poor prognosis in SARS-CoV-2 infections [22].

Preventing SARS-CoV-2 infection is yet the best strategy to avoid virus dissemination. Blockade of ACE2 constitute an important way to prevent viral invasion, inhibitors of this receptor and monoclonal antibodies have been studied in clinical trials [18, 23].

## *CD147 and CD209, Additional Mechanisms of Infection*

CD147 is a transmembrane glycoprotein that belongs to the immunoglobulin superfamily, a group of proteins with at least one Ig domain which play an essential role in intracellular communication and various physiological and pathological processes [24]. CD147, also known as basigin (BSG) or extracellular matrix metalloproteinase inducer (EMMPRIN), is expressed in various tissues and progressively overexpressed during tumor development. In fact, in tumor cells it triggers the production and/or release of metalloproteinases, contributing to tumor invasion [25]. In addition, CD147 may be important for bacterial and virus infection, such as HIV, and it is an essential receptor for the invasion of *Plasmodium falciparum*, which causes malaria [26].

It has been shown that CD147 is a multifunctional protein related to inflammatory processes. The affinity for cyclophilins increases the migration of inflammatory leukocytes and acts as a receptor for cyclophilin A. Similarly, previous studies have shown that the nucleocapsid (N) protein of SARS-CoV, linked to cyclophilin A (CyPA), interacts with CD147, facilitating SARS-CoV infection [27]. Based on this study, possible interactions of CD147 with SARS-CoV-2 proteins were also investigated.

The direct interaction of CD147 with the SARS-CoV-2S protein was identified by Wang et al. [28]. That study showed that the loss of CD147 or its blockage by Meplazumab inhibits the replication of SARS-CoV-2. On the other hand, CD147 overexpression facilitates virus infection. These results reveal a potential receptor for SARS-CoV-2 entry and highlight the importance of developing drugs that block this pathway [28]. Actually, CD147 levels are significantly higher than ACE2 levels in human bronchial epithelial BEAS-2B cells, which are particularly susceptible to SARS-CoV-2 infection. Moreover, expression of ACE2 has not been detected in these lung cells, further supporting a role for CD147 and ACE2 levels in SARS-CoV-2 infection [28].

CD147 has been identified as a marker of lymphocyte activation, whereas ACE2 is not expressed in these cells. SARS-CoV-2 infection compromises lung cells and triggers an inflammatory storm, including T cell immune responses. The decline of CD8+ T cells by SARS-CoV-2 infection has been associated to poor prognosis in patients with COVID-19. Current evidence suggests that CD147 can mediate SARS-CoV-2 infection in CD4+ and CD8+ T cells, significantly impacting on prognosis of infected patients [29]. Importantly, anti-CD147 antibodies block the development of infectious diseases mentioned above. At last, experimental models have revealed that this strategy may be a promising therapy for other CD147-dependent diseases [30, 31].

A recent study has identified CD209 and CD209L proteins as receptors for SARS-CoV-2 entry into human cells. CD209 is expressed on dendritic cells and alveolar macrophages and CD209L is mainly expressed on lung and liver cells. Both proteins belong to the C-type lectin superfamily. SARS-CoV-2S protein binds to CD209L and CD209, mediating its entry into these cells. A mutual cooperative role for both proteins in virus entry and infection has been described in all tissues where CD209L and ACE2 proteins are expressed. These studies suggest that CD147, CD209 and CD209L are putative receptors that may be promising targets for developing novel therapies for COVID-19 [32].

## Bradykinin and Kinin–Kallikrein System

Bradykinin (BK) is a potent regulator of blood pressure and has been considered an extension of the renin–angiotensin–aldosterone system (RAAS) [33]. BK is a peptide produced from an inactive preprotein kininogen through activation by two types of serine proteases called kallikreins, which constitute the kallikrein–kinin system (KKS), a part of innate inflammation (Fig. 3.1). Kallikreins can be divided in plasma and tissue kallikreins. Tissue kallikrein cleaves low-molecular weight kininogen (LMWK) to release Lys-bradykinin (Lys-BK). Plasma kallikrein processes high-molecular-weight kininogen (HMWK) into BK. Both BK and Lys-BK are the

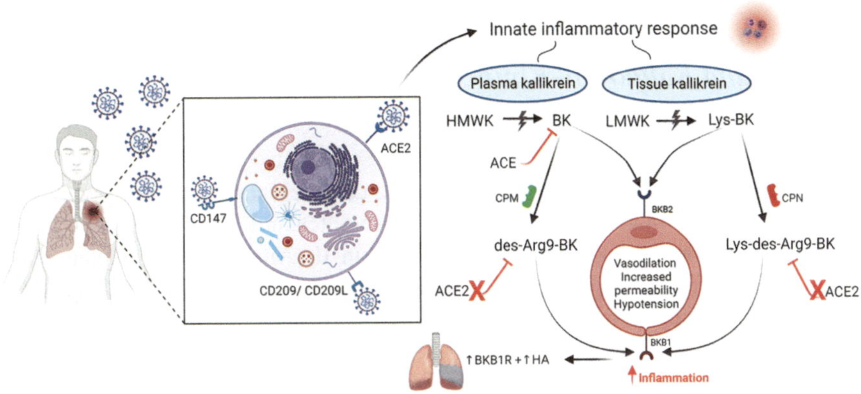


**Fig. 3.1** Schematic representation of the SARS-CoV-2 receptors and involvement of kallikrein–kinin system on the COVID-19. SARS-CoV-2 can bind to three main receptors on host cells: angiotensin-converting enzyme 2 (ACE2), CD147, and CD209. This interaction between spike from virus and these receptors on the host cell is the first step for SARS-CoV-2 invasion, intracellular infection cycle and, posteriorly, dissemination of virus among other cells starting the immune answer. BK is a peptide produced from an inactive preprotein kininogen through activation by two types of serine proteases called kallikreins, which constitute the kallikrein–kinin system (KKS). Tissue kallikrein cleaves low-molecular weight kininogen (LMWK) to release Lys-bradykinin (Lys-BK). Plasma kallikrein processes high-molecular-weight kininogen (HMWK) into BK. Both BK and Lys-BK are the ligands for the constitutively expressed kinin receptor type 2 (B2R) on the endothelial cells, and its binding results in vasodilation, increased blood vessel permeability, natriuresis, and hypotension. BK is degraded primarily by angiotensin-converting enzyme (ACE), a dipeptidase participating in RAAS that removes the C-terminal phe-arg, which inactivates it, followed by removal of ser-pro. In addition, carboxypeptidase M (CPM) and carboxypeptidase N (CPN) can further process BK and Lys-BK into des-Arg9-BK and Lys-des-Arg9-BK, respectively. These peptides are ligands for kinin receptor type 1 (B1R), a receptor present on endothelial cells that also mediates vasodilation and vascular permeability, particularly during inflammation, as observed in COVID-19

ligands for the constitutively expressed kinin receptor type 2 (B2R) on the endothelial cells, and its binding results in vasodilation, increased blood vessel permeability, natriuresis, and hypotension [34–36]. BK is degraded primarily by Angiotensin-converting enzyme (ACE), a dipeptidase participating in RAAS that removes the C-terminal phe-arg, which inactivates it, followed by removal of ser-pro [36, 37]. In addition, carboxypeptidase M (CPM) and carboxypeptidase N (CPN) can further process BK and Lys-BK into des-Arg9-BK and Lys-des-Arg9-BK, respectively. These peptides are ligands for kinin receptor type 1 (B1R), a receptor present on endothelial cells that also mediates vasodilation and vascular permeability, particularly during inflammation, a condition in which these receptors are upregulated [35, 38].

In addition to its role in pressure and fluid homeostasis, BK induces neutrophil recruitment, increases vascular permeability, and induces pain via stimulation of B1R [39]. BK has also been associated with a range of different pathophysiological conditions, including angioedema, asthma, autoimmunity, vasculitis, acute brain injury, and neuroinflammation [40].

## *Functional Relation Between Angiotensin-Converting Enzyme-2 (ACE2) and Kallikrein–Kinin System: Implications in COVID-19*

It has already been mentioned that ACE2 is a cell membrane receptor involved in SARS-CoV-2 internalization. ACE2 cleaves Angiotensin I (Ang I) into a nonapeptide, Angiotensin$_{1-9}$ (Ang 1–9), and Angiotensin II (Ang II) into a heptapeptide, Angiotensin$_{1-7}$ (Ang 1–7) [41]. Despite their structural homology, ACE2 and ACE have divergent physiological functions. Whereas ACE regulates the RAAS, which is a critical regulator of blood volume and systemic vascular resistance, ACE2 counterbalances the effects of the RAAS/ACE/Ang II pathway. This occurs through its action with the ACE2/Ang 1–7 axis that activates MAS/G receptor, which has been implicated in cell survival [42].

Under physiological conditions, there is a balance between ACE and ACE2 receptor activity, which is lost after SARS-CoV-2 infection. To gain entry to endothelial cells of the lungs, this virus binds to ACE2 via its viral S protein that is cleaved by a transmembrane serum protease (TMPRSS2) [9]. This process leads to shedding of ACE2 and loss of its protective function that, in turn, prevents production of Ang 1–9 and Ang 1–7. Thus, the protective functions of Ang 1–7 are lost, including vasodilation, and cell protection both at the epithelial and endothelial sites by activating the MAS/G receptor. In addition, the diminishing in ACE2 function leads to a substantial imbalance and unchecked effects of Ang II and upregulation of RAAS/Ang II pathway. Therefore, the SARS-CoV-2-mediated downregulation of ACE2 and the resulting increased overall ratio of Ang II to Ang 1–7 leads to important physiological effects, such as vasoconstriction, thrombophilia and microthrombosis [41]. Moreover, the increase in Ang II can lead to deterioration of the pulmonary function and acute lung injury [43] which have been attributed to exacerbated vasoconstriction, oxidative stress, inflammation, atrophy, fibrosis and endothelial dysfunction through cyclooxygenase-2 (COX-2) activation. All these events, along with the loss of the modulating effect of Ang 1–7 via its binding to MAS/G receptor may be further contributing factors to the hyperinflammation status of the late phase in COVID-19 patients [44, 45].

Therefore, based on the described mechanisms, it is clear that in addition to its protective role in the RAAS, ACE2 has a direct protective effect on alveolar epithelial cells, preventing lung injury. In this sense, there is a race to better understand the relationship between RAAS, viral infection and lung injury [46]. Recent studies have shed new light on the role of ACE2 in the pathophysiology of COVID-19 through the KKS [47, 48]. The association of ACE2 downregulation with severe angioedema, together with the prominent lung edema seen in SARS-CoV-2-infected patients, has directed special attention to the prominent role of BK in the pathogenesis of the pulmonary dysfunction of COVID-19, which is linked in part to changes in the RAAS. BK is tightly integrated with the RAAS as BK receptor signaling is increased by Ang 1–9, likely by resensitization of the B2R, and also because BK is degraded by ACE [37].

The KKS is a hormonal system that plays a key role in the regulation of physiological processes such as inflammation, blood pressure control, coagulation, and pain. Following the viral invasion, the understanding of the main cellular and molecular alterations responsible by symptoms observed in COVID-19 patients is fundamental. Although many times neglected in current studies, it was evidenced that the KKS plays an essential role in regulating the inflammatory process. In this context, recent analyses of samples from COVID-19 patients demonstrate extreme imbalance in KKS, revealing upregulation of multiple components that lead to BK production and downregulation of factors that control the process [1].

As previously mentioned, both BK and Lys-BK are further processed into des-Arg9-BK and Lys-des-Arg9-BK by carboxypeptidases. These kinins have potent vasopermeable and vasodilatory capacity and need to be controlled to prevent angioedema. Both ACE and ACE2 have roles in inactivating the ligands for BK receptors. The expression of ACE is downregulated in SARS-CoV-2 so that BK would not be inactivated normally, which has been associated to systemic angioedema since it can lead to an exacerbated presence of BK. On the other hand, under normal conditions, ACE2 protects against pulmonary edema by inactivating des-Arg9-BK and Lys-des-Arg9-BK, which are potent ligand of the B1R in the lung. It is known that SARS-CoV-2 binding to ACE2 limits its enzymatic activity, which would likely impair the inactivation of these two kinins. Consequently, they would be free to activate the endothelial B1R, leading to extra vascular leakage, resulting in pulmonary edema, inflammation, and oxidative stress in COVID-19 [39, 47]. Altogether, it is evidenced that an upregulation and overactivation of BK receptors take place in COVID-19 patients. B2R was increased 207-fold and the B1R 2945-fold, and this markedly augmented BK receptors production may result in the so-called bradykinin storm [36].

Therefore, it is easy to note that RAAS and KKS are functionally related, suggesting that any intervention aiming to treat COVID-19 patients by only triggering one system and ignoring the other may not be adequately effective in limiting the state of hyperinflammation typical of severe cases of SARS-CoV-2 infection.

## *Bradykinin Storm*

After SARS-CoV-2 invasion, a cascade of events occurs in the host, and the severity of COVID-19 is associated with a "cytokine storm", since inflammatory mechanisms and pro-inflammatory cytokines are fundamentally associated with progression of the disease [44]. However, more recent studies have evidenced the BK and its dysregulated signaling, so-called "Bradykinin Storm", as a primary mechanism likely responsible for most of the observed COVID-19 symptoms, which also explain COVID-19-related complications [1]. It is worth mentioning that the "Bradykinin storm" is the result of extreme imbalance in the KKS, and BK is close associated to RAAS, which is linked to many of the COVID-19 outcomes. Firstly, the decrease ACE expression induced by SARS-CoV-2 infection resulted in the impairment of BK degradation, leading to an exacerbation of BK-effects, such as pain sensitization and increased vascular permeability in tissues that have been infected by the virus. In addition, despite the negative regulation of ACE2 has a direct effect in the upregulation of Ang II, the decreased function of ACE2 has also a straight role in the KKS imbalance. ACE2 does not inactivate BK, but can cleave the terminal residue of des-arg9-BK and Lys-des-arg9-BK, rendering them unable to interact with B1R [35, 37, 49]. Therefore, ACE2 downregulation observed on COVID-19 suppresses the immunomodulatory effects, leading to accentuation of the cytokine levels. Therefore, the resulted KKS imbalance will overactivate the des-arg9-BK/Lys-des-arg9-BK/B1R receptor axis, resulting in pulmonary edema [48]. The B1R has low expression in physiological conditions, but is upregulated in pro-inflammatory events, like what occurs in COVID-19. In the lungs, B1R is expressed on bronchiolar exocrine cells and pneumocytes type II and signaling through this receptor can induce fluid extravasation and recruitment of leucocytes to the lungs [39]. Unlike B1R, B2R is expressed continuously, and BK binding leads to vasodilation, inflammation, and capillary extravasation, triggering angioedema, that is, intravascular fluid extravasation [36]. Considering that both receptors take part in the occurrence of edema, it is suggested that the blockage of B1R in the inflammatory state is just as important as blocking B2R to prevent edema in COVID-19 patients [2].

Concomitantly with the "bradykinin storm," there is an exacerbated release of hyaluronic acid (HA). HA is present in most connective tissues and can hold water at about 1000 times its weight. This means that when it is exposed to water, the HA molecules form a gel. Similar to what happens in the RAAS and KKS, the genes that code for HA are positively regulated, increasing its production, in contrast to the genes that code for the HA degradation receptor and the gene that codes hyaluronidase (enzyme that degrades HA), which are negatively regulated. The association of these events increases the amount of HA in the bronchoalveolar space which, added to the increase in vascular permeability caused by BK, constitutes a gel that impairs gas exchange [1].

The link of the KKS in the pulmonary manifestations in COVID-19 patients was supported by research findings in bronchoalveolar lavage (BAL), where positive regulation of genes related to BK, its precursor, and enzymes that degrade BK and its analogues was found. In the same study, ACE2 expression was reported to be increased in COVID-19 patients, which may be explained by increased soluble ACE2 along with decreased membrane surface ACE2 in COVID-19 patients [1].

## Purinergic System as Target in the Modulation of Immune System Triggered by SARS-CoV-2

### *Purinergic Signalling*

During SARS-CoV-2 infection intense cell death occurs. This event promotes intracellular content overflow together the virus particles, activating immune response. ATP (adenosine triphosphate) is one of these intracellular molecules that trigger inflammation by activating a specific signalling system, named purinergic system [50].

It was long believed that ATP role was limited to provide intracellular energy source for biochemical reactions. However, in 1972, Geoffrey Burnstock proposed that ATP could act as a neurotransmitter beyond the adrenergic and cholinergic nerves and then the term "purinergic" was coined [51]. This hypothesis was gradually accepted in the field of scientific research until 1976, when Burnstock defined purinergic receptors [52]. Soon after, in 1978, he proposed a basis to differentiate two types of purinoceptor, identified as P1 (for adenosine) and P2 (for ATP/ADP) [53]. These receptors are further subclassified into several subtypes, which are diffusely expressed in tissues and modulate important biological processes, including muscle contraction, immune response, inflammation, platelet aggregation, pain, and neurotransmission [54, 55].

P1 receptors are G protein-coupled receptors and sensitive to adenosine in the extracellular environment. They can be described in four subtypes: $A_1$, $A_{2a}$, $A_{2b}$, and $A_3$, with different pharmacological properties between them [55]. P2 receptors can be further divided into type ligand-gated ion channels (P2X) and as well as P1 receptors, P2Y are G protein-coupled [56]. To date, seven members belong to the P2X receptor Family ($P2X_{1-7}$) and eight members belong to the P2Y receptors ($P2Y_{1,2,4,6,11-14}$) [57, 58].

Ectonucleotidases are a family of enzymes that hydrolyze the nucleotides present in the extracellular environment that control the signalling of extracellular nucleotides and the interaction with their respective receptors. For instance, ectonucleoside triphosphate diphosphohydrolase (NTPDase) and ecto-5′-nucleotidase/CD73 (ecto-5′NT/CD73) promote the hydrolysis of ATP into adenosine, respectively, and are involved in the balance of extracellular nucleotides in physiological and pathological conditions [59, 60].

## *Involvement of Purinergic Signalling on the Modulation of Inflammatory Process Generated by SARS-CoV-2 Infection*

SARS-CoV-2 infection is clinically defined by different manifestations and may present, in milder cases, fever, dry cough, fatigue, gastrointestinal infections, and dyspnea, while in critical situations it can lead to multiple organ failure, hyperinflammation, deranged coagulation, exuberant release of cytokines, profound and progressive hypoxia, characterized as acute respiratory distress syndrome (ARDS) [61]. This disorder of pro-inflammatory cytokines can trigger neuroinflammation, thrombotic events, oxidative stress, dysregulation of the hypothalamic–pituitary–adrenal axis and other natural mechanisms. Thus, although inflammation is physiologically a protective strategy for the organism, the lack of control caused by the virus makes it harmful to the organism as a whole.

In that regard, purinergic signalling, which was thought to be an essential signalling pathway only in the nervous system, is also considered even more important in the immune and inflammatory systems [62]. Purinergic system has main functions in inflammation, promotion of immune cells, and chemotaxis of inflammatory cells [63]. Thus, it is understood why the modulation of this system can reduce cytokine storm damage and return inflammatory or stressed environments to homeostasis. From this perspective, many studies have highlighted purinergic modulation for its therapeutic potential.

Among them are studies that analyze the role of P2X7R in the pathology of COVID-19 [64], the therapeutic potential of different purinergic receptors in cardiovascular diseases mediated by COVID-19 [65], the protective action of adenosine in hypoxia and pulmonary inflammation [66], as well as its relationship in neuroinflammation and ATP signalling in Guillain–Barré syndrome, a neurodegenerative disease associated with SARS-CoV-2 infection [67]. In addition, the purinergic system has been highlighted as a therapeutic target for the treatment of immune-mediated inflammatory diseases [68]. From this perspective, one realizes that the pathophysiology of previous diseases revolves around the lack of control of inflammation, promoted and exacerbated by the COVID-19 cytokine storm. Thus, understanding how purinergic modulation would act on this generalized inflammation allows us to understand its potentials and use this knowledge specifically in diseases triggered by SARS-CoV-2 infection.

Characterized by a complex immune system response, which can be initiated by infections, irradiation, tissue damage, and toxic compounds, inflammation is an essential natural mechanism to contain harmful stimuli and initiate the repair and healing process [63]. In its acute phase, in the extravascular space or at the site of injury/infection, there is an accumulation of fluid, inflammatory cells and pro-inflammatory mediators that will act directly on the inflammatory process for eventual restoration of homeostasis. Among these components, immune cells such as neutrophils, macrophages, natural killer (NK) cells [69] and pro-inflammatory mediators such as interleukins (IL), colony stimulating factors, interferons (IFNs), tumor necrosis factors (TNFs), chemokines, histamine, kinins stand out, clotting factors, complement factors, nitric oxide, and pro-inflammatory eicosanoids such as prostaglandins and leukotrienes [69].

In addition, a wide variety of anti-inflammatory molecular mechanisms and cellular interactions come into effect to minimize the extent of tissue damage [63]. Among the anti-inflammatory mediators, IL-10, transforming growth factors (TGFs), carbon monoxide, and glucocorticoids act directly and significantly in this restoration, which will be finalized by the mechanisms of inflammatory resolution, which is mediated by anti-inflammatory eicosanoids, such as lipoxins, as well as resolvins, protectins, and maresins [70]. Thus, in addition to the components described above, purines also orchestrate the onset, duration, magnitude, and resolution of the inflammatory picture by extracellular signalling from purinergic receptors, which are widely expressed in the involved cells [68, 71–77].

In this perspective, purinergic enzymatic activity can also be modulated, given that the increased activity of CD39 and CD73 contribute, respectively, to the reduction of ATP levels and the increase in the amount of adenosine at the site of infection. Thus, inflammation that results in cell injury, as well as ischemia–reperfusion injury in pulmonary involvement [78], is capable of releasing ATP and other inflammatory mediators (Fig. 3.2). This extracellular ATP can trigger an immune response [79] by serving as a chemotactic signal to phagocytes and other inflammatory cells. In addition, it is able to activate P2X7R and promote the release of cytokines (IL-1β) and activation of the NLRP3 inflammasome, as well as the release of cytokines (IL-1β, IL-6, and TNF-α) [80] and damage to the pulmonary epithelium by P2Y6R [81]. In addition, it acts on platelet aggregation by activating P2Y12, P2Y1, and P2X1 [82–84], and this activation is a positive feedback mechanism, further exacerbating the inflammation generated by the cytokine storm in COVID-19 (Fig. 3.2).

The research by Ahmadi et al. [85], a control group study that analyzed the expression pattern of CD39 and CD73 in CD4+ T, CD8+ T, natural killer T (NKT) cells in patients with COVID-19, showed a correlation between the absence of CD73 from CD8+ and NKT T cells, as well as increased secretion of inflammatory molecules. Considering that overexpressed CD39 negatively regulates the NLRP3 inflammasome and decreases the release of reactive oxygen species (ROS) [86], the lack of these enzymes in the framework of COVID-19 and other diseases leads to increased inflammation and lack of control of this condition, increasing the severity and lethality of the disease.

In contrast, by attenuating hypoxia-induced inflammation, extracellular adenosine has been highlighted in the literature for its anti-inflammatory role [87]. Thus, the extracellular conversion of ATP to adenosine plays a central role in attenuating sterile inflammation during ischemia–reperfusion injury, as demonstrated in

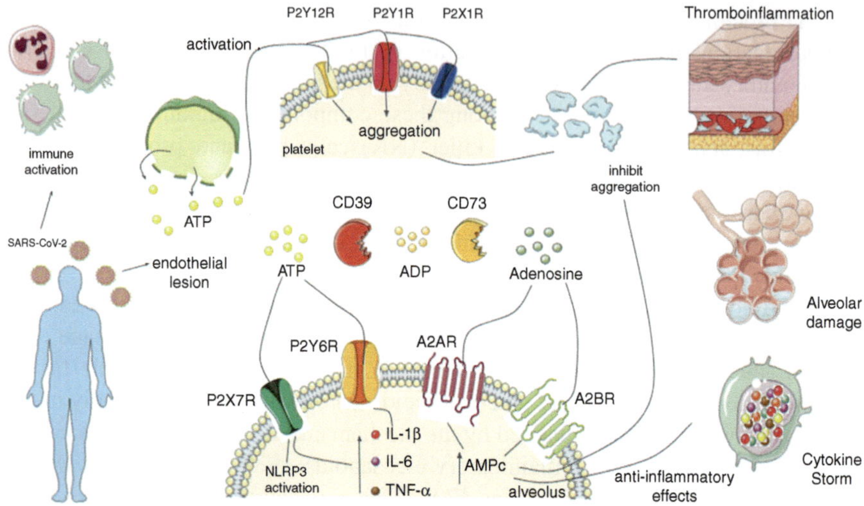


**Fig. 3.2** Schematic representation of the involvement of purinergic signalling on the modulation of inflammatory process generated by SARS-CoV-2 infection. Inflammation that results in cell injury after SARS-CoV-2 infection, is capable of releasing ATP and other inflammatory mediators. This extracellular ATP can trigger an immune response by serving as a chemotactic signal to phagocytes and other inflammatory cells. In addition, it is able to activate P2X7R and promote the release of cytokines and activation of the NLRP3 inflammasome, as well as the release of cytokines and damage to the pulmonary epithelium by P2Y6R. In addition, it acts on platelet aggregation by activating P2Y12, P2Y1, and P2X1 and this activation is a positive feedback mechanism, further exacerbating the inflammation generated by the cytokine storm in COVID-19. Purinergic enzymatic activity can also be modulated, given that the increased activity of CD39 and CD73 contribute, respectively, to the reduction of ATP levels and the increase in the amount of adenosine at the site of infection

experimental pharmacological studies [88–90]. Thus, the increase in adenosine levels after ATP degradation, adenosine acts on receptors, coupled to G protein, A2A and A2B, which increases the intracellular concentration of cyclic adenosine monophosphate (cAMP) , produces anti-inflammatory effects in several tissue and inhibits platelet activation [91, 92].

## *Pharmacological Approaches*

Targeting the BK system by either inhibiting BK production or blocking BK receptors may open new therapeutic options to control COVID-19–induced pulmonary edema. Icatibant, ecallantide, and lanadelumab all target the BK system and may open new therapeutic options. Icatibant, a selective peptidomimetic B2R antagonist, is suggested as a useful drug to alleviate the inflammatory symptoms by inhibiting B2R. Preliminary observations indicated that it improved oxygenation and thus may be a possible therapy for the severe pulmonary manifestations of COVID-19 [36,

48]. Lanadelumab is a long-acting agent that blocks plasma kallikrein and has been suggested as a therapeutic strategy for COVID-19 by inhibiting BK production. Ecallantide also blocks kallikrein and thus its use in COVID-19 patients has been suggested as a possible pharmacological approach to inhibit BK production and, consequently, inflammatory and coagulation pathways [1, 2].

A better understanding of adenosine nucleotides and nucleosides, as well as the signalling of their respective receptors and enzymatic action, can support different studies and potential therapies for several inflammatory diseases, such as COVID-19. However, applying these concepts in in vitro and in vivo studies is essential to enable the application of drugs with these mechanisms of action.

**Acknowledgments** This work was supported by Rio Grande do Sul Research Foundation (FAPERGS proj. No. 21/2551-0001982-4). MMP further acknowledges grant support from FAPERGS and Marylou Ingram Scholarship 2021-2025 from International Society for Advancement of Cytometry (ISAC). JBS, JDL, JCMC, and JLBS are grateful for the doctoral fellowship grant by CAPES. CFM and MDB acknowledge grant support from National Council of Technological and Scientific Development (CNPq).

## References

1. Garvin MR, Alvarez C, Miller JI, Prates ET, Walker AM, Amos BK, Mast AE, Justice A, Aronow B, Jacobson D. A mechanistic model and therapeutic interventions for covid-19 involving a ras-mediated bradykinin storm. Elife. 2020;9:1–16. https://doi.org/10.7554/eLife.59177.
2. Zwaveling S, Gerth van Wijk R, Karim F. Pulmonary edema in COVID-19: explained by bradykinin? J Allergy Clin Immunol. 2020;146(6):1454–5. https://doi.org/10.1016/j.jaci.2020.08.038.
3. Li W, Moore MJ, Vasllieva N, Sui J, Wong SK, Berne MA, Somasundaran M, Sullivan JL, Luzuriaga K, Greeneugh TC, Choe H, Farzan M. Angiotensin-converting enzyme 2 is a functional receptor for the SARS coronavirus. Nature. 2003;426(6965):450–4. https://doi.org/10.1038/nature02145.
4. Sieńko J, Kotowski M, Bogacz A, Lechowicz K, Drożdżal S, Rosik J, Sietnicki M, Sieńko M, Kotfis K. COVID-19: the influence of ACE genotype and ACE-I and ARBs on the course of SARS-CoV-2 infection in elderly patients. Clin Interv Aging. 2020;15:1231. https://doi.org/10.2147/CIA.S261516.
5. Tai W, He L, Zhang X, Pu J, Voronin D, Jiang S, Zhou Y, Du L. Characterization of the receptor-binding domain (RBD) of 2019 novel coronavirus: implication for development of RBD protein as a viral attachment inhibitor and vaccine. Cell Mol Immunol. 2020;17(6):613–20. https://doi.org/10.1038/s41423-020-0400-4.
6. Li F. Structure, function, and evolution of coronavirus spike proteins. Annu Rev Virol. 2016;3:237–61. https://doi.org/10.1146/annurev-virology-110615-042301.
7. Shang J, Wan Y, Luo C, Ye G, Geng Q, Auerbach A, Li F. Cell entry mechanisms of SARS-CoV-2. Proc Natl Acad Sci U S A. 2020;117(21):11727. https://doi.org/10.1073/pnas.2003138117.
8. Hoehl S, Ciesek S. The virology of SARS-CoV-2. Internist. 2020;61(8):789–92. https://doi.org/10.1007/s00108-020-00853-6.
9. Zhou P, Yang X-L, Wang X-G, Hu B, Zhang L, Zhang W, Si H-R, Zhu Y, Li B, Huang C-L, Chen H-D, Chen J, Luo Y, Guo H, Jiang R-D, Liu M-Q, Chen Y, Shen X-R, Wang X, Shi

Z-L. A pneumonia outbreak associated with a new coronavirus of probable bat origin. Nature. 2020;579:270–3. https://doi.org/10.1038/s41586-020-2012-7.
10. Wrapp D, Wang N, Corbett KS, Goldsmith JA, Hsieh C-L, Abiona O, Graham BS, McLellan JS. Cryo-EM structure of the 2019-nCoV spike in the prefusion conformation. BioRxiv: The Preprint Server for Biology. 2020 https://doi.org/10.1101/2020.02.11.944462.
11. Ortega JT, Serrano ML, Pujol FH, Rangel HR. Role of changes in SARS-CoV-2 spike protein in the interaction with the human ACE2 receptor: an in silico analysis. EXCLI J. 2020;19:410–7. https://doi.org/10.17179/excli2020-1167.
12. Bourgonje AR, Abdulle AE, Timens W, Hillebrands J-L, Navis GJ, Gordijn SJ, Bolling MC, Dijkstra G, Voors AA, Osterhaus AD, van der Voort PH, Mulder DJ, van Goor H. Angiotensin-converting enzyme 2 (ACE2), SARS-CoV-2 and the pathophysiology of coronavirus disease 2019 (COVID-19). J Pathol. 2020;251:228–48. https://doi.org/10.1002/path.5471.
13. Li Y, Zhou W, Yang L, You R. Physiological and pathological regulation of ACE2, the SARS-CoV-2 receptor. Pharmacol Res. 2020b;157:104833. https://doi.org/10.1016/j.phrs.2020.104833.
14. Mendoza Torres E, Oyarzún A, Mondaca Ruff D, Azocar A, Chiong M, Castro PF, Jalil JE, Lavandero S, Ocaranza MP. ACE2 and vasoactive peptides: novel players in cardiovascular/renal remodeling and hypertension. Ther Adv Cardiovasc Dis. 2015;9(4):217–37. https://doi.org/10.1177/1753944715597623.
15. Hamming I, Timens W, Bulthuis MLC, Lely AT, Navis GJ, van Goor H. Tissue distribution of ACE2 protein, the functional receptor for SARS coronavirus. A first step in understanding SARS pathogenesis. J Pathol. 2004;203(2):631–7. https://doi.org/10.1002/path.1570.
16. Glowacka I, Bertram S, Muller MA, Allen P, Soilleux E, Pfefferle S, Steffen I, Tsegaye TS, He Y, Gnirss K, Niemeyer D, Schneider H, Drosten C, Pohlmann S. Evidence that TMPRSS2 activates the severe acute respiratory syndrome coronavirus spike protein for membrane fusion and reduces viral control by the humoral immune response. J Virol. 2011;85(9):4122–34. https://doi.org/10.1128/jvi.02232-10.
17. Hoffmann M, Kleine-Weber H, Schroeder S, Krüger N, Herrler T, Erichsen S, Schiergens TS, Herrler G, Wu NH, Nitsche A, Müller MA, Drosten C, Pöhlmann S. SARS-CoV-2 cell entry depends on ACE2 and TMPRSS2 and is blocked by a clinically proven protease inhibitor. Cell. 2020;181(2):271–280.e8. https://doi.org/10.1016/j.cell.2020.02.052.
18. Beyerstedt S, Casaro EB, Rangel ÉB. COVID-19: angiotensin-converting enzyme 2 (ACE2) expression and tissue susceptibility to SARS-CoV-2 infection. Eur J Clin Microbiol Infect Dis. 2021;40(5):905–19. https://doi.org/10.1007/s10096-020-04138-6.
19. Aksoy H, Karadag AS, Wollina U. Angiotensin II receptors: impact for COVID-19 severity. Dermatol Ther. 2020;33(6):e13989. https://doi.org/10.1111/dth.13989.
20. Kuba K, Imai Y, Penninger JM. Multiple functions of angiotensin-converting enzyme 2 and its relevance in cardiovascular diseases. Circ J. 2013;77(2):301–8. https://doi.org/10.1253/circj.CJ-12-1544.
21. Kuba K, Imai Y, Rao S, Gao H, Guo F, Guan B, Huan Y, Yang P, Zhang Y, Deng W, Bao L, Zhang B, Liu G, Wang Z, Chappell M, Liu Y, Zheng D, Leibbrandt A, Wada T, Penninger JM, et al. A crucial role of angiotensin converting enzyme 2 (ACE2) in SARS coronavirus-induced lung injury. Nat Med. 2005;11(8):875–9. https://doi.org/10.1038/nm1267.
22. Verdecchia P, Cavallini C, Spanevello A, Angeli F. The pivotal link between ACE2 deficiency and SARS-CoV-2 infection. Eur J Intern Med. 2020;76:14–20. https://doi.org/10.1016/j.ejim.2020.04.037.
23. Dalan R, Bornstein SR, El-Armouche A, Rodionov RN, Markov A, Wielockx B, Beuschlein F, Boehm BO. The ACE-2 in COVID-19: foe or friend? Horm Metab Res. 2020;52(5):257–63. https://doi.org/10.1055/a-1155-0501.
24. Miyauchi T, Kanekura T, Yamaoka A, Ozawa M, Miyazawa S, Muramatasu T. Basigin, a new, broadly distributed member of the immunoglobulin superfamily, has strong homology with both the immunoglobulin V domain and the β-chain of major histocompatibility complex class

II antigen. J Biochem. 1990;107(2):316–23. https://doi.org/10.1093/oxfordjournals.jbchem.a123045.
25. Lu M, Wu J, Hao ZW, Shang YK, Xu J, Nan G, Li X, Chen ZN, Bian H. Basolateral CD147 induces hepatocyte polarity loss by E-cadherin ubiquitination and degradation in hepatocellular carcinoma progress. Hepatology. 2018;68(1):317–32. https://doi.org/10.1002/hep.29798.
26. Crosnier C, Bustamante LY, Bartholdson SJ, Bei AK, Theron M, Uchikawa M, Mboup S, Ndir O, Kwiatkowski DP, Duraisingh MT, Rayner JC, Wright GJ. Basigin is a receptor essential for erythrocyte invasion by *plasmodium falciparum*. Nature. 2011;480(7378):534–7. https://doi.org/10.1038/nature10606.
27. Chen Z, Mi L, Xu J, Yu J, Wang X, Jiang J, Xing J, Shang P, Qian A, Li Y, Shaw PX, Wang J, Duan S, Ding J, Fan C, Zhang Y, Yang Y, Yu X, Feng Q, Zhu P, et al. Function of HAb18G/CD147 in invasion of host cells by severe acute respiratory syndrome coronavirus. J Infect Dis. 2005;191(5):755–60. https://doi.org/10.1086/427811.
28. Wang K, Chen W, Zhang Z, Deng Y, Lian JQ, Du P, Wei D, Zhang Y, Sun XX, Gong L, Yang X, He L, Zhang L, Yang Z, Geng JJ, Chen R, Zhang H, Wang B, Zhu YM, Chen ZN. CD147-spike protein is a novel route for SARS-CoV-2 infection to host cells. Signal Transduct Target Ther. 2020;5(1):283. https://doi.org/10.1038/s41392-020-00426-x.
29. Urra JM, Cabrera CM, Porras L, Ródenas I. Selective CD8 cell reduction by SARS-CoV-2 is associated with a worse prognosis and systemic inflammation in COVID-19 patients. Clin Immunol. 2020;217:108486. https://doi.org/10.1016/j.clim.2020.108486.
30. Muramatsu T. Basigin: A multifunctional membrane protein with an emerging role in infections by malaria parasites. Expert Opin Ther Targets. 2012;16(10):999–1011. https://doi.org/10.1517/14728222.2012.711818.
31. Ulrich H, Pillat MM. CD147 as a target for COVID-19 treatment: suggested effects of azithromycin and stem cell engagement. Stem Cell Rev Rep. 2020;16(3):434–40. https://doi.org/10.1007/s12015-020-09976-7.
32. Amraei R, Yin W, Napoleon M, Suder E, Berrigan J, Zhao Q, Olejnik J, Chandler KB, Xia C, Feldman J, Hauser B, Caradonna T, Schmidt A, Gummuluru S, Mühlberger E, Chitalia V, Costello C, Rahimi N. CD209L/L-SIGN and CD209/DC-SIGN act as receptors for SARS-CoV-2 and are differentially expressed in lung and kidney epithelial and endothelial cells. BioRxiv: The Preprint Server for Biology; 2020. p. 2020.06.22.165803. https://doi.org/10.1101/2020.06.22.165803.
33. Schmaier AH. The plasma kallikrein–kinin system counterbalances the renin-angiotensin system. J Clin Investig. 2002;109(8):1007–9. https://doi.org/10.1172/jci15490.
34. Abassi Z, Skorecki K, Hamo-Giladi DB, Kruzel-Davila E, Heyman SN. Kinins and chymase: the forgotten components of the renin-angiotensin system and their implications in COVID-19 disease. Am J Physiol Lung Cell Mol Physiol. 2021;320(3):L422–9. https://doi.org/10.1152/AJPLUNG.00548.2020.
35. Gangnus T, Burckhardt BB. Sensitive mass spectrometric determination of kinin–kallikrein system peptides in light of COVID-19. Sci Rep. 2021;11(1):3061. https://doi.org/10.1038/s41598-021-82191-7.
36. Kaplan AP, Ghebrehiwet B. Pathways for bradykinin formation and interrelationship with complement as a cause of edematous lung in COVID-19 patients. J Allergy Clin Immunol. 2021;147(2):507–9. https://doi.org/10.1016/j.jaci.2020.10.025.
37. Gouda AS, Mégarbane B. Snake venom-derived bradykinin-potentiating peptides: A promising therapy for COVID-19? Drug Dev Res. 2021;82(1):38–48. https://doi.org/10.1002/ddr.21732.
38. Jurado-Palomo J, Caballero T. Pathophysiology of bradykinin-mediated angioedema: the role of the complement system. In: A comprehensive review of urticaria and angioedema. London: IntechOpen; 2017. https://doi.org/10.5772/67704.
39. Sodhi CP, Wohlford-Lenane C, Yamaguchi Y, Prindle T, Fulton WB, Wang S, McCray PB, Chappell M, Hackam DJ, Jia H. Attenuation of pulmonary ACE2 activity impairs inactivation of des-arg9 bradykinin/BKB1R axis and facilitates LPS-induced neutrophil infiltra-

tion. Am J Physiol Lung Cell Mol Physiol. 2018;314(1):L17–31. https://doi.org/10.1152/ajplung.00498.2016.
40. Karamyan VT. Between two storms, vasoactive peptides or bradykinin underlie severity of COVID-19? Physiol Rep. 2021;9(5):e14796. https://doi.org/10.14814/phy2.14796.
41. Samavati L, Uhal BD. ACE2, much more than just a receptor for SARS-COV-2. Front Cell Infect Microbiol. 2020;10:317. https://doi.org/10.3389/fcimb.2020.00317.
42. de Kloet AD, Krause EG, Woods SC. The renin angiotensin system and the metabolic syndrome. Physiol Behav. 2010;100(5):525–34. https://doi.org/10.1016/j.physbeh.2010.03.018.
43. Razeghian-Jahromi I, Zibaeenezhad MJ, Lu Z, Zahra E, Mahboobeh R, Lionetti V. Angiotensin-converting enzyme 2: a double-edged sword in COVID-19 patients with an increased risk of heart failure. Heart Fail Rev. 2021;26(2):371–80. https://doi.org/10.1007/s10741-020-10016-2.
44. Mahmudpour M, Roozbeh J, Keshavarz M, Farrokhi S, Nabipour I. COVID-19 cytokine storm: the anger of inflammation. Cytokine. 2020;133:155151. https://doi.org/10.1016/j.cyto.2020.155151.
45. Scialo F, Daniele A, Amato F, Pastore L, Matera MG, Cazzola M, Castaldo G, Bianco A. ACE2: the major cell entry receptor for SARS-CoV-2. Lung. 2020;198:867–77. https://doi.org/10.1007/s00408-020-00408-4.
46. Simko F, Hrenak J, Adamcova M, Paulis L. Renin–angiotensin–aldosterone system: friend or foe—the matter of balance. Insight on history, therapeutic implications and covid-19 interactions. Int J Mol Sci. 2021;22(6):1–8. https://doi.org/10.3390/ijms22063217.
47. Roche JA, Roche R. A hypothesized role for dysregulated bradykinin signaling in COVID-19 respiratory complications. FASEB J. 2020;34(6):7265–9. https://doi.org/10.1096/fj.202000967.
48. van de Veerdonk FL, Netea MG, van Deuren M, van der Meer JWM, de Mast Q, Brüggemann RJ, van der Hoeven H. Kallikrein-kinin blockade in patients with covid-19 to prevent acute respiratory distress syndrome. Elife. 2020;9:e57555. https://doi.org/10.7554/ELIFE.57555.
49. Bernard I, Limonta D, Mahal LK, Hobman TC. Endothelium infection and dysregulation by sars-cov-2: evidence and caveats in covid-19. Viruses. 2021;13(1):29. https://doi.org/10.3390/v13010029.
50. Cekic C, Linden J. Purinergic regulation of the immune system. Nat Rev Immunol. 2016;16(3):177–92. https://doi.org/10.1038/nri.2016.4.
51. Burnstock G. Purinergic nerves. Pharmacol Rev. 1972;24(3):509–81. https://pubmed.ncbi.nlm.nih.gov/4404211/.
52. Burnstock G. Do some nerve cells release more than one transmitter? Neuroscience. 1976;1(4):239–48. https://doi.org/10.1016/0306-4522(76)90054-3.
53. Burnstock G. A basis for distinguishing two types of purinergic receptor. In: Straub RW, Sods L, editors. Cell membrane receptors for drugs and hormones: a multidisciplinary approach, vol. 103. New York: Raven Press; 1978. p. 107–18. https://doi.org/10.1016/0014-5793(79)81367-8.
54. Sträter N. Ecto-5′-nucleotidase: structure function relationships. Purinergic Signal. 2006;2:343–50. https://doi.org/10.1007/s11302-006-9000-8.
55. Ralevic V, Burnstock G. Receptors for purines and pyrimidines. Pharmacol Rev. 1998;50(3):413–92. https://doi.org/10.1007/978-3-642-28863-0_5.
56. Khakh BS, Burnstock G, Kennedy C, King BF, North RA, Séguéla P, Voigt M, Humphrey PPA. International union of pharmacology. XXIV. Current status of the nomenclature and properties of P2X receptors and their subunits. Pharmacol Rev. 2001;53(1):107–18.
57. Abbracchio MP, Burnstock G, Verkhratsky A, Zimmermann H. Purinergic signalling in the nervous system: an overview. Trends Neurosci. 2009;32(1):19–29. https://doi.org/10.1016/j.tins.2008.10.001.
58. Volonté C, Amadio S, D'Ambrosi N, Colpi M, Burnstock G. P2 receptor web: complexity and fine-tuning. Pharmacol Ther. 2006;112(1):264–80. https://doi.org/10.1016/j.pharmthera.2005.04.012.
59. Zimmermann H. Extracellular metabolism of ATP and other nucleotides. Naunyn Schmiedebergs Arch Pharmacol. 2000;362(4–5):299–309. https://doi.org/10.1007/s002100000309.

60. Zimmermann H, Zebisch M, Sträter N, Zimmermann H, Zebisch M, Sträter N. Cellular function and molecular structure of ecto-nucleotidases Madin-Darby canine kidney MS mass spectrometry NDP nucleoside diphosphate NLD nuclease-like domain NMP nucleoside monophosphate NMN nicotinamide mononucleotide NMR nuclear magnetic resonance NPP nucleotide pyrophosphatase/ phosphodiesterase NR nicotinamide riboside NTP nucleoside triphosphate. Purinergic Signal. 2012;8:437–502. https://doi.org/10.1007/s11302-012-9309-4.
61. Huang C, Wang Y, Li X, Ren L, Zhao J, Hu Y, Zhang L, Fan G, Xu J, Gu X, Cheng Z, Yu T, Xia J, Wei Y, Wu W, Xie X, Yin W, Li H, Liu M, Cao B. Clinical features of patients infected with 2019 novel coronavirus in Wuhan, China. Lancet. 2020;395(10223):497–506. https://doi.org/10.1016/S0140-6736(20)30183-5.
62. Di Virgilio F. P2X receptors and inflammation. Curr Med Chem. 2015;22(7):866–77. https://doi.org/10.2174/0929867322666141210155311. PMID: 25524252.
63. Di Virgilio F, Sarti AC, Coutinho-Silva R. Purinergic signaling, DAMPs, and inflammation. Am J Physiol Cell Physiol. 2020a;318(5):C832–5. https://doi.org/10.1152/ajpcell.00053.2020.
64. Di Virgilio F, Tang Y, Sarti AC, Rossato M. A rationale for targeting the P2X7 receptor in coronavirus disease 19. Br J Pharmacol. 2020b;177(21):4990–4. https://doi.org/10.1111/bph.15138.
65. Dos Anjos F, Simões JLB, Assmann CE, Carvalho FB, Bagatini MD. Potential therapeutic role of purinergic receptors in cardiovascular disease mediated by SARS-CoV-2. J Immunol Res. 2020;2020:8632048. https://doi.org/10.1155/2020/8632048.
66. Li X, Berg NK, Mills T, Zhang K, Eltzschig HK, Yuan X. Adenosine at the interphase of hypoxia and inflammation in lung injury. Front Immunol. 2021;11:604944. https://doi.org/10.3389/fimmu.2020.604944.
67. Simões JLB, Bagatini MD. Purinergic signaling of ATP in COVID-19 associated Guillain-Barré syndrome. J Neuroimmune Pharmacol. 2021;16(1):48–58. https://doi.org/10.1007/s11481-020-09980-1.
68. Antonioli L, Blandizzi C, Pacher P, Haskó G. The purinergic system as a pharmacological target for the treatment of immune-mediated inflammatory diseases. Pharmacol Rev. 2019;71(3):345–82. https://doi.org/10.1124/pr.117.014878.
69. Chen L, Deng H, Cui H, Fang J, Zuo Z, Deng J, Li Y, Wang X, Zhao L. Inflammatory responses and inflammation-associated diseases in organs. Oncotarget. 2017;9(6):7204–18. https://doi.org/10.18632/oncotarget.23208.
70. Serhan CN, Levy BD. Resolvins in inflammation: emergence of the pro-resolving superfamily of mediators. J Clin Investig. 2018;128(7):2657–69. https://doi.org/10.1172/JCI97943.
71. Burnstock G, Boeynaems JM. Purinergic signalling and immune cells. Purinergic Signal. 2014;10(4):529–64. https://doi.org/10.1007/s11302-014-9427-2.
72. Csóka B, Himer L, Selmeczy Z, Vizi ES, Pacher P, Ledent C, Deitch EA, Spolarics Z, Németh ZH, Haskü G. Adenosine A 2A receptor activation inhibits T helper 1 and T helper 2 cell development and effector function. FASEB J. 2008;22(10):3491–9. https://doi.org/10.1096/fj.08-107458.
73. Csóka B, Németh ZH, Rosenberger P, Eltzschig HK, Spolarics Z, Pacher P, Selmeczy Z, Koscsó B, Himer L, Vizi ES, Blackburn MR, Deitch EA, Haskó G. A 2B adenosine receptors protect against sepsis-induced mortality by dampening excessive inflammation. J Immunol. 2010;185(1):542–50. https://doi.org/10.4049/jimmunol.0901295.
74. Csóka B, Németh ZH, Szabó I, Davies DL, Varga ZV, Pálóczi J, Falzoni S, Di Virgilio F, Muramatsu R, Yamashita T, Pacher P, Haskó G. Macrophage P2X4 receptors augment bacterial killing and protect against sepsis. JCI Insight. 2018;3(11):e99431. https://doi.org/10.1172/jci.insight.99431.
75. Csóka B, Németh ZH, Töro G, Idzko M, Zech A, Koscsó B, Spolarics Z, Antonioli L, Cseri K, Erdélyi K, Pacher P, Haskó G. Extracellular ATP protects against sepsis through macrophage P2X7 purinergic receptors by enhancing intracellular bacterial killing. FASEB J. 2015a;29(9):3626–37. https://doi.org/10.1096/fj.15-272450.

76. Csóka B, Németh ZH, Töro G, Koscsó B, Kókai E, Robson SC, Enjyoji K, Rolandelli RH, Erdélyi K, Pacher P, Haskó G. CD39 improves survival in microbial sepsis by attenuating systemic inflammation. FASEB J. 2015b;29(1):25–36. https://doi.org/10.1096/fj.14-253567.
77. Csóka B, Selmeczy Z, Koscsó B, Németh ZH, Pacher P, Murray PJ, Kepka-Lenhart D, Morris SM, Gause WC, Leibovich SJ, Haskó G. Adenosine promotes alternative macrophage activation via A2A and A2B receptors. FASEB J. 2012;26(1):376–86. https://doi.org/10.1096/fj.11-190934.
78. Eltzschig HK, Eckle T. Ischemia and reperfusion-from mechanism to translation. Nat Med. 2011;17(11):1391–401. https://doi.org/10.1038/nm.2507.
79. Ravichandran KS. Beginnings of a good apoptotic meal: the find-me and eat-me signaling pathways. Immunity. 2011;35(4):445–55. https://doi.org/10.1016/j.immuni.2011.09.004.
80. Li G, Fan Y, Lai Y, Han T, Li Z, Zhou P, Pan P, Wang W, Hu D, Liu X, Zhang Q, Wu J. Coronavirus infections and immune responses. J Med Virol. 2020a;92(4):424–32. https://doi.org/10.1002/jmv.25685.
81. Cicko S, Köhler TC, Ayata CK, Müller T, Ehrat N, Meyer A, Hossfeld M, Zech A, Di Virgilio F, Idzko M. Extracellular ATP is a danger signal activating P2X7 receptor in a LPS mediated inflammation (ARDS/ALI). Oncotarget. 2018;9(55):30635–48. https://doi.org/10.18632/oncotarget.25761.
82. Anyanwu AC, Kanthi Y, Fukase K, Liao H, Mimura T, Desch KC, Gruca M, Kaskar S, Sheikh-Aden H, Chi L, Zhao R, Yadav V, Wakefield TW, Hyman MC, Pinsky DJ. Tuning the Thromboinflammatory response to venous flow interruption by the Ectonucleotidase CD39. Arterioscler Thromb Vasc Biol. 2019;39(4):e118–29. https://doi.org/10.1161/ATVBAHA.119.312407.
83. Covarrubias R, Chepurko E, Reynolds A, Huttinger ZM, Huttinger R, Stanfill K, Wheeler DG, Novitskaya T, Robson SC, Dwyer KM, Cowan PJ, Gumina RJ. Role of the CD39/CD73 purinergic pathway in modulating arterial thrombosis in mice. Arterioscler Thromb Vasc Biol. 2016;36(9):1809–20. https://doi.org/10.1161/ATVBAHA.116.307374.
84. Hechler B, Gachet C. Purinergic receptors in thrombosis and inflammation. Arterioscler Thromb Vasc Biol. 2015;35(11):2307–15. https://doi.org/10.1161/ATVBAHA.115.303395.
85. Ahmadi P, Hartjen P, Kohsar M, Kummer S, Schmiedel S, Bockmann JH, Fathi A, Huber S, Haag F, Schulze Zur Wiesch J. Defining the CD39/CD73 Axis in SARS-CoV-2 infection: the CD73- phenotype identifies Polyfunctional cytotoxic lymphocytes. Cell. 2020;9(8):1750. https://doi.org/10.3390/cells9081750.
86. Yang M, Lu L, Kang Z, Ma T, Wang Y. Overexpressed CD39 mitigates sepsis-induced kidney epithelial cell injury via suppressing the activation of NLR family pyrin domain containing 3. Int J Mol Med. 2019;44(5):1707–18. https://doi.org/10.3892/ijmm.2019.4349.
87. Grenz A, Homann D, Eltzschig HK. Extracellular adenosine: a safety signal that dampens hypoxia-induced inflammation during ischemia. Antioxid Redox Signal. 2011;15(8):2221–34. https://doi.org/10.1089/ars.2010.3665.
88. Grenz A, Zhang H, Hermes M, Eckle T, Klingel K, Huang DY, Müller CE, Robson SC, Osswald H, Eltzschig HK. Contribution of E-NTPDasel (CD39) to renal protection from ischemia-reperfusion injury. FASEB J. 2007;21(11):2863–73. https://doi.org/10.1096/fj.06-7947com.
89. Hart ML, Gorzolla IC, Schittenhelm J, Robson SC, Eltzschig HK. SP1-dependent induction of CD39 facilitates hepatic ischemic preconditioning. J Immunol. 2010;184(7):4017–24. https://doi.org/10.4049/jimmunol.0901851.
90. Köhler D, Eckle T, Faigle M, Grenz A, Mittelbronn M, Laucher S, Hart ML, Robson SC, Müller CE, Eltzschig HK. CD39/ectonucleoside triphosphate diphosphohydrolase 1 provides myocardial protection during cardiac ischemia/reperfusion injury. Circulation. 2007;116(16):1784–94. https://doi.org/10.1161/CIRCULATIONAHA.107.690180.
91. Di Virgilio F, Vuerich M. Purinergic signaling in the immune system. In: Autonomic neuroscience: basic and clinical, vol. 191. Amsterdam: Elsevier; 2015. p. 117–23. https://doi.org/10.1016/j.autneu.2015.04.011.
92. Johnston-Cox HA, Yang D, Ravid K. Physiological implications of adenosine receptor-mediated platelet aggregation. J Cell Physiol. 2011;226(1):46–51. https://doi.org/10.1002/jcp.22379.

# Chapter 4
# Genetics and Biological Characteristics of SARS-CoV-2

**Mahnaz Norouzi, Mark A. Miles, and Shaghayegh Norouzi**

## Introduction

Coronaviruses (CoVs) are hypermutable viruses that have rapidly evolved over the past years to give rise to many related and unrelated strains. They belong to the order *Nidovirales*, suborder *Cornidovirineae*, and family *Coronaviridae*, which are characterized by their roughly spherical shapes and corona-like spike (S protein) appearance. This family is also subdivided into *Othocoronaviridae and Torovirinae*, the latter of which is distinguishable based on their helical doughnut-shaped nucleocapsid. The *Orthocoronaviridae* are genetically classified into four genera: *Alphacoronavirus* (αCoV) and *Betacoronavirus* (βCoV), which primarily infect mammals (including humans and bats); and *Gammacoronavirus* (γCoV) and *Deltacoronavirus* (δCoV), which typically infect birds [1]. About 60 CoVs have been isolated from bats, most of which comprise βCoV, and these mammals act as large and highly mobile reservoirs for CoVs [2]. Genetic recombination of the viral genome has allowed CoVs to adapt and infect humans as new hosts, and as such all human CoVs (HCoV) have evolved from animal origins. Zoonotic transmission of CoVs from bats to humans typically occur through intermediate hosts: civets for

M. Norouzi
Department of Genetics, Faculty of Sciences, Shahid Chamran University of Ahvaz, Ahvaz, Iran

M. A. Miles
School of Health and Biomedical Sciences, RMIT University, Bundoora, VIC, Australia
e-mail: mark.miles@rmit.edu.au

S. Norouzi (✉)
School of Health and Biomedical Sciences, RMIT University, Bundoora, VIC, Australia

College of Medicine, Markey Cancer Centre, University of Kentucky, Lexington, KY, USA
e-mail: sharni.norouzi@uky.edu


S. Adibi et al. (eds.), *Frontiers of COVID-19*,
https://doi.org/10.1007/978-3-031-08045-6_4

SARS-CoV and the dromedary camel for MERS-CoV. Other domestic animals can suffer disease and also transmit the virus to humans [3]. SARS-CoV, MERS-CoV, HCoV-NL63, and HCoV-229E are believed to have originated from bats while HCoV-OC43 and HKU1 were likely derived from rodents [4–6]. The first reported case of HCoV in 1960 was associated with the common cold and from then the evolution and expansion of the virus into different strains (most of them belonging to the βCoVs genera) led to more large-scale respiratory and enteric illness [7]. The year 2002 witnessed an outbreak of SARS-CoV (lineage B βCoV) in China resulting in serious respiratory distress and many casualties [8]. Another highly pathogenic virus strain MERS-CoV (lineage C βCoV) appeared in the Middle East 10 years later, also leading to substantial loss of life [9]. In December 2019, a novel CoV (SARS-CoV-2) was identified in a group of patients with pneumonia in Wuhan, China, and has since disseminated to over 200 countries leading to widespread outbreaks and over seven million cases reported globally [10]. Similar to SARS-CoV, SARS-CoV-2 was found to induce respiratory infectious disease in humans, ranging from minor to severe, and is the infectious agent responsible for the COVID-19 global pandemic [11].

## SARS-CoV-2 Genome and Replication

### *Genomic Structure*

CoVs form nonsegmented, enveloped, spherical viral particles that encapsulate positive-sense single stranded RNA. CoV genomes range from 26 to 32 kb long and include between 6 and 11 open reading frames (ORFs) making it the largest genome among RNA viruses. Most of the genome (around 67%) is encoded by ORF1 (consisting of two overlapping regions: ORF1a and ORF1ab) which encodes 16 nonstructural proteins (nsps). The remaining third of the genome consists of additional ORFs that encode accessory and structural proteins. The SARS-CoV-2 genome follows this structure (Fig. 4.1) and contains 14 ORFs encoding 27 proteins [12]. The 5′ terminus contains a flanking untranslated region (UTR) followed by ORF1a (encoding polyprotein1a, pp1a) and ORF1ab (encoding polyprotein1ab, pp1ab) which together comprise 15 nsps: nsp1-nsp10 and nsp12-nsp16 (nsp11 has an identical sequence to nsp12). ORF1 products are important for RNA replication and further in vitro analysis revealed that the frameshift between ORF1a and ORF1b induces a pause in the production of pp1ab, resulting in enhanced pp1a expression [13]. Proteases cleave these polyproteins to generate their respective nsps, which are key components of the viral replication and transcription complexes (RTCs). This is also known as the replicase allowing for viral RNA to attach to host cell ribosomes to enable subsequent transcription and replication of viral RNA [14, 15].

The proteolytic release of nsp1 is known to happen quickly to target the host cell translation machinery. Nsps2–11 is thought to aid in viral RTC accommodation by

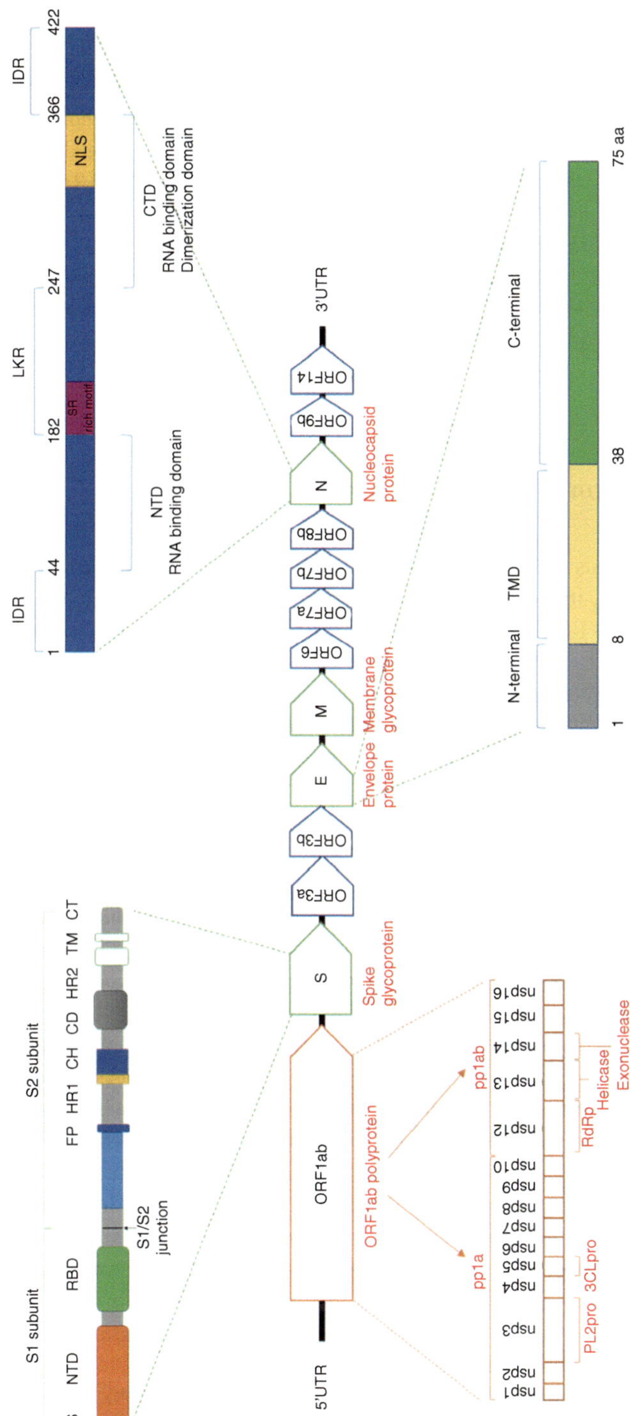


**Fig. 4.1** Genome structure of SARS-CoV-2. See text for detail on genes encoding nonstructural and structural components

modulating intracellular membranes, evading host immune defences, and supplying replication cofactors. Nsp3 and nsp5, respectively, encode the cysteine proteases PL2pro and 3CLpro, which cleave pp1a and pp1ab to generate the 15 nsp replicase products that are subsequently translated [16]. Meanwhile, the core enzymatic functions of RNA replication, modification, and proofreading are promoted by nsp12–16 [17]. These key nsps include RNA-dependent RNA polymerase (RdRp) encoded by nsp12, helicase by nsp13, and exonuclease by nsp14. The 3′ terminus also contains a flanking UTR as well as genes encoding 4 structural proteins: Spike (S), Envelope (E), Membrane (M), and Nucleocapsid (N), and 8 accessory proteins derived from subgenomic RNA: 3a, 3b, p6, 7a, 7b, 8b, 9b, and ORF14 [18]. As discussed below, these proteins are important for viral–host cell receptor binding, virion assembly, and viral release from the host cell [19].

## *Viral Replication*

Viral RNA synthesis takes place in double-membrane vesicles where the RTC complex forms. RdRp, its cofactors, and nsp7 and nsp8 mainly carry out synthesis of SARS-CoV-2 viral RNA. The complex transcribes the virus genome to the negative-sense template of both the progeny genome and subgenomic RNA. Both progeny and subgenomic RNA transcripts are first transcribed into negative-strand intermediates which are subsequently converted to the positive-sense counterparts by RdRp [20]. Thus, RdRp plays a crucial role in the initial stages of viral replication. The newly positive strands could then be used to generate more nsps and RTCs, or they may be packaged into new viruses. The 5′ end of the viral genome includes a leader sequence that harbors multiple stem–loop structures required for RNA replication and transcription. Furthermore, most ORFs in the 3′ one-third of the SARS-CoV-2 genome contain transcriptional regulatory sequences (TRSs) at their upstream [21]. TRSs are necessary for viral gene expression and can prevent RTC during negative-strand RNA synthesis. The stopped negative-strand RNA is reinitiated at the TRS adjacent to a leader sequence to add a copy of the leader sequence to the nascent RNA and complete the synthesis [22, 23]. These discontinuous RNA synthesis steps produce a series of negative-strand subgenomic RNAs that are used as templates to generate a distinct range of positive-sense nested mRNAs. Positive-sense nested subgenomic mRNAs are then translated into structural and accessory proteins (discussed below). These proteins are subsequently insulated in the endoplasmic reticulum before being transferred to the endoplasmic reticulum–Golgi intermediate compartment (ERGIC). Meanwhile, the previously replicated genome will directly bind to the N protein, forming a nucleocapsid that will then transfer into the ERGIC. In this site, nucleocapsids bind to the other structural proteins forming small vesicles that contain the necessary components to form mature virions, which are then exocytosed from the host cell [20].

Novel and existing antiviral treatments that target RdRp of SARS-Cov-2 are currently being tested [24]. Nucleoside analogs like remdesivir and favipiravir compete with endogenous nucleosides during RdRp-mediated RNA synthesis resulting in its termination, and have shown promising preclinical in vitro and in vivo antiviral activity in hamster models of SARS-CoV-2 [25–27]. Remdesivir was shown to reduce the recovery time in patients suffering from severe COVID-19 and is to date the only approved antiviral for treating COVID-19 [28]. In contrast, other repurposed drugs targeting non-RdRp stages in the SARS-CoV-2 life cycle, such as hydroxychloroquine, have shown good in vitro antiviral potential, although this is yet to be conclusively translated to clinical efficacy [24]. Conclusions from current and future clinical trials of these potential anti-SARS-CoV-2 drugs will provide more insight into the efficacy of targeting other components of SARS-CoV-2.

## *Key Structural Proteins*

### Spike (S)

The attachment of the virus to the host cell-surface receptor is the first step during infection. CoVs use the S glycoprotein on the envelope to bind to host receptors and enable fusion of the virus with the cell membrane [29, 30]. Electron microscopy revealed that the SARS-CoV-2 outer surface is studded with distinctive 9 to 12 nm long S glycoproteins and form homotrimers protruding from the viral surface [31]. This gives the virus the appearance of a solar corona, hence its classed name. The ability of S proteins to detect and interact with host receptors determines viral tropism and pathogenicity. Indeed, a fitness advantage incurred by the amino acid change D614G within the S protein sequence of SARS-CoV-2 enhances its virulence resulting in this strain being the most prevalent variant in the current pandemic [32]. Therefore, S protein structure is an important factor for host and cross-species transmission [33], and given its surface location is a key target for neutralizing antibodies and therapeutic antiviral and vaccine design [34].

S glycoprotein is a type-I transmembrane protein and consist of three segments: a large ectodomain, a single-pass transmembrane domain, and a cytoplasmic tail [31]. The ectodomain of the S protein contains two functional subunits: the S1 subunit, which composes of the N-terminal domain (NTD) and a receptor-binding domain (RBD), and the S2 subunit which acts as a fusion protein to help in the fusion of the virus with the host cell membrane, and contains a fusion peptide (FP), heptad repeat 1 (HR1), central helix (CH), connector domain (CD), heptad repeat 2 (HR2), transmembrane domain (TM), and cytoplasmic tail (CT) (Fig. 4.1). A unique furin cleavage site exists at the S1/S2 boundary of SARS-CoV-2 to facilitate conformation change and membrane fusion [34, 35]. Interestingly, this cleavage site is absent in other B lineages of the βCoV genus and possibly facilitates the high pathogenicity of SARS-CoV-2 [36]. An additional cleavage event at the S2′ site (upstream of the fusion peptide) by host proteases "activates" the S protein via an irreversible conformational change that further enables the fusion of virus with the host cell. SARS-CoV-2 and SARS-CoV recognize the same receptor in humans:

angiotensin-converting enzyme 2 (ACE2) (and alternatively CD209L) [37, 38]. ACE2 is a surface exposed receptor primarily expressed in respiratory tissues such as alveoli. The RBD of the S1 subunit directly interacts with the ACE2 receptor making it critical for viral infection and transmission as, along with the S2 subunit, ensures close proximity of the viral and host cell membranes to allow fusion to occur. MERS-CoV binds to a different host receptor, dipeptidylpeptidase 4 (DPP4), via different RBDs although bioinformatic evidence suggests that the SARS-CoV-2 may also have affinity for this receptor [39]. The S glycoprotein can exist in either a closed or open state. In the closed state, the three ACE2 recognition motifs lack protrusion from the interface formed by three S protein protomers meaning interaction with the ACE2 receptor does not occur [40]. Conversely, the RBD is in the "up" conformation in the open state allowing for receptor binding [30]. The open state is necessary for the fusion of the SARS-CoV-2 and the host cell membranes, thereby facilitating its entry into host cells. Once bound to the ACE2 receptor, the host transmembrane Serine Protease 2 (TMPRSS-2) transmembrane protease cleaves SARS-CoV-2S proteins at S2′ to facilitate receptor-mediated endocytosis, plasma membrane fusion and release of genetic material into the host cell. Indeed, serine protease inhibitors that blocked TMPRSS-2 activity also blocked SARS-CoV-2 infection in lung cells [41].

### Envelope (E)

The E protein is a minor component of the viral membrane, but it is regarded as one of the essential structural proteins of the virus. Once internalized, it localizes to the ER and Golgi complex of host cells and plays a significant role in viral morphogenesis and assembly, budding, and release of progeny viruses [42]. The E protein is a short 75 residue viroporin-like protein consisting of a hydrophilic N-terminus (NTD), a hydrophobic transmembrane domain (TMD) and a long hydrophilic C-terminus (CTD) (Fig. 4.1). The TMD hydrophobic region has a lipid-bilayer-based structure [43] and possesses at least one predicted amphipathic α-helix that oligomerizes to form a pentameric cation-selective channel across the ERGIC membrane, which is important for virus pathogenicity [44, 45]. The importance of E proteins in SARS-CoV-2 is illustrated by its sequence conservation among other species-specific CoVs, although there are some minor modifications when compared to other SARS-CoVs. For instance, a Glu/Gln substitution at position 69 with positively charged Arg and a deletion that flanks this position [46]. It is not yet clear whether these modifications occur on the external or internal sides of the viral membrane, though they are likely to critically impact the conformational properties and possibly the protein–protein interactions. In silico modelling of the conformation and docking of the E protein suggests these changes enhance tissue binding and inflammatory response in comparison to SARS-CoV [47]. It is also possible that these changes affect the process of oligomerization which is necessary for the formation of the transmembrane ion-conductive pore/channel [48].

### Membrane (M)

The M protein is a transmembrane protein and more prevalent within the virus membrane. It is the most abundant structural protein of the virus and plays a major role in RNA packaging, virion assembly and budding process given it interacts with all other structural proteins. Homotypic interactions between M proteins also define the shape of the viral envelope. During virus assembly, M protein interacts with the N, E, S, and M glycoprotein itself, importantly cooperating with S proteins during cell attachment and entry [49]. Its N-terminus is exposed on the viral surface and as such mutations could alter host cell interactions to boost pathogenicity in different variants [48]. SARS-CoV-2 M protein has also been reported to antagonize the production of type I and III IFNs by targeting RIG-I/MDA-5 signaling, allowing for immune evasion [50, 51]. Clinical trials administering type I and III IFNs in combination with other antiviral drugs show effective suppression of SARS-CoV-2 infection indicating that mitigating the immune suppression by M proteins is critical for treatment [52].

### Nucleocapsid (N)

The N protein is a 46 kDa phosphoprotein that is the most abundant protein within the infected host cell and is important for the packaging of viral RNA into ribonucleocapsid. Its N-terminal and C-terminal domains act independently and do not interact with one another. There are three intrinsically disordered regions: N-arm (residues 1–44), linker region (LKR) (residues 182–247), and C-tail (residues 248–365) (Fig. 4.1). These regions lack a defined tertiary structure in the native state but have critical roles in biological processes including macromolecular interactions.

N proteins are the only structural proteins of the virus that bind to the RNA genome, binding at multiple sites to form a ribonucleoprotein (RNP) complex called the nucleocapsid. Based on EM studies, RNPs are helical consisting of coils ranging between 9 and 16 nm in diameter and a hollow interior of approximately 3 to 4 nm, located within 25 nm of the inner face of the membrane. The RNP complex organizes the essential template for replication by the RdRp complex. Localization of N to the ER–Golgi region suggests additional functions in assembly and budding [53]. A nuclear localization signal (NLS) is also present and alterations to enhance nuclear localization of N proteins may be associated with the emergence of more pathogenic strains [54]. The structural plasticity of N proteins facilitates the RNA packaging process and viral self-assembly, in addition to its other roles within the cell such as chaperon activity, cell cycle regulation, cell stress responses, and signal transduction [55].

## Genetic Diversity of SARS-CoV-2

### *SARS-CoV-2 Classification*

Different nomenclatures are used for SARS-CoV-2 variant naming which uses a certain identifier for each genotype of the virus depending on its mutations. These subtypes are often referred to as clades, a term used in virology to classify viruses that are genetically identical and can be tracked using phylogeny studies [56]. According to data from the Global Initiative on Sharing All Influenza Data (GISAID) public database, SARS-CoV-2 sequenced genomes can be classified into seven main clades. Clade L includes the SARS-CoV-2 virus reference strain (GenBank accession number NC_045512, GISIAD accession ID: EPI ISL 402124), from which the other clades: S, V, G, GH, GR, and GV show few variation. The O clade represents other SARS-CoV-2 strains that do not fall into any of these major clades [57]. The Phylogenetic Assignment of Named Global Outbreak Lineages (PANGOLIN) software team proposed classification containing six main lineages: A, B, B.1, B.1.1, B.1.177, and B.1.1.7, which divide into further clades. A is the original strain considered to be the reference sequence in the PANGOLIN system, equivalent to the GISAID S clade [58]. Nextstrain [59] categorizes the SARS-CoV-2 variants as 19A, 19B, 20A, 20B, 20C, 20D, 20E, 20F, 20G, 20H, 20I, and 20 J. The initial reference strain within these clades is 19B. The presence of various terminology frameworks can imply that a similar variation has numerous names, which can be confusion for health authorities, the media and the general population. Under another naming framework recently reported by the World health organization (WHO), Greek letters were utilized only for simplicity of communication. WHO additionally groups SARS-CoV-2 variations as variations of concern (VOCs) and variations of interest (VOIs) (Table 4.1) [60].

Since the SARS-CoV-2 genome databases contain a relatively limited number of sequenced genomes, clades are categorized based on the unique set of the currently observed mutations. These clades were named based on the mutations that caused them to branch and can be further characterized by discovering additional mutations, likely diverging the network even further as time goes on [56]. Forster et al. [61] developed an early phylogenetic network of SARS-CoV-2 and denoted 3 main lineage clusters based on amino acid changes, with the root cluster (lineage A) obtained from the SARS-like bat CoV RaTG13. Lineage A is subdivided into further clusters based on common SNPs. Lineage B is derived from A by 2 distinct mutations (T8782C and C28144T) and are almost exclusive to East Asia. Further mutations exist in the genomes of B lineage identified outside of East Asia suggesting here the need for the virus to adapt in order to propagate and survive outside this region. A third lineage C is derived from B and has a large European demographic. The branching and evolution of this network to generate new (and more virulent) strains derives from the inherent ability of RNA viruses to alter their genomes and adapt to new hosts.

**Table 4.1** The corresponding nomenclature of the most prevalent variants of SARS-CoV-2

| WHO label[a] | Genomic changes of Spike protein[a] | GISAID clade/ variant[a] | Nextstrain clade[a] | Pango lineage[a] | Variant type[a] | Country of first detection |
|---|---|---|---|---|---|---|
| Alpha | 69del, 70del, 144del, (E484K), (S494P), N501Y, A570D, D614G | GRY (formerly GR/501Y. V1) | 20I/501Y.V1 | B.1.1.7 | VOC | UK |
| Beta | D80A, D215G, 241del, 242del, 243del, K417N, E484K, N501Y, D614G, A701V | GH/501Y. V2 | 20H (V2) | B.1.351 | VOC | South Africa |
| Gamma | L18F, T20N, P26S, D138Y, R190S, K417T, E484K, N501Y, D614G, H655Y, T1027I | GR/501Y. V3 | 20 J (V3) | P.1 | VOC | Brazil |
| Delta | T19R, (G142D), 156del, 157del, R158G, L452R, T478K, D614G, P681R, D950N | G/478 K.V1 | 21A | B.1.617.2 | VOC | India |
| Epsilon | L452R, D614G | GH/452R. V1 | 21C | B.1.427/B.1.429 | VOC/ VOI | USA |
| Zeta | E484K, (F565L), D614G, V1176F | GR/484 K. V2 | 20B/S.484 K | P.2 | VOI | Brazil |
| Eta | A67V, 69del, 70del, 144del, E484K, D614G, Q677H, F888L | G/484 K.V3 | 21D | B.1.525 | VOI | Multiple countries |
| Lota | (L5F), T95I, D253G, (S477N), (E484K), D614G, (A701V) | GH/253G. V1 | 21F | B.1.526 | VOI | USA |
| Kappa | G142D, E154K, L452R, E484Q, D614G, P681R, Q1071H | G/452R.V3 | 21B | B.1.617.1 | VOI | India |

[a]Data were collected based on the latest update of https://www.who.int/en/activities/tracking-SARS-CoV-2-variants/ and https://www.cdc.gov/coronavirus/2019-ncov/variants on 23 June 2021

## *Evidence of Genetic Recombination*

The genome of SARS-CoV-2 is highly similar to other SARS-CoV and SARS-like viruses. Next generation sequencing and PCR was first used to identify the full-length genome sequences of novel SARS-CoV-2 from 5 patients, demonstrating it shares the greatest sequence similarity to the SARS-like bat CoV RaTG13 (96% similarity) followed by SARS-CoV (79.5% similarity to the BJ01 isolate) and MERS-CoV (55% similarity) [38]. From this, SARS-CoV-2 belongs to the βCoV genus along with SARS-like bat CoV, SARS-CoV and MERS-CoV. Interestingly, SARS-CoV-2 appears to transmit in parallel to SARS-like bat CoV but not with SARS-CoV, which is directly derived from SARS-like bat CoV, and least aligned to MERS-CoV [12]. This indicates a fundamental difference in disease spectrum and propagation efficiency between the two human viruses. The estimated distance between SARS-CoV-2 and SARS-CoV differs among various studies depending on the unit of measurement (nucleotide or amino acid) and size of the selected genomic region. Accordingly, there is no agreement yet on the exact taxonomic position of SARS-CoV-2 within the βCoV genus [62] but consensus indicates bats as the possible host of origin for SARS-CoV-2 [31]. Supporting this, the genome sequences of key encoding genes pp1ab, pp1a, E, matrix, accessory protein 7a, and N share closest sequence similarity to SARS-like bat CoV.

The S protein of SARS-CoV-2 showed 93.1% nucleotide identity to RaTG13, but was highly divergent from other CoVs indicating variable origins to SARS-CoV. On the other hand, the amino acid sequence of the replicase domains of ORF1ab from SARS-CoV and SARS-CoV-2 were 94.4% identical, further demonstrating these viruses belong to the same species [38]. The overall amino acid sequence of SARS-CoV-2 is similar to that of SARS-CoV and SARS-like bat CoV with around 380 amino acid substitutions identified in SARS-CoV-2. These differences are mainly in nsp2, nsp3, and S protein (including the RBD and subdomain). Genetic comparative analysis revealed that the majority of the S protein of SARS-CoV-2 probably originated from a SARS-like bat CoV while the RBD came from SARS-CoV, suggesting viral genetic recombination leading to the structural rearrangement of the S protein in SARS-CoV-2 [63]. It is likely this event occurred to facilitate binding to human host cells, although some of these amino acid changes within the SARS-CoV-2 RBD were identified in regions that did not directly interact with the ACE2 receptor. Instead, structural analysis identified two binding sites in the RBD-ACE2 interface that provided a more compact confirmation and increased ACE2-binding affinity than SARS-CoV RBD, probably enhancing viral infectivity [64]. Even though the whole genome sequence of SARS-CoV-2 is highly similar to SARS-like bat CoV, there is no evidence of yet for any SARS-like bat virus harbouring all proteins encoded by SARS-CoV-2 further implying genetic recombination in the genesis of this novel virus.

## *Genetic Mutations of SARS-CoV-2*

RNA viruses are extremely mutable viruses that can mutate and evolve a million times higher than their hosts evolve [65]. This high mutation rate correlates with their virulence modulation that is thought to be beneficial for viral adaptation and rapid evolution. The mutagenesis rate of CoVs can be up to $10^{-4}$ substitutes per bp per year, which is moderately high compared to other ssRNA viruses [6]. CoVs are therefore highly adaptive and this is a contributing factor as to why effective therapeutic intervention against CoV-mediated disease has been less successful than other viral diseases [66]. The SARS-CoV genome mutation rate was estimated to be up to $2.4 \times 10^{-3}$ substitutions per site per year and mutations can be generated during each replication cycle [6]. The adaptability of SARS-CoV-2 to combat recent human interventions against the pandemic (such as pan-antivirals) and ensure propagation throughout the population is imperative to its survival. Analysis of 63 isolated strains of SARS-CoV-2 showed low sequence variation and a random distribution of mutations [67]. Interestingly, mutation hot spots identified in at least 5 samples that altered the amino acid sequence were identified in ORF1a, S, ORF8 and N, suggesting those regions of the genome are critical for viral survival [67].

Many of these mutations are located in the S protein that targets the ACE2 receptor. Notably, the D614G mutation that alters ACE2-binding conformation to increase viral transmission is found in SARS-CoV-2 strains from G, GH, GR, and GV clades [68, 69]. Apart from the S protein D614G mutation, amino acid changes that affect the nsp12 (P323L and P314L) and RdRp were also observed in the whole datasets [70]. These mutations are intriguingly important since RdRp is a key component of the replication/transcription machinery, and its fidelity determines the mutagenic capabilities of the virus [70–72]. Moreover, other mutations that alter protein sequence of the N protein and the less characterized ORF3a, ORF8, nsp2, nsp6, and nsp13 proteins are the other reported common mutations in the SARS-CoV-2 genome databases [70, 71, 73]. These mutational events mainly include nonsynonymous mutations that lead to amino acid exchanges, followed by nonsynonymous single nucleotide polymorphism (SNPs) (Table 4.1). While silent events do not directly affect protein sequences, they do have consequences because they greatly affect the biological functions of the proteins. Nonsynonymous SNPs in the 5′UTR may affect viral transcription, replication rates and the folding of the genomic RNA although the direct mutational effects here are not yet fully defined [21, 70]. Furthermore, other mutations, including deletions, may have physiological importance because they escape the proofreading function of the SARS-CoV-2 RdRp and may accelerate its evolution [74].

Clade-wise analysis indicated that there is a low relative heterogeneity across different SARS-CoV-2 clades. According to these findings, the most commonly mutated amino acids in various clades are Glu and Ser that are often replaced by His and Leu, respectively [72]. Nevertheless, it is unclear if diversity in fatality rates and the speed of transmission observed in different countries are due to varying virulence of different clades [75, 76]. Global distribution studies of SARS-CoV-2 indicate that clade GR is dominant in Africa, India, and Russia. Conversely, the predominant clade in North America is clade GH with the highest reported deleterious mutation load. In Europe, both GR and the recently emerged GV clade are the most common variant groups of SARS-CoV-2 [57, 70]. It has been proposed that the diverse pathogenicity and virulence among different clades may be linked to the genomic heterogeneity that changes the structure or stability of SARS-CoV-2 proteins coming from different countries. On the other hand, it is possible that the high frequency of polymorphisms within the human genome could contribute to the fatality of the disease [70].

While low, SARS-CoV-2 mutation frequencies have increased over time and novel mutations have arisen as the virus spread geographically around the globe [71]. For instance, a RdRp mutation (position 14,408, NC_045512) surfaced mainly in European populations after the virus escaped from East Asia and the location of this mutation (probably due to its impact on RdRp function) resulted in the simultaneous occurrence of other point mutations [71]. A distinct mutational pattern has therefore emerged that represents the geographic area with which the virus has propagated. Of particular importance to the general population is the Alpha variant of SARS-CoV-2 (named B.1.17 variant, formerly "UK strain") that emerged in late 2020, which displays a 64% higher mortality rate and greater transmissibility than previously circulating strains [77, 78]. More than half of the mutations in this strain are located within the S gene and probably increase ACE2 binding affinity (N501Y, within the RBD). Other key mutations enable better immune evasion (69–70 del) and increased viral infectivity (P681H, occurring close to the furin cleavage site at the S1/S2 junction) [79]. Other current variants of interest including the B.1.351 (emerged in South Africa) and P.1 (emerged in Brazil) variants also contain mutations that increase infectivity (eg. N439K) and viral fitness, and compromise immunity and vaccine efficacy (E484K, K417N/T) [80–82].The more recent Delta variant (named B.1.617.2) that was first detected in India is 60% more transmissible than the Alpha variant and has been linked to a resurgence of COVID-19 in Nepal, southeast Asia, the UK, and the USA [83]. Research is currently underway to identify the key mutations that make this particular variant responsible for a new wave of the current pandemic.

## Concluding Remarks

Coronaviruses display a continuous pattern of evolution and this has challenged mankind to invent new strategies to overcome their impacts on health. The gaps in knowledge, lack of specific antiviral interventions, and often confusing circulating information about the newly emerged SARS-CoV-2 has not only made it difficult to control and manage the COVID-19 pandemic but it can cause drastic misconceptions in the future. Genetic recombination of the viral genome has historically allowed for novel CoVs to emerge, so it will be necessary to share the latest research progress to make available accurate and crucial information about SARS-CoV-2 in order to provide the best global opportunities to combat this disease. In the present chapter, we have reviewed the key areas of the SARS-CoV-2 genome structure and defined the encoded proteins responsible for viral replication, propagation and diversity. Based on the currently available data, SARS-CoV-2 has a high tendency for genetic mutations that affect antigenicity and other aspects of the virus biology, and this is a matter of immediate concern particularly given the severe impact that newer variants have on our current measures to reduce viral transmission and lower mortality rates. It is imperative that we continue to track and report the research about significant SARS-CoV-2 variants if we hope to implement targeted control measures, such as facilitating the automated detection of the potential variants of concern and establish several alternative pathways to inhibit viral proliferation. An essential part of this process will be identifying the key data that help in the development and success of tailored vaccines and treatments against these variants. Overall, the containment of SARS-CoV-2 remains a robust public health problem that needs comprehensive investigation about the genetic and biological characteristics of the CoVs family members to limit the adverse consequence of current and future viral pandemics.

## References


1. Woo PCY, Huang Y, Lau SKP, Yuen K-Y. Coronavirus genomics and bioinformatics analysis. Viruses. 2010;2(8):1804–20.
2. Payne S. Chapter 17. Family Coronaviridae. In: Payne S, editor. Viruses. New York: Academic Press; 2017. p. 149–58.
3. Cui J, Li F, Shi Z-L. Origin and evolution of pathogenic coronaviruses. Nat Rev Microbiol. 2019;17(3):181–92.
4. Forni D, Cagliani R, Clerici M, Sironi M. Molecular evolution of human coronavirus genomes. Trends Microbiol. 2017;25(1):35–48.
5. Lacroix A, Duong V, Hul V, San S, Davun H, Omaliss K, Chea S, Hassanin A, Theppangna W, Silithammavong S, Khammavong K, Singhalath S, Greatorex Z, Fine AE, Goldstein T, Olson S, Joly DO, Keatts L, Dussart P, Afelt A, Frutos R, Buchy P. Genetic diversity of coronaviruses in bats in Lao PDR and Cambodia. Infect Genet Evol. 2017;48:10–8.
6. Su S, Wong G, Shi W, Liu J, Lai ACK, Zhou J, Liu W, Bi Y, Gao GF. Epidemiology, genetic recombination, and pathogenesis of coronaviruses. Trends Microbiol. 2016;24(6):490–502.
7. Helmy YA, Fawzy M, Elaswad A, Sobieh A, Kenney SP, Shehata AA. The COVID-19 pandemic: a comprehensive review of taxonomy, genetics, epidemiology, diagnosis, treatment, and control. J Clin Med. 2020;9(4):1225.
8. Drosten C, Günther S, Preiser W, van der Werf S, Brodt HR, Becker S, Rabenau H, Panning M, Kolesnikova L, Fouchier RA, Berger A, Burguière AM, Cinatl J, Eickmann M, Escriou N, Grywna K, Kramme S, Manuguerra JC, Müller S, Rickerts V, Stürmer M, Vieth S, Klenk HD, Osterhaus AD, Schmitz H, Doerr HW. Identification of a novel coronavirus in patients with severe acute respiratory syndrome. N Engl J Med. 2003;348(20):1967–76.
9. Zaki AM, van Boheemen S, Bestebroer TM, Osterhaus AD, Fouchier RA. Isolation of a novel coronavirus from a man with pneumonia in Saudi Arabia. N Engl J Med. 2012;367(19):1814–20.
10. Sanyaolu A, Okorie C, Hosein Z, Patidar R, Desai P, Prakash S, Jaferi U, Mangat J, Marinkovic A. Global Pandemicity of COVID-19: situation report as of June 9, 2020. Infect Dis Res Treat. 2021;14:1178633721991260.

11. Chen N, Zhou M, Dong X, Qu J, Gong F, Han Y, Qiu Y, Wang J, Liu Y, Wei Y, Xia J, Yu T, Zhang X, Zhang L. Epidemiological and clinical characteristics of 99 cases of 2019 novel coronavirus pneumonia in Wuhan, China: a descriptive study. Lancet. 2020;395(10223):507–13.
12. Wu A, Peng Y, Huang B, Ding X, Wang X, Niu P, Meng J, Zhu Z, Zhang Z, Wang J, Sheng J, Quan L, Xia Z, Tan W, Cheng G, Jiang T. Genome composition and divergence of the novel coronavirus (2019-nCoV) originating in China. Cell Host Microbe. 2020;27(3):325–8.
13. Finkel Y, Mizrahi O, Nachshon A, Weingarten-Gabbay S, Morgenstern D, Yahalom-Ronen Y, Tamir H, Achdout H, Stein D, Israeli O, Beth-Din A, Melamed S, Weiss S, Israely T, Paran N, Schwartz M, Stern-Ginossar N. The coding capacity of SARS-CoV-2. Nature. 2021;589(7840):125–30.
14. Thoms M, Buschauer R, Ameismeier M, Koepke L, Denk T, Hirschenberger M, Kratzat H, Hayn M, Mackens-Kiani T, Cheng J, Straub JH, Stürzel CM, Fröhlich T, Berninghausen O, Becker T, Kirchhoff F, Sparrer KMJ, Beckmann R. Structural basis for translational shutdown and immune evasion by the Nsp1 protein of SARS-CoV-2. Science. 2020;369(6508):1249–55.
15. Ziebuhr J. The coronavirus replicase. Curr Top Microbiol Immunol. 2005;287:57–94.
16. Sun L, Xing Y, Chen X, Zheng Y, Yang Y, Nichols DB, Clementz MA, Banach BS, Li K, Baker SC, Chen Z. Coronavirus papain-like proteases negatively regulate antiviral innate immune response through disruption of STING-mediated signaling. PLoS One. 2012;7(2):e30802.
17. Schubert K, Karousis ED, Jomaa A, Scaiola A, Echeverria B, Gurzeler L-A, Leibundgut M, Thiel V, Mühlemann O, Ban N. SARS-CoV-2 Nsp1 binds the ribosomal mRNA channel to inhibit translation. Nat Struct Mol Biol. 2020;27(10):959–66.
18. Naqvi AAT, Fatima K, Mohammad T, Fatima U, Singh IK, Singh A, Atif SM, Hariprasad G, Hasan GM, Hassan MI. Insights into SARS-CoV-2 genome, structure, evolution, pathogenesis and therapies: structural genomics approach. Biochim Biophys Acta. 2020;1866(10):165878.
19. Siu YL, Teoh KT, Lo J, Chan CM, Kien F, Escriou N, Tsao SW, Nicholls JM, Altmeyer R, Peiris JS, Bruzzone R, Nal B. The M, E, and N structural proteins of the severe acute respiratory syndrome coronavirus are required for efficient assembly, trafficking, and release of virus-like particles. J Virol. 2008;82(22):11318–30.
20. Haque SM, Ashwaq O, Sarief A, Mohamed AKAJ. A comprehensive review about SARS-CoV-2. Futur Virol. 2020;15(9):625–48.
21. Kim D, Lee JY, Yang JS, Kim JW, Kim VN, Chang H. The architecture of SARS-CoV-2 transcriptome. Cell. 2020;181(4):914–921.e910.
22. Fehr AR, Perlman S. Coronaviruses: an overview of their replication and pathogenesis. Methods Mol Biol. 2015;1282:1–23.
23. V'kovski P, Kratzel A, Steiner S, Stalder H, Thiel V. Coronavirus biology and replication: implications for SARS-CoV-2. Nat Rev Microbiol. 2021;19(3):155–70.
24. Simonis A, Theobald SJ, Fätkenheuer G, Rybniker J, Malin JJ. A comparative analysis of remdesivir and other repurposed antivirals against SARS-CoV-2. EMBO Mol Med. 2021;13(1):e13105.
25. Kaptein SJF, Jacobs S, Langendries L, Seldeslachts L, Ter Horst S, Liesenborghs L, Hens B, Vergote V, Heylen E, Barthelemy K, Maas E, De Keyzer C, Bervoets L, Rymenants J, Van Buyten T, Zhang X, Abdelnabi R, Pang J, Williams R, Thibaut HJ, Dallmeier K, Boudewijns R, Wouters J, Augustijns P, Verougstraete N, Cawthorne C, Breuer J, Solas C, Weynand B, Annaert P, Spriet I, Vande Velde G, Neyts J, Rocha-Pereira J, Delang L. Favipiravir at high doses has potent antiviral activity in SARS-CoV-2-infected hamsters, whereas hydroxychloroquine lacks activity. Proc Natl Acad Sci U S A. 2020;117(43):26955–65.
26. Rattanaumpawan P, Jirajariyavej S, Lerdlamyong K, Palavutitotai N, Saiyarin J. Real-world experience with Favipiravir for treatment of COVID-19 in Thailand: results from a Multicenter Observational Study. medRxiv. 2020. p. 2020.2006.2024.20133249.
27. Ye ZW, Yuan S, Chan JF, Zhang AJ, Yu CY, Ong CP, Yang D, Chan CC, Tang K, Cao J, Poon VK, Chan CC, Cai JP, Chu H, Yuen KY, Jin DY. Beneficial effect of combinational methylprednisolone and remdesivir in hamster model of SARS-CoV-2 infection. Emerg Microbes Infect. 2021;10(1):291–304.

28. Wang Y, Zhang D, Du G, Du R, Zhao J, Jin Y, Fu S, Gao L, Cheng Z, Lu Q, Hu Y, Luo G, Wang K, Lu Y, Li H, Wang S, Ruan S, Yang C, Mei C, Wang Y, Ding D, Wu F, Tang X, Ye X, Ye Y, Liu B, Yang J, Yin W, Wang A, Fan G, Zhou F, Liu Z, Gu X, Xu J, Shang L, Zhang Y, Cao L, Guo T, Wan Y, Qin H, Jiang Y, Jaki T, Hayden FG, Horby PW, Cao B, Wang C. Remdesivir in adults with severe COVID-19: a randomised, double-blind, placebo-controlled, multicentre trial. Lancet. 2020c;395(10236):1569–78.
29. Ou X, Liu Y, Lei X, Li P, Mi D, Ren L, Guo L, Guo R, Chen T, Hu J, Xiang Z, Mu Z, Chen X, Chen J, Hu K, Jin Q, Wang J, Qian Z. Characterization of spike glycoprotein of SARS-CoV-2 on virus entry and its immune cross-reactivity with SARS-CoV. Nat Commun. 2020;11(1):1620.
30. Wang M-Y, Zhao R, Gao L-J, Gao X-F, Wang D-P, Cao J-M. SARS-CoV-2: structure, biology, and structure-based therapeutics development. Front Cell Infect Microbiol. 2020b;10:587269.
31. Mittal A, Manjunath K, Ranjan RK, Kaushik S, Kumar S, Verma V. COVID-19 pandemic: insights into structure, function, and hACE2 receptor recognition by SARS-CoV-2. PLoS Pathog. 2020;16(8):e1008762.
32. Korber B, Fischer WM, Gnanakaran S, Yoon H, Theiler J, Abfalterer W, Hengartner N, Giorgi EE, Bhattacharya T, Foley B, Hastie KM, Parker MD, Partridge DG, Evans CM, Freeman TM, de Silva TI, McDanal C, Perez LG, Tang H, Moon-Walker A, Whelan SP, LaBranche CC, Saphire EO, Montefiori DC. Tracking changes in SARS-CoV-2 spike: evidence that D614G increases infectivity of the COVID-19 virus. Cell. 2020;182(4):812–827.e819.
33. Hulswit RJ, de Haan CA, Bosch BJ. Coronavirus spike protein and tropism changes. Adv Virus Res. 2016;96:29–57.
34. Walls AC, Park Y-J, Tortorici MA, Wall A, McGuire AT, Veesler D. Structure, function, and antigenicity of the SARS-CoV-2 spike glycoprotein. Cell. 2020;181(2):281-292. e286.
35. Millet JK, Whittaker GR. Host cell proteases: critical determinants of coronavirus tropism and pathogenesis. Virus Res. 2015;202:120–34.
36. Coutard B, Valle C, de Lamballerie X, Canard B, Seidah NG, Decroly E. The spike glycoprotein of the new coronavirus 2019-nCoV contains a furin-like cleavage site absent in CoV of the same clade. Antiviral Res. 2020;176:104742.
37. Lan J, Ge J, Yu J, Shan S, Zhou H, Fan S, Zhang Q, Shi X, Wang Q, Zhang L, Wang X. Structure of the SARS-CoV-2 spike receptor-binding domain bound to the ACE2 receptor. Nature. 2020;581(7807):215–20.
38. Zhou P, Yang X-L, Wang X-G, Hu B, Zhang L, Zhang W, Si H-R, Zhu Y, Li B, Huang C-L, Chen H-D, Chen J, Luo Y, Guo H, Jiang R-D, Liu M-Q, Chen Y, Shen X-R, Wang X, Zheng X-S, Zhao K, Chen Q-J, Deng F, Liu L-L, Yan B, Zhan F-X, Wang Y-Y, Xiao G-F, Shi Z-L. A pneumonia outbreak associated with a new coronavirus of probable bat origin. Nature. 2020;579(7798):270–3.
39. Li Y, Zhang Z, Yang L, Lian X, Xie Y, Li S, Xin S, Cao P, Lu J. The MERS-CoV receptor DPP4 as a candidate binding target of the SARS-CoV-2 spike. iScience. 2020;23(6):101160.
40. Li F, Li W, Farzan M, Harrison SC. Structure of SARS coronavirus spike receptor-binding domain complexed with receptor. Science. 2005;309(5742):1864–8.
41. Hoffmann M, Kleine-Weber H, Schroeder S, Krüger N, Herrler T, Erichsen S, Schiergens TS, Herrler G, Wu NH, Nitsche A, Müller MA, Drosten C, Pöhlmann S. SARS-CoV-2 cell entry depends on ACE2 and TMPRSS2 and is blocked by a clinically proven protease inhibitor. Cell. 2020;181(2):271–280.e278.
42. Li S, Yuan L, Dai G, Chen RA, Liu DX, Fung TS. Regulation of the ER stress response by the Ion Channel activity of the infectious bronchitis coronavirus envelope protein modulates Virion release, apoptosis, viral fitness, and pathogenesis. Front Microbiol. 2019;10:3022.
43. Surya W, Li Y, Torres J. Structural model of the SARS coronavirus E channel in LMPG micelles. Biochim Biophys Acta Biomembr. 2018;1860(6):1309–17.
44. Mandala VS, McKay MJ, Shcherbakov AA, Dregni AJ, Kolocouris A, Hong M. Structure and drug binding of the SARS-CoV-2 envelope protein transmembrane domain in lipid bilayers. Nat Struct Mol Biol. 2020;27(12):1202–8.

45. Schoeman D, Fielding BC. Coronavirus envelope protein: current knowledge. Virol J. 2019;16(1):1–22.
46. Hassan SS, Choudhury PP, Roy B. SARS-CoV2 envelope protein: non-synonymous mutations and its consequences. Genomics. 2020;112(6):3890–2.
47. De Maio F, Lo Cascio E, Babini G, Sali M, Della Longa S, Tilocca B, Roncada P, Arcovito A, Sanguinetti M, Scambia G, Urbani A. Improved binding of SARS-CoV-2 envelope protein to tight junction-associated PALS1 could play a key role in COVID-19 pathogenesis. Microbes Infect. 2020;22(10):592–7.
48. Bianchi M, Benvenuto D, Giovanetti M, Angeletti S, Ciccozzi M, Pascarella S. Sars-CoV-2 envelope and membrane proteins: structural differences linked to virus characteristics? Biomed Res Int. 2020;2020:4389089.
49. Alsaadi EA, Jones IM. Membrane binding proteins of coronaviruses. Futur Virol. 2019;14(4):275.
50. Mantlo E, Bukreyeva N, Maruyama J, Paessler S, Huang C. Antiviral activities of type I interferons to SARS-CoV-2 infection. Antiviral Res. 2020;179:104811.
51. Zheng Y, Zhuang M-W, Han L, Zhang J, Nan M-L, Zhan P, Kang D, Liu X, Gao C, Wang P-H. Severe acute respiratory syndrome coronavirus 2 (SARS-CoV-2) membrane (M) protein inhibits type I and III interferon production by targeting RIG-I/MDA-5 signaling. Signal Transduct Target Ther. 2020;5(1):299.
52. Hung IF, Lung KC, Tso EY, Liu R, Chung TW, Chu MY, Ng YY, Lo J, Chan J, Tam AR, Shum HP, Chan V, Wu AK, Sin KM, Leung WS, Law WL, Lung DC, Sin S, Yeung P, Yip CC, Zhang RR, Fung AY, Yan EY, Leung KH, Ip JD, Chu AW, Chan WM, Ng AC, Lee R, Fung K, Yeung A, Wu TC, Chan JW, Yan WW, Chan WM, Chan JF, Lie AK, Tsang OT, Cheng VC, Que TL, Lau CS, Chan KH, To KK, Yuen KY. Triple combination of interferon beta-1b, lopinavir-ritonavir, and ribavirin in the treatment of patients admitted to hospital with COVID-19: an open-label, randomised, phase 2 trial. Lancet. 2020;395(10238):1695–704.
53. Saraste J, Prydz K. Assembly and cellular exit of coronaviruses: hijacking an unconventional secretory pathway from the pre-Golgi intermediate compartment via the Golgi ribbon to the extracellular space. Cell. 2021;10(3):503.
54. Gussow AB, Auslander N, Faure G, Wolf YI, Zhang F, Koonin EV. Genomic determinants of pathogenicity in SARS-CoV-2 and other human coronaviruses. Proc Natl Acad Sci. 2020;117(26):15193–9.
55. Su M, Chen Y, Qi S, Shi D, Feng L, Sun D. A mini-review on cell cycle regulation of coronavirus infection. Front Vet Sci. 2020;7:586826.
56. Guan Q, Sadykov M, Mfarrej S, Hala S, Naeem R, Nugmanova R, Al-Omari A, Salih S, Mutair AA, Carr MJ, Hall WW, Arold ST, Pain A. A genetic barcode of SARS-CoV-2 for monitoring global distribution of different clades during the COVID-19 pandemic. Int J Infect Dis. 2020;100:216–23.
57. Hamed SM, Elkhatib WF, Khairalla AS, Noreddin AM. Global dynamics of SARS-CoV-2 clades and their relation to COVID-19 epidemiology. Sci Rep. 2021;11(1):8435.
58. Rambaut A, Holmes EC, O'Toole Á, Hill V, McCrone JT, Ruis C, du Plessis L, Pybus OG. A dynamic nomenclature proposal for SARS-CoV-2 lineages to assist genomic epidemiology. Nat Microbiol. 2020;5(11):1403–7.
59. Hadfield J, Megill C, Bell SM, Huddleston J, Potter B, Callender C, Sagulenko P, Bedford T, Neher RA. Nextstrain: real-time tracking of pathogen evolution. Bioinformatics. 2018;34(23):4121–3.
60. Konings F, Perkins MD, Kuhn JH, Pallen MJ, Alm EJ, Archer BN, Barakat A, Bedford T, Bhiman JN, Caly L, Carter LL, Cullinane A, de Oliveira T, Druce J, El Masry I, Evans R, Gao GF, Gorbalenya AE, Hamblion E, Herring BL, Hodcroft E, Holmes EC, Kakkar M, Khare S, Koopmans MPG, Korber B, Leite J, MacCannell D, Marklewitz M, Maurer-Stroh S, Rico JAM, Munster VJ, Neher R, Munnink BO, Pavlin BI, Peiris M, Poon L, Pybus O, Rambaut A, Resende P, Subissi L, Thiel V, Tong S, van der Werf S, von Gottberg A, Ziebuhr J, Van

Kerkhove MD. SARS-CoV-2 variants of interest and concern naming scheme conducive for global discourse. Nat Microbiol. 2021;6:821.
61. Forster P, Forster L, Renfrew C, Forster M. Phylogenetic network analysis of SARS-CoV-2 genomes. Proc Natl Acad Sci. 2020;117(17):9241–3.
62. Gorbalenya AE, Baker SC, Baric RS, de Groot RJ, Drosten C, Gulyaeva AA, Haagmans BL, Lauber C, Leontovich AM, Neuman BW, Penzar D, Perlman S, Poon LLM, Samborskiy DV, Sidorov IA, Sola I, Ziebuhr J. The species severe acute respiratory syndrome-related coronavirus: classifying 2019-nCoV and naming it SARS-CoV-2. Nat Microbiol. 2020;5(4):536–44.
63. Jia Y, Shen G, Zhang Y, Huang KS, Ho HY, Hor WS, Yang CH, Li C, Wang WL. Analysis of the mutation dynamics of SARS-CoV-2 reveals the spread history and emergence of RBD mutant with lower ACE2 binding affinity. bioRxiv. 2020. p. 2020.2004.2009.034942.
64. Shang J, Ye G, Shi K, Wan Y, Luo C, Aihara H, Geng Q, Auerbach A, Li F. Structural basis of receptor recognition by SARS-CoV-2. Nature. 2020;581(7807):221–4.
65. Duffy S. Why are RNA virus mutation rates so damn high? PLoS Biol. 2018;16(8):e3000003.
66. Han YJ, Lee KH, Yoon S, Nam SW, Ryu S, Seong D, Kim JS, Lee JY, Yang JW, Lee J, Koyanagi A, Hong SH, Dragioti E, Radua J, Smith L, Oh H, Ghayda RA, Kronbichler A, Effenberger M, Kresse D, Denicolò S, Kang W, Jacob L, Shin H, Shin JI. Treatment of severe acute respiratory syndrome (SARS), Middle East respiratory syndrome (MERS), and coronavirus disease 2019 (COVID-19): a systematic review of in vitro, in vivo, and clinical trials. Theranostics. 2021;11(3):1207–31.
67. Wang C, Liu Z, Chen Z, Huang X, Xu M, He T, Zhang Z. The establishment of reference sequence for SARS-CoV-2 and variation analysis. J Med Virol. 2020a;92(6):667–74.
68. Plante JA, Liu Y, Liu J, Xia H, Johnson BA, Lokugamage KG, Zhang X, Muruato AE, Zou J, Fontes-Garfias CR, Mirchandani D, Scharton D, Bilello JP, Ku Z, An Z, Kalveram B, Freiberg AN, Menachery VD, Xie X, Plante KS, Weaver SC, Shi P-Y. Spike mutation D614G alters SARS-CoV-2 fitness. Nature. 2021;592(7852):116–21.
69. Yurkovetskiy L, Wang X, Pascal KE, Tomkins-Tinch C, Nyalile T, Wang Y, Baum A, Diehl WE, Dauphin A, Carbone C, Veinotte K, Egri SB, Schaffner SF, Lemieux JE, Munro J, Rafique A, Barve A, Sabeti PC, Kyratsous CA, Dudkina N, Shen K, Luban J. SARS-CoV-2 Spike protein variant D614G increases infectivity and retains sensitivity to antibodies that target the receptor binding domain. bioRxiv: the preprint server for biology. 2020. p. 2020.2007.2004.187757.
70. Mercatelli D, Giorgi FM. Geographic and genomic distribution of SARS-CoV-2 mutations. Front Microbiol. 2020;11:1800.
71. Pachetti M, Marini B, Benedetti F, Giudici F, Mauro E, Storici P, Masciovecchio C, Angeletti S, Ciccozzi M, Gallo RC, Zella D, Ippodrino R. Emerging SARS-CoV-2 mutation hot spots include a novel RNA-dependent-RNA polymerase variant. J Transl Med. 2020;18(1):179.
72. Sengupta A, Hassan SS, Choudhury PP. Clade GR and clade GH isolates of SARS-CoV-2 in Asia show highest amount of SNPs. Infect Genet Evol. 2021;89:104724.
73. Zhang L, Lin D, Sun X, Curth U, Drosten C, Sauerhering L, Becker S, Rox K, Hilgenfeld R. Crystal structure of SARS-CoV-2 main protease provides a basis for design of improved α-ketoamide inhibitors. Science. 2020;368(6489):409–12.
74. Wu A, Wang L, Zhou H-Y, Ji C-Y, Xia SZ, Cao Y, Meng J, Ding X, Gold S, Jiang T, Cheng G. One year of SARS-CoV-2 evolution. Cell Host Microbe. 2021;29(4):503–7.
75. Ceraolo C, Giorgi FM. Genomic variance of the 2019-nCoV coronavirus. J Med Virol. 2020;92(5):522–8.
76. Lu R, Zhao X, Li J, Niu P, Yang B, Wu H, Wang W, Song H, Huang B, Zhu N, Bi Y, Ma X, Zhan F, Wang L, Hu T, Zhou H, Hu Z, Zhou W, Zhao L, Chen J, Meng Y, Wang J, Lin Y, Yuan J, Xie Z, Ma J, Liu WJ, Wang D, Xu W, Holmes EC, Gao GF, Wu G, Chen W, Shi W, Tan W. Genomic characterisation and epidemiology of 2019 novel coronavirus: implications for virus origins and receptor binding. Lancet. 2020;395(10224):565–74.
77. Challen R, Brooks-Pollock E, Read JM, Dyson L, Tsaneva-Atanasova K, Danon L. Risk of mortality in patients infected with SARS-CoV-2 variant of concern 202012/1: matched cohort study. BMJ. 2021;372:n579.

78. Davies NG, Abbott S, Barnard RC, Jarvis CI, Kucharski AJ, Munday JD, Pearson CAB, Russell TW, Tully DC, Washburne AD, Wenseleers T, Gimma A, Waites W, Wong KLM, van Zandvoort K, Silverman JD, Diaz-Ordaz K, Keogh R, Eggo RM, Funk S, Jit M, Atkins KE, Edmunds WJ. Estimated transmissibility and impact of SARS-CoV-2 lineage B.1.1.7 in England. Science. 2021;372(6538):eabg3055.
79. Ramírez JD, Muñoz M, Patiño LH, Ballesteros N, Paniz-Mondolfi A. Will the emergent SARS-CoV2 B.1.1.7 lineage affect molecular diagnosis of COVID-19? J Med Virol. 2021;93(5):2566–8.
80. Planas D, Bruel T, Grzelak L, Guivel-Benhassine F, Staropoli I, Porrot F, Planchais C, Buchrieser J, Rajah MM, Bishop E, Albert M, Donati F, Prot M, Behillil S, Enouf V, Maquart M, Smati-Lafarge M, Varon E, Schortgen F, Yahyaoui L, Gonzalez M, De Sèze J, Péré H, Veyer D, Sève A, Simon-Lorière E, Fafi-Kremer S, Stefic K, Mouquet H, Hocqueloux L, van der Werf S, Prazuck T, Schwartz O. Sensitivity of infectious SARS-CoV-2 B.1.1.7 and B.1.351 variants to neutralizing antibodies. Nat Med. 2021;27:917–24.
81. Thomson EC, Rosen LE, Shepherd JG, Spreafico R, da Silva Filipe A, Wojcechowskyj JA, Davis C, Piccoli L, Pascall DJ, Dillen J, Lytras S, Czudnochowski N, Shah R, Meury M, Jesudason N, De Marco A, Li K, Bassi J, O'Toole A, Pinto D, Colquhoun RM, Culap K, Jackson B, Zatta F, Rambaut A, Jaconi S, Sreenu VB, Nix J, Zhang I, Jarrett RF, Glass WG, Beltramello M, Nomikou K, Pizzuto M, Tong L, Cameroni E, Croll TI, Johnson N, Di Iulio J, Wickenhagen A, Ceschi A, Harbison AM, Mair D, Ferrari P, Smollett K, Sallusto F, Carmichael S, Garzoni C, Nichols J, Galli M, Hughes J, Riva A, Ho A, Schiuma M, Semple MG, Openshaw PJM, Fadda E, Baillie JK, Chodera JD, Rihn SJ, Lycett SJ, Virgin HW, Telenti A, Corti D, Robertson DL, Snell G. Circulating SARS-CoV-2 spike N439K variants maintain fitness while evading antibody-mediated immunity. Cell. 2021;184(5):1171–1187.e1120.
82. Wibmer CK, Ayres F, Hermanus T, Madzivhandila M, Kgagudi P, Oosthuysen B, Lambson BE, de Oliveira T, Vermeulen M, van der Berg K, Rossouw T, Boswell M, Ueckermann V, Meiring S, von Gottberg A, Cohen C, Morris L, Bhiman JN, Moore PL. SARS-CoV-2 501Y.V2 escapes neutralization by south African COVID-19 donor plasma. Nat Med. 2021;27(4):622–5.
83. Bolze A, Cirulli ET, Luo S, White S, Cassens T, Jacobs S, Nguyen J, Ramirez JM, Sandoval E, Wang X, Wong D, Becker D, Laurent M, Lu JT, Isaksson M, Washington NL, Lee W. Rapid displacement of SARS-CoV-2 variant B.1.1.7 by B.1.617.2 and P.1 in the United States. medRxiv. 2021. p. 2021.2006.2020.21259195.

# Chapter 5
# COVID-19 Impact on Host at Pathophysiological and Cellular Level

**Omkar Indari, Shweta Jakhmola, Dharmendra Kashyap, Budhadev Baral, Tarun Prakash Verma, Khushboo Jain, and Hem Chandra Jha**

## Introduction

Coronavirus disease 2019 (COVID-19), caused by severe acute respiratory syndrome coronavirus-2 (SARS-CoV-2), affected the entire world and has given rise to novel challenges in every possible sector of life. The COVID-19 pandemic first appeared in Wuhan, China in December 2019 [1]. Although the SARS-CoV-2 showed similarity to the earlier CoV associated outbreaks, it affected comparatively larger populations and geographic areas. SARS-CoV-2 is a large single-stranded RNA virus. It encodes Spike (S), membrane (M), envelope (E), and nucleocapsid (N) proteins along with some nonstructural proteins (nsp) which are important for the development of its structure and infection [2]. SARS-CoV-2 through its S protein interacts with angiotensin-converting enzyme 2 (ACE2), and the virus shows 10- to 20-fold higher affinity toward ACE2 compared to SARS-CoV [3]. ACE2 is widely expressed in various organs and different types of human body cells like the heart, kidneys, gastrointestinal tract, and testes, which makes them possible sites for SARS-CoV-2 infection.

The cascade of SARS-CoV-2 infection is initiated when the viral particles from the surrounding environment enter into the respiratory system by various direct or indirect routes [4]. The virus first causes the infection of the upper respiratory tract and ultimately propagates into the infected cells, and bursts out to infect nearby

Omkar Indari and Shweta Jakhmola are equal contributors.

O. Indari · S. Jakhmola · D. Kashyap · B. Baral · T. P. Verma · K. Jain · H. C. Jha (✉)
Infection Bio-Engineering Group, Department of Biosciences and Biomedical Engineering, Indian Institute of Technology Indore, Indore, Madhya Pradesh, India
e-mail: hemcjha@iiti.ac.in


S. Adibi et al. (eds.), *Frontiers of COVID-19*,
https://doi.org/10.1007/978-3-031-08045-6_5

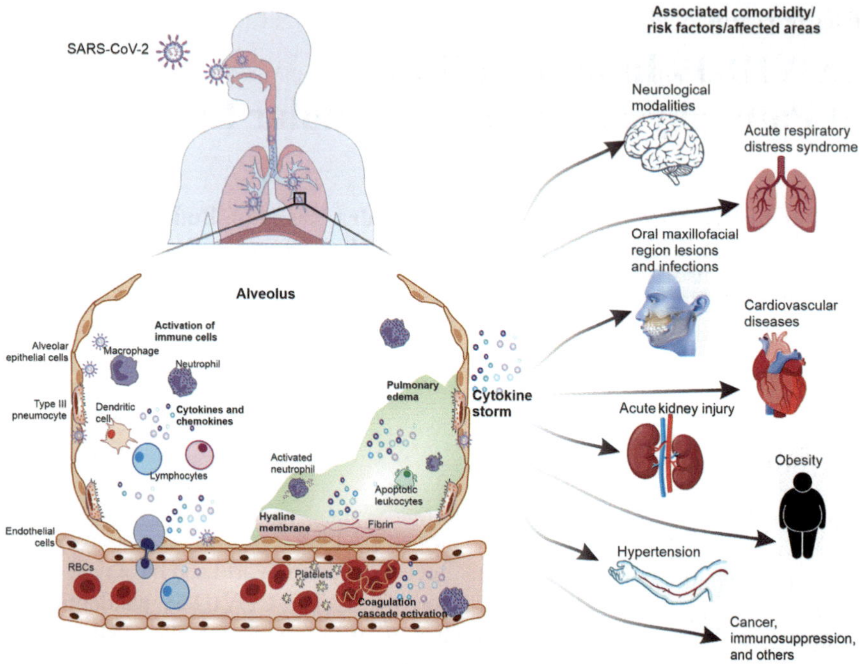


**Fig. 5.1** Illustration of impacts of COVID-19 and associated comorbidities, risk factors and possible affected areas. Virus particles from the surrounding environment enter the body through oronasal routes. After infecting the cells of the upper respiratory system the virus travels to infect cells of lower respiratory system. It infects alveolar epithelial cells and macrophages. The infected cells produce cytokines and chemokines. The antigen presenting cells like dendritic cells recognize and phagocytose infected cells. They display antigens to T cells. Further cytotoxic T cells attack infected cells and helper T cells activate B cells. Through an immune cascade, all the nearby immune cells get activated. In case of severe infection, immune dysregulation occurs causing the pneumocyte desquamation and apoptosis of nearby cells including immune cells. This leads to pulmonary edema, hyaline membrane formation, and ARDS. The nearby immune cells get activated and more immune cells from the circulatory system are transported at the infection site. Due to altered immune response, cytokine storms are developed. Coagulation dysfunction is also initiated at the nearby circulatory system. The conditions generated on virus infection affect different body parts thus increasing the severity in patients with comorbidities

cells. Further, it travels to the lower respiratory system and targets epithelial cells of bronchi, alveoli, and alveolar macrophages for infection [5] (Fig. 5.1). Due to the subsequent host defense mechanism, the infected cells become apoptotic. The antigen-presenting cells (APCs) eventually phagocytose these cells. APCs further present antigens to T-lymphocytes. CD8+ T-lymphocytes then can attack virus infected cells and CD4+ T-lymphocytes induce activation of B lymphocytes which can produce antibodies against the virus. Lung biopsies of COVID-19 patients have shown the presence of immune cell infiltrates with a major proportion of lymphocytes [6]. As a consequence of the progression of infection, pneumocyte desquamation has been observed [6]. Additionally, pulmonary edema along with hyaline membrane formation and subsequent acute respiratory distress syndrome (ARDS) was observed [7–9].

Dysregulated inflammation post–COVID-19 development has been observed to cause severe complications. Pathological features of COVID-19 patients have shown drastically increased cytokines, leading to the generation of a cytokine storm [10]. Further, these cytokine storms are related to poor outcomes and mortality in COVID-19 patients [10]. The viral infection, cytokine storm, and dysregulated inflammation can have impacts on various systems of the body.

The people with underlying comorbidities may show higher complications than healthy ones [11]. Cardiovascular diseases (CVD), diabetes, and hypertension are the major underlying conditions observed in the worldwide population. During the pandemic, people with these conditions remained at greater risk of developing complications due to existing status. Many studies investigated and reported the associated risks and repercussions of various comorbidities in these individuals due to COVID-19. Other conditions like obesity, immunosuppression, and chronic diseases like kidney diseases were also investigated by researchers to check their association with COVID-19 morbidity and mortality. Obesity is observed to be widespread in the global population. Obese individuals showed limited truncal expansion, hence have an increased risk of alleviated respiratory airflow and poor breathing. Hence, it was important to study this condition in regard to COVID-19. In patients with cancer and individuals on immunosuppressants, an additional healthcare burden was prevalent as there was a hindrance in providing necessary treatments during the pandemic. Researchers demonstrated the impacts of COVID-19 on these patients in various reports. The SARS-CoV-2 infection has shown to develop neurological complications too. It has also been observed that the disease develops oral and maxillofacial manifestations. The infection and impacts on oral and maxillofacial regions have been linked to the possible route of SARS-CoV-2 entry into the central nervous system (CNS). The impacts of underlying conditions like diabetes, steroid treatments, and altered immune system have been shown to make people prone to secondary infections, at oral and maxillofacial regions, like mucormycosis. Overall, all the studies addressing these comorbid conditions and repercussions provided valuable inputs considering COVID-19 patients. However, there is currently a lack of studies that provide a detailed mechanism involved in the severe disease progression in people with different comorbidities. Hence, there is a requirement of dedicated research on each comorbidity and its manifestations. The available crucial information related to this is scattered into various important reports. Here, we provide a comprehensive account of various aspects regarding COVID-19 like the associated comorbidities.

Additionally, severe inflammation is the central point which affects the COVID-19 patients. Various cellular pathways are involved in driving the exaggerated immune response and inflammation post–SARS-CoV-2 infection. Studies have shown the involvement of Nuclear factor kappa-light-chain-enhancer of activated B cells (NFκB), p38 mitogen-activated protein kinase (MAPK), interferon (IFN) regulatory factor (IRF), and Janus kinase (JAK)-signal transducer and activator of transcription factor (STAT) associated pathways. These pathways were found to regulate numerous immune responses associated with genes contributing to cytokine storms observed in COVID-19. Interestingly, many SARS-CoV-2 associated proteins have also shown to alter these pathways in distinct ways. There could be various proteins from these pathways which can be therapeutic targets to reduce the inflammation as well as the progression of infection. We have discussed the details of these molecular pathways in SARS-CoV-2 infection. Further, we believe that assorted information provided in this chapter highlights various key points which would help researchers and physicians to look into various therapeutic challenges collectively for providing healthcare solutions.

## Cardiovascular Diseases

SARS-CoV-2 has the potential to cause multiorgan damage including the heart thereby causing cardiovascular issues [10]. SARS-CoV-2 may influence the prevailing cardiac complications which include conditions like ischemic/inflammatory heart disease, ventricular arrhythmias, conduction disturbances, thrombotic events at the level of the lungs, and systemic activation of the coagulation cascade, configuring the scenario of disseminated intravascular coagulation [11]. Several meta-analysis studies have related CVD with COVID-19 [12, 13]. The initial symptoms of implications of the cardiovascular system include arrhythmias, palpitations, chest tightness and pain [14, 15]. A report by Liu et al. suggested that 7.3% of patients have palpitation as initial signs and further 2% experienced chest pain [16]. Also, Wang et al. found that 16.7% of patients with COVID-19 had arrhythmias [17]. According to the Centers for Disease Control and Prevention, USA (CDC) or World Health Organization (WHO), it has been estimated that approximately 12.8% of the COVID-19 patients developed hypertension and 4% had CVD. According to the American Heart Association (AHA) among COVID-19 patients, 40% had cardiovascular and cerebrovascular diseases [18]. Also the mortality rate of patients with cardiac ailments was higher compared to patients with no comorbidities. Accumulating evidence showed the presence of cardiac necrosis biomarkers in the serum which mark varying degrees of myocardial tissue damage. Interestingly, this damage is noticed more in the severe and deceased COVID-19 patients unlike the patients with mild COVID-19 symptoms [19]. Also, CVD was found to be prevalent in older (age range 57 to 91 years) individuals and patients with multiple comorbid conditions like diabetes, renal disorders, and immunodeficiency [20]. More reports suggest that hypertension, diabetes, coronary heart disease, chronic renal disease, and chronic obstructive pulmonary disease (COPD) are more common in the deceased COVID-19 patients than in the survivors. It is also reported that patients with CVD had higher chances of developing dysfunctional liver, inflated levels of serum creatinine and lactate dehydrogenase. Overall, the study demonstrated that COVID-19 patients with CVD were more vulnerable to injury and damage. There exists an interrelation of CVD and COVID-19; however, the specific mechanisms of interaction are yet to be elucidated.

It is predicted that the myocardial damage may be direct, that is, a result of upregulation of heart ACE2 induced by SARS-CoV-2 or may arise due to hyperactivated immune response to the viral infection. ACE2 the master regulator of the renin–angiotensin–aldosterone system (RAAS) pathway has a critical role in regulating systemic and pulmonary hypertension, cardiac failure, myocardial infarction, and cardiovascular complications arising due to diabetes [21, 22]. ACE2 is abundantly expressed by the cardiac epithelial cells [22, 23]. Also, Chen et al. reported enhanced expression of ACE2 in the cardiac pericytes made them possible virus targets [24]. It is hypothesized that the damage caused by the virus could instigate capillary endothelial and microvascular cell dysfunction. The patients with cardiac failure exhibited elevated ACE2 transcript and proteins thus increased their risk of SARS-CoV-2 infection [25]. Moreover, reports suggested that angiotensin receptor blockers (ARBs) can increase ACE2 expression in animal models. The study underlines the high dosage of ARBs necessary for inducing the upregulation of ACE2. However, currently there is insufficient data that could explain that the usage of ARBs facilitated SARS-CoV-2 entry and COVID-19.

In addition, the physiological functions of the heart and lungs are inseparable. Complications in the heart may increase the risk of pneumonia, while lung injury may aggravate prevailing heart problems like blood pressure, heart failure, and myocardial infarction. The infected host may exhibit vivid signs of severe coronary artery disease or myocarditis regardless of the earlier history [26, 27]. In particular, the hypoxic conditions generated as an outcome of respiratory failure in COVID-19 may also cause damage to the heart [14]. Hypoxemia induced by the damage of the lung cells is known to decrease the oxygen saturation and increase the amounts of harmful bi-products such as oxygen free radicals, and lactic acid which through circulation reach the myocardial cells and may lead to myocardial injury [18]. Additionally, due to poor oxygen supply in the body, the pumping of blood is intensified, which may increase the chances of heart failure. Nonetheless, hypoxemia is also a known trigger of inflammatory reactions. The inflammatory reactions induced by SARS-CoV-2 upon invasion of the lung cells can cause inflammation, degeneration, and necrosis of cardiac muscle cells. An increase in levels of inflammatory molecules like c-reactive protein (CRP), interleukin (IL)-1, and IL-6 is described in SARS-CoV-2 infection [28]. Inflammation also causes the release of stress factors like catecholamine, which may cause direct myocardial toxicity, which in turn may culminate in microcirculation disturbance, vasospasm, and arrhythmia. Often COVID-19 patients with heart ailments need active life support treatment, including mechanical ventilation, intra-aortic balloon counterpulsation (IABP), extracorporeal membrane pulmonary oxygenation (ECMO), and temporary implantation of a pacemaker. Further the myocardial damage and cardiovascular inflammation may upregulate the levels of serum creatine kinase and troponin. Nonetheless, hypercoagulability is observed in COVID-19 patients due to an altered coagulation cascade [29, 30]. Among 94 COVID-19 patients the levels of antithrombin III were significantly reduced, while clotting factors like D-dimer and fibrinogen were found to be elevated in comparison to healthy controls. Also, to compensate for the elevated body temperature observed in COVID-19 the body's response includes activation of sympathetic nerves and increased heart rate and cardiac output [31]. It is also important to mention that no specific therapeutic interventions exist for the treatment of CVD caused by SARS-CoV-2. Individuals with preexisting heart conditions must strictly follow the doctor's advice on uptake of statins, beta-blockers, and ACE inhibitors (ACEI).

## Hypertension

The systolic blood pressure (BP) ≥130 or diastolic BP ≥80 $mm^3$ is considered as hypertension as per the guideline of the American College of Cardiology (ACC) and AHA [32]. In COVID-19, hypertension has been associated with an increased risk of infection [33]. Moreover, it has also been associated with high chances of severity and subsequent death [33]. To be specific, hypertension (27%), diabetes (19%), and CVD (6%) were the most associated comorbidities in severe COVID-19 patients with ARDS [33]. Another report also showed hypertension (30%), diabetes (19%), and coronary heart disease (8%) as most associated comorbidities with respect to COVID-19 [34]. Several other studies also demonstrated that hypertension was a commonly found preexisting condition in patients with COVID-19 patients [35, 36]. An initial large scale (44,672 confirmed COVID-19 cases) study from China demonstrated an overall increased case fatality rate of 6.0% for people with hypertension compared to 2.3% observed in people without hypertension [37]. Contrastingly, another large epidemiological cohort study involving 17 million health records from England, suggested that hypertension was not associated with COVID-19 disease outcome. However, sensitivity analyses showed that hypertension was associated with slightly increased risk (Hazard Ratio (HR) 1.07, 95% CI 1.00–1.15) while high blood pressure (≥140/90 mmHg) at the most recent measurement was associated with lower risk (HR 0.61, CI 0.56–0.67) [38]. Shi et al., and Guo et al. showed an increased prevalence of hypertension (59.8–63.5%) among COVID-19 patients, which was accompanied by a higher chance of in-hospital mortality [39, 40]. However, it has not been established whether hypertension alone significantly increases susceptibility to SARS-CoV-2. In a retrospective study by Zhou et al., the presence of hypertension in patients with COVID-19 patients was correlated with an elevation in the odds ratio (OR) for death by 3.05 (95% CI 1.57–5.92) [41]. These associations may, however, be greatly confounded by the higher prevalence of hypertension in older individuals, as they show comparatively poorer clinical outcomes and greater mortality rate post–COVID-19 infection as opposed to younger people. Hypertensive adults over 60 years of age appeared to be at a higher risk when infected with SARS-CoV-2 [42].

Hypertension involves immune dysregulation and is correlated with high circulating lymphocyte counts [43, 44]. Hypertensive patients exhibited CD8+ T cell dysfunction [45]. These immunosenescent CD8+ T cells showed incapability to battle viral infections effectively and may subsequently lead to excessive cytokine production, presenting a probable connection between COVID-19 infection and increased complications in hypertensive patients [46].

It remains unclear whether hypertension alone increases susceptibility for COVID-19. However, one of the key players intensely being debated lately for poor disease prognosis is the use of antihypertensive agents in COVID-19 hypertensive patients. Underlying hypertension in COVID-19 patients is often treated with ACEIs and ARBs. Questions are being raised regarding the effects of these agents in relation to susceptibility and COVID-19 disease outcome; whether they are beneficial or harmful for the patients [47, 48]. In contrast to these findings, however, some studies have reported no change in expression of ACE2 in response to these antihypertensive drugs [49–52]. The work by Reynolds et al. demonstrated that among 12,594 patients who were tested positive for COVID-19, there was no association between any ACEIs/ARBs and the likelihood of testing positive or risk of a severe COVID-19 infection [53]. Another population-based study reported (after adjusting for confounders) that there was no independent association for the use of ACEIs/ARBs with the risk or susceptibility for COVID-19 infection [54]. In hospitalized COVID-19 patients having hypertension, people taking ACEIs/ARBs demonstrated a lower risk of mortality than the people not consuming ACEs/ARBs [55]. Nevertheless, higher ACE2 expression driven by the use of these drugs can in principle increase the chance of cellular SARS-CoV-2 entry, but it is also conceivable that RAAS inhibition can have a protective effect against respiratory infection [56, 57].

Inappropriately discontinuing drugs with well-defined and scientifically proven health benefits would increase cardiovascular risk. Many cases of myocardial infarction, myocarditis, and cardiomyopathy have been seen in patients with COVID-19, and a break in taking cardioprotective medications, including RAAS inhibitors, could show deterioration clinical status of these individuals [58–60]. Tocilizumab (IL-6 antagonist) is being administered to severe COVID-19 patients, and in a study evaluating post-tocilizumab (post-TCZ) toxicities, hypertension was an observed toxicity in 8% of the total patients receiving tocilizumab [61]. However, the lopinavir–ritonavir combination is being used for the treatment of SARS-CoV-2 infection, and high BP is one of its very rare side effects. A study, however, reports that treatment with lopinavir/ritonavir associates significantly with elevated blood pressure, which is mediated through an increase in body mass index (BMI) [62]. Also, concomitant use of sildenafil with lopinavir/ritonavir in patients of pulmonary arterial hypertension (PAH) is not advised, due to the potential of sildenafil-associated serious adverse events [63].

Use of corticosteroid to severe COVID-19 patients is recommended by WHO [64]. Systemic corticosteroids such as dexamethasone may cause elevated blood pressure [65]. The increase in blood pressure is dose-dependent. Chronic dexamethasone use has been associated with the development of hypertension [66]. Moreover, dexamethasone induced hypertension has also been linked to impacts from other hypertension related systems or factors like plasma volume, RAAS, sympathetic activity, vasopressor, and vasodepressor systems [66]. Hence, the use of corticosteroids in COVID-19 patients with hypertension should be cautious.

## Diabetes

Diabetes is one of the important COVID-19–associated risk factors that cause rapid disease progression and badly interfere with COVID-19 disease prognosis [67]. Interestingly, a case study of 191 COVID-19 patients from China had shown that 48% of the SARS-CoV-2 infected patients were associated with different comorbidity while 19% of patients were affected by diabetes [68]. A study showed that among 26 COVID-19 deceased individuals from Wuhan, 42.3% had diabetes [33, 69]. Moreover, reports suggested that diabetes is a high-risk factor in patients who developed ARDS. Notably, among 41.8% of ARDS cases 19% and 5.1% non-ARDS patients respectively had developed diabetes as second most common comorbidity [33]. Furthermore, the largest cohort study of 72,314 COVID-19 patients from China, showed that patients with diabetes had higher lethality rates (7.3%) in comparison to the overall population (2.3%) [70]. Importantly, diabetic patients were more susceptible to various pathogen associated diseases, such as tuberculosis, pneumonia, or influenza thus accounting for greater mortality [71]. Study have shown that infection of SARS-CoV-2 increased the severity of COVID-19 in patients having diabetes mellitus [72, 73]. Besides SARS-CoV-2 infection also predisposes the patients to hyperglycemia which further modulates the immune and inflammatory responses leading to lethal outcomes [72]. However, some limited evidence is now available on type 1 diabetes mellitus and COVID-19.

When the diabetic disorder is left untreated, it may cause various severe lethal complications such as kidney dysfunctioning and failure, blindness, or heart related disease [74]. Less insulin production by the pancreas or lack of insulin receptor on respective cells is one of the reasons behind this metabolic disorder [75]. Therefore, tight control of blood glucose levels in patients with diabetes is crucial to decrease diabetes associated mortality [76]. ACE2 and ACE1 exert their function to maintain systemic blood pressure [68]. Studies reported that ACE2 directly affects the pancreas and plays a role in the improvement of glucose levels, by the stimulation of insulin release [52, 77]. In diabetes, ACE2 favored the development of renal and cardiovascular complications thus it could be a potential therapeutic target for the cure of diabetes [72]. Importantly, it is well established that SARS-CoV-2 infection ephemerally damages the pancreas, and due to its excessive binding affinity to ACE2 it may enhance the infectivity; thus, it is a major concern to hyperglycemia and recovery of diabetic patients [68, 78].

## Obesity

WHO defines overweight and obesity as abnormal or excessive fat accumulation that can jeopardize a person's health. They state that a BMI greater than 25 is considered overweight, and greater than 30 is obese [79]. However, the WHO expert consultation has added that Asians generally tend to have a higher percentage of body fat as compared to white people of the same sex, age, and BMI [80]. The cutoff point for observed risk ranges from 22 kg/m$^2$ to 25 kg/m$^2$ in different Asian populations. Moreover, obesity has been characterized as an epidemic, and in 2016, more than 1.9 billion people (39% of the global population) were overweight and over 650 million people (13% of the total population) were obese [81]. In 2018, 40 million children below the age of 5 were overweight or obese. Obesity is massively widespread in the global population, and should not be neglected as it is a serious underlying factor associated with increased morbidity and mortality rates [82]. Mechanistically, obese patients tend to have limited truncal expansion, which increases the risk of reduced airflow and poor breathing [83]. This diminished airflow and oxygen consumption can predispose obese patients to a greater requirement of oxygen support after respiratory infections like COVID-19 [83]. Furthermore, these patients present a serious problem for intubation (as the additional adipose tissue on the larynx increases the difficulty in intubation). Thus, the physical challenges involved in obesity may exacerbate the disease risks and outcomes of COVID-19 infections.

Several independent studies have observed that people with obesity are at a greater risk of severe disease and death due to COVID-19. The World Obesity Federation and the CDC propound that obesity-related conditions increase the risk of severe COVID-19 [84, 85]. An analysis demonstrated that individuals with obesity were more prone to test positive for COVID-19 (>46.0% higher), and even more likely to be hospitalized (113% higher, OR = 2.13; $p < 0.0001$) while 74% exhibited a higher risk for ICU admission, (OR = 1.74) and 48% developed an increased mortality risk (OR = 1.48; $p < 0.001$) [86]. A study by Simonnet et al. involving obese and normal-weight patients reported that obese COVID-19 (BMI 31.1 kg/m$^2$) patients required invasive mechanical ventilation. According to the study, individuals with a BMI of 30–35 kg/m$^2$ and ≥35 kg/m$^2$ (severe obesity) required mechanical ventilation three and six times more often, respectively, than normal-weight individuals [87].

In addition to myriad smaller studies, obesity may be an independent factor, predicting disease outcome and increasing the risk of mortality (and of requiring intensive care) in SARS-CoV-2 infected patients [88–90]. High BMI has particularly been found to be an important indicator of disease severity in patients, including individuals younger than 60 years of age [87, 91]. However, BMI is an indirect indicator of excess body fat and does not describe the distribution of body fat. Body composition of excess fat changes in older adults with lower muscle mass—subcutaneous fat shifts to visceral adipose tissue (VAT) and total fat is increased in them [92, 93]. Thus, the degree of VAT accumulation is a better marker of obesity status, and a meta-analysis demonstrates that its levels were significantly higher in severe COVID-19 patients [94]. Also, patients with central obesity (a state of excessive VAT accumulation), assessed by waist circumference or waist-to-hip ratio, were more likely to develop severe COVID-19 ($P<0.001$) according to a large population-based cohort [95, 96]. However, there is no substantial evidence regarding whether significant weight loss in people with obesity, especially massive weight loss after bariatric surgery, influences outcomes of COVID-19. Interestingly, obesity was also a striking risk factor for severe influenza morbidity and mortality in H1N1 influenza patients, wherein obese patients were at a higher risk of hospitalization [97, 98]. A correlation between obesity and COVID-19 susceptibility in individuals, however, is yet to be established.

## *Obesity-Related Complications and COVID-19: Immune Dysfunction and Adipose Inflammation*

High levels of inflammation with high C-reactive protein (CRP) and circulating pro-inflammatory cytokines were observed in patients with severe COVID-19 [99]. Obesity represents a state of low-grade inflammation. The dipose tissue-derived inflammatory cytokines; TNFα, IL-1β, IL-6. TNFα may be involved in insulin resistance and diabetes, causing hyperglycemia [81, 100]. Macrophage accumulation in adipose tissue induces proinflammatory cytokines. This further facilitates multiple metabolic consequences of obesity [101].

Leptin acts as an inhibitory signal, or alarm, to the body, to decrease caloric consumption and return to a steady state [81]. Also, leptin resistance greatly impacts the proper development and activity of immune cells thus, increasing the risk of COVID-19 in obese COVID-19 [102, 103].

## *Thrombosis in Obese COVID-19 Patients*

A low-grade chronic inflammatory status of obesity is contributed by the complement system proteins [104]. Adipocytes act as a major source of many components of the complement system proteins [104]. Complement deposition is observed in the endothelium in many obese individuals, which correlates with the formation of microthrombi [105]. This indicates that COVID-19 may lead to a state of alveolar hypoperfusion due to thrombotic pulmonary angiopathy. Multiple studies have further demonstrated that obesity is associated with a hypercoagulable state and obese individuals have higher levels of prothrombin factors and reduced levels of anti-thrombin molecules [106, 107]. Since severely ill COVID-19 patients are often associated with coagulopathy/thrombosis, obesity could potentially aggravate it.

Additionally, obesity involves increased activation of local systemic and adipose tissue RAAS [108, 109]. The expression of several RAAS components is elevated in adipose tissue of obese people, and angiotensin 2 has adverse effects on multiple organs [108]. Thus, it is not far-fetched to postulate that ACE2 in adipose tissue may play a critical role in increasing susceptibility to and severity of COVID-19 in people with obesity and noncommunicable diseases (NCDs).

## *COVID-19 and the Obesity Paradox*

Obese patients are more vulnerable to developing pneumonia; however, ironically, obese patients with pneumonia have lower mortality as compared to nonobese individuals. This phenomenon is called the "Obesity survival paradox" and has been discussed in several independent studies [110–112]. Obesity survival paradox has been challenged by COVID-19 and is still a matter of debate. A meta-analysis of ten cohort studies on mortality reported the existence of the obesity paradox for patients with pneumonia [113, 114]. Mechanistically, it has been suggested that obesity induces preconditioning to inflammatory cues, inducing a higher resistance to the high influx of inflammatory cytokines under ARDS or heart failure conditions in obese patients [115]. However, a majority of the studies have reported that obese subjects are at an increased risk of severe disease and increased mortality due to COVID-19, as discussed earlier [103, 116, 117]. This high mortality among obese patients with SARS-CoV-2 infection prompts the notion that SARS-CoV-2 has disproved the obesity paradox in ARDS [118].

## Neurological Modalities

Several neurological manifestations in COVID-19 patients hint toward the involvement of the nervous system; these include headache, dizziness, altered consciousness, rhabdomyolysis, neuralgia, and myalgia [119]. Severe conditions like meningitis, encephalopathy, meningoencephalitis, Guillain–Barre syndrome (GBS), acute hemorrhagic necrotizing encephalitis, and cerebral venous thrombosis are also associated with SARS-CoV-2 infection [119–121]. Although most RT-PCR studies report the presence of SARS-CoV-2 in the nasopharyngeal swab samples and absence of the virions in the cerebrospinal fluid (CSF) of COVID-19 patients, some studies stand as exceptions. Antibody response against SARS-CoV-2 was detected in the CSF of the infected patients suggesting an immune response to viral infection [122]. Additionally, there exists an association between appearance of various neurological complications and COVID-19 severity. According to a correspondence by Helms et al., 84% of COVID-19 patients with neurological manifestations like agitation (69%), confusion (65%), corticospinal tract signs (67%), and dysexecutive syndrome (33%) required intensive care [123]. Yet another study from Britain highlighted the appearance of neurological alterations like septic or parainfectious encephalopathy, autoimmune encephalitis including acute disseminated encephalomyelitis (ADEM), and GBS in severe cases of COVID-19 [124, 125]. Nevertheless, microgliosis and astrogliosis have been identified in the brains of COVID-19 patients [126]. However, neither microgliosis nor chronic inflammation is related to COVID-19 severity. Also, microglial activation, perivascular lymphocytosis, and leptomeningeal lymphocytic infiltration are reported in the brain of COVID-19 patients and the control brain specimens (septic patients) [127]. Some

COVID-19 studies present findings similar to viral meningoencephalitis, like the clustering of the lymphocytes near the activated microglia. Phagocytosis of the neurons related to histiocytic and lymphocytic parenchymal infiltration is also reported in some studies [126, 128]. A study by von Weyhern et al. revealed that the COVID-19 patients manifested perivascular and parenchymal lymphocytosis with neuronal loss and axonal degeneration in the brainstem, concluding SARS-CoV-2 induced viral encephalitis. Also, it is reported that the majority of cases of meningitis appeared in children between 5 and 10 years old. Also, over 30 cases of GBS have been reported in COVID-19 to date.

In a study, among the 113 patients considered in the survey, CSF protein was elevated in 100% of the fatal cases [129]. Moreover, CSF protein was high in 68.6% of severe COVID-19 patients. Nonetheless, stroke appeared in 1.1% of 3218 COVID-19 patients [130]. It was investigated through neuroimaging analysis that 68.5% of strokes were ischemic and 24% were hemorrhagic. Interestingly SARS-CoV-2 virions have been identified in the nasal neuroepithelium and olfactory bulb; however, the exact mechanism of olfactory dysfunction in COVID-19 remains elusive.

Investigations report the expression of ACE2 on brain endothelium, vascular pericytes and smooth muscle cells, neurons, and glial cells [131, 132]. Other receptors like basigin (BSG; CD147) [133], neuropilin-1 (NRP1), transmembrane serine protease 2 and 4 (TMPRSS2/4) [134, 135], and cathepsin L (CTSL) [136] are also utilized by the virus to gain entry into the cells of the nervous system. Predominantly ACE2 is expressed on the oligodendrocytes, while TMPRSS2/4, CTSL, and NRP1 are majorly expressed on the neurons, microglia, and endothelial cells, respectively. Thus, SARS-CoV-2 can plausibly infect various CNS and peripheral nervous system (PNS) cells. It is predicted that the virus may enter the CNS through three major routes: (1) the olfactory sensory neurons, (2) hidden in the infiltered peripheral immune cells, and (3) across the blood–brain barrier (BBB). Anosmia and ageusia strengthen the theory that the virus may reach the brain regions upon initial infection of the neuroepithelial cells in the mucosa of the nasal cavity. The sustentacular cells and the stem cells of the nasal olfactory epithelium express ACE2. SARS-CoV-2 is detected in the olfactory epithelial through immunohistochemistry of the infected tissue samples and electron microscopic analysis of the nasal mucosa at autopsy [137]. Also, like many viruses (human immunodeficiency virus (HIV), herpes simplex virus, etc.), SARS-CoV-2 may enter into the CNS through trojan horse mechanisms, that is, hidden in the peripheral blood mononuclear cells. Leucocytes, lymphocytes, and monocytes are known to express ACE2 receptors [138, 139]. However, an explicit mention of infected lymphocytes in the inflicted area is a subject of further investigation. The virus may also traverse across the BBB upon infection of the cells of the blood vessel. Staining techniques to target the virus and its inclusion bodies have successfully identified SARS-CoV-2 around the edges of subcortical white matter microinfarcts [140]. However, more studies to conclude the direct role of SARS-CoV-2 in inducing nervous system damage are yet to be conducted.

There are several proposed mechanisms that explain the fatalistic characteristics of the virus on the CNS. One such hypothesis elucidates the effect of pro-inflammatory chemical modulators like IL-6 and IL-1β, released as a response to SARS-CoV-2 infection, in demyelination and axonal damage [137]. The exaggerated immune response in COVID-19 also marks the release of antibodies that may target the gangliosides, leading to peripheral neuropathy. Additionally, the hypercoagulable state induced by the virus in the host may result in central venous thrombosis (CVT) [141]. Thus, there exists a need to investigate further the role of hypercoagulable states on the CNS. Another pathological change, namely, acute hemorrhagic necrotizing encephalopathy characterized by multifocal symmetric brain lesions in COVID-19 patients, may be caused by the virus upon disrupting the BBB through intracranial cytokine storms. IL-6 can be associated with increased vascular permeability, which along with viral endotheliopathy, may result in COVID-19–associated coagulopathy [142, 143]. Hypercoagulability in COVID-19 may further result in microthrombi, infarcts, and hemorrhages. Moreover, IL-1β majorly responsible for forming "neutrophilic plugs," a dense mesh containing DNA-rich material, neutrophils, and platelets, is observed in infected organs like the brain, lungs, heart, kidneys, and liver of COVID-19 patients [144]. The principal outcomes of COVID-19, pneumonia, and ARDS may induce hypoxia, further contributing to cerebral infarcts. Involvement of the nervous system in COVID-19 further complicates the course of disease diagnosis and treatment.

## Cancer

Cancer is a deadly disease and its co-occurrence with COVID-19 can worsen the outcomes. Cancer patients are vulnerable to SARS-CoV-2 infection and its associated severity. People suffering from cancers could be immunocompromised due to antineoplastic therapy, supportive medications such as steroids, and the immunosuppressive properties of cancer itself. Further, the population is often older (i.e., aged $\geq$60 years) with one or more major comorbidities. Multiple studies have suggested increased mortality of the cancer-COVID-19 patients compared to only COVID-19 patients and the general population. In addition, multiorgan failure is reported in cancer patients compared to the patients without cancer [145]. One of the early studies suggested that the virus clearance in cancer patients is longer than noncancer patients [146]. Among the cancer types the patients with hematological malignancies are reported to have higher mortality among all the cancer types. Further, the location and stage of cancer play a crucial role in the severity of COVID [147]. Patients with lung cancer are susceptible to severe COVID-19 due to involvement of the organ in COVID-19 as well [147]. Further people with cancer have an adverse start in the fighting of COVID-19 due to preexisting T cell defects [148]. Metastasis or stage IV carcinoma patients are more susceptible to severe forms of COVID-19 than those with localized cancer [148, 149].

Due to the already altered physiology, the drugs used in COVID-19 treatment may act differently in cancer patients. One of the preliminary studies by Luo et al. has demonstrated the use of hydroxychloroquine in COVID-19 patients with lung cancer did not affect the final outcome in the patients [150]. Another study suggested that hydroxychloroquine or azithromycin or its combination is not effective in reducing the COVID-19 related illness in cancer patients [151]. Further a study by Zhang et al. showed that patients who had received anticancer therapy had poor response to COVID-19 treatment and are at increased risk of developing severe events [152]. Drugs like dexamethasone are recommended in cancer patients to reduce inflammation and lower the immune response of the body. These immune checkpoint inhibitors are also used in COVID-19 treatment and are associated with better clinical outcomes in the infected patients [149].

As cancer is also closely associated with inflammation some clinically approved anti-inflammatory anticancer drugs are used in cancer treatment [149]. These drugs can be used in the treatment of severe COVID-19 patients as well. Ruxolitinib which inhibits the activation of a broad range of pro-inflammatory cytokines and growth factors by inhibiting the c-Jun N-terminal kinases (JNK) pathway had shown to significantly reduce inflammation and related parameters in the COVID-19 patients [153]. Another anti-neoplastic drug acalabrutinib, known to inhibit Bruton tyrosine kinase (BTK) signaling, proved to be effective in treating severe COVID-19 cases [149]. Further antiproliferative drugs like IFN-α-2b, showed a positive effect on the recovery of COVID-19 patients possibly due to its antiviral properties [149].

## Immunocompromised Status

Immunocompromised patients with SARS-CoV-2 infection could develop severe conditions due to the altered immunity within the body. These patients, compared to the immunocompetent ones, are prone to catch secondary bacterial or fungal infections as well and hence are at risk during the pandemic. But considering the involvement of increased inflammation in COVID-19 progression and severity, the immunocompromised status of an individual may actually aid in controlling the disease severity [1]. The individuals suffering from any type of cancer, HIV infection, solid organ transplant (SOT) procedures, patients taking immunity suppressing drugs like steroids or anti-rheumatic drugs, and so on are considered as an immunocompromised population. Out of these correlations, cancer and COVID-19 have already been described earlier, while others are discussed below. However, looking at the development of immunosuppressed conditions due to COVID-19, the reports are rare.

The individuals undergoing SOT procedure are given immunosuppressive therapy to decrease the possibilities of occurrence of graft rejection to transplanted organs. Various reports mentioned the requirement of mechanical ventilation by high proportions of COVID-19 patients who underwent kidney SOT. A New York City–based study [154] denoted 39% while another study conducted in Iran [155] denoted 75% of the kidney SOT patients with COVID-19 required mechanical ventilation. On comparing various types of SOT patients it was observed that mortality rates ranged from 5% to 67%. Among these, a study including the highest number of patients (90) from New York considering liver, kidney, lung, heart SOT patients recorded 18% mortality [156]. During the pandemic, there was heterogeneity in therapies prescribed to SOT patients in different countries. Overall, the decrease in immunosuppressive treatments was followed in most cases. The break in antimetabolite therapy was also prescribed in many studies. The treatments followed to control COVID-19 progression in patients also differed as per region. Majorly, hydroxychloroquine was used as antiviral and tocilizumab was utilized to control inflammation. Additionally, boosted protease inhibitors as anti-SARS-CoV-2 along with intravenous immunoglobulins were widely used. Few other interesting studies included transplant patients with HIV and SARS-CoV-2 positive status. In HIV- and SARS-CoV-2–positive kidney SOT patients, mild COVID-19 without hospitalization was reported [157].

Many studies of SARS-CoV-2 infection in HIV-positive individuals have been reported worldwide [158–164]. Anti-HIV drugs were initially widely considered against COVID-19. Hence, it was considered that the HIV patients may get protection from severe COVID-19. However, reports have shown different outcomes. Various targeted disease modifying antirheumatic drugs like JAK inhibitors or biologics (anti-TNF inhibitors, vedolizumab, or ustekinumab) are a continuous requirement of patients with rheumatological diseases. Conditions of COVID-19 patients taking these medicines have also been investigated. An investigation that focused on patients with inflammatory bowel disease noticed not antirheumatic medicines (biologics) but active disease status, age factor, and related comorbidities were responsible for poor outcomes [165]. An interesting analysis carried out by the international registry included 525 inflammatory bowel disease patients suffering from COVID-19. The patients were from 33 different countries and 63% of them were taking biologics while 2% took JAK inhibitors. In these patients, only 3% mortality was observed and it also depicted that utilization of TNF antagonists had no correlation with COVID-19 severity [166]. Together, these studies revealed only 25 cases of COVID-19 with ~50% hospitalization requirement and no occurrence of mortality. Twelve of these patients required hospitalization and no deaths were reported; 22 of the cases occurred in patients taking biologics of JAK inhibitors. Overall existing reports denoted that there is no correlation between intake of biologics or antirheumatic drugs and severe COVID-19.

## Oral and Maxillofacial Manifestations

The oral cavity, nasal cavity, and nasopharynx, comprising the upper respiratory tract, are the sites of high viral load in COVID-19 patients [167]. SARS-CoV-2 is secreted in the saliva and mucosal discharge of the respiratory tract in COVID-19 patients [168]. The viral contagion occurs through the salivary and nasal discharge by direct contact or in the form of aerosol and minute droplets. Its presence in the saliva, nasal and nasopharyngeal discharge is important for the diagnosis of COVID-19. The current diagnostic method includes the collection of samples from these sites for the identification of viral antigen by rapid antigen test or by real-time PCR [169]. Among the various methods and sites of sample collection, it has been found that the viral load is high in nasopharyngeal secretions. However, some studies suggest that saliva serves better for the detection of SARS-CoV-2.

Dysfunction in taste (ageusia or dysgeusia) and olfactory alterations (anosmia or hyposmia) were the most common findings reported in patients infected with early strains of SARS-CoV-2 with taste alterations considered to be the early and most relevant manifestation of COVID-19 [170]. However, the B.1.1.7 variant is less likely to cause loss of sense of smell or taste [171]. Reports suggest that 33.9% of the COVID-19 patients presented either olfactory or taste alterations while 18.6% presented both. Another study found the prevalence of taste alteration in COVID-19 patients was 45%, with 38% presented dysgeusia, 35% presented hypogeusia, while 24% presented ageusia [172]. It has been found that these alterations were due to SARS-CoV-2 infection to nonneuronal cells [132]. The impairment in the RAAS may play some role in the pathophysiology of anosmia and ageusia during the initial presentation of SARS-CoV-2 infection [173]. However, the exact pathophysiology of altered gustatory and olfactory sensations is less understood. The difference in the occurrence of anosmia may be due to genetic differences causing variations in the binding affinity of the ACE2 receptor for the virus that may lead to varied chemosensory defects.

## *Oral Mucosal Lesions Associated with COVID-19*

Several oral lesions were found to be associated with COVID-19. The commonly reported conditions are xerostomia, vesiculobullous lesions, and aphthous-like lesions [174]. The oral manifestations of COVID-19 include erosions, ulcers, vesicles, gingival swelling, bleeding gums, and so on [175]. White and erythematous plaques, desquamative gingivitis, stomatopyrosis, pseudomembranous candidiasis at commissure, and angular cheilitis have also been reported to be associated with COVID-19. The occurrence of these oral lesions in COVID-19 may be attributed to the comorbidities like stress, insufficient oral hygiene, nutritional deficiency, immunosuppression, hyperinflammatory response, and other systemic diseases like diabetes mellitus and HIV infection.

These lesions were found to be symptomatic in about 68% of the cases with the most common sites of involvement as the tongue in 38% of the cases. The labial mucosa was involved in 26%, and palate in 22% of the cases. The severity of these lesions is found to be associated with older age and COVID-19 severity [175]. No gender predilection has been reported in lesions due to COVID-19.

## *Effect of Poor Oral Hygiene and Periodontal Diseases on COVID-19*

Gingivitis and periodontitis, which are inflammatory diseases of the supporting tissues of the teeth, are caused by poor oral hygiene and an alteration in the microflora of dental plaque [176]. It has been reported that the dental plaque of the COVID-19 patients can harbor SARS-CoV-2 [177]. Moreover, increased severity of COVID-19 has also been found to be associated with periodontitis. Reports suggested increased levels of hematological markers linking both diseases. It is a well-established fact that the pathogenesis of periodontitis is rooted in cytokine response. Moreover, COVID-19 has also been reported to show adverse outcomes due to a cytokine storm [178]. Thus, coinfection of periodontal pathogens and the SARS-CoV-2 along with other established comorbidities and risk factors like diabetes mellitus, obesity, and various hematological disorders, may play a role in the enhanced inflammation. Due to this, the adverse outcomes of COVID-19 are frequently observed in patients with poor oral hygiene. Researchers have also studied the effects of the regulatory circadian genes, like *Bmal1*, viral infections including COVID-19 as well as in periodontitis. It suggests that both the diseases share common pathogenesis via the NFκB pathway.

## *Effect of Nasal Irrigation and Antimicrobial Oral Rinses on COVID-19 Disease Outcome*

It has been suggested that nasal irrigation with hypertonic saline and antimicrobial oral rinses may reduce the viral load locally and prevent its transmission [179]. Its usage by the healthcare workers has been advocated as a preventive measure while treating COVID-19 patients; however, there is a lack of supporting evidence. Moreover, these modalities as therapeutics in COVID-19 have also been cautioned by the WHO due to limited evidence. The efficacy of oral rinses in reducing the viral load may be questionable, but it surely lowers the circulating cytokine levels by reducing periodontal inflammation. Hence, the usage of oral rinses as adjunctive therapy improves the patient outcome in COVID-19 and reduces the repercussions at the systemic level [180].

## COVID-19–Associated Mucormycosis

The clinical similarity of COVID-19 with many other flu-like syndromes tends to cause negligence in the diagnosis of other infections in patients. This could have happened frequently due to potential suspicions of COVID-19 in the patients and the burden of handling an excessive number of patients during the pandemic.

Moreover, during handling of the burden, the chances of the development of secondary infections increased in the patients. This was more likely to be observed in critically ill patients, especially those who were admitted to the ICU and required mechanical ventilation or had a longer duration of hospital stays [181].

Many studies have put forth the association of fungal infections in COVID-19 patients. It is not surprising as it has earlier been observed in previous SARS outbreak as well [182]. Studies investigating abundance of fungal infections in SARS patients observed that 14–27% of patients may encounter fungal infections [183, 184]. Moreover, the incidents were observed to be higher in ill patients. Additionally, the fungal infection was predicted to be a major factor associated with mortality in SARS patients, accounting for 25–73% in other causes of mortality [185]. With respect to lung pathologies, factors like severe viral pneumonia, dysfunction in immune responses, and immunosuppressive therapies like corticosteroids are linked to the chances of invasive fungal infections (IFIs) like aspergillosis and mucormycosis [186]. Recently a mass increase in cases of mucormycosis, as a catastrophic infection, in COVID-19 patients has been observed in India. Mucormycosis, also known as zygomycosis or phycomycosis, is an angioinvasive disease caused by fungi of the order Mucorales [187]. This infection quickly spreads in the body and, if not readily diagnosed and treated, may lead to poor prognosis [187]. People with diabetes, patients undergoing immunosuppressive treatments, systemic corticosteroid use, patients with neutropenia and hematologic malignancies, stem cell transplant patients and immunocompromised individuals are prone to the development of mucormycosis [188]. The spores of mucormycetes are widely observed to be present in natural surroundings, like in soil and decaying organic matter and leaves [189]. The fungal spores may get inhaled by an individual through paranasal sinuses. In an immunocompetent individual the macrophages can instantly recognize and phagocytose the spores [190]. The neutrophils can act on hyphae and may initiate a further immune response. With help of immune machinery including lymphocytes and other cells of the immune cascade the infection could be controlled in a healthy individual [190].

Recently, many case studies and case series from different regions of the world have reported COVID-19 association with mucormycosis. As expected with respect to risk factors, COVID-19–associated mucormycosis was prevalent in patients on steroid treatments and also with underlying diabetic condition [191]. Few cases have identified the development of this fungal disease in COVID-19 patients without diabetes as well, so the use of steroids remains as the only risk factor [191]. In diabetic patients mostly rhino-orbital and rhino-orbital-cerebral presentation was observed [192]. *Rhizopus* was found to be commonly involved [186, 193]. In very rare cases the presence of *Aspergillus* was noted (2 out of 41 cases) [193]. In a recent report, a compiled analysis of various cases published till now has been performed [193]. Among these cases, 71% were observed to be from India. In India, per 1000 individuals approximately 0.14 cases of mucormycosis were found [188]. This proportion is 80 times greater than that observed in developed countries [188].

Various hypotheses have been put forth by scientists to explain the occurrence of COVID-19 associated with mucormycosis. Severe forms of COVID-19 have been shown to cause diffuse alveolar damage, inflammatory exudation, endothelial damage, and microvascular thrombosis [194]. This may give invasive fungus an upper hand for easy invasive progression. Lymphocytopenia with reduced levels of cytotoxic and helper T cells is commonly observed in severe cases of COVID-19 [195]. This may alter innate immunity increasing propensity for secondary fungal infections. Use of steroids is approved in severe conditions of COVID-19 and has been found to be effective in several trials [196]. Hence, it is widely used in treating hospitalized patients with severe conditions. Most of the hospitalized patients have comorbidities which may aid in dampening the immune response in various ways and open the gateways for secondary infection [197]. Diabetes mellitus has been identified as one of the major comorbidities associated with hospitalized and severe COVID-19 patients. Hence, most of the patients who are COVID-19 positive or recovered, have diabetes and/or undergoing immunosuppressive treatments (steroids) can be prone to mucormycosis and associated severe outcome. Figure 5.2 illustrates the development and impact of mucormycosis in immunocompetent and COVID-19 patients.

Studies have shown diabetes mellitus as the most common risk factor in India. India tops at second position in the world in case of diabetes with around 77 million patients affected and another 36.5 million with prediabetes condition [188]. Hence, the occurrence of mucormycosis in Indian COVID-19 patients can be correlated to prevalence of the fungal infection in general as well as the proportion diabetic population. In a meta-analysis of around 600 studies with more than 800 cases, diabetes mellitus has been observed as an independent factor involved in rhino-orbital-cerebral mucormycosis [198]. The *Rhizopus* species were found to be more prevalent in the cause and mortality is observed in around 46% of the mucormycosis cases [198]. Being invasive in nature, the involvement of the fungi in causing vascular damage, inflammation and endothelial dysfunction is observed. And it develops the chances of endotheliitis in various organs which may lead to severe outcomes in patients with diabetes mellitus. These patients had to undergo adjunct surgery. The overall mortality was observed to be 49% [198]. Hence, the occurrence of increased mucormycosis in Indian COVID-19 patients can be correlated to the prevalence of the fungal infection in general as well as the proportion diabetic population.

Recently physicians have tried to correlate the involvement of excess zinc supplementation in the generation of mucormycosis to COVID-19 patients. The total zinc content in the human body amounts to 2–4 g (plasma concentration—12–16 μM) [199]. The recommended daily intake of zinc is 11 mg/day for adult males and 8 mg/day for adult females, with a tolerable upper intake of 40 mg/day [200, 201]. Zinc supplementation of 50–150 mg/day can cause disturbance in copper metabolism, reduced iron function, neutropenia, and excess cellular zinc can generate an imbalance in oxidative metabolism [202]. Zinc supplementation can downregulate inflammatory cytokines, inhibit NFκB activation, and at very high concentrations (>100 μM), zinc can cause increased cytokine production in some cell types [203, 204]. Zinc-depleting conditions have been shown to reduce fungal growth, and host cells can employ sequestration of zinc to hinder fungal development [205]. The mechanism of fungal zinc homeostasis in the model *Saccharomyces cerevisiae*

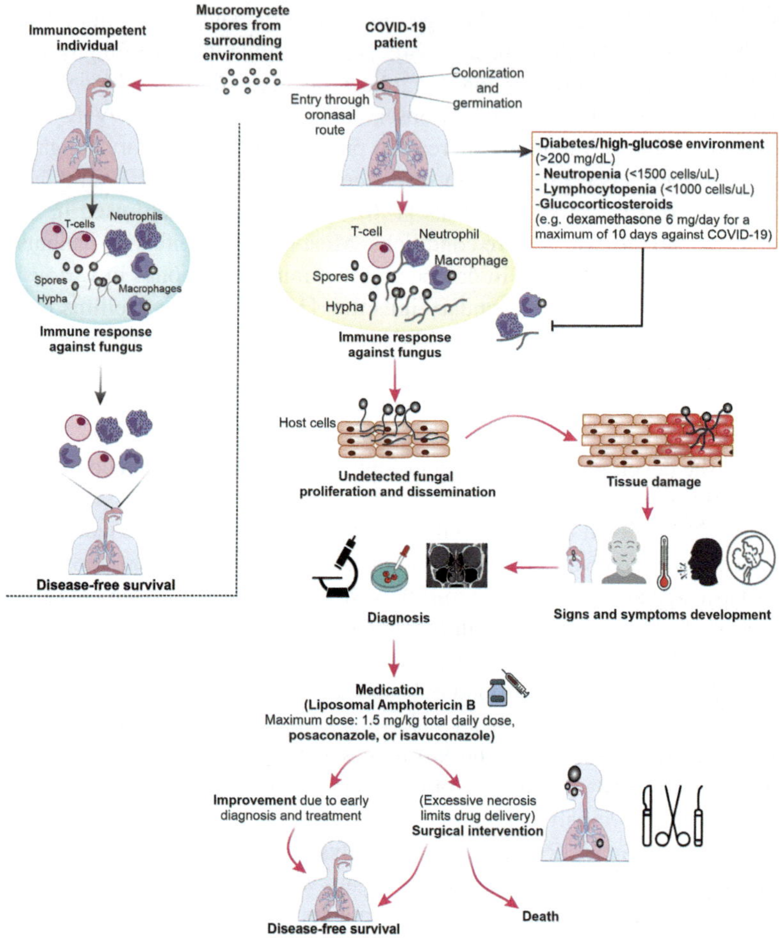


**Fig. 5.2** Schematics of mucormycosis progression in immunocompetent and COVID-19 individuals. Mucormycetes spores can enter the body through oronasal routes and enter into paranasal sinuses. Immune cells like macrophages and neutrophils can instantly recognize the foreign pathogen and phagocytose the spores. Neutrophils act on the fungal hyphae. In the immunocompetent individuals, further infection may not progress due to suppressed immune response and could show disease-free survival. However, in COVID-19 patients the risk factors like altered immune response, lymphocytopenia, neutropenia, underlying conditions like diabetes, or immunosuppressive drugs given in treatment could limit the immune response against the mucormycetes spores. The undetected spores then germinate, proliferate, and disseminate in nearby cells and further lead to tissue damage. Meanwhile, the person develops signs and symptoms like fever, swelling in the infected area, black lesions on the infected area, cough, and shortness of breath. The infection can be diagnosed using microscopic examination and fungal culture, and progression can be assessed using CT scan. After confirmation, antifungal medication by providing liposomal amphotericin B can be initiated. If the infection is diagnosed early, it can be cured using medication. In severe infection cases, excessive tissue necrosis limits drug delivery and hence surgical intervention is required. There could either be improvement in health and disease-free survival is achieved. In cases of severely disseminated infection and progressed disease conditions, the patient may die

includes zinc uptake, mediated by the plasma membrane transporters Zrt1 and Zrt2, under Zap1 regulon [206]. Zap1 is a transcriptional activator that senses zinc depletion and controls zinc homeostasis [207, 208]. These membrane transporters or zinc-binding proteins that mediate zinc uptake or storage, help maintain the zinc quota in organisms. Many fungal pathogens have shown decreased infectivity upon deletion of their respective Zap1 ortholog, hinting toward the requirement of zinc uptake for establishing infection in the host [209]. For instance, *C. albicans* possesses a dedicated zinc scavenging system consisting of the secreted "zincophore" protein, Pra1, and the Zrt1 transporter [210]. Moreover, *Rhizopus delemar*, belonging to the subphylum Mucoromycotina, and of particular interest during mucormycosis, is known to encode three cell surface zinc importers [211]. Thus continued zinc administration might have an associated risk of creating a zinc microenvironment that is more favorable for fungal growth. This is particularly notable in the context of India, where prolonged zinc supplementation could be an underlying contributor to the rising mucormycosis cases.

Monitoring and controlling hyperglycemia, early treatment with antifungals, and surgical operations are crucial for managing mucormycosis successfully [212]. The patients suffering from COVID-19–associated mucormycosis are usually treated with liposomal Amphotericin B treatment as direct use of amphotericin B is found to be nephrotoxic [213]. Moreover, liposomal amphotericin-B can stay longer in circulation [212]. The mild COVID-19 cases without hypoxaemia should not be treated with glucocorticoids, or at least higher doses should be avoided. A delay of even 6 days in initiating treatment doubles the 30-day mortality from 35% to 66%. Therefore, vigilant and prior as well as continuous monitoring of patients is necessary. Early diagnosis, especially in patients associated with risk factors, should be preceded with the help of a multidisciplinary team including ophthalmology, otorhinolaryngology, infectious diseases, neurosurgery, critical care, microbiology, and pathology department [214]. Visual prognosis (vision, pupil, ocular motility, and sinus tenderness) has low chances of confirming the presence of mucormycosis in the patient. Thus, a high index of suspicion for fungal coinfection in patients with COVID-19 presenting with comorbidities is important [214]. The patients showing signs and symptoms of mucormycosis should immediately undergo pathological and imaging studies and the management team should always be prepared for surgical intervention.

## Kidney Injury

SARS-CoV-2 infection is lethal to patients with severe renal dysfunction especially individuals with chronic kidney disease. COVID-19–associated kidney disease deaths in various European countries have been observed [215]. AKI is common among critically ill COVID-19 patients; >40% of cases have revealed anomalous proteinuria at hospital admission and it affects about 20–40% of patients admitted to intensive care from the observation in Europe and the USA [216, 217].

Furthermore, increased D-dimer and lower platelet count correlated with severe outcomes while, some patients with COVID-19 apparently confirmed microangiopathy in other organ systems, such as splenic infarction hematuria and renal infarction. COVID-19 related renal injury increased the serum creatinine causing proteinuria, hematuria in the kidney. The study put forth that hypercoagulation is one of the characteristic complications of COVID-19 patients which may lead to irreversible kidney failure [218, 219]. The interstitium of the kidney showed edema and related inflammatory infiltrates, which predominantly consisted of immune cells such as plasma cells and lymphocytes with scattered eosinophils [220]. Importantly, due to the expression of ACE2 on lymphocytes, SARS-CoV-2 could also bind to this receptor which may lead to the lymphocytes activation and hence activation induced cell death decrease the $CD4^+$ and $CD8^+$ T cell populations [99].

Interstitial and renal parenchyma could be more prone to damage but higher injury has been reported in the glomerular interstitium [220]. Kidney autopsy revealed the damage of brush border and nonisometric vacuolation which may be responsible for proteinuria [216]. The glomerular lesions are minor and showed various structural changes which lead to hypertension and diabetic nephropathy [221, 222]. Kidney endothelial cell injury activates the complement system by activating C3 complex formation confirmed by indirect immunofluorescence staining [223]. Importantly, SARS-CoV-2 infection is commonly associated with high-risk apolipoprotein L1 (APOL1) in African patients [224, 225]. Moreover, the expression of ACE2 is prominent in proximal tubular cells confirmed by ACE2 staining, particularly at the sight of severe injury [226]. Kidney epithelial cells also prominently express ACE2; however, it was comparatively less in podocytes [227]. Presence of SARS-CoV-2 RNA confirmed by quantitative real time PCR (qRT-PCR) [228]. Presence of spherical viral particles in podocytes has been also confirmed by electron microscopy [227]. Indirect fluorescence of tissues revealed the nuclear or cytoplasmic marking in kidney tubules in presence of SARS-CoV-2 nucleoprotein antigens [229].

SARS-CoV-2 infection is associated with enhanced kidney injury related to lipid metabolic disorder, altered immune cell clearance, endothelium-mediated vasculitis, hyperimmunity-related disorder, thrombogenesis, and it also creates the hypoxic cellular milieu [220]. Furthermore, alterations in the kidney play an important role in the regulation of the RAAS. Juxtaglomerular cells in the kidneys convert the precursor prorenin into renin and secrete it directly into circulation. This renin formulates conversion of angiotensin to angiotensin 1. Further ACE converts this to angiotensin 2. The angiotensin 2 later induces the release of aldosterone, which acts on the kidney and increases sodium absorption. This leads to increased blood pressure. In aberrant conditions like in the case of COVID-19, dysregulation of this system subsequently can affect kidney as well as cardiovascular functions. ACE2 is a homolog of ACE and functions both in a peptidase-dependent and a peptidase-independent manner. It negatively regulates the RAAS to regulate the various functions of ACE [220]. Importantly, the binding of SARS-CoV-2 to its host receptor causes cleavage of the external domain of ACE2, which further downregulates the expression of ACE2 and thus increases the Angiotensin 2 levels. Hence, ACE2 receptor could also be associated with renal injury in SARS-CoV-2 infected patients. Increased Angiotensin 2 levels further stimulate the cytokine storm which lead to severe complications and are lethal to the patients [230].

In COVID-19 patients, SARS-CoV-2 infectivity is one of the major etiologies of kidney dysfunction. Infection of SARS-CoV-2 directly can cause renal injury or it may exert its role through the systemic mechanism in which it promotes the deposition of immune cells in renal glomerulus and hypercoagulation.

## Molecular Pathways Involved in the Development of COVID-19 Pathology

Virus intelligently takes advantage of host machinery for its survival and dissemination. After viral entry into the body, various molecular pathways inside the infected cells get triggered as a natural defense response. Throughout the virus life cycle inside the cell, various cellular components can interact with numerous viral factors. These interactions can drive the host defense response and expression of important immune response genes. Subsequently, immune response molecules get expressed and dispersed in the vicinity of infected cells which further develop cross talk with nearby cells to fight against the virus. NFκB, IRF, and Activator protein-1 (AP-1) associated pathways are important genes that get triggered by respective cellular sensors (Fig. 5.3). These pathways induce the production of various cytokines and chemokines. Subsequently, components associated with these receptors, like JAK, can initiate the downstream cascade to induce further immune response associated genes (Fig. 5.3). Interestingly, the virus smartly utilizes its machinery to modulate these pathways either for better survival or transmission. We have discussed details of the important cellular pathways which can generate an immune response at the molecular level and further initiate inflammation.

### *NFκB Signaling*

NFκB is a family of transcription factors closely associated with inflammatory signaling. During the infection scenario, it enhances the expression of multiple molecules. The pathway is triggered by the binding of ligands or antigens to receptors like cytokine receptors and toll-like receptors (TLRs). Further, the cascade of interactions phosphorylates important kinases—IκB kinases (IKK), which include IKKα and IKKβ, which take part in the phosphorylation of IκB protein. IκB is an unstimulated state bound to p50 and p65 NFκB subunits and plays the role of an inhibitor. IKK induced phosphorylation of IκB leads to its ubiquitin mediated proteasomal degradation, thus allowing the nuclear translocation of p50/p65 dimers. In the nucleus, the dimer binds to specific enhancer regions that mediate the expression of κB-responsive genes [231].

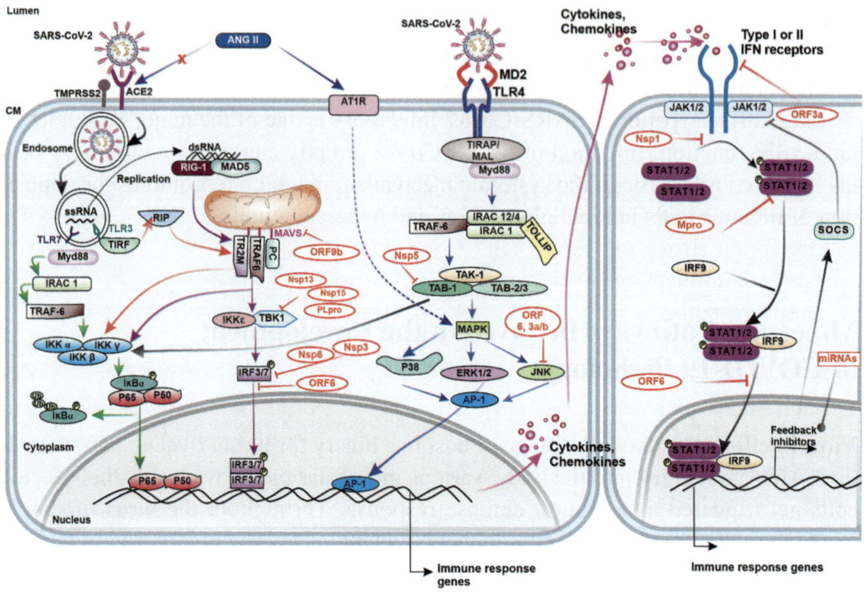


**Fig. 5.3** Molecular pathways involved in SARS-CoV-2 infection and subsequent inflammation. SARS-CoV-2 enters into the cell using the ACE2 receptor followed by direct entry through cleavage from TMPRSS2 or by endosomal pathway. When the viral RNA is released into the cell, TLR7 and TLR3 can recognize the ssRNA. TLR7 activates downstream molecules like Myd88, IRAC-1, TRAF-6, and IKK, and initiates the NFκB pathway. By detecting ssRNA, TLR3 induces TIRF, RIP and activates MAVS components. This further drives IKK induction and NFκB activation. The replicated viral dsRNA can be recognized by RIG-1 and MAD5 molecules which also activate the MAVS complex. The complex can then initiate the IRF pathway by inducing IKKε and TBK1. IRF3/7 can then get induced, translocated to the nucleus, and induce transcription of various genes. SARS-CoV-2 protein ORF9b has been shown to indirectly interact with the host MAVS protein via mitochondrial outer membrane component Tom70 and further can modulate the signaling. Other SARS-CoV-2 proteins Nsp13, Nsp15 and $PL_{pro}$ can inhibit TBK1 activation, while Nsp3, Nsp6, and ORF6 can hinder IRF nuclear translocation. RIG-1/MDA-5 can also induce the NFκB pathway through the MAVS complex. TLR4 can also recognize the viral component that activates downstream molecules to induce the MAPK pathway. SARS-CoV-2 protein Nsp5 may alter MAPK pathway by interacting with TAB1. MAPK can further initiate activation of AP-1 through pathways including either p38, ERK, or JNK. Due to ACE2 masking by SARS-CoV-2, Ang II can accumulate and hence interact with the AT1R receptor. This can activate MAPK and downstream pathways. Ultimately, NFκB, IRF, and AP-1 molecules induce the expression of molecules like cytokines and chemokines involved in the immune response. The cytokines especially IFN can cross-talk with nearby cells and make them aware of the infection. IFN or respective cytokines can bind IFN receptors and initiate the JAK-STAT pathway. Various SARS-CoV-2 components like ORF3a, Nsp6, ORF6, and $M_{pro}$ can interact with factors of the JAK-STAT pathway to cause the inhibition of this pathway. Also, various SARS-CoV-2 components induce feedback control molecules of the JAK-STAT pathway

During SARS-CoV-2 infection pattern recognition molecules recognize the virus. Further TLRs like TLR 3 and TLR 7/8 activate the downstream pathway with the help of adaptor proteins TIR-domain-containing adapter-inducing IFN-β (TRIF) and myeloid differentiation primary response 88 (MyD88). The TRIF and MyD88 activate TNF-receptor associated factor 6 (TRAF6) transforming growth factor-β-activated kinase-1 (TAK1), resulting in activation of the IKK complex enabling NFκB nuclear translocation [232]. Furthermore, TLR4 and endoplasmic reticulum stress-induced NFκB activation was also reported in SARS-CoV-2 infected cells [232].

The pathogenesis of COVID-19 is similar to some previously reported viruses like MERS, and varicella. It has been observed that the SARS-CoV-2 infection may lead to brain stroke due to a heightened immune response. The NFκB signaling plays a multidimensional role in the development and maintenance of the nervous system. The pathway gets activated by downstream signaling of a lipopolysaccharide receptor complex. Moreover, the NFκB pathway regulates the inflammatory reaction around the neuronal microenvironment by regulating different fractions of the glial cells and astrocytes. The upregulated proinflammatory genes may also result in the generation of excessive ROS which can cause cerebellar damage and neuropathogenic dysregulation associated with neurotransmitters [233].

Dual-specificity phosphatases (DUSP) are negative regulators for both p38-MAPK and NFκB. During SARS-CoV-2 infection the level of DUSP5 and DUSP1 is decreased, leading to upregulation of pro-inflammatory genes such as TNF-α, IL-1β, IL-1A, IL-6, IL-8, and IL-23 [234]. Importantly treatment with medications like chloroquine, theophylline, and anti-inflammatory and immune-modulatory medications such as colchicine, diclofenac, cyclosporine, and azathioprine has shown to increase the level of these DUSPs [234]. A recent study suggested that SARS-CoV-2 nsp13 can regulate the NFκB mediated inflammatory response by interacting with several transducin-like enhancer (TLE) family proteins. Further, SARS-CoV-2 encoded ORF9c can modulate the IκB kinase activity and the NFκB signaling by interacting with NDFIP2, NLRX1, F2RL1 [235]. The cellular interactome study of SARS-CoV2-PLpro revealed that it decreases the phosphorylation of TANK Binding Kinase 1 (TBK1) and strongly attenuates degradation of IκB-α. This led to reduced nuclear translocation of NFκB. TBK1 is known to activate the NFκB pathway, causing upregulation of inflammatory signaling after phosphorylation [236]. Another cellular component, mitochondrial antiviral signaling protein (MAVS) is also known to activate the NFκB pathway. The SARS-CoV-2 ORF9b has been shown to indirectly interact with the host MAVS protein via mitochondrial outer membrane component Tom70 [232]. This may further impel downstream pathway activation.

## *The p38 MAPK Signaling*

MAPK is a protein kinase that is specific to serine and threonine amino acids and has a role in cell differentiation, proliferation, and death in response to various stimuli [237]. The p38 MAPK signaling pathway is responsible for cell death via p53, transforming growth factor (TGF)-β1, and syntenin in SARS-CoV infection [238]. It is also found to be involved in various aspects of the progression of COPD like inflammation of the respiratory tract, overproduction of mucus, fibrosis, and infiltration of immune cells. Similarly, SARS-CoV-2 is also likely to use p38 MAPK signaling to induce apoptosis and lung damage [235]. Therefore, it may serve as a putative drug target even in COVID-19.

The p38 can regulate the transcription of genes encoding various cytokines and cell surface receptors [231]. During the SARS-CoV-2 infection, the virus binds to ACE2. ACE2 is required for conversion of Angiotensin 2 to Angiotensin 1–7 [25]. Angiotensin 2 mediates its effects through p38 MAPK activation. Angiotensin 1–7 decreases p38 MAPK activation to reduce inflammation. Aberrant MAPK activation promotes inflammatory mediators production and thus helps in the development of cytokine storm, which is a characteristic of severe respiratory viral diseases [239]. During the SARS-CoV-2 infection, the p38 MAPK pathway is upregulated disproportionately due to the loss of ACE2 activity after the viral entry. Moreover, p38 activation also upregulated the ADAM17 factor, which is known to cleave the ACE2 ectodomain [240]. It is known that p38 can phosphorylate other protein kinases, such as MAP kinase activated protein kinase 2 (MK2), activating transcription factors (ATF1/2/6), and p53 [231].

Growth factor signaling inhibition through the MAPK signaling pathway has been shown to modulate SARS-CoV-2 replication [241]. SARS-CoV-2 infection also leads to the induction of phosphatidylinositol 3-kinase (PI3K) along with MAPK signaling events. Together, these signaling events help in higher intracellular viral replication; however, inhibition of any one of the pathways will lead to decreased replication inside the host cells [242]. The inhibition of the PI3K pathway can be carried out by pictilisib, or omapalisib. While inhibition of the MAPK pathway can be carried out by sorafenib, RP5126766, or lonafarnib [242].

### *JNK Pathway*

C-Jun NH2-terminal kinase (JNK) cascade is another important pathway that could activate the various processes at cellular levels such as hyperactivation of immune cells, prolonged cell survival, cell proliferation, and reduce cell death [243]. JNK signaling works downstream of MAPK which is activated via phosphorylation through MAP kinase (MKK)-7 and MKK4 [244]. JNK signaling pathways lastly stimulates transcription factor AP-1 [245]. This further binds to respective genomic elements involved in the expression of antiviral and Th1 cytokines (pro-inflammatory cytokines) [246]. Various studies have shown that JNKs are one of the important kinases which activate the innate immunity against viral infection [235, 247]. While doing so JNKs signaling activates several important cytokines like interleukins (IL-1β, IL-2, IL-4) and IFN-γ [248]. Studies revealed that influenza A virus and respiratory syncytial virus enhance the JNK/AP-1 signaling cascade [235]. Apart from this study, it has been suggested that the proinflammatory responses of S1 subunit S protein from SARS-CoV-2 in human and murine macrophages [249]. Meanwhile, vulnerability to the S1 subunit of S protein may further activate JNK and NFκB signaling cascade [250]. Adversely, pro-inflammatory cytokine induction by S1 was suppressed by selective inhibitors of NFκB and JNK pathways [249]. Moreover, Ken et al. showed that exotic knockdown of TLR4 via siRNA attenuated the pro-inflammatory cytokine production and inhibited the S1 medicated TLR4 signaling cascade [249]. On the contrary, TLR2 neutralizing antibodies could not abrogate the S1-induced pro-inflammatory cytokine induction in either RAW264.7 or THP-1 cell-derived macrophages [249]. Hence, TLR4 receptor mediated signaling cascade is very crucial for the activation of Th1 responses in humans and mice macrophages [251]. Therefore, TLR4 signaling in macrophages may be a potential target for regulating excessive inflammation in COVID-19 patients [249, 252].

Coronavirus induced apoptosis in H1299 cells through the activation of JNK signaling pathway. Viral pathogenesis does not directly activate the JNK signaling. It does it via mediator signaling molecules like MKK7. Importantly, suppression of the JNK cascade during viral infection in Huh-7 cells through SP600125 inhibitors reduced the inhibitory effect of JNK signaling on antiapoptotic protein Bcl2. In case of SARS-CoV infection of Vero cells exotic expression of Bcl-2 was observed. However, subsequent viral induced apoptosis was not observed in the cells. Another study observed that the HCoV-229E also activated the JNK signaling pathway and promoted cell survival through increased production of anti-apoptotic Bcl-2 family proteins [235, 253]. Moreover activated JNK signaling ultimately regulated innate immunity by increasing the production and secretion of proinflammatory cytokines such as IFN-β and IL-8 [235]. Furthermore, studies revealed that there is a phosphorylation of proteins in the upstream cascade of JNK signaling during the viral infection hence, JNK signaling played a very crucial role in SARS-CoV-2 infection. Another study in Vero E6 cells revealed that the N protein of SARS-CoV could also phosphorylate the PI3K/AKT and JNK signaling cascade which led to the establishment of persistent SARS-CoV infection [254, 255]. Previously it has been shown that SARS-CoV associated N protein in the absence of growth factors was involved in the activation JNK and p38 MAPK signaling cascade and simultaneously inhibited the programmed cell death in COS-1 monkey kidney cells [256]. Notably, SARS-CoV-2 showed a higher degree of sequence similarity of various antigenic proteins such as N, S, E, and RNA-dependent RNA polymerase with SARS-CoV; hence, SARS-CoV-2 may activate the AP1 in a similar way to SARS-CoV, which further can activate the Th1 responses [248]. In another study by Mizutani et al, Vero E6 and HEK293 cells showed that the SARS-CoV encoded ORF6, 3a and 7a induced apoptosis through the JNK-dependent as well as caspase-3-mediated ER stress pathways [257]. Moreover, another protein, 3b of SARS-CoV-2, upregulated the AP-1 through the stimulation of ERK and JNK signaling cascade in Huh7 cells [258].

## *IRF Involved Signaling*

Severe COVID-19 characterized by hypercytokinemia and ARDS arises due to the virus's ability to antagonize the host immune response. Nonetheless, coagulopathy observed in severe COVID-19 cases is related to impaired production of Type I IFN

(IFN-I) [259]. IFN-1 is crucial for imparting antiviral response triggers the expression of numerous IFN-stimulated genes (ISGs) through various transcription factors [259]. The transcription of downstream genes modulates the inflammatory responses through the regulation of proinflammatory cytokines which in turn modulate viral replication and recruitment of immune cells [259]. In a study, a delayed antiviral response, marked by reduced expressions of IFN-β and ISG56, during the initial hours of infection was observed which was predicted to provide a window to virus replication [260]. Interestingly, significant amounts of viral transcripts were observed prior to the induction of IFN in SARS-CoV-2-infected cells [260]. SARS-CoV-2 encoded ORF6 was predicted to alter IFN production and associated downstream signaling [261].

ORF6 of SARS-CoV-2, which is ~66% similar to SARS-CoV-1 ORF6, has a two amino acid truncation at the C terminus of the protein [260]. Both the proteins perform similar functions, that is, exhibit the ability to inhibit IRF3 activation and STAT-1 nuclear translocation [261, 262]. It has been demonstrated that the amino acids at the C terminus tail of ORF6, DEEQPMEID, were accountable for ORF6's function in blocking IRF3 and STAT1 activation [260]. Nonetheless, protein–protein interaction study showed that ORF6 interacted with nucleoporin (NUP)-98 and RAE1, to form a nuclear pore complex [263]. Thus, it is believed that ORF6 could block STAT1 nuclear translocation by interacting with these proteins.

Following recognition in the cytoplasm by retinoic acid-inducible gene-I (RIG-I) and melanoma differentiation-associated protein 5 (MDA5), the caspase activation recruitment domains (CARD) of these two proteins get associated with the mitochondrial antiviral signaling protein (MAVS) [264, 265]. MAVS result in the recruitment of a complex consisting of the TRAF3/TANK/TBK1/IKKϵ (TNF receptor associated factor 3/ TRAF family member-associated NFκB activator-binding kinase 1/ inhibitor of nuclear factor κB (IκB) kinase-ε). Subsequently the complex generates phosphorylated IRF-3 and IRF-7 [266, 267]. The dimerized IRF-3 and IRF-7 move into the nucleus and initiate the transcription of IFN-I and ISGs. Then henceforth produced IFN-1 can bind to the IFN receptors α and β, comprising the IFNAR1 and IFNAR2 subunits, thereby resulting in activation of JAK-STAT pathway [267]. The phosphorylated STAT components of JAK-STAT pathway and IRF9 form the IFN-stimulated growth factor 3 (ISGF3) complex [268]. Also, SARS-CoV-2 nsp1 is known to bind to the subunits of 40S ribosome causing mRNA translation inhibition of the host including IFN-I [269]. Additionally, it is proven that SARS-CoV-2 ORF9b interacted with MAVS by interacting with Tom70, thus influencing the IFN-1 pathway [267]. Importantly, SARS-CoV-2 nsp13 and nsp15 associated with TBK1 and the TBK1 activator protein 41 (RNF41)/Nrdp1, respectively [270]. Studies have validated the interaction between SARS-CoV-2 nsp15 and TBK1 [263].

Moreover, SARS-CoV-1 structural proteins like M and N may sequester the IFN response [267]. The SARS-CoV-1 N protein on binding to the tripartite motif protein 25 (TRIM25) E3 ubiquitin ligase may cause interference in the binding of TRIM25 with RIG-I [271]. Moreover, the M protein was shown to alter TRAF3/

TANK/TBK1/IKKϵ formation, which is crucial for IRF3/IRF7 signaling [266]. Due to the high structural similarity between the SARS-CoV-1 and -2 proteins, it is believed that SARS-CoV-2 proteins may function similarly to SARS-CoV-1. SARS-CoV-2 ORF3b protein retains the ability to inhibit IFN-1 signaling like that of SARS-CoV-1. Intriguingly, SARS-CoV-2 ORF3b has been found to suppress the IFN production more efficiently than the SARS-CoV ORF3b [261]. Studies have researched variants of SARS-CoV-2 sequences and interestingly a longer version of ORF3b displayed a potentially greater inhibitory activity. On the other hand, SARS-CoV-2 S protein and nsp2 showed stimulatory effects on IFN production [260].

SARS-CoV-2 encoded proteases, which are the nsp3/papain-like protease and nsp5/3C-like protease, are crucial for viral replication and can also cleave proteins of the host innate immune system [272]. In a study, it was identified that three host proteins, namely, IRF-3, NLR Family Pyrin Domain Containing 12 (NLRP12), and TGF-β activated kinase 1 binding protein 1 (TAB1), were selectively cleaved by nsp3 and nsp5, the former cleaving IRF-3 and the latter cleaving both NLRP12 and TAB1 [272]. Cleavage of IRF-3 by nsp3 resulted in altered type-I IFN responses, and nsp5-mediated NLRP12 and TAB1 cleavage resulted in enhanced cytokines production through the NFκB pathway [272]. Additionally, NLRP12 cleavage by nsp5 could influence the assembly of NLRP3 inflammasome leading to an enhanced production of IL-1β [272]. Nonetheless the deubiquitinase and deISGylation activity of the Orf1a/b, PLpro result in inhibited IRF3 activity [272, 273]. Also, it is shown that ubiquitin-like protein ISG15 cleavage can be induced by PLpro of SARS-CoV-2 [236].

## *JAK-STAT Pathway*

The JAK-STAT pathway is involved in communicating the signals received by nearby cells by driving the expression of numerous response genes such as ISGs [274]. The pathway plays a vital role in the regulation of immune responses against viral pathogens [275]. JAK is associated with various cytokines receptors, most importantly with IFN receptors. The virus infected cells release IFNs which makes nearby cells aware of infection by binding to the IFN receptors present on them. IFN-I and IFN-II receptors are ubiquitously found; however, IFN-III receptors are present exclusively on cells lining the epithelial barrier [259]. On receiving the signal, the JAK gets phosphorylated which in turn phosphorylates adjacent JAKs. Any of the four JAKs, namely, JAK1, JAK2, JAK3, and JAK4, can be involved as per the respective receptor [274]. The cascade then proceeds with phosphorylation of STAT molecules. STAT has various isomers (STAT1, STAT2, STAT3, STAT4, STAT5A, STAT5B, and STAT6) which can form hetero- or homodimers after phosphorylation. The STAT dimers then get displaced in the nucleus where it binds to the respective promoter of ISGs. Viruses try to hinder this important pathway, for their own benefit, through various mechanisms [275]. In COVID-19 cases with high viral load, an upregulation of JAK-STAT pathway components especially JAK2, STAT1, and STAT2 have been noted [276]. The study demonstrated a dampened level of various cytokines in STAT2 knockout hamsters infected with SARS-CoV-2 when compared to that of uninfected animals. Moreover, the severe pathological effects of SARS-CoV-2 infection observed in wild type hamsters were not observed in STAT2 knockout hamsters. This highlighted the importance of STAT in SARS-CoV-2 infection aftermath [277].

Luo et al., in the case of SARS-CoV as well as SARS-CoV-2 infection, observed that components of signaling pathways of ACE2 and JAK-STAT are significantly correlated. It further provided the probability of involvement of the JAK-STAT signaling pathway in the downstream action of the overactivation of ACE2 [278]. A study noted the muted expression of JAK/STAT and some interleukin pathways in a subset of early mild–moderate infections. This was permissive to hypoinflammatory responses. However, in severely ill subjects increased interleukin and IFN pathway activation was observed [279]. An interesting investigation demonstrated a reduction in IFN-triggered phosphorylated STAT1 level post–SARS-CoV-2 infection. Additionally, viral Mpro was found to interact with STAT1 with the plausible ability of STAT-1 autophagic degradation [280]. This indicated employment of additional strategies to alter JAK-STAT signaling by SARS-CoV-2 [280]. Investigation of the effects of SARS-CoV-2 miRNA on cellular pathways informed that the viral miRNA targeted JAK1 and JAK2 wild STAT3, STAT4, STAT5B, and STAT6 were targeted by SARS-CoV-2 miRNAs. It has been shown that viruses increase the suppressor of cytokine signaling cellular genes (SOCS) that regulate this pathway by a feedback mechanism. In this study, some of the viral miRNA were found to induce SOCS [281]. Xia et al. analyzed the potency of various SARS-CoV-2 proteins to alter components associated with the JAK-STAT pathway. The results showed interesting findings that nsp1, nsp6, nsp13, ORF3a, M, ORF7a, and ORF7b inhibited STAT1 and/or STAT2 phosphorylation as well as nuclear translocation. Further, ORF6 was found to interact with nuclear transporter protein KPNA2 which led to suppression of STAT1 nuclear translocation [282]. In another study, ORF6, ORF8 and N protein of SARS-CoV-2 were found to inhibit type I IFN signaling. These factors were demonstrated to inhibit ISRE promoter [283, 284]. N protein was observed to cause a reduction in phosphorylated STAT1 and STAT2 by directly interacting with these molecules. Moreover, the N protein is also found to inhibit the nuclear translocation of STAT1 and STAT2 induced by IFN. This indicated that N protein could inhibit phosphorylation of these STAT molecules and could antagonize IFN-I signaling [284]. In another study, ORF7a was also found to suppress STAT2 phosphorylation and nuclear translocation [285]. In this study ubiquitination of ORF7a by the host system was also demonstrated to be important to perform this action. This indicates the use of the one host machinery by the viral system in antagonism of another molecular pathway.

## Conclusion

The COVID-19 pandemic has given rise to serious public health concerns. Individuals with underlying health conditions like CVD, hypertension, diabetes, AKI, and obesity are prone to risk of severe manifestations. Often, increased hospitalization time, severity, delayed viral clearance, or increased mortality are observed in patients with one of these comorbidities. The large-scale or worldwide studies investigating different comorbidities and associated risk factors with respect to COVID-19 may provide a clearer picture of important risk factors. Current studies have clarified that the withdrawal of necessary medications like ACEI, RAAS inhibitors, and antirheumatic drugs should be avoided during COVID-19. The withdrawal could actually aid in worsening many preexisting conditions. The specific mechanisms of interaction of various factors related to abovementioned comorbidities and COVID-19 are yet to be elucidated. Moreover, some comorbidities like obesity or repercussions like secondary infections with respect to COVID-19 still remain underexplored. Moreover, due to COVID-19 as well as its aftermath, many people become susceptible to secondary deadly infections like bacterial infections in the oral cavity and fungal infections mucormycosis. During and after COVID-19, every sign and symptoms should be cautiously observed and diagnostic tests for susceptive conditions should be carried out without delay. This may help in controlling progression of secondary infections like mucormycosis. This demands further investigation for understanding and management of the disease progression and severity in patients with underlying conditions or with COVID-19 repercussions.

Furthermore, investigation of modulation in cellular activities upon SARS-CoV-2 infection need to be conducted. Some studies have shown that viral infection can trigger various molecular pathways inside the cells. Most of the reports have put forth involvement of NFκB, IRF, and JAK-STAT pathways which ultimately lead to activation of immune response genes. Overactivation of these pathways are correlated to cytokine storms prevalently seen in COVID-19 patients. Effects of approved inhibitors of proteins involved in these pathways should be investigated in COVID-19 disease models. Various SARS-CoV-2 proteins have also shown to interact with components of these pathways which further could modulate the cellular responses against infection. Further research can reveal effective small molecule or peptide inhibitors to target SARS-CoV-2 protein to hinder any alterations in the host system.

**Acknowledgments** We thank the Ministry of Human Resource Development, Govt. of India for a fellowship to Shweta Jakhmola and Tarun Prakash Verma; Department of Biotechnology, Govt. of India for a fellowship to Omkar Indari; Council of Scientific and Industrial Research, Govt. of India for a fellowship to Dharmendra Kashyap; University Grant Commission, Govt. of India for a fellowship to Budhadev Baral, all in the form of research stipends. We appreciate our lab colleagues for insightful discussions and advice. We gratefully acknowledge Indian Institute of Technology Indore for providing facilities and support.

## References


1. Jakhmola S, Indari O, Kashyap D, Varshney N, Rani A, Sonkar C, et al. Recent updates on COVID-19: a holistic review. Heliyon. 2020;6(12):e05706.
2. Jakhmola S, Indari O, Kashyap D, Varshney N, Das A, Manivannan E, et al. Mutational analysis of structural proteins of SARS-CoV-2. Heliyon. 2021;7(3):e06572.
3. Zheng J. SARS-CoV-2: an Emerging Coronavirus that Causes a Global Threat. Int J Biol Sci. 2020;16(10):1678–85.
4. Anand U, Adelodun B, Pivato A, Suresh S, Indari O, Jakhmola S, et al. A review of the presence of SARS-CoV-2 RNA in wastewater and airborne particulates and its use for virus spreading surveillance. Environ Res. 2021;196:110929.
5. Mason RJ. Pathogenesis of COVID-19 from a cell biology perspective. Eur Respir J. 2020;55(4):2000607. https://doi.org/10.1183/13993003.00607-2020.
6. Carsana L, Sonzogni A, Nasr A, Rossi RS, Pellegrinelli A, Zerbi P, et al. Pulmonary post-mortem findings in a series of COVID-19 cases from northern Italy: a two-centre descriptive study. Lancet Infect. 2020;20(10):1135–40.
7. Xu Z, Shi L, Wang Y, Zhang J, Huang L, Zhang C, et al. Pathological findings of COVID-19 associated with acute respiratory distress syndrome. Lancet Respir Med. 2020;8(4):420–2.
8. Wiersinga WJ, Rhodes A, Cheng AC, Peacock SJ, Prescott HC. Pathophysiology, transmission, diagnosis, and treatment of coronavirus disease 2019 (COVID-19): a review. JAMA. 2020;324(8):782–93.
9. Batah SS, Fabro AT. Pulmonary pathology of ARDS in COVID-19: a pathological review for clinicians. Respir Med. 2021;176:106239.
10. Zaim S, Chong JH, Sankaranarayanan V, Harky A. COVID-19 and multiorgan response. Curr Probl Cardiol. 2020;45(8):100618.
11. Mai F, Del Pinto R, Ferri C. COVID-19 and cardiovascular diseases. J Cardiol. 2020;76(5):453–8.
12. Bae S, Kim SR, Kim M-N, Shim WJ, Park S-M. Impact of cardiovascular disease and risk factors on fatal outcomes in patients with COVID-19 according to age: a systematic review and meta-analysis. Heart. 2021;107(5):373–80.
13. Rodriguez-Morales AJ, Cardona-Ospina JA, Gutiérrez-Ocampo E, Villamizar-Peña R, Holguin-Rivera Y, Escalera-Antezana JP, et al. Clinical, laboratory and imaging features of COVID-19: a systematic review and meta-analysis. Travel Med Infect Dis. 2020;34:101623.
14. Wang D, Hu B, Hu C, Zhu F, Liu X, Zhang J, et al. Clinical Characteristics of 138 Hospitalized Patients With 2019 Novel Coronavirus-Infected Pneumonia in Wuhan, China. JAMA. 2020;323(11):1061–9.
15. Chen N, Zhou M, Dong X, Qu J, Gong F, Han Y, et al. Epidemiological and clinical characteristics of 99 cases of 2019 novel coronavirus pneumonia in Wuhan, China: a descriptive study. Lancet. 2020;395(10223):507–13.
16. Liu K, Fang Y-Y, Deng Y, Liu W, Wang M-F, Ma J-P, et al. Clinical characteristics of novel coronavirus cases in tertiary hospitals in Hubei Province. Chin Med J (Engl). 2020;133(9):1025–31.
17. Zhao M, Wang M, Zhang J, Ye J, Xu Y, Wang Z, et al. Advances in the relationship between coronavirus infection and cardiovascular diseases. Biomed Pharmacother. 2020;127:110230.
18. Li G, Hu R, Gu X. A close-up on COVID-19 and cardiovascular diseases. Nutr Metab Cardiovasc Dis. 2020;30(7):1057–60.
19. Yang X, Yu Y, Xu J, Shu H, Xia J, Liu H, et al. Clinical course and outcomes of critically ill patients with SARS-CoV-2 pneumonia in Wuhan, China: a single-centered, retrospective, observational study. Lancet Respir Med. 2020;8(5):475–81.
20. Li Y, Li M, Wang M, Zhou Y, Chang J, Xian Y, et al. Acute cerebrovascular disease following COVID-19: a single center, retrospective, observational study. Stroke Vasc Neurol. 2020;5(3):279–84.

21. Nishiga M, Wang DW, Han Y, Lewis DB, Wu JC. COVID-19 and cardiovascular disease: from basic mechanisms to clinical perspectives. Nat Rev Cardiol. 2020;17(9):543–58.
22. Zheng Y-Y, Ma Y-T, Zhang J-Y, Xie X. COVID-19 and the cardiovascular system. Nat Rev Cardiol. 2020;17(5):259–60.
23. Jiang F, Yang J, Zhang Y, Dong M, Wang S, Zhang Q, et al. Angiotensin-converting enzyme 2 and angiotensin 1-7: novel therapeutic targets. Nat Rev Cardiol. 2014;11(7):413–26.
24. Chen L, Li X, Chen M, Feng Y, Xiong C. The ACE2 expression in human heart indicates new potential mechanism of heart injury among patients infected with SARS-CoV-2. Cardiovasc Res. 2020;116(6):1097–100.
25. Patel VB, Zhong J-C, Grant MB, Oudit GY. Role of the ACE2/angiotensin 1-7 axis of the renin-angiotensin system in heart failure. Circ Res. 2016;118(8):1313–26.
26. Clerkin KJ, Fried JA, Raikhelkar J, Sayer G, Griffin JM, Masoumi A, et al. COVID-19 and cardiovascular disease. Circulation. 2020;141(20):1648–55.
27. Fried JA, Ramasubbu K, Bhatt R, Topkara VK, Clerkin KJ, Horn E, et al. The variety of cardiovascular presentations of COVID-19. Circulation. 2020;141(23):1930–6.
28. Dinh QN, Drummond GR, Sobey CG, Chrissobolis S. Roles of inflammation, oxidative stress, and vascular dysfunction in hypertension. Biomed Res Int. 2014;2014:406960.
29. Han H, Yang L, Liu R, Liu F, Wu K-L, Li J, et al. Prominent changes in blood coagulation of patients with SARS-CoV-2 infection. Clin Chem Lab Med. 2020;58(7):1116–20.
30. Tang N, Bai H, Chen X, Gong J, Li D, Sun Z. Anticoagulant treatment is associated with decreased mortality in severe coronavirus disease 2019 patients with coagulopathy. J Thromb Haemost. 2020;18(5):1094–9.
31. Deussen A. Hyperthermia and hypothermia. Effects on the cardiovascular system. Anaesthesist. 2007;56(9):907–11.
32. Arnett DK, Blumenthal RS, Albert MA, Buroker AB, Goldberger ZD, Hahn EJ, et al. 2019 ACC/AHA guideline on the primary prevention of cardiovascular disease: a report of the American college of cardiology/American heart association task force on clinical practice guidelines. J Am Coll Cardiol. 2019;74(10):e177–232.
33. Wu C, Chen X, Cai Y, Xia J, Zhou X, Xu S, et al. Risk factors associated with acute respiratory distress syndrome and death in patients with coronavirus disease 2019 pneumonia in Wuhan, China. JAMA Intern Med. 2020;180(7):934–43.
34. Huang C, Wang Y, Li X, Ren L, Zhao J, Hu Y, et al. Clinical features of patients infected with 2019 novel coronavirus in Wuhan, China. Lancet. 2020;395(10223):497–506.
35. Zhang J-J, Dong X, Cao Y-Y, Yuan Y-D, Yang Y-B, Yan Y-Q, et al. Clinical characteristics of 140 patients infected with SARS-CoV-2 in Wuhan, China. Allergy. 2020;75(7):1730–41.
36. Wang Z, Yang B, Li Q, Wen L, Zhang R. Clinical Features of 69 Cases With Coronavirus Disease 2019 in Wuhan, China. Clin Infect Dis. 2020;71(15):769–77.
37. Epidemiology Working Group for NCIP Epidemic Response, Chinese Center for Disease Control and Prevention. The epidemiological characteristics of an outbreak of 2019 novel coronavirus diseases (COVID-19) in China. Zhonghua Liu Xing Bing Xue Za Zhi. 2020;41(2):145–51.
38. The OpenSAFELY Collaborative, Williamson E, Walker AJ, Bhaskaran K, Bacon S, Bates C, et al. OpenSAFELY: factors associated with COVID-19-related hospital death in the linked electronic health records of 17 million adult NHS patients [Internet]. bioRxiv. medRxiv; 2020. http://medrxiv.org/lookup/doi/10.1101/2020.05.06.20092999.
39. Shi S, Qin M, Shen B, Cai Y, Liu T, Yang F, et al. Association of cardiac injury with mortality in hospitalized patients with COVID-19 in Wuhan, China. JAMA Cardiol. 2020;5(7):802–10.
40. Guo T, Fan Y, Chen M, Wu X, Zhang L, He T, et al. Cardiovascular implications of fatal outcomes of patients with coronavirus disease 2019 (COVID-19). JAMA Cardiol. 2020;5(7):811–8.
41. Zhou F, Yu T, Du R, Fan G, Liu Y, Liu Z, et al. Clinical course and risk factors for mortality of adult inpatients with COVID-19 in Wuhan, China: a retrospective cohort study. Lancet. 2020;395(10229):1054–62.

42. Mills KT, Stefanescu A, He J. The global epidemiology of hypertension. Nat Rev Nephrol. 2020;16(4):223–37.
43. Guzik TJ, Mohiddin SA, Dimarco A, Patel V, Savvatis K, Marelli-Berg FM, et al. COVID-19 and the cardiovascular system: implications for risk assessment, diagnosis, and treatment options. Cardiovasc Res. 2020;116(10):1666–87.
44. Siedlinski M, Jozefczuk E, Xu X, Teumer A, Evangelou E, Schnabel RB, et al. White blood cells and blood pressure: a Mendelian Randomization Study. Circulation. 2020;141(16):1307–17.
45. Youn J-C, Yu HT, Lim BJ, Koh MJ, Lee J, Chang D-Y, et al. Immunosenescent CD8+ T cells and C-X-C chemokine receptor type 3 chemokines are increased in human hypertension. Hypertension. 2013;62(1):126–33.
46. Kamyshnyi A, Krynytska I, Matskevych V, Marushchak M, Lushchak O. Arterial hypertension as a risk comorbidity associated with COVID-19 pathology. Int J Hypertens. 2020;4(2020):8019360.
47. Li XC, Zhang J, Zhuo JL. The vasoprotective axes of the renin-angiotensin system: physiological relevance and therapeutic implications in cardiovascular, hypertensive and kidney diseases. Pharmacol Res. 2017;125(Pt A):21–38.
48. Ferrario CM, Jessup J, Chappell MC, Averill DB, Brosnihan KB, Tallant EA, et al. Effect of angiotensin-converting enzyme inhibition and angiotensin II receptor blockers on cardiac angiotensin-converting enzyme 2. Circulation. 2005;111(20):2605–10.
49. Burchill LJ, Velkoska E, Dean RG, Griggs K, Patel SK, Burrell LM. Combination renin-angiotensin system blockade and angiotensin-converting enzyme 2 in experimental myocardial infarction: implications for future therapeutic directions. Clin Sci. 2012;123(11):649–58.
50. Takeda Y, Zhu A, Yoneda T, Usukura M, Takata H, Yamagishi M. Effects of aldosterone and angiotensin II receptor blockade on cardiac angiotensinogen and angiotensin-converting enzyme 2 expression in Dahl salt-sensitive hypertensive rats. Am J Hypertens. 2007;20(10):1119–24.
51. Burrell LM, Risvanis J, Kubota E, Dean RG, MacDonald PS, Lu S, et al. Myocardial infarction increases ACE2 expression in rat and humans. Eur Heart J. 2005;26(4):369–75; discussion 322–4.
52. Tikellis C, Bialkowski K, Pete J, Sheehy K, Su Q, Johnston C, et al. ACE2 deficiency modifies renoprotection afforded by ACE inhibition in experimental diabetes. Diabetes. 2008;57(4):1018–25.
53. Reynolds HR, Adhikari S, Pulgarin C, Troxel AB, Iturrate E, Johnson SB, et al. Renin-angiotensin-aldosterone system inhibitors and risk of Covid-19. N Engl J Med. 2020;382(25):2441–8.
54. Mancia G, Rea F, Ludergnani M, Apolone G, Corrao G. Renin-angiotensin-aldosterone system blockers and the risk of Covid-19. N Engl J Med. 2020;382(25):2431–40.
55. Zhang P, Zhu L, Cai J, Lei F, Qin J-J, Xie J, et al. Association of inpatient use of angiotensin-converting enzyme inhibitors and Angiotensin II receptor blockers with mortality among patients with hypertension hospitalized with COVID-19. Circ Res. 2020;126(12):1671–81.
56. Kuba K, Imai Y, Rao S, Gao H, Guo F, Guan B, et al. A crucial role of angiotensin converting enzyme 2 (ACE2) in SARS coronavirus-induced lung injury. Nat Med. 2005;11(8):875–9.
57. Imai Y, Kuba K, Rao S, Huan Y, Guo F, Guan B, et al. Angiotensin-converting enzyme 2 protects from severe acute lung failure. Nature. 2005;436(7047):112–6.
58. Vaduganathan M, Vardeny O, Michel T, McMurray JJV, Pfeffer MA, Solomon SD. Renin-angiotensin-aldosterone system inhibitors in patients with Covid-19. N Engl J Med. 2020;382(17):1653–9.
59. Zeng J-H, Liu Y-X, Yuan J, Wang F-X, Wu W-B, Li J-X, et al. First case of COVID-19 complicated with fulminant myocarditis: a case report and insights. Infection. 2020;48(5):773–7.
60. Arentz M, Yim E, Klaff L, Lokhandwala S, Riedo FX, Chong M, et al. Characteristics and outcomes of 21 critically ill patients with COVID-19 in Washington State. JAMA. 2020;323(16):1612–4.

61. Pettit NN, Nguyen CT, Mutlu GM, Wu D, Kimmig L, Pitrak D, et al. Late onset infectious complications and safety of tocilizumab in the management of COVID-19. J Med Virol. 2021;93(3):1459–64.
62. Crane HM, Van Rompaey SE, Kitahata MM. Antiretroviral medications associated with elevated blood pressure among patients receiving highly active antiretroviral therapy. AIDS. 2006;20(7):1019–26.
63. Agarwal S, Agarwal SK. Lopinavir-Ritonavir in SARS-CoV-2 infection and drug-drug interactions with cardioactive medications. Cardiovasc Drugs Ther. 2021;35(3):427–40.
64. Coronavirus disease (COVID-19): Dexamethasone [Internet]. [cited 2021 Jun 8]. https://www.who.int/news-room/q-a-detail/coronavirus-disease-covid-19-dexamethasone.
65. Grossman E, Messerli FH. Drug-induced hypertension: an unappreciated cause of secondary hypertension. Am J Med. 2012;125(1):14–22.
66. Sharon LHO, Yi Z, Judith AW. Mechanisms of dexamethasone-induced hypertension. Curr Hypertens Rev. 2009;5(1):61–74.
67. Apicella M, Campopiano MC, Mantuano M, Mazoni L, Coppelli A, Del Prato S. COVID-19 in people with diabetes: understanding the reasons for worse outcomes. Lancet Diabetes Endocrinol. 2020;8(9):782–92.
68. Cristelo C, Azevedo C, Marques JM, Nunes R, Sarmento B. SARS-CoV-2 and diabetes: new challenges for the disease. Diabetes Res Clin Pract. 2020;164:108228.
69. Shaw K. The impact of diabetes on COVID -19 infection. Pract Diabetes. 2020;37(3):79–81.
70. Abdi A, Jalilian M, Sarbarzeh PA, Vlaisavljevic Z. Diabetes and COVID-19: A systematic review on the current evidences. Diabetes Res Clin Pract. 2020;166:108347.
71. Hulme KD, Gallo LA, Short KR. Influenza virus and glycemic variability in diabetes: a killer combination? Front Microbiol. 2017;22(8):861.
72. Lim S, Bae JH, Kwon H-S, Nauck MA. COVID-19 and diabetes mellitus: from pathophysiology to clinical management. Nat Rev Endocrinol. 2021;17(1):11–30.
73. Holman N, Knighton P, Kar P, O'Keefe J, Curley M, Weaver A, et al. Risk factors for COVID-19-related mortality in people with type 1 and type 2 diabetes in England: a population-based cohort study. Lancet Diabetes Endocrinol. 2020;8(10):823–33.
74. Deshpande AD, Harris-Hayes M, Schootman M. Epidemiology of diabetes and diabetes-related complications. Phys Ther. 2008;88(11):1254–64.
75. Wilcox G. Insulin and insulin resistance. Clin Biochem Rev. 2005;26(2):19–39.
76. Ceriello A. Hyperglycemia and COVID-19: What was known and what is really new? Diabetes Res Clin Pract. 2020;167:108383.
77. Batlle D, Jose Soler M, Ye M. ACE2 and diabetes: ACE of ACEs? Diabetes. 2010;59(12):2994–6.
78. Liu F, Long X, Zou W, Fang M, Wu W, Li W, et al. Highly ACE2 expression in pancreas may cause pancreas damage after SARS-CoV-2 infection [Internet]. bioRxiv. medRxiv; 2020. https://doi.org/10.1101/2020.02.28.20029181.
79. Lampard AM. Obesity. In: Encyclopedia of feeding and eating disorders. Singapore: Springer; 2015. p. 1–5.
80. WHO Expert Consultation. Appropriate body-mass index for Asian populations and its implications for policy and intervention strategies. Lancet. 2004;363(9403):157–63.
81. Michalakis K, Ilias I. SARS-CoV-2 infection and obesity: Common inflammatory and metabolic aspects. Diabetes Metab Syndr. 2020;14(4):469–71.
82. Michalakis K, Goulis DG, Vazaiou A, Mintziori G, Polymeris A, Abrahamian-Michalakis A. Obesity in the ageing man. Metabolism. 2013;62(10):1341–9.
83. Ryan DH, Ravussin E, Heymsfield S. COVID 19 and the patient with obesity—the editors speak out. Obesity. 2020;28(5):847.
84. Obesity & COVID-19 [Internet]. [cited 2021 Jun 8]. https://www.worldobesity.org/resources/policy-dossiers/obesity-covid-19.
85. [No title] [Internet]. [cited 2021 Jun 10]. https://www.cdc.gov/coronavirus.

86. Popkin BM, Du S, Green WD, Beck MA, Algaith T, Herbst CH, et al. Individuals with obesity and COVID-19: a global perspective on the epidemiology and biological relationships. Obes Rev. 2020;21(11):e13128.
87. Simonnet A, Chetboun M, Poissy J, Raverdy V, Noulette J, Duhamel A, et al. High prevalence of obesity in severe acute respiratory syndrome Coronavirus-2 (SARS-CoV-2) requiring invasive mechanical ventilation. Obesity. 2020;28(7):1195–9.
88. Zheng KI, Gao F, Wang X-B, Sun Q-F, Pan K-H, Wang T-Y, et al. Letter to the Editor: Obesity as a risk factor for greater severity of COVID-19 in patients with metabolic associated fatty liver disease. Metabolism. 2020;108:154244.
89. Yang J, Tian C, Chen Y, Zhu C, Chi H, Li J. Obesity aggravates COVID-19: an updated systematic review and meta-analysis. J Med Virol. 2021;93(5):2662–74.
90. Rottoli M, Bernante P, Belvedere A, Balsamo F, Garelli S, Giannella M, et al. How important is obesity as a risk factor for respiratory failure, intensive care admission and death in hospitalised COVID-19 patients? Results from a single Italian centre. Eur J Endocrinol. 2020;183(4):389–97.
91. Sales-Peres SHC, de Azevedo-Silva LJ, Bonato RCS, Sales-Peres MC, Pinto AC, Santiago Junior JF. Coronavirus (SARS-CoV-2) and the risk of obesity for critically illness and ICU admitted: Meta-analysis of the epidemiological evidence. Obes Res Clin Pract. 2020;14(5):389–97.
92. Batsis JA, Mackenzie TA, Bartels SJ, Sahakyan KR, Somers VK, Lopez-Jimenez F. Diagnostic accuracy of body mass index to identify obesity in older adults: NHANES 1999-2004. Int J Obes (Lond). 2016;40(5):761–7.
93. Watanabe M, Caruso D, Tuccinardi D, Risi R, Zerunian M, Polici M, et al. Visceral fat shows the strongest association with the need of intensive care in patients with COVID-19. Metabolism. 2020;111:154319.
94. Huang Y, Lu Y, Huang Y-M, Wang M, Ling W, Sui Y, et al. Obesity in patients with COVID-19: a systematic review and meta-analysis. Metabolism. 2020;113:154378.
95. Ohkawara K, Tanaka S, Miyachi M, Ishikawa-Takata K, Tabata I. A dose-response relation between aerobic exercise and visceral fat reduction: systematic review of clinical trials. Int J Obes (Lond). 2007;31(12):1786–97.
96. Zhu Z, Hasegawa K, Ma B, Fujiogi M, Camargo CA Jr, Liang L. Association of obesity and its genetic predisposition with the risk of severe COVID-19: analysis of population-based cohort data. Metabolism. 2020;22(112):154345.
97. Louie JK, Acosta M, Samuel MC, Schechter R, Vugia DJ, Harriman K, et al. A novel risk factor for a novel virus: obesity and 2009 pandemic influenza A (H1N1). Clin Infect Dis. 2011;52(3):301–12.
98. Van Kerkhove MD, Vandemaele KAH, Shinde V, Jaramillo-Gutierrez G, Koukounari A, Donnelly CA, et al. Risk factors for severe outcomes following 2009 influenza A (H1N1) infection: a global pooled analysis. PLoS Med. 2011;8(7):e1001053.
99. Chen G, Wu D, Guo W, Cao Y, Huang D, Wang H, et al. Clinical and immunological features of severe and moderate coronavirus disease 2019. J Clin Invest. 2020;130(5):2620–9.
100. Lockhart SM, O'Rahilly S. When two pandemics meet: why is obesity associated with increased COVID-19 mortality? Med (N Y). 2020;1(1):33–42.
101. Weisberg SP, McCann D, Desai M, Rosenbaum M, Leibel RL, Ferrante AW Jr. Obesity is associated with macrophage accumulation in adipose tissue. J Clin Invest. 2003;112(12):1796–808.
102. Rebello CJ, Kirwan JP, Greenway FL. Obesity, the most common comorbidity in SARS-CoV-2: is leptin the link? Int J Obes (Lond). 2020;44(9):1810–7.
103. Mohammad S, Aziz R, Al Mahri S, Malik SS, Haji E, Khan AH, et al. Obesity and COVID-19: what makes obese host so vulnerable? Immun Ageing. 2021;18(1):1.
104. Vlaicu SI, Tatomir A, Boodhoo D, Vesa S, Mircea PA, Rus H. The role of complement system in adipose tissue-related inflammation. Immunol Res. 2016;64(3):653–64.

105. Magro C, Mulvey JJ, Berlin D, Nuovo G, Salvatore S, Harp J, et al. Complement associated microvascular injury and thrombosis in the pathogenesis of severe COVID-19 infection: a report of five cases. Transl Res. 2020;220:1–13.
106. Targher G, Zoppini G, Moghetti P, Day CP. Disorders of coagulation and hemostasis in abdominal obesity: emerging role of fatty liver. Semin Thromb Hemost. 2010;36(1):41–8.
107. Abdollahi M, Cushman M, Rosendaal FR. Obesity: risk of venous thrombosis and the interaction with coagulation factor levels and oral contraceptive use. Thromb Haemost. 2003;89(3):493–8.
108. Goossens GH, Blaak EE, van Baak MA. Possible involvement of the adipose tissue renin-angiotensin system in the pathophysiology of obesity and obesity-related disorders. Obes Rev. 2003;4(1):43–55.
109. Engeli S, Negrel R, Sharma AM. Physiology and pathophysiology of the adipose tissue renin-angiotensin system. Hypertension. 2000;35(6):1270–7.
110. Braun N, Hoess C, Kutz A, Christ-Crain M, Thomann R, Henzen C, et al. Obesity paradox in patients with community-acquired pneumonia: Is inflammation the missing link? Nutrition. 2017;33:304–10.
111. Corrales-Medina VF, Valayam J, Serpa JA, Rueda AM, Musher DM. The obesity paradox in community-acquired bacterial pneumonia. Int J Infect Dis. 2011;15(1):e54–7.
112. Cho WH, Oh JY, Yeo HJ, Han J, Kim J, Hong S-B, et al. Obesity survival paradox in pneumonia supported with extracorporeal membrane oxygenation: analysis of the national registry. J Crit Care. 2018;48:453–7.
113. Nie W, Zhang Y, Jee SH, Jung KJ, Li B, Xiu Q. Obesity survival paradox in pneumonia: a meta-analysis. BMC Med. 2014;12:61.
114. Stefan N, Birkenfeld AL, Schulze MB, Ludwig DS. Obesity and impaired metabolic health in patients with COVID-19. Nat Rev Endocrinol. 2020;16(7):341–2.
115. Petrakis D, Margină D, Tsarouhas K, Tekos F, Stan M, Nikitovic D, et al. Obesity—a risk factor for increased COVID-19 prevalence, severity and lethality (review). Mol Med Rep. 2020;22(1):9–19.
116. Pettit NN, MacKenzie EL, Ridgway JP, Pursell K, Ash D, Patel B, et al. Obesity is associated with increased risk for mortality among hospitalized patients with COVID-19. Obesity. 2020;28(10):1806–10.
117. Tartof SY, Qian L, Hong V, Wei R, Nadjafi RF, Fischer H, et al. Obesity and mortality among patients diagnosed with COVID-19: results from an Integrated Health Care Organization. Ann Intern Med. 2020;173(10):773–81.
118. Jose RJ, Manuel A. Does coronavirus disease 2019 disprove the obesity paradox in acute respiratory distress syndrome? Obesity. 2020;28(6):1007.
119. Jakhmola S, Baral B, Muduli K, Suar M, Das P, Patnaik PK, et al. The interrelation of COVID-19 and neurological modalities. Neurol Sci. 2021;42(6):2157–60.
120. Moriguchi T, Harii N, Goto J, Harada D, Sugawara H, Takamino J, et al. A first case of meningitis/encephalitis associated with SARS-Coronavirus-2. Int J Infect Dis. 2020;94:55–8.
121. Poyiadji N, Shahin G, Noujaim D, Stone M, Patel S, Griffith B. COVID-19-associated acute hemorrhagic necrotizing encephalopathy: imaging features. Radiology. 2020; 296(2):E119–20.
122. Alexopoulos H, Magira E, Bitzogli K, Kafasi N, Vlachoyiannopoulos P, Tzioufas A, et al. Anti-SARS-CoV-2 antibodies in the CSF, blood-brain barrier dysfunction, and neurological outcome: Studies in 8 stuporous and comatose patients. Neurol Neuroimmunol Neuroinflamm. 2020;7(6):e893. https://doi.org/10.1212/NXI.0000000000000893.
123. Helms J, Kremer S, Merdji H, Clere-Jehl R, Schenck M, Kummerlen C, et al. Neurologic features in severe SARS-CoV-2 infection. N Engl J Med. 2020;382(23):2268–70.
124. Paterson RW, Brown RL, Benjamin L, Nortley R, Wiethoff S, Bharucha T, et al. The emerging spectrum of COVID-19 neurology: clinical, radiological and laboratory findings. Brain. 2020;143(10):3104–20.
125. Mao L, Jin H, Wang M, Hu Y, Chen S, He Q, et al. Neurologic manifestations of hospitalized patients with coronavirus disease 2019 in Wuhan, China. JAMA Neurol. 2020;77(6):683–90.

126. Matschke J, Lütgehetmann M, Hagel C, Sperhake JP, Schröder AS, Edler C, et al. Neuropathology of patients with COVID-19 in Germany: a post-mortem case series. Lancet Neurol. 2020;19(11):919–29.
127. Deigendesch N, Sironi L, Kutza M, Wischnewski S, Fuchs V, Hench J, et al. Correlates of critical illness-related encephalopathy predominate postmortem COVID-19 neuropathology. Acta Neuropathol. 2020;140(4):583–6.
128. Jaunmuktane Z, Mahadeva U, Green A, Sekhawat V, Barrett NA, Childs L, et al. Microvascular injury and hypoxic damage: emerging neuropathological signatures in COVID-19. Acta Neuropathol. 2020;140(3):397–400.
129. Tandon M, Kataria S, Patel J, Mehta TR, Daimee M, Patel V, et al. A comprehensive systematic review of CSF analysis that defines neurological manifestations of COVID-19. Int J Infect Dis. 2021;104:390–7.
130. Jain R, Young M, Dogra S, Kennedy H, Nguyen V, Jones S, et al. COVID-19 related neuroimaging findings: a signal of thromboembolic complications and a strong prognostic marker of poor patient outcome. J Neurol Sci. 2020;414:116923.
131. Xia H, Lazartigues E. Angiotensin-converting enzyme 2 in the brain: properties and future directions. J Neurochem. 2008;107(6):1482–94.
132. Brann DH, Tsukahara T, Weinreb C, Lipovsek M, Van den Berge K, Gong B, et al. Non-neuronal expression of SARS-CoV-2 entry genes in the olfactory system suggests mechanisms underlying COVID-19-associated anosmia. Sci Adv. 2020;6(31):eabc5801. https://doi.org/10.1126/sciadv.abc5801.
133. Wang K, Chen W, Zhou Y-S, Lian J-Q, Zhang Z, Du P, et al. SARS-CoV-2 invades host cells via a novel route: CD147-spike protein [Internet]. bioRxiv. 2020 [cited 2021 Jun 8]. p. 2020.03.14.988345. https://www.biorxiv.org/content/10.1101/2020.03.14.988345v1.
134. Hoffmann M, Kleine-Weber H, Schroeder S, Krüger N, Herrler T, Erichsen S, et al. SARS-CoV-2 cell entry depends on ACE2 and TMPRSS2 and is blocked by a clinically proven protease inhibitor. Cell. 2020;181(2):271–80.e8.
135. Zang R, Gomez Castro MF, McCune BT, Zeng Q, Rothlauf PW, Sonnek NM, et al. TMPRSS2 and TMPRSS4 promote SARS-CoV-2 infection of human small intestinal enterocytes. Sci Immunol. 2020;5(47):eabc3582. https://doi.org/10.1126/sciimmunol.abc3582.
136. Ou X, Liu Y, Lei X, Li P, Mi D, Ren L, et al. Characterization of spike glycoprotein of SARS-CoV-2 on virus entry and its immune cross-reactivity with SARS-CoV. Nat Commun. 2020;11(1):1620.
137. Lou JJ, Movassaghi M, Gordy D, Olson MG, Zhang T, Khurana MS, et al. Neuropathology of COVID-19 (neuro-COVID): clinicopathological update. Free Neuropathol. 2021;2:2. https://doi.org/10.17879/freeneuropathology-2021-2993.
138. Trojanowicz B, Ulrich C, Kohler F, Bode V, Seibert E, Fiedler R, et al. Monocytic angiotensin-converting enzyme 2 relates to atherosclerosis in patients with chronic kidney disease. Nephrol Dial Transplant. 2017;32(2):287–98.
139. Salamanna F, Maglio M, Landini MP, Fini M. Body localization of ACE-2: on the trail of the keyhole of SARS-CoV-2. Front Med. 2020;7:594495.
140. Song E, Zhang C, Israelow B, Lu-Culligan A, Prado AV, Skriabine S, et al. Neuroinvasion of SARS-CoV-2 in human and mouse brain. bioRxiv [Internet]. 2020. https://doi.org/10.1101/2020.06.25.169946
141. Cavalcanti DD, Raz E, Shapiro M, Dehkharghani S, Yaghi S, Lillemoe K, et al. Cerebral venous thrombosis associated with COVID-19. AJNR Am J Neuroradiol. 2020;41(8):1370–6.
142. Song P, Li W, Xie J, Hou Y, You C. Cytokine storm induced by SARS-CoV-2. Clin Chim Acta. 2020;509:280–7.
143. Thachil J, Tang N, Gando S, Falanga A, Cattaneo M, Levi M, et al. ISTH interim guidance on recognition and management of coagulopathy in COVID-19. J Thromb Haemost. 2020;18(5):1023–6.

144. Schurink B, Roos E, Radonic T, Barbe E, Bouman CSC, de Boer HH, et al. Viral presence and immunopathology in patients with lethal COVID-19: a prospective autopsy cohort study. Lancet Microbe. 2020;1(7):e290–9.
145. Tian J, Yuan X, Xiao J, Zhong Q, Yang C, Liu B, et al. Clinical characteristics and risk factors associated with COVID-19 disease severity in patients with cancer in Wuhan, China: a multicentre, retrospective, cohort study. Lancet Oncol. 2020;21(7):893–903.
146. Avanzato VA, Matson MJ, Seifert SN, Pryce R, Williamson BN, Anzick SL, et al. Case study: prolonged infectious SARS-CoV-2 shedding from an asymptomatic immunocompromised individual with cancer. Cell. 2020;183(7):1901–12.e9.
147. Dai M, Liu D, Liu M, Zhou F, Li G, Chen Z, et al. Patients with cancer appear more vulnerable to SARS-CoV-2: a multicenter study during the COVID-19 outbreak. Cancer Discov. 2020;10(6):783–91.
148. Derosa L, Melenotte C, Griscelli F, Gachot B, Marabelle A, Kroemer G, et al. The immuno-oncological challenge of COVID-19. Nat Cancer. 2020;1(10):946–64.
149. Pathania AS, Prathipati P, Abdul BA, Chava S, Katta SS, Gupta SC, et al. COVID-19 and cancer comorbidity: therapeutic opportunities and challenges. Theranostics. 2021;11(2):731–53.
150. Luo J, Rizvi H, Preeshagul IR, Egger JV, Hoyos D, Bandlamudi C, et al. COVID-19 in patients with lung cancer. Ann Oncol. 2020;31(10):1386–96.
151. Rivera DR, Peters S, Panagiotou OA, Shah DP, Kuderer NM, Hsu C-Y, et al. Utilization of COVID-19 treatments and clinical outcomes among patients with cancer: a COVID-19 and Cancer Consortium (CCC19) Cohort Study. Cancer Discov. 2020;10:1514–27.
152. Zhang L, Zhu F, Xie L, Wang C, Wang J, Chen R, et al. Clinical characteristics of COVID-19-infected cancer patients: a retrospective case study in three hospitals within Wuhan, China. Ann Oncol. 2020;31(7):894–901.
153. La Rosée F, Bremer HC, Gehrke I, Kehr A, Hochhaus A, Birndt S, et al. The Janus kinase 1/2 inhibitor ruxolitinib in COVID-19 with severe systemic hyperinflammation. Leukemia. 2020;34(7):1805–15.
154. Akalin E, Azzi Y, Bartash R, Seethamraju H, Parides M, Hemmige V, et al. Covid-19 and kidney transplantation. N Engl J Med. 2020;382(25):2475–7.
155. Abrishami A, Samavat S, Behnam B, Arab-Ahmadi M, Nafar M, Sanei TM. Clinical course, imaging features, and outcomes of COVID-19 in kidney transplant recipients. Eur Urol. 2020;78(2):281–6.
156. Pereira MR, Mohan S, Cohen DJ, Husain SA, Dube GK, Ratner LE, et al. COVID-19 in solid organ transplant recipients: initial report from the US epicenter. Am J Transplant. 2020;20(7):1800–8.
157. Kumar RN, Tanna SD, Shetty AA, Stosor V. COVID-19 in an HIV-positive kidney transplant recipient. Transpl Infect Dis. 2020;22(5):e13338.
158. Okoh AK, Bishburg E, Grinberg S, Nagarakanti S. COVID-19 pneumonia in patients with HIV: a case series. J Acquir Immune Defic Syndr. 2020;85(1):e4–5.
159. Vizcarra P, Pérez-Elías MJ, Quereda C, Moreno A, Vivancos MJ, Dronda F, et al. Description of COVID-19 in HIV-infected individuals: a single-centre, prospective cohort. Lancet HIV. 2020;7(8):e554–64.
160. Altuntas Aydin O, Kumbasar Karaosmanoglu H, Kart YK. HIV/SARS-CoV-2 coinfected patients in Istanbul, Turkey. J Med Virol. 2020;92(11):2288–90.
161. Gervasoni C, Meraviglia P, Riva A, Giacomelli A, Oreni L, Minisci D, et al. Clinical features and outcomes of patients with human immunodeficiency virus with COVID-19. Clin Infect Dis. 2020;71(16):2276–8.
162. Ridgway JP, Farley B, Benoit J-L, Frohne C, Hazra A, Pettit N, et al. A case series of five people living with HIV hospitalized with COVID-19 in Chicago, Illinois. AIDS Patient Care STDS. 2020;34(8):331–5.
163. Härter G, Spinner CD, Roider J, Bickel M, Krznaric I, Grunwald S, et al. COVID-19 in people living with human immunodeficiency virus: a case series of 33 patients. Infection. 2020;48(5):681–6.

164. Shalev N, Scherer M, LaSota ED, Antoniou P, Yin MT, Zucker J, et al. Clinical characteristics and outcomes in people living with human immunodeficiency virus hospitalized for coronavirus disease 2019. Clin Infect Dis. 2020;71(16):2294–7.
165. Bezzio C, Saibeni S, Variola A, Allocca M, Massari A, Gerardi V, et al. Outcomes of COVID-19 in 79 patients with IBD in Italy: an IG-IBD study. Gut. 2020;69(7):1213–7.
166. Brenner EJ, Ungaro RC, Gearry RB, Kaplan GG, Kissous-Hunt M, Lewis JD, et al. Corticosteroids, but not TNF antagonists, are associated with adverse COVID-19 outcomes in patients with inflammatory bowel diseases: results from an International Registry. Gastroenterology. 2020;159(2):481–91.e3.
167. Yuki K, Fujiogi M, Koutsogiannaki S. COVID-19 pathophysiology: a review. Clin Immunol. 2020;215:108427.
168. Huang N, Pérez P, Kato T, Mikami Y, Okuda K, Gilmore RC, et al. SARS-CoV-2 infection of the oral cavity and saliva. Nat Med. 2021;27(5):892–903.
169. Chaimayo C, Kaewnaphan B, Tanlieng N, Athipanyasilp N, Sirijatuphat R, Chayakulkeeree M, et al. Rapid SARS-CoV-2 antigen detection assay in comparison with real-time RT-PCR assay for laboratory diagnosis of COVID-19 in Thailand. Virol J. 2020;17(1):177.
170. de Sousa FACG, Paradella TC. Considerations on oral manifestations of COVID-19. J Med Virol. 2021;93(2):667–8.
171. Graham MS, Sudre CH, May A, Antonelli M, Murray B, Varsavsky T, et al. Changes in symptomatology, reinfection, and transmissibility associated with the SARS-CoV-2 variant B.1.1.7: an ecological study. Lancet Public Health. 2021;6(5):e335–45.
172. Amorim Dos Santos J, Normando AGC, Carvalho da Silva RL, Acevedo AC, De Luca CG, Sugaya N, et al. Oral manifestations in patients with COVID-19: a living systematic review. J Dent Res. 2021;100(2):141–54.
173. Luchiari HR, Giordano RJ, Sidman RL, Pasqualini R, Arap W. Does the RAAS play a role in loss of taste and smell during COVID-19 infections? Pharmacogenomics J. 2021;21(2):109–15.
174. Díaz Rodríguez M, Jimenez Romera A, Villarroel M. Oral manifestations associated with COVID-19. Oral Dis. 2020. https://doi.org/10.1111/odi.13555.
175. Iranmanesh B, Khalili M, Amiri R, Zartab H, Aflatoonian M. Oral manifestations of COVID-19 disease: a review article. Dermatol Ther. 2021;34(1):e14578.
176. Papapanou PN, Sanz M, Buduneli N, Dietrich T, Feres M, Fine DH, et al. Periodontitis: Consensus report of workgroup 2 of the 2017 World Workshop on the classification of periodontal and peri-implant diseases and conditions. J Periodontol. 2018;89(Suppl 1):S173–82.
177. Gomes SC, Fachin S, da Fonseca JG, Angst PDM, Lamers ML, da Silva ISB, et al. Dental biofilm of symptomatic COVID-19 patients harbours SARS-CoV-2. J Clin Periodontol. 2021;48(7):880–5.
178. Hajizadeh F, Houshmand B, Ekhlasmandkermani M, Khazaei S, Kheiri A. Cytokine profiles in periodontitis and COVID-19. Dent Hypotheses. 2021;12(1):36.
179. Stathis C, Victoria N, Loomis K, Nguyen SA, Eggers M, Septimus E, et al. Review of the use of nasal and oral antiseptics during a global pandemic. In: Future microbiology, vol. 16. London: Future Medicine; 2021. p. 119–30. https://www.ncbi.nlm.nih.gov/pmc/articles/PMC7842245/.
180. Liu R, Yi S, Zhang J, Lv Z, Zhu C, Zhang Y. Viral load dynamics in sputum and nasopharyngeal swab in patients with COVID-19. J Dent Res. 2020;99(11):1239–44.
181. Feldman C, Anderson R. The role of co-infections and secondary infections in patients with COVID-19. Pneumonia. 2021;13(1):5.
182. Song G, Liang G, Liu W. Fungal co-infections associated with global COVID-19 pandemic: a clinical and diagnostic perspective from China. Mycopathologia. 2020;185(4):599–606.
183. Zhang Y, Li WX, Huang KW, Cao ZX, Hao JY. Hospital acquired pneumonia occurring after acute stage of the serious sars and its treating strategies. Chin J Nosoconmiol. 2003;11(13):1081–7. https://en.cnki.com.cn/Article_en/CJFDTotal-ZHYY200311042.htm.

184. Yin C, Wang C, Tang Z, et al. Clinical analysis of 146 patients with critical sever acute respiratory syndrome in Beijing areas. J Emerg Med. 2004;1:12–4.
185. Li C-S, Pan S-F. Analysis and causation discussion of 185 severe acute respiratory syndrome dead cases. Zhongguo Wei Zhong Bing Ji Jiu Yi Xue. 2003;15(10):582–4.
186. Ahmadikia K, Hashemi SJ, Khodavaisy S, Getso MI, Alijani N, Badali H, et al. The double-edged sword of systemic corticosteroid therapy in viral pneumonia: a case report and comparative review of influenza-associated mucormycosis versus COVID-19 associated mucormycosis. Mycoses. 2021. https://doi.org/10.1111/myc.13256.
187. Waness A, Dawsari GA, Al JH. The rise of an opportunistic infection called "Invasive Zygomycosis". J Glob Infect. 2009;1(2):131–8.
188. Prakash H, Chakrabarti A. Global epidemiology of mucormycosis. J Fungi. 2019;5:26. https://doi.org/10.3390/jof5010026.
189. Richardson M. The ecology of the Zygomycetes and its impact on environmental exposure. Clin Microbiol Infect. 2009;15(Suppl 5):2–9.
190. Ghuman H, Voelz K. Innate and adaptive immunity to mucorales. J Fungi. 2017;3(3):48. https://doi.org/10.3390/jof3030048.
191. Sharma S, Grover M, Bhargava S, Samdani S, Kataria T. Post coronavirus disease mucormycosis: a deadly addition to the pandemic spectrum. J Laryngol Otol. 2021;135:442–7.
192. Verma DK, Bali RK. COVID-19 and mucormycosis of the craniofacial skeleton: causal, contributory or coincidental? J Maxillofac Oral Surg. 2021;20:165–6.
193. John TM, Jacob CN, Kontoyiannis DP. When uncontrolled diabetes mellitus and severe COVID-19 converge: the perfect storm for mucormycosis. J Fungi. 2021;7(4):298. https://doi.org/10.3390/jof7040298.
194. Bösmüller H, Matter M, Fend F, Tzankov A. The pulmonary pathology of COVID-19. Virchows Arch. 2021 Jan;478(1):137–50.
195. Tavakolpour S, Rakhshandehroo T, Wei EX, Rashidian M. Lymphopenia during the COVID-19 infection: What it shows and what can be learned. Immunol Lett. 2020;225:31–2.
196. RECOVERY Collaborative Group, Horby P, Lim WS, Emberson JR, Mafham M, Bell JL, et al. Dexamethasone in Hospitalized Patients with Covid-19. N Engl J Med. 2021;384(8):693–704.
197. Anjorin AA, Abioye AI, Asowata OE, Soipe A, Kazeem MI, Adesanya IO, et al. Comorbidities and the COVID-19 pandemic dynamics in Africa. Trop Med Int Health. 2021;26(1):2–13.
198. Jeong W, Keighley C, Wolfe R, Lee WL, Slavin MA, Kong DCM, et al. The epidemiology and clinical manifestations of mucormycosis: a systematic review and meta-analysis of case reports. Clin Microbiol Infect. 2019;25(1):26–34.
199. Rink L, Gabriel P. Zinc and the immune system. Proc Nutr Soc. 2000 Nov;59(4):541–52.
200. of Medicine I. In: Otten JJ, Hellwig JP, Meyers LD, editors. Dietary reference intakes: the essential guide to nutrient requirements. Washington, DC: The National Academies Press; 2006.
201. Institute of Medicine (US) Panel on Micronutrients. Zinc. Washington, DC: National Academies Press (US); 2001.
202. Pagani MA, Casamayor A, Serrano R, Atrian S, Ariño J. Disruption of iron homeostasis in Saccharomyces cerevisiae by high zinc levels: a genome-wide study. Mol Microbiol. 2007;65(2):521–37.
203. Chang K-L, Hung T-C, Hsieh B-S, Chen Y-H, Chen T-F, Cheng H-L. Zinc at pharmacologic concentrations affects cytokine expression and induces apoptosis of human peripheral blood mononuclear cells. Nutrition. 2006;22(5):465–74.
204. Prasad AS, Bao B, Beck FWJ, Kucuk O, Sarkar FH. Antioxidant effect of zinc in humans. Free Radic Biol Med. 2004;37(8):1182–90.
205. Lulloff SJ, Hahn BL, Sohnle PG. Fungal susceptibility to zinc deprivation. J Lab Clin Med. 2004;144(4):208–14.
206. Lyons TJ, Gasch AP, Gaither LA, Botstein D, Brown PO, Eide DJ. Genome-wide characterization of the Zap1p zinc-responsive regulon in yeast. Proc Natl Acad Sci U S A. 2000;97(14):7957–62.

207. Herbig A, Bird AJ, Swierczek S, McCall K, Mooney M, Wu C-Y, et al. Zap1 activation domain 1 and its role in controlling gene expression in response to cellular zinc status. Mol Microbiol. 2005;57(3):834–46.
208. Wang Z, Feng LS, Matskevich V, Venkataraman K, Parasuram P, Laity JH. Solution structure of a Zap1 zinc-responsive domain provides insights into metalloregulatory transcriptional repression in Saccharomyces cerevisiae. J Mol Biol. 2006;357(4):1167–83.
209. Ballou ER, Wilson D. The roles of zinc and copper sensing in fungal pathogenesis. Curr Opin Microbiol. 2016;32:128–34.
210. Citiulo F, Jacobsen ID, Miramón P, Schild L, Brunke S, Zipfel P, et al. Candida albicans scavenges host zinc via Pra1 during endothelial invasion. PLoS Pathog. 2012;8(6):e1002777.
211. Wilson D. An evolutionary perspective on zinc uptake by human fungal pathogens. Metallomics. 2015;7(6):979–85.
212. Mohamed MS, Abdel-Motaleb HY, Mobarak FA. Management of rhino-orbital mucormycosis. Saudi Med J. 2015;36(7):865–8.
213. Moorthy A, Gaikwad R, Krishna S, Hegde R, Tripathi KK, Kale PG, et al. SARS-CoV-2, uncontrolled diabetes and corticosteroids-an unholy trinity in invasive fungal infections of the maxillofacial region? A retrospective, multi-centric analysis. J Maxillofac Oral Surg. 2021;20:418–25.
214. Sen M, Lahane S, Lahane TP, Parekh R, Honavar SG. Mucor in a viral land: a tale of two pathogens. Indian J Ophthalmol. 2021;69(2):244–52.
215. Jakhmola S, Indari O, Baral B, Kashyap D, Varshney N, Das A, et al. Comorbidity assessment is essential during COVID-19 treatment. Front Physiol. 2020;11:984.
216. Ronco C, Reis T, Husain-Syed F. Management of acute kidney injury in patients with COVID-19. Lancet Respir Med. 2020;8(7):738–42.
217. Richardson S, Hirsch JS, Narasimhan M, Crawford JM, McGinn T, Davidson KW, et al. Presenting characteristics, comorbidities, and outcomes among 5700 patients hospitalized with COVID-19 in the New York City Area. JAMA. 2020;323(20):2052–9.
218. Tang N, Li D, Wang X, Sun Z. Abnormal coagulation parameters are associated with poor prognosis in patients with novel coronavirus pneumonia. J Thromb Haemost. 2020;18(4):844–7.
219. Batlle D, Soler MJ, Sparks MA, Hiremath S, South AM, Welling PA, et al. Acute kidney injury in COVID-19: emerging evidence of a distinct pathophysiology. J Am Soc Nephrol. 2020;31(7):1380–3.
220. Wang M, Xiong H, Chen H, Li Q, Ruan XZ. Renal injury by SARS-CoV-2 infection: a systematic review. Kidney Dis (Basel). 2021;7(2):100–10.
221. Tervaert TWC, Mooyaart AL, Amann K, Cohen AH, Cook HT, Drachenberg CB, et al. Pathologic classification of diabetic nephropathy. J Am Soc Nephrol. 2010;21(4):556–63.
222. López-Novoa JM, Rodríguez-Peña AB, Ortiz A, Martínez-Salgado C, López Hernández FJ. Etiopathology of chronic tubular, glomerular and renovascular nephropathies: clinical implications. J Transl Med. 2011;9:13.
223. Pfister F, Vonbrunn E, Ries T, Jäck H-M, Überla K, Lochnit G, et al. Complement activation in kidneys of patients with COVID-19. Front Immunol. 2020;11:594849.
224. Meliambro K, Li X, Salem F, Yi Z, Sun Z, Chan L, et al. Molecular analysis of the kidney from a patient with COVID-19-associated collapsing glomerulopathy. Kidney Med. 2021;3:653–8. https://doi.org/10.1016/j.xkme.2021.02.012.
225. Nlandu YM, Makulo J-RR, Pakasa NM, Sumaili EK, Nkondi CN, Bukabau JB, et al. First case of COVID-19-associated collapsing glomerulopathy in Sub-Saharan Africa. Case Rep Nephrol Urol. 2020;2020:8820713.
226. Dong M, Zhang J, Ma X, Tan J, Chen L, Liu S, et al. ACE2, TMPRSS2 distribution and extrapulmonary organ injury in patients with COVID-19. Biomed Pharmacother. 2020;131:110678.
227. Su H, Yang M, Wan C, Yi L-X, Tang F, Zhu H-Y, et al. Renal histopathological analysis of 26 postmortem findings of patients with COVID-19 in China. Kidney Int. 2020;98(1):219–27.
228. ACP Journals [Internet]. [cited 2021 Jun 13]. https://doi.org/10.7326/M20-2003.

229. Diao B, Wang C, Wang R, Feng Z, Tan Y, Wang H, et al. Human kidney is a target for novel severe acute respiratory syndrome Coronavirus 2 (SARS-CoV-2) infection [Internet]. bioRxiv. medRxiv; 2020. https://doi.org/10.1101/2020.03.04.20031120.
230. Gheblawi M, Wang K, Viveiros A, Nguyen Q, Zhong J-C, Turner AJ, et al. Angiotensin-converting enzyme 2: SARS-CoV-2 receptor and regulator of the renin-angiotensin system: celebrating the 20th anniversary of the discovery of ACE2. Circ Res. 2020;126(10):1456–74.
231. Battagello DS, Dragunas G, Klein MO, Ayub ALP, Velloso FJ, Correa RG. Unpuzzling COVID-19: tissue-related signaling pathways associated with SARS-CoV-2 infection and transmission. Clin Sci. 2020;134(16):2137–60.
232. Dong Y, Dai T, Wei Y, Zhang L, Zheng M, Zhou F. A systematic review of SARS-CoV-2 vaccine candidates. Signal Transduct Target Ther. 2020;5(1):237.
233. Bhandari R, Khanna G, Kaushik D, Kuhad A. Divulging the intricacies of crosstalk between NF-Kb and Nrf2-Keap1 pathway in neurological complications of COVID-19. Mol Neurobiol. 2021;58:3347–61. https://doi.org/10.1007/s12035-021-02344-7.
234. More SA, Patil AS, Sakle NS, Mokale SN. Network analysis and molecular mapping for SARS-CoV-2 to reveal drug targets and repurposing of clinically developed drugs. Virology. 2021;555:10–8.
235. Hemmat N, Asadzadeh Z, Ahangar NK, Alemohammad H, Najafzadeh B, Derakhshani A, et al. The roles of signaling pathways in SARS-CoV-2 infection; lessons learned from SARS-CoV and MERS-CoV. Arch Virol. 2021;166(3):675–96.
236. Shin D, Mukherjee R, Grewe D, Bojkova D, Baek K, Bhattacharya A, et al. Papain-like protease regulates SARS-CoV-2 viral spread and innate immunity. Nature. 2020;587(7835):657–62.
237. Keyse SM. Protein phosphatases and the regulation of mitogen-activated protein kinase signalling. In: Current opinion in cell biology, vol. 12. London: Current Biology; 2000. p. 186–92. https://doi.org/10.1016/S0955-0674(99)00075-7.
238. Mizutani T. Signal transduction in SARS-CoV-infected cells. Ann N Y Acad Sci. 2007;1102:86–95.
239. Yu J, Sun X, Goie JYG, Zhang Y. Regulation of host immune responses against influenza a virus infection by mitogen-activated protein kinases (Mapks). Microorganisms. 2020;8:1067. https://www.ncbi.nlm.nih.gov/pmc/articles/PMC7409222/.
240. Grimes JM, Grimes KV. p38 MAPK inhibition: a promising therapeutic approach for COVID-19. J Mol Cell Cardiol. 2020;144:63–5.
241. Schmidt N, Lareau CA, Keshishian H, Ganskih S, Schneider C, Hennig T, et al. The SARS-CoV-2 RNA-protein interactome in infected human cells. Nat Microbiol. 2021;6(3):339–53.
242. Klann K, Bojkova D, Tascher G, Ciesek S, Münch C, Cinatl J. Growth Factor Receptor Signaling Inhibition Prevents SARS-CoV-2 Replication. Mol Cell. 2020;80(1):164–74.e4.
243. Johnson GL, Nakamura K. The c-jun kinase/stress-activated pathway: regulation, function and role in human disease. Biochim Biophys Acta. 2007;1773(8):1341–8.
244. Park JG, Aziz N, Cho JY. MKK7, the essential regulator of JNK signaling involved in cancer cell survival: a newly emerging anticancer therapeutic target. Ther Adv Med Oncol. 2019;11:1758835919875574.
245. Gazon H, Barbeau B, Mesnard J-M, Peloponese J-M Jr. Hijacking of the AP-1 signaling pathway during development of ATL. Front Microbiol. 2017;8:2686.
246. Zhang Y-Y, Li B-R, Ning B-T. The comparative immunological characteristics of SARS-CoV, MERS-CoV, and SARS-CoV-2 coronavirus infections. Front Immunol. 2020;11:2033.
247. Qu F, Xu W, Deng Z, Xie Y, Tang J, Chen Z, et al. Fish c-Jun N-Terminal Kinase (JNK) pathway is involved in bacterial MDP-induced intestinal inflammation. Front Immunol. 2020;11:459.
248. Costela-Ruiz VJ, Illescas-Montes R, Puerta-Puerta JM, Ruiz C, Melguizo-Rodríguez L. SARS-CoV-2 infection: the role of cytokines in COVID-19 disease. Cytokine Growth Factor Rev. 2020;54:62–75. https://www.ncbi.nlm.nih.gov/pmc/articles/PMC7265853/.

249. Shirato K, Kizaki T. SARS-CoV-2 spike protein S1 subunit induces pro-inflammatory responses via toll-like receptor 4 signaling in murine and human macrophages. Heliyon. 2021;7(2):e06187.
250. Zhang H, Li L, Wang Y, Dong F, Chen X, Liu F, et al. NF-κB signaling maintains the survival of cadmium-exposed human renal glomerular endothelial cells. Int J Mol Med. 2016;38(2):417–22.
251. Swanson L, Katkar GD, Tam J, Pranadinata RF, Chareddy Y, Coates J, et al. TLR4 signaling and macrophage inflammatory responses are dampened by GIV/Girdin. Proc Natl Acad Sci U S A. 2020;117(43):26895–906.
252. Aboudounya MM, Heads RJ. COVID-19 and Toll-Like Receptor 4 (TLR4): SARS-CoV-2 may bind and activate TLR4 to increase ACE2 expression, facilitating entry and causing hyperinflammation. Mediators Inflamm. 2021;2021:8874339.
253. Fung TS, Liu DX. Activation of the c-Jun NH2-terminal kinase pathway by coronavirus infectious bronchitis virus promotes apoptosis independently of c-Jun. Cell Death Dis. 2017;8(12):3215.
254. Mizutani T, Fukushi S, Ishii K, Sasaki Y, Kenri T, Saijo M, et al. Mechanisms of establishment of persistent SARS-CoV-infected cells. Biochem Biophys Res Commun. 2006;347(1):261–5.
255. Mizutani T, Fukushi S, Saijo M, Kurane I, Morikawa S. JNK and PI3k/Akt signaling pathways are required for establishing persistent SARS-CoV infection in Vero E6 cells. Biochim Biophys Acta. 2005;1741(1–2):4–10.
256. Surjit M, Liu B, Jameel S, Chow VTK, Lal SK. The SARS coronavirus nucleocapsid protein induces actin reorganization and apoptosis in COS-1 cells in the absence of growth factors. Biochem J. 2004;383(Pt 1):13–8.
257. Diemer C, Schneider M, Schätzl HM, Gilch S. Modulation of host cell death by SARS coronavirus proteins. In: Lal SK, editor. Molecular biology of the SARS-coronavirus. Berlin, Heidelberg, Springer; 2010. p. 231–45.
258. Varshney B, Lal SK. SARS-CoV accessory protein 3b induces AP-1 transcriptional activity through activation of JNK and ERK pathways. Biochemistry. 2011;50(24):5419–25.
259. Matsuyama T, Kubli SP, Yoshinaga SK, Pfeffer K, Mak TW. An aberrant STAT pathway is central to COVID-19. Cell Death Differ. 2020;27(12):3209–25.
260. Lei X, Dong X, Ma R, Wang W, Xiao X, Tian Z, et al. Activation and evasion of type I interferon responses by SARS-CoV-2. Nat Commun. 2020;11(1):3810.
261. Kopecky-Bromberg SA, Martínez-Sobrido L, Frieman M, Baric RA, Palese P. Severe acute respiratory syndrome coronavirus open reading frame (ORF) 3b, ORF 6, and nucleocapsid proteins function as interferon antagonists. J Virol. 2007;81(2):548–57.
262. Frieman M, Yount B, Heise M, Kopecky-Bromberg SA, Palese P, Baric RS. Severe acute respiratory syndrome coronavirus ORF6 antagonizes STAT1 function by sequestering nuclear import factors on the rough endoplasmic reticulum/Golgi membrane. J Virol. 2007;81(18):9812–24.
263. Gordon DE, Jang GM, Bouhaddou M, Xu J, Obernier K, White KM, et al. A SARS-CoV-2 protein interaction map reveals targets for drug repurposing. Nature. 2020;583(7816):459–68.
264. Kawai T, Takahashi K, Sato S, Coban C, Kumar H, Kato H, et al. IPS-1, an adaptor triggering RIG-I- and Mda5-mediated type I interferon induction. Nat Immunol. 2005;6(10):981–8.
265. Seth RB, Sun L, Ea C-K, Chen ZJ. Identification and characterization of MAVS, a mitochondrial antiviral signaling protein that activates NF-kappaB and IRF 3. Cell. 2005;122(5):669–82.
266. Siu K-L, Kok K-H, Ng M-HJ, Poon VKM, Yuen K-Y, Zheng B-J, et al. Severe acute respiratory syndrome coronavirus M protein inhibits type I interferon production by impeding the formation of TRAF3.TANK.TBK1/IKKepsilon complex. J Biol Chem. 2009;284(24):16202–9.
267. Sa Ribero M, Jouvenet N, Dreux M, Nisole S. Interplay between SARS-CoV-2 and the type I interferon response. PLoS Pathog. 2020;16(7):e1008737.
268. Schindler C, Levy DE, Decker T. JAK-STAT signaling: from interferons to cytokines *. J Biol Chem. 2007;282(28):20059–63.

269. Thoms M, Buschauer R, Ameismeier M, Koepke L, Denk T, Hirschenberger M, et al. Structural basis for translational shutdown and immune evasion by the Nsp1 protein of SARS-CoV-2. Science. 2020;369(6508):1249–55.
270. Yuen C-K, Lam J-Y, Wong W-M, Mak L-F, Wang X, Chu H, et al. SARS-CoV-2 nsp13, nsp14, nsp15 and orf6 function as potent interferon antagonists. Emerg Microbes Infect. 2020;9(1):1418–28.
271. Hu Y, Li W, Gao T, Cui Y, Jin Y, Li P, et al. The severe acute respiratory syndrome coronavirus nucleocapsid inhibits type I interferon production by interfering with TRIM25-mediated RIG-I ubiquitination. J Virol. 2017;91(8):e02143. https://doi.org/10.1128/JVI.02143-16.
272. Moustaqil M, Ollivier E, Chiu H-P, Van Tol S, Rudolffi-Soto P, Stevens C, et al. SARS-CoV-2 proteases PLpro and 3CLpro cleave IRF3 and critical modulators of inflammatory pathways (NLRP12 and TAB1): implications for disease presentation across species. Emerg Microbes Infect. 2021;10(1):178–95.
273. Frieman M, Ratia K, Johnston RE, Mesecar AD, Baric RS. Severe acute respiratory syndrome coronavirus papain-like protease ubiquitin-like domain and catalytic domain regulate antagonism of IRF3 and NF-kappaB signaling. J Virol. 2009;83(13):6689–705.
274. Seif F, Khoshmirsafa M, Aazami H, Mohsenzadegan M, Sedighi G, Bahar M. The role of JAK-STAT signaling pathway and its regulators in the fate of T helper cells. Cell Commun Signal. 2017;15(1):23.
275. Nan Y, Wu C, Zhang Y-J. Interplay between Janus Kinase/Signal Transducer and activator of transcription signaling activated by type I interferons and viral antagonism. Front Immunol. 2017;8:1758.
276. Desai N, Neyaz A, Szabolcs A, Shih AR, Chen JH, Thapar V, et al. Temporal and spatial heterogeneity of host response to SARS-CoV-2 pulmonary infection. Nat Commun. 2020;11(1):6319.
277. Boudewijns R, Thibaut HJ, Kaptein SJF, Li R, Vergote V, Seldeslachts L, et al. STAT2 signaling restricts viral dissemination but drives severe pneumonia in SARS-CoV-2 infected hamsters. Nat Commun. 2020;11(1):5838.
278. Luo J, Lu S, Yu M, Zhu L, Zhu C, Li C, et al. The potential involvement of JAK-STAT signaling pathway in the COVID-19 infection assisted by ACE2. Gene. 2021;768:145325.
279. McClain MT, Constantine FJ, Henao R, Liu Y, Tsalik EL, Burke TW, et al. Dysregulated transcriptional responses to SARS-CoV-2 in the periphery. Nat Commun. 2021;12(1):1079.
280. Wu Y, Ma L, Zhuang Z, Cai S, Zhao Z, Zhou L, et al. Main protease of SARS-CoV-2 serves as a bifunctional molecule in restricting type I interferon antiviral signaling. Signal Transduct Target Ther. 2020;5(1):221.
281. Aydemir MN, Aydemir HB, Korkmaz EM, Budak M, Cekin N, Pinarbasi E. Computationally predicted SARS-COV-2 encoded microRNAs target NFKB, JAK/STAT and TGFB signaling pathways. Gene Rep. 2021;22:101012.
282. Xia H, Cao Z, Xie X, Zhang X, Chen JY-C, Wang H, et al. Evasion of Type I Interferon by SARS-CoV-2. Cell Rep. 2020;33(1):108234.
283. Li J-Y, Liao C-H, Wang Q, Tan Y-J, Luo R, Qiu Y, et al. The ORF6, ORF8 and nucleocapsid proteins of SARS-CoV-2 inhibit type I interferon signaling pathway. Virus Res. 2020;286:198074.
284. Mu J, Fang Y, Yang Q, Shu T, Wang A, Huang M, et al. SARS-CoV-2 N protein antagonizes type I interferon signaling by suppressing phosphorylation and nuclear translocation of STAT1 and STAT2. Cell Discov. 2020;6:65.
285. Cao Z, Xia H, Rajsbaum R, Xia X, Wang H, Shi P-Y. Ubiquitination of SARS-CoV-2 ORF7a promotes antagonism of interferon response. Cell Mol Immunol. 2021;18(3):746–8.

289. Thoms M, [illegible] M, [illegible] (2020) Structural basis for translational shutdown and immune evasion by the Nsp1 protein of SARS-CoV-2. Science [illegible]

290. [illegible]

# Chapter 6
# Identification of the COVID-19 Droplet Deposition Path and Its Effects on the Human Respiratory Tract Before and After the Disease: A Scoping Novel Respiratory Mask Design

**Hamidreza Mortazavy Beni, Hamed Mortazavi, Maryam Mansoori, and Fatemeh Aghaei**

## Introduction

Coronavirus was first identified in 1965, with an average size of 0.15–0.08 μm [1]. At the time, no one thought that the virus could change its genetic structure, and appears as COVID-19 and could plunge the world into crisis in 2020. According to the World Health Organization, the death rate from the coronavirus is 10 times higher than the swine flu, which was common from 2009 to 2010. Until now, it was thought that the virus was transmitted through contact and droplet outputs from the airways during cough and sneezing. But recently, with the help of high-sensitivity laser cameras, researchers have found that even in normal conversations, these viruses with a diameter smaller than 10 μm can float in the air for a long time. Moreover, microdroplets with a diameter smaller than 5 μm can also be easily transmitted through inhalation to other people's airways in longer paths [2].

Coronavirus belongs to the large, positive, and single-strand RNA viruses [3]. This virus is one of the subbranches of acute respiratory syndrome virus, SARS,

H. M. Beni (✉) · H. Mortazavi
Department of Biomedical Engineering, Arsanjan Branch, Islamic Azad University, Arsanjan, Iran
e-mail: HRM.Beni@iau.ac.ir

M. Mansoori
Department of Molecular Medicine, Faculty of Advanced Technologies, Iran University of Medical Sciences, Tehran, Iran

F. Aghaei
Department of Immunology, Shiraz University of Medical Sciences, Shiraz, Iran


S. Adibi et al. (eds.), *Frontiers of COVID-19*,
https://doi.org/10.1007/978-3-031-08045-6_6

which is associated with clinical symptoms in the lower and upper respiratory tract. One of the most important transmitting ways for the virus is through the air, which can be transported on air paths inside the room. During respiratory activity, the size of the droplets increases, and the actual size distribution of these droplets depends on parameters such as expiratory air velocity, fluid viscosity, and flow path [4]. Lippmann [5] concluded that the deposition efficiency of aerosol particles with an aerodynamic diameter greater than 2 μm depends on the Stokes number. Nowak et al. [6] used a simulation model of CT scans and found that in airway intersections, the deposition mechanism was more prevalent. On the other hand, Matida et al. [7] used the eddy interaction model to particles deposition and concluded that the kinetic velocity of the flow turbulent plays a major role in the particles deposition. In the human respiratory system, Heyder [8] concluded that due to the inlet air forces applied to inhaled particles, their path differs from that of airflow lines. Also, the most important mechanical forces applied to them include gravity, inertia and impact transfer from molecular collisions. Therefore, the particles move from the flow lines and deposit on the surfaces of the respiratory tract.

Zhang and Kleinstreuer [9], in a model of the upper human airway, analyzed the transfer and deposition of nanoparticles in a steady flow. Like Heyder [8], they concluded that the regional deposition of nanoparticles in the 0.001–0.15 μm range could depends on the flow rate of inhalation, particle size, and geometric length scale. Mahesh et al. [10] developed a numerical algorithm to perform large eddy simulation (LES) in very complex geometries such as the respiratory system geometry. This algorithm is very efficient for very fine mesh with high Reynolds numbers. Zhou and Cheng [11] also found that deposition efficiency, in addition to stock numbers subordination, similar to Lipmann's research [5] depends on the other parameters, including the angle of intersection and the diameter of the tract. Also, the deposition of particles in the trachea depends on the type of flow in this area which is turbulent, and is due to the laryngeal jet. Jin et al. [12] simulated the deposition of inhaled particles in the human upper respiratory tract by LES method. Then, they modeled a steady flow with three types of flow rates of 30, 60, and 90 L/min. The results showed that the growth of diameter and density of particles and the intensity of respiration increased the deposition of particles in the upper human respiratory tract. Farkas et al. [13] found that nanoparticle deposition patterns were more uniform than microparticles in the entire respiratory tract at all flow rates. They also observed that the deposition of nanoparticles in the airway decreases with flow velocity increasing. However, in the case of microparticles, deposition increases at high flow velocities. Xi and Longest [14], using a real model, concluded that the low Reynolds number k-omega turbulent model was suitable for simulating particles with a diameter of 1 to 31 μm in a simplified geometry of the respiratory system. They also found that real geometries provided the best predictions of regional deposition compared to experimental data as a function of particle diameter. Shi et al. [15] studied the inertial particles in the diameter range of 1 to 50 μm, considering the steady laminar flow rate of 7.5 and 20 L/min, and concluded that the most deposition occurs in the anterior part of the nasal cavity. The results of the simulation of Li et al. [16], like other researchers [7, 9] in the upper human airway, demonstrate that the specific inlet velocities affect the particle deposition. They also found that kinematic upstream effects are very important for particle deposition, although they have less effect on flow field. Also, due to the structures of the tracheal ring, the highest deposition occurs at a higher flow rate. The results of Lin et al. [17], as other studies [11], showed that a turbulent jet flow in the larynx occurs, while the intensity of turbulence in other airways is weaker. Jayaraju et al. [18] set the inhalation rate at 15, 30 and 60 L/min with a particle diameter between 2 and 20 μm. Their results revealed that heavier particles at very low flow rates cause more deposition than sediments at higher flow rates. Oral inhalation (15, 30, and 60 L/min) along with the deposition of aerosols with a diameter of 1–30 μm calculated by computational fluid dynamics (CFD) using the K-epsilon turbulent model by Ma and Lutchen [19] similar to Jayaraju et al. method [18]. They found that more deposition were obtained from micrometer sized aerosol particles [19]. Mihai et al. [20] exploited two stable strategies to model the flow including steady Reynolds-averaged Navier–Stokes (RANS) and LES. The greatest differences in static pressure distribution in the air walls between LES and RANS data were observed at the cross-sectional area of the pharynx. An analysis of Shanley et al. [21] in a steady laminar flow illustrated that a simple uniform flow occurs in the nose with a peak in the speed, and a peak immediately occurs in the posterior part in the size of a vorticity. The results of particle accumulation smaller than 10 μm through the Lagrangian method depicted that the deposition increases with higher particle size and flow velocity. In other studies conducted by Kleinstreuer and Zhang [22], the flows of a respiratory system can include flows such as turbulent jet with substantially pressure drop, while breathing in the airways. It was also found that micron particles were modeled in the Lagrange-Euler framework and nanoparticles were modeled based on the Euler-Euler approach preferably. Inthavong et al. [23] found that there was an upsurge in deposition in the nasal cavity for nanoparticles. Huang and Zhang [24] concluded that the deposition is highly dependent on the rate of respiration and is less dependent on the turbulence of the flow. Particles are mainly distributed in high-velocity axial regions and basically follow the secondary flow. Frank et al. [25] recognized that speeds of more than 3 m/s slowed down particle deposition in the respiratory system. Philip and Wang [26] believe that the complex geometry of the airway of the human respiratory system itself creates a stable hydrodynamic flow. The Li et al. [27] findings indicate that the efficacy of microparticle deposition is much higher than that of nanoparticles. Because the diameter of nanoparticles is less important than that of microparticles in particle deposition. Yousefi et al. [28], like other researchers [11, 12, 17], found that the most particles deposition exist in the larynx, where the airways have a smaller cross-sectional area. Also, as Mihai et al. [20] showed, particle deposition patterns in airways depend on their initial inlet position at the mouth inlet. Varghese and Gangamma [29] believe that the presence of water droplet in the inhale can alter the size of inhaled aerosols. Therefore, they could change the deposition profile of inhaled airborne particles in the lungs. However, the analytical method applied for particles with diameter more than 1 μm and at high concentrations has a high computational error. Basu et al. [30] simulated airflow during respiration through a steady, viscous, and laminar model and found that such a method demonstrates a relative insensitivity to input disturbances. Islam et al. [31] in the studies of sediment pattern showed that most aerosol particles are placed on the tracheal wall instead of the carina angle. At low flow velocity, particle density is mostly in the middle of the trachea. At higher flow velocity, particle density increases at the top region and in the path change region. Like other studies [12, 14, 18, 27], they concluded that particle diameter and fluid flow velocity affect the deposition pattern. Using the CFD simulation, they found that the effects of turbulence on deposition were more effective for larger diameter particles and less effective for smaller diameter particles. Using the CT-based model, they found that a significant amount of particle deposition settles on the tracheal wall, whereas in the simulation it was observed that more particles precipitate at the carnival angle in the unreal model [32]. In another numerical study, they depicted that neither Euler-Lagrange (E-L) nor Euler-Euler (E-E) methods influence the sedimentary patterns of nanoparticles with diameter of 50 nm and the flow rate of 25 L/min [33]. Ma et al. [34] exploited a standard DPM method for particle deposition, and the results showed how particle deposition is affected by throat narrow path so that the reduction of the cross-sectional area of the pharynx in the epiglottis has a great impact on the flow field in the airways and in the case of oral inhalation has an effect on the deposition of the regional sediment. Kayhani et al. [35] found that in the main nasal route, the highest velocity of inhaled air alongside the nasal floor occurred below the lower turbinate. Another low peak also occurs in the middle of the airway, between the lower and middle turbinate and the septum. About 30% of the inhaled volume flow rate passes under the lower turbinate and about 10% passes through the olfactory airway. Horschler et al. [36] presented the results of numerical simulation of flow in a model of the human nasal cavity in a multiblock structural grid and compared it with experimental data. Calculations for inhalation and exhalation at rest state were performed with the Reynolds numbers Re = 1560 and Re = 1230, respectively, in the nostrils. Grgic et al. [37] illustrated that aerosol deposition is more common in the larynx and trachea and is caused by morphological limitations of the pharynx, glottal, and flow jets. Also, it was found that the deposition efficiency is related to the inertia parameter. Even if, the Stokes number is kept constant, due to the change in the velocity profile, the accumulation efficiency increases with increasing Reynolds flow. In another study they showed that both total and regional deposition have a large differences, as well as a significant difference in intersubjectivity [38]. The results of Heenan et al. [39] showed that there is a strong relationship between local deposition and local fluid velocity field. The level of local deposition is strongly related to the velocity and curvature of the flow. Shi et al. [40] found that very small particles, smaller than 5 nanometers in diameter, have a particular importance because they were absorbed more rapidly. Therefore, as opposed to the larger particles, have higher toxicity or therapeutic effect. Xi and Longest [41] examined the particles with 1 nanometer size up to 1 μm and an inhalation flow rate of 4–30 L/min. Under these circumstances, the turbulence was visible only in the area of the nasal valve and the posterior part of the nasopharynx. They also found that many of the main parts of the nose have a linear flow. Chen et al. [42] found that secondary flow may contribute to the deposition of particles in the filled airways for actual inhalation. The results obtained by Nicolaou and Zaki [43] provide an insight into how the geometry changes affect the aerosol deposition and the dispersion of the deposition data. The assessment of flow fields in different mouth and throat geometries allows to investigate the source of the deposition dependence on Reynolds number. The results of Shinneeb and Pollard [44] showed that the nature of the flow in the respiratory system is definitely three-dimensional and is associated with the recirculation as well as jet-like and sink-like form flows. In general, it can be understood from the above researches that there is a great deal of difference in the findings, due to the complex geometry of the respiratory system and the computational method used for particle deposition. As very little information is available on droplet deposition in the respiratory system, employing of the FSI method, if more complicated, generates accurate answer.

Microdroplets are a subcategory of aerosols; nevertheless, not only are there no investigations toward viral effects of droplets smaller than 10 μm diameter, but even in vitro studies investigations to determine the exact deposition location of these droplets in the upper human respiratory system have also not been carried out. These small microdroplets are also able to pass through ordinary respirator masks and can infect people, if the permitted distance is not observed. However, it should be noted that ordinary masks are more effective for droplets larger than 10 μm [45]. As mentioned in the literature review, avoiding the real model in the respiratory system can immensely affect the results of particle deposition. Not only is real geometry very important in modeling, but computational methods based on actual body performance also can affect the results. Unlike previous researches, which examined the motion of particles by CFD, in this study, the FSI model is used. Because the physiological conditions of the body behave as FSI manner.

## Methods

### *Computational Model*

The model used in this study is related to a 30-year-old healthy man who has been reviewed and approved in the past research in terms of CFD [46] and FSI [47] and has a very high level of reliability. In this model, the three-dimensional (3D) model of the upper airway is extracted using CT technology. Then, three-dimensional geometry is constructed, which includes the nostril entrance to the carina (nasal cavity, pharynx, larynx, and trachea). It is very carefully segmented and meshed to create a computational grid, considering the appropriate boundary layer. This model, after examining the independence of the grid, has been made with an approximate number of 2.6 million computational nodes for mesh production. This computational grid has very good quality which could accurately predict the behavior of thyroid cartilage failure as well as brain damage in respiratory reflexes.

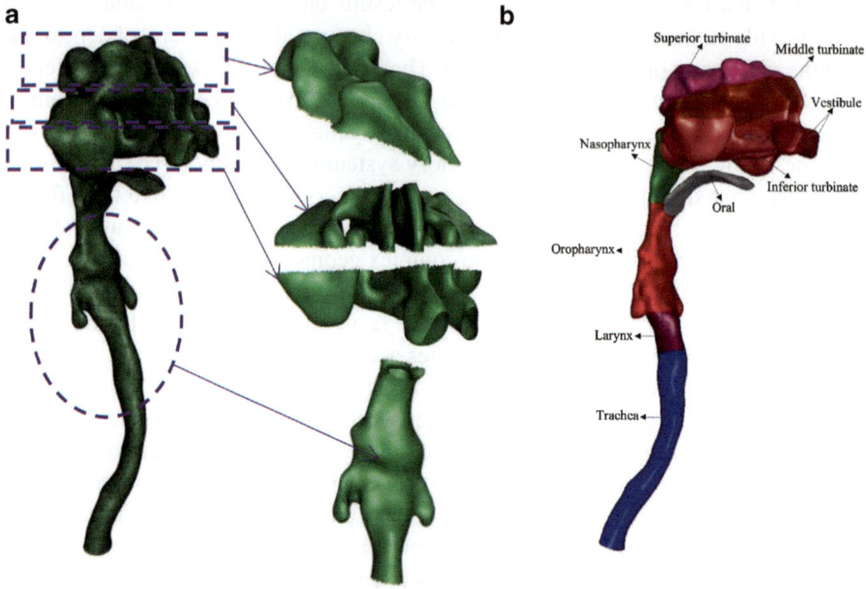


**Fig. 6.1** Computational model geometry and meshing. (**a**) Numerical model meshing. (**b**) Geometry of the 3-D model

Details of reconstruction of geometry and meshing of this model has been presented in details, in Mortazavy et al. study [46], and it is not mentioned here again. Figure 6.1 shows the meshed geometry of the computational model. It should be noted that in this figure, the nasal cavity was divided into three parts: superior, middle and inferior turbinate. The volume of each area is increasing from top to bottom, so that the superior turbinate has the most and the inferior turbinate has the least volume. These areas have a special importance, so that they play the important role on heat transfer, increase moisture, and filter inhalation air. What makes this division salient, is that these areas are full of blood vessels which their vastness have changed with slight changes in temperature, humidity, physical activity, body position, and hormonal changes.

## *Governing Equations*

Air is considered as a viscous and incompressible fluid. The governing equations for the viscous, incompressible, and steady state in the human respiratory system in the state of turbulent flow are the Navier-Stokes, and continuity equations. These equations include the following.

$$\frac{\partial U_i}{\partial x_i} = 0 \tag{6.1}$$

$$U_i \frac{\partial U_j}{\partial x_i} = -\frac{1}{\rho}\frac{\partial P}{\partial x_i} + \frac{\partial}{\partial x_i}\left[ v\left( \frac{\partial U_i}{\partial x_j} + \frac{\partial U_j}{\partial x_i} \right) - \overline{U_i' U_j'} \right] + G_i \tag{6.2}$$

In these equations, the parameters $U$, $\rho$, $P$, $v$, and $G_i$ for air fluid represent speed, density, pressure, kinematic viscosity, and gravity term, respectively. Also $i$ and $j$ represent Cartesian coordinates. Based on Kleinstreuer and Zhang [22], the E-L method was selected as the best method to investigate the microdroplet particles movement along with fluid. The equation of motion for the microdroplet is as follows.

$$\frac{du_i^P}{dt} = \left( \frac{18\mu}{\rho^P d^2 C_c} \right)\left( U_i - u_i^P \right) + g_i + F_x \tag{6.3}$$

Also $\mu$, $\rho^P$, $d$, $g_i$, and $F_x$ are viscosity, density, particle diameter, gravity term, and, Brownian Force, respectively. Furthermore, in this equation, $\frac{dx_i}{dt} = u_i^P$ . Also $C_c$ is the Cunningham correction factor, which is equal to

$$C_c = 1 + \frac{2\lambda}{d}\left( 1.257 + 0.4e^{-\frac{1.1d}{2\lambda}} \right). \tag{6.4}$$

In this equation $\lambda$ is the average molecular distance for air and is assumed to be 0.065 μm. The Stokes number is used to calculate the ratio of the relaxation time of the droplet per the characteristic time scale of the flow, and is defined as follows.

$$St^P = \frac{\tau u_f}{d_c} \tag{6.5}$$

In which $\tau$ is the relaxation time, $u_f$ is the velocity of the fluid, and $d_c$ is the hydraulic diameter of the tract through which the fluid passes. By putting the value of relaxation time, the following equation is obtained.

$$St^P = \frac{\rho^P d^2 u_f}{18\mu d_c} \tag{6.6}$$

The walls of the airway are considered as an elastic wall. It is also assumed that the droplets are absorbed at the first encounter with the wall. In the FSI boundary condition, the equilibrium force between the fluid and solid is determined as the following equation.

$$\sigma_{ij}^{f} n = -\sigma_{ij}^{s} n, \tag{6.7}$$

where, $\sigma_{ij}^{f}$ is fluid stress tensor, $\sigma_{ij}^{s}$ is solid stress tensor, and $n$ is the outward vector perpendicular to the surface of the FSI facing. More details on the governing equations of FSI mentioned in the Mortazavy et al. study [47]. The difference is that in the present model, the input of the flow rate is from the nostril or mouth, and its output is from the end of trachea (carina zone) as the boundary condition. It is noticeable that when the entrance is from the nose, the boundary condition of the wall is applied to the entrance of the mouth, and vice versa.

## *Numerical Solution and Method Verification*

In order to solve the numerical equations, the geometry was entered to the fluent 6.3 software (ANSYS, USA). Fluent software converts and solves the governing equations into algebraic equations by the finite volume method. In this study, the second-order upwind scheme was used to the momentum equation discretization, and the SIMPLE algorithm was used to couple the pressure and velocity equations. The k-epsilon turbulence model is a subcategory of the RANS group, which has been shown to have viable results in the use of DPM in the study of deposition mapping in the human respiratory system [19]. In the present study, this method was used, and according to Fig. 6.2, the reliability of this method was confirmed.

Air enters the computational model at 25 °C from the nasal or oral tract. Given that the COVID-19 virus is related to Betacoronavirus family, and the density of Betacoronaviruses is approximately $\rho = 1240\,\text{kg/m}^3$ [48]. Thus, considering $\rho_1 = 998\,\text{kg/m}^3$ for pure water density, $\rho_2 = 1119\,\text{kg/m}^3$ equivalent to 50% water +50% virus (average density), finally $\rho_3 = 1240\,\text{kg/m}^3$ was assumed for net virus droplet. Also, the range of droplet diameter changes was considered from 1 to 10 μm for normal conversation. For the respiratory wall, the expansion of the yang modules was considered in the range of $0.51\ \text{kpa} \leq E \leq 100.64\ \text{kpa}$, which the lowest value is in the uvula area and the highest value is in contact with the hard palate [49]. In order to validate the present study, the results obtained by Cheng [50] in the field of high-density solid aerosol (Fig. 6.2a), and the findings from Heyder study [8] regarding particle deposition with water density (Fig. 6.2b) were used. As can be seen in Fig. 6.2, the results show a similar trend. Of course, according to Fig. 6.2b due to the similarity between the type of boundary conditions and the air flow with the droplet type, a better match has been obtained in the results. The reason for the incomplete overlap in the results can be described in the difference of the analyzed geometries.

# Results

In this study, in two different input states to the model, the fluid flow, and droplet parameters along with wall deformation analysis were investigated: (**A**) flow inlet from the nose with the closed mouth and (**B**) flow inlet from the mouth with the closed nose. In both groups, three flow rates of 6, 15, and 30 L/min were entered to

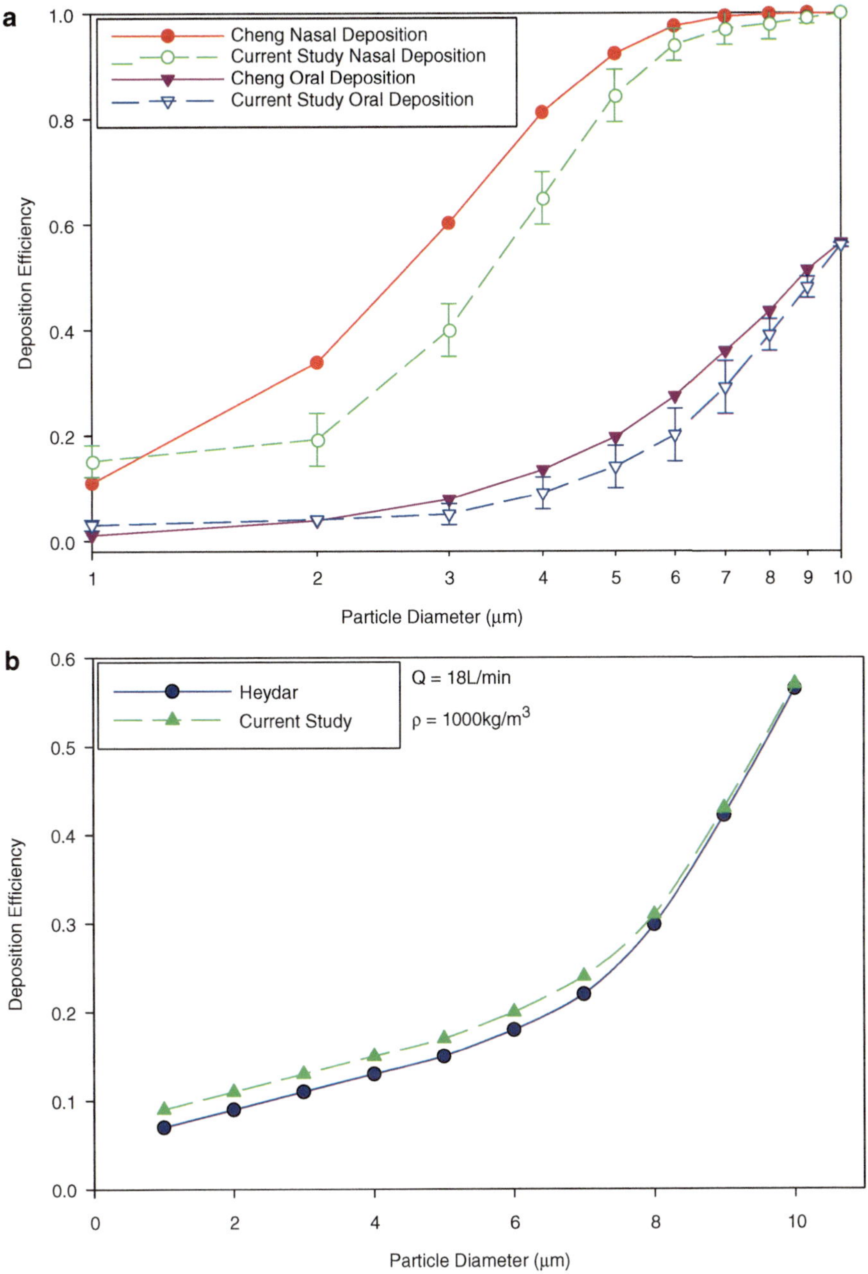


**Fig. 6.2** Comparison of deposition efficiency toward particle diameter for the Cheng and Heyder results with the present model. (**a**) particles deposition in the inhalation through the nose with the closed mouth and vice versa with an input flow rate of 30 L/min in Cheng's study. (**b**) Water droplet deposition in the oral inhalation at an inlet flow rate of 18 L/min in the Heyder study

the model along with the droplet diameter change, and based on this, the performance of the upper respiratory system was evaluated from different aspects. Meanwhile, the flow rate of 6, and the 5 μm droplet diameter are the basis for comparisons. It should be noted that during normal breathing, a man in a state of rest breathes about 500 $cm^3$ of air per inhalation, which is the same as tidal volume at rest [51]. This number is exactly in concordance with the model presented in this study after spirometry testing during patient health in the database [47]. Therefore, the inlet flow rate in the model was considered to be 6 L/min in rest mode.

## *The Flow Enters from the Nose with the Closed Mouth—Group* A

### Simulated Airflow and Droplet Transport and Deposition

According to Fig. 6.3a, the highest droplet deposition occurred in the nasal cavity at rest position. On the other hand, by growth of the droplet density, the amount of deposition is increased in the nasal cavity. The deposition efficiency is always smaller than 5%, and after the nasal cavity, the highest droplet deposition occurs in the nasopharynx, oropharynx, trachea, and larynx, respectively. Nasal deposition rate is several times more than other parts of the respiratory tract. Thus, if just Fig. 6.3b has been considered for investigation of droplet deposition level in three basic parts of the nasal cavity, it is clear that the efficiency of deposition is always smaller than 2.5%. The highest droplet deposition is in the inferior region and the lowest deposition is in the superior turbinate (olfactory zone). Also, with the growth of droplet density, the droplet deposition increases in the olfactory region.

Now, if we evaluate the droplet relaxation time parameter in the respiratory system, similar to contour with transparent face wall in Fig. 6.4, it can be seen that the most relaxation time of the particles is in the nasal part, especially in the olfactory and maxillary sinus area. Due to the geometric conditions in these areas, the flow is recirculated and the droplet get stuck. After these two regions, we should mention the recirculating turbulence flow and relaxation value in the oropharynx zone, which although it is not to the extent of nasal part, but is relatively noticeable throughout the breathing path from the nasopharynx to the trachea. High relaxation of the viral droplet in the superior turbinate, and on the other hand, the presence of the virus receptors in the olfactory epithelium [52] leads to the neurologic attack manifestations in more than 30% of COVID-19 patients [53]. As, taste and odor impairment was observed in the studied subject.

In order to obtain a more significant relationship between the density, the diameter, and the flow rate changes in the whole scope of the droplets study, according to Fig. 6.5, the deposition efficiency curve was plotted according Stokes number. Based on Fig. 6.5a, with the growth of Stokes number, the rate of deposition efficiency increases exponentially in different parts of the respiratory system, so that the changes rate in the Stokes number is smaller than one, and the rate of deposition

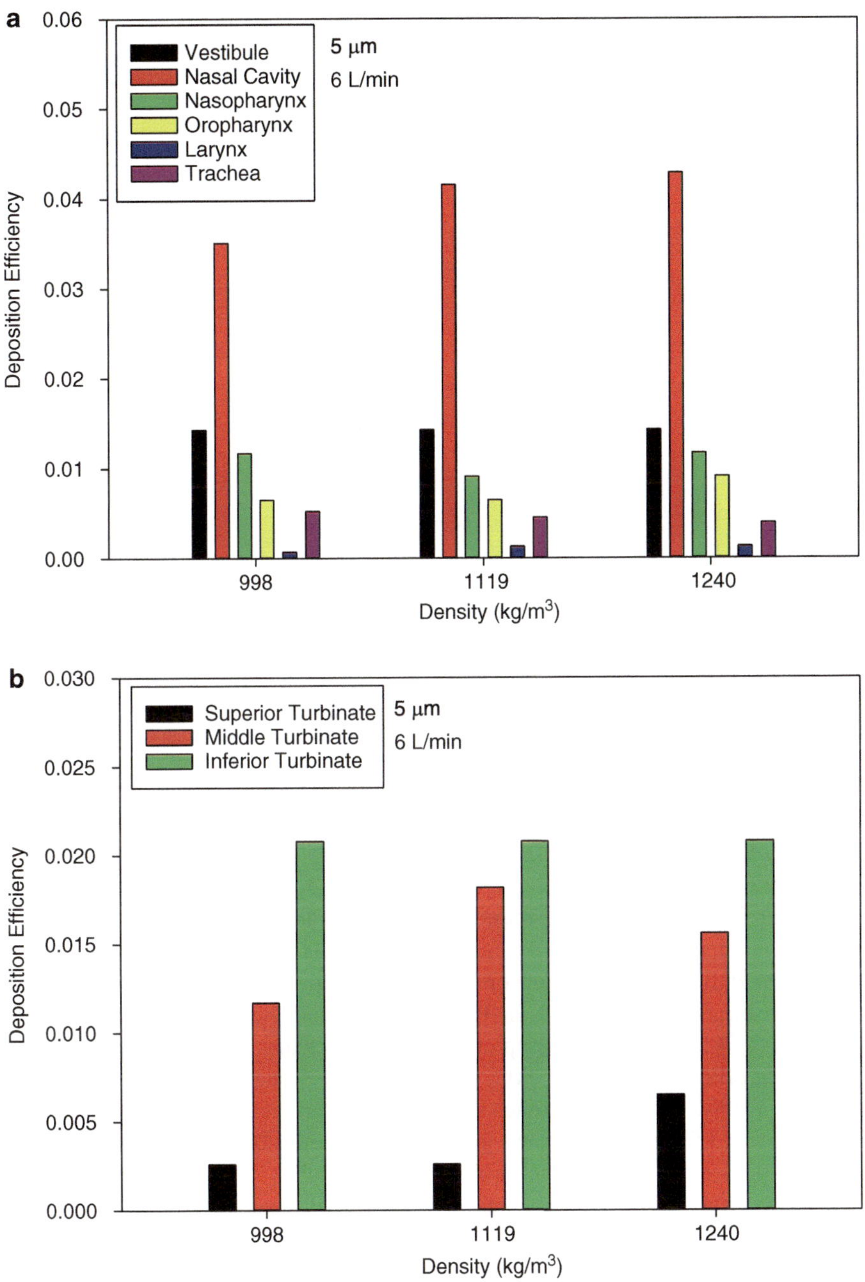


**Fig. 6.3** Droplet deposition in the upper respiratory tract in average density at 5 μm, and 6 L/min condition for the inhalation from the nostril entrance with closed mouth. (**a**) In the entire upper airway. (**b**) Only in the nasal cavity

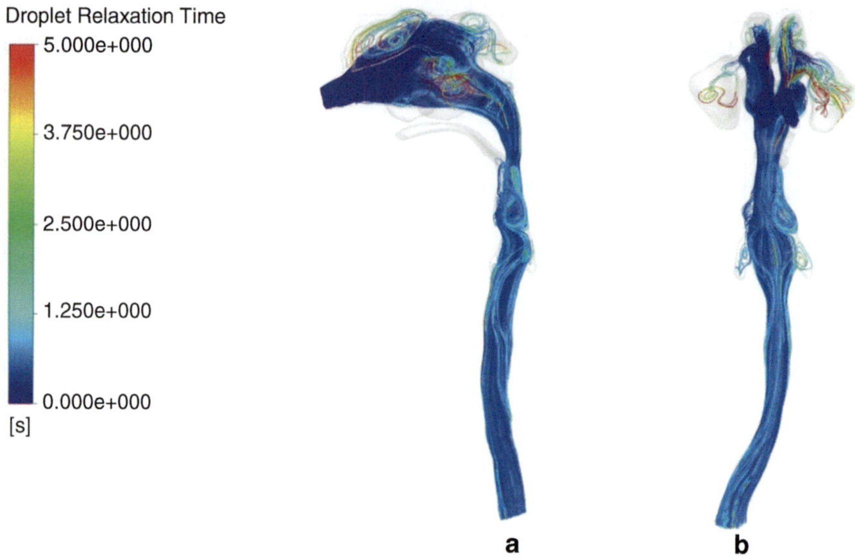


**Fig. 6.4** Droplet relaxation contour with average density at 5 μm, and 6 L/min for Group **A**. (**a**) Anterior droplet relaxation time tracking. (**b**) Posterior droplet relaxation time tracking

does not exceed 40%. The highest report in the amount of deposition is in oropharynx and the lowest amount of deposition in trachea.

Now, according to Fig. 6.5b, if the deposition changes per stokes number considered in the nasal cavity, it could be perceived that the highest droplet deposition occurs in the inferior turbinate which is smaller than 10%, and the lowest deposition is obtained in the superior turbinate.

Figure 6.6a shows the effect of changes in flow rate and droplet diameter on the deposition in the respiratory system. In general, with the growth of diameter or flow rate the amount of deposition efficiency increases. As the drop diameter increases, the effect of flow rate elevation on the droplet deposition enlarged much more. Although the flow rate doubles in 10 μm droplet diameter and flow rate changes from 15 to 30; however, the droplet deposition escalates almost 5 times and the deposition efficiency increases 90%. Figure 6.6b illustrates the same trend only in the nasal cavity, with the difference that deposition efficiency does not exceed 5%. As can be seen from this curve, the greatest deposition is often in the inferior turbinate and the least in the superior turbinate

Droplet deposition is a superficial phenomenon. If the concentration of droplets in the volume has been taken into consideration, the contour of Fig. 6.7 is obtained. It is obvious in this figure that the droplet concentration in the nasal cavity, carina zone, and the oropharynx is higher than other areas, respectively. In other words, in some parts of the respiratory system where geometric curves are complexed, the droplets concentration are trapped.

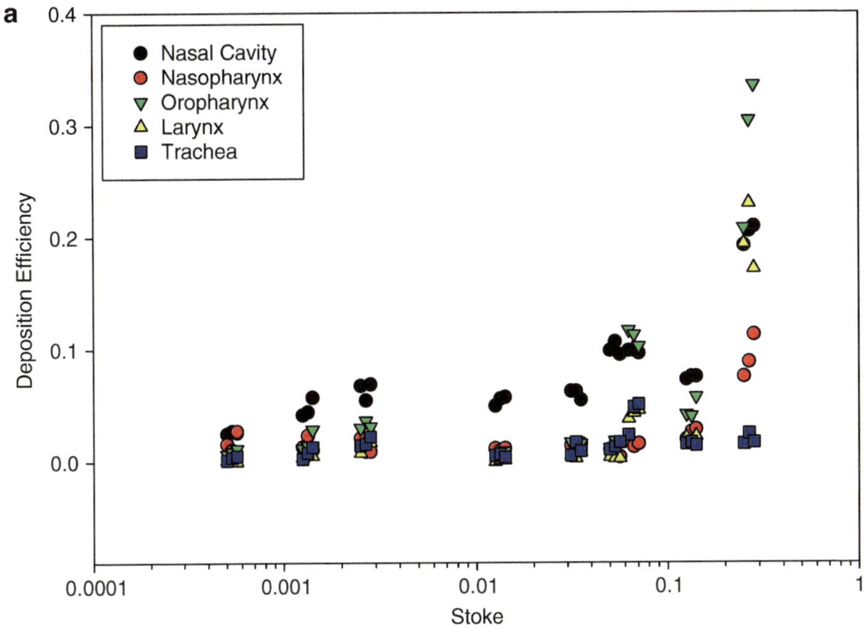


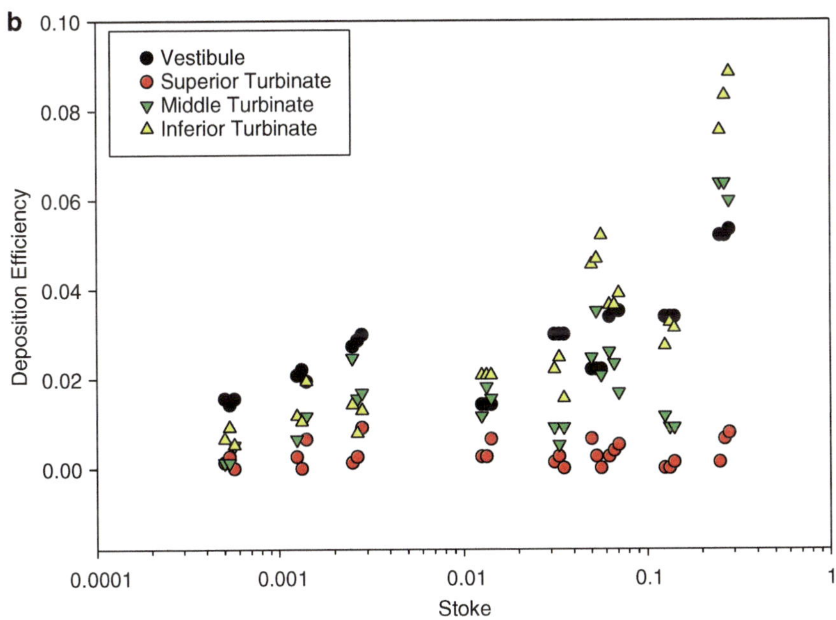


**Fig. 6.5** Deposition efficiency change according to stokes number for Group **A**. (**a**) In the whole respiratory airway. (**b**) In the different zone of the nasal cavity

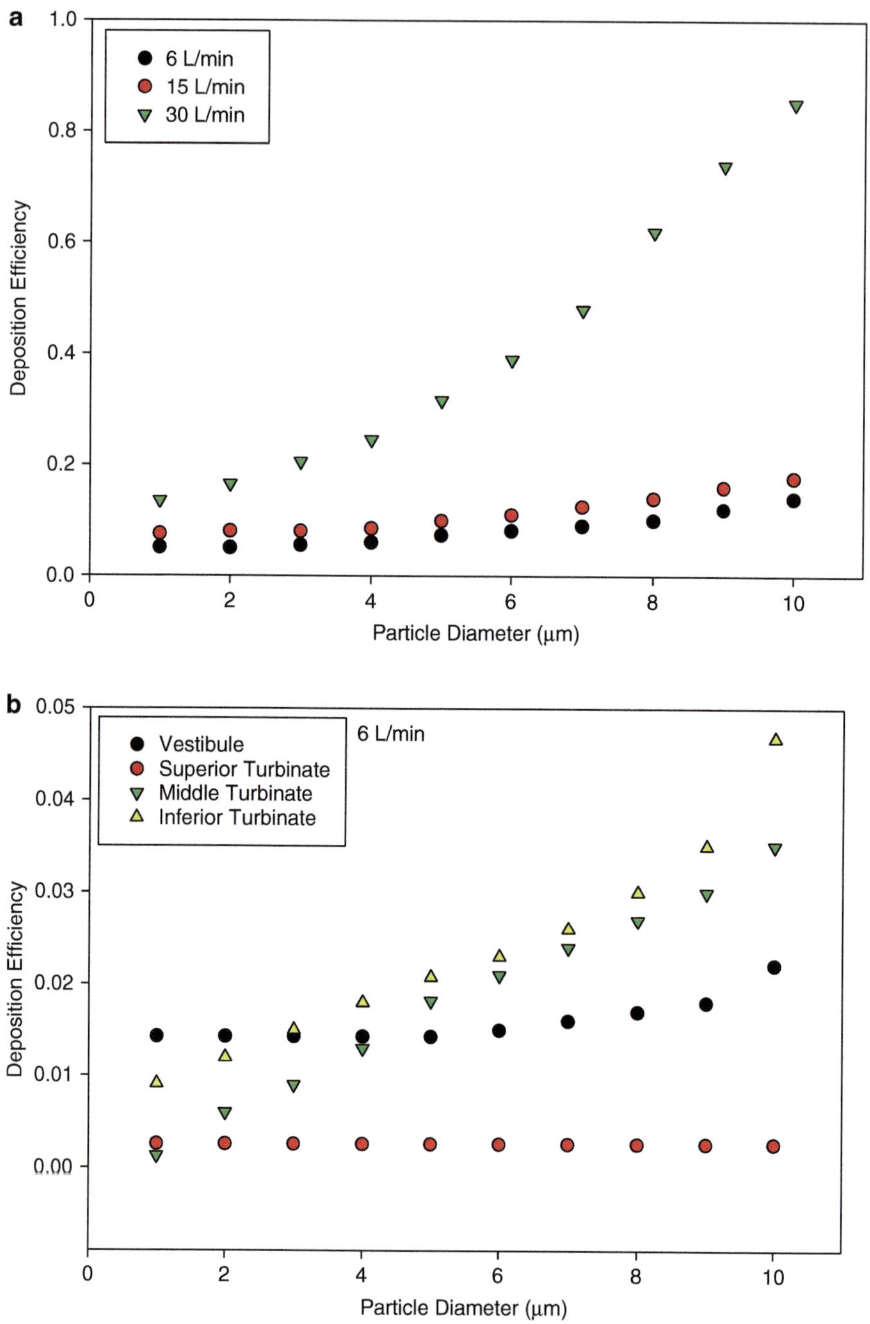


**Fig. 6.6** The effect of diameter on deposition efficiency with average droplet density and 5 μm diameter. (**a**) In the entire inhalation path at the different inlet nostril flow rates. (**b**) In the different nasal cavity zone at a flow rate of 6 L/min

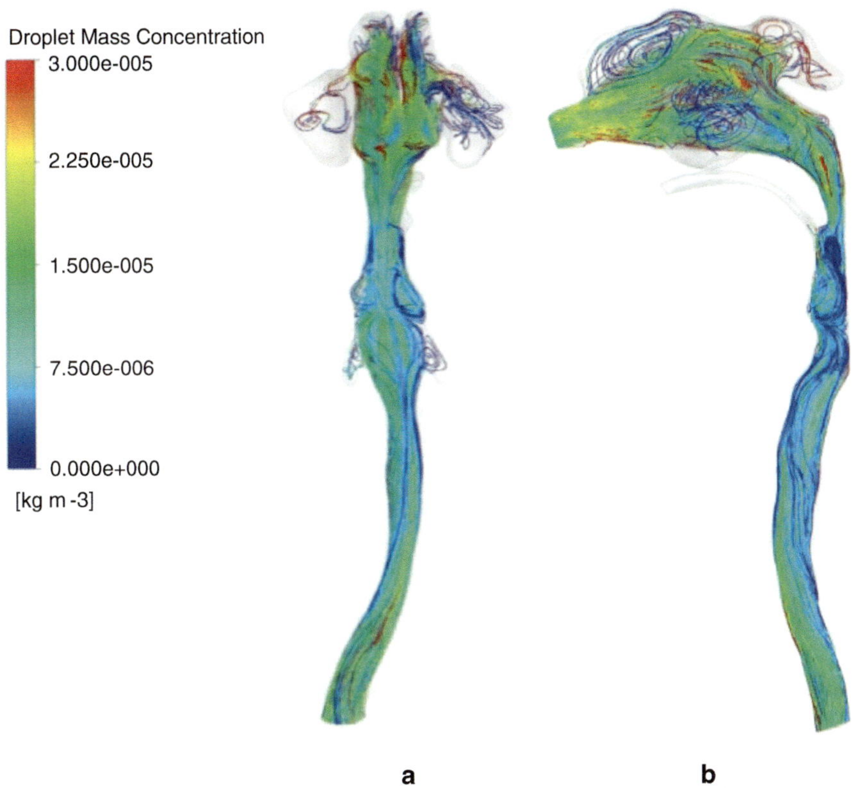


**Fig. 6.7** Concentration droplet contour at average density in 6 L/min, and 5 μm for Group **A**. (**a**) Anterior concentration on the respiratory tract. (**b**) Posterior concentration on the respiratory tract

## Simulated Solid Domain Deformation

As to last analysis of the inhalation through the nose, the deformation contour in the respiratory system is extracted as Fig. 6.8. In this figure, the most deformation is related to the trachea at carina zone. Also, the most deformed part of the nasal cavity is the olfactory zone. In other words, in places where deformation increases, according to the Fig. 6.5, the deposition rate depicts a significant decrease. The maximum deformation rate at flow rates of 15 and 30 L/min is 5 and 21 times higher than the flow rate of 6 L/min, respectively. Additionally, the maximum increase percentage in deformation is several times greater than the rate of flow rate increase.

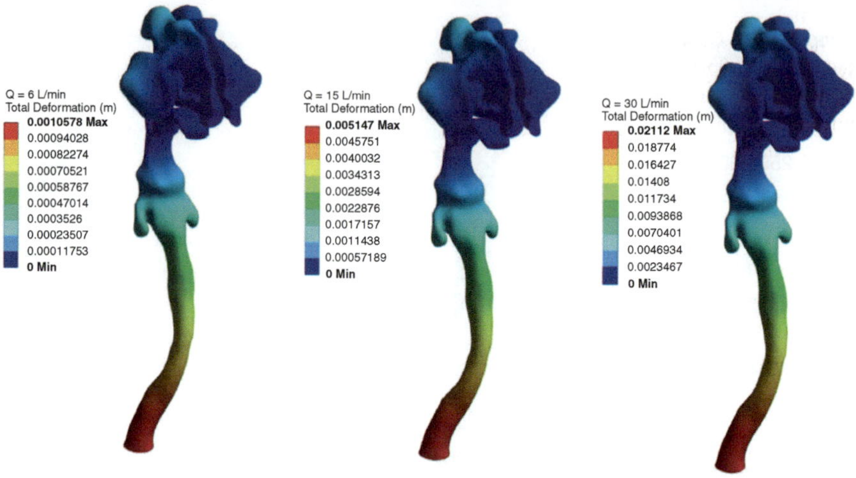


**Fig. 6.8** Deformity contour at average density for different nostril flow rates with closed mouth in droplet diameter of 5 μm

## *The Flow Enters from the Mouth with Closed Nose—Group* B

### Simulated Airflow with Droplet Transport and Deposition

As discussed in section "Simulated Airflow and Droplet Transport and Deposition", nasal breathing can greatly increase transmission of the coronavirus through the olfactory nerve receptor; in other words, the nasal cavity is high-risk area. Whereas, if the inhalation is done just through the mouth, based on the results of Fig. 6.9, the highest droplet deposition in the different density changes occurs in the oral, oropharynx, and trachea, respectively. The deposition efficiency is smaller than 6%, which in the mouth is at least several times greater than the trachea.

The most relaxation time according to Fig. 6.10 has a similar trend as Fig. 6.4, so that it has the highest value in the superior turbinate during the mouth inhalation, with the difference in the number of droplet entering this upper area of the nasal cavity, which is very small. After this area, we should mention the amount of relaxation time in the trachea region, which is relatively significant. The most interesting issue is that relaxation time in oral and oropharynx is almost zero. Also, in general, it can be assumed that the amount of relaxation time is very small, except in the nasal cavity.

According to Fig. 6.11, the highest droplet deposition in oral inhalation occurs in the oral, and oropharynx, why the lowest in the larynx, and trachea, respectively. The amount of deposition in the mouth is significant, and is often several times that of other respiratory areas. For small Stokes numbers (St << 1), the droplet relaxation time is very short, and is almost equal to the fluid response time. Therefore, droplets almost follow the same as air flow field.

Deposition efficiency changes based on droplet diameter at different flow rates for average density are shown in Fig. 6.12. As can be seen, the amount of deposition

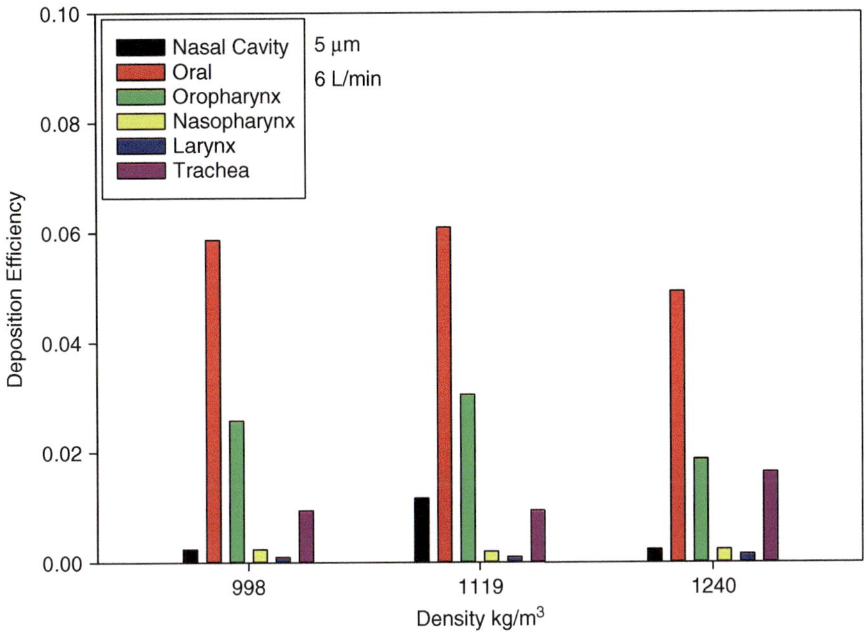


**Fig. 6.9** Droplet deposition in the upper respiratory system regarding density for Group **B** at 5 μm, 6 L/min

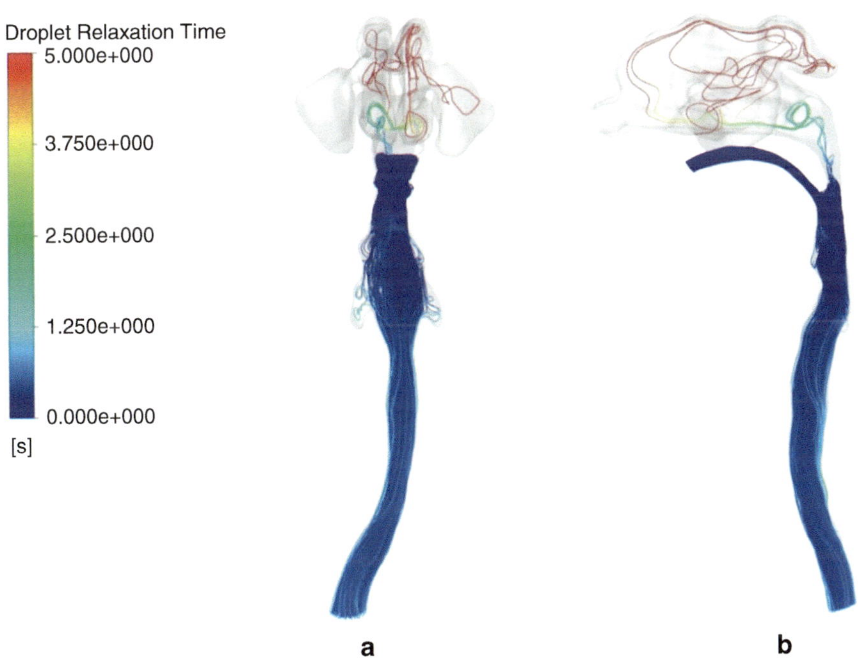


**Fig. 6.10** Droplet relaxation time contour with average density at 5 μm, and 6 L/min for Group **B**. (**a**) Anterior tracking view, (**b**) Posterior tracking view

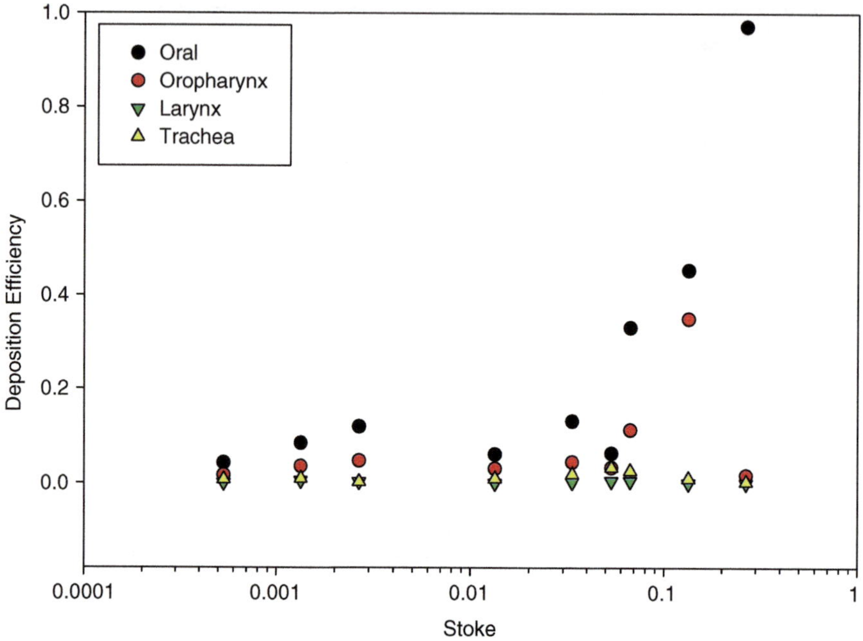


**Fig. 6.11** Droplet deposition efficiency in different stokes numbers for Group **B**

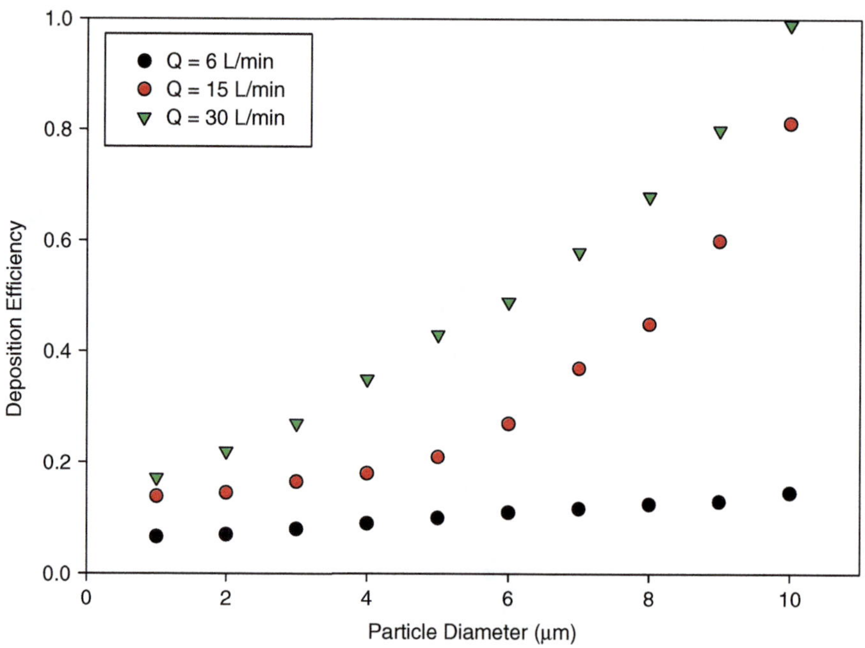


**Fig. 6.12** Deposition efficiency in different droplet diameter, and flow rates for Group **B** at average density

increases with diameter or flow rate elevation. At a flow rate of 6 L/min, the total deposition efficiency in the range of droplet diameter changes from 1 to 10 μm is smaller than 20%, and the incremental slope of the curve is very slow. However, at the flow rates between 15 and 30 L/min, with growth of droplet diameter, the deposition efficiency substantially increases. Such a way that, deposition efficiency is about 100% in 30 L/min flow rate, and 10 μm diameter; in other words, no droplet enters to the lung.

Meanwhile, it is important to study the contours of the droplet mass concentration, as shown in Fig. 6.13, for accurate observation of droplet gathering regions. As can be seen from this figure, in mouth inhalation with closed nose, the nasal cavity is filled with a very small concentration of droplet at the beginning of the flow. This low concentration can also cause deposition due to high relaxation in the olfactory area and maxillary sinus (see Fig. 6.10).

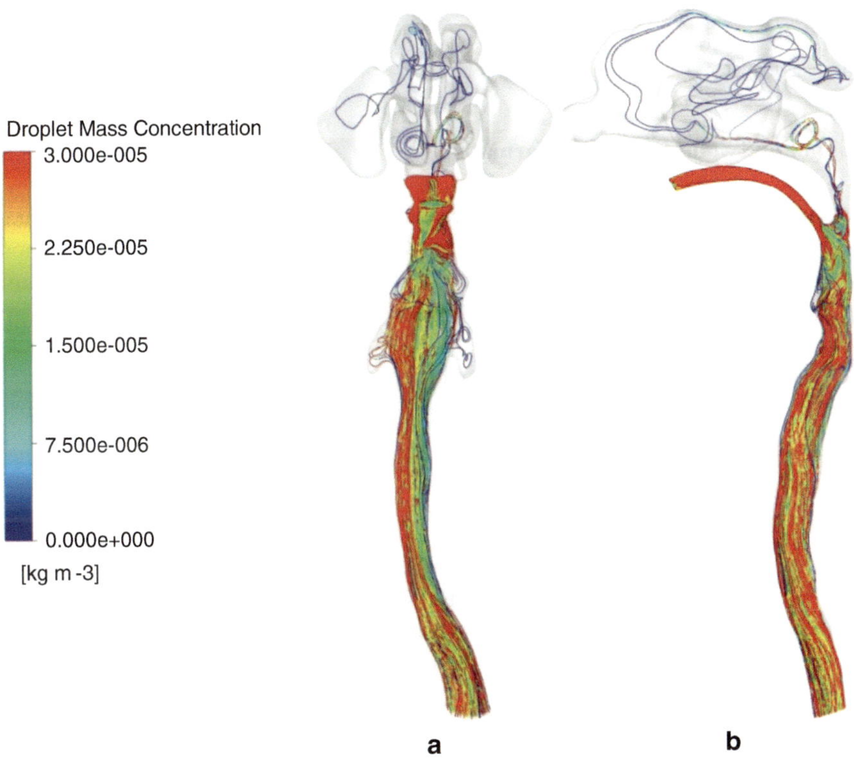


**Fig. 6.13** Droplet mass concentration tracking contour for average density at 5 μm, and 6 L/min. (**a**) Anterior tracking view, (**b**) Posterior tracking view

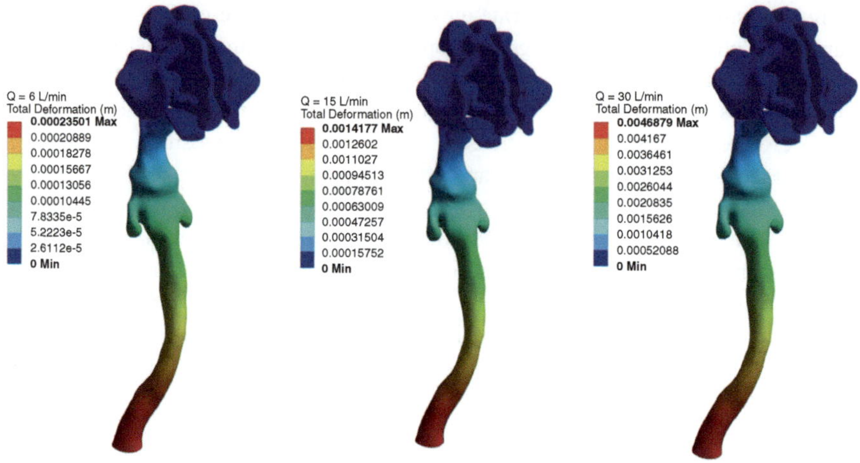


**Fig. 6.14** Deformation contour at average density for different flow rates in Group **B** at 5 μm droplet diameter

### Simulated Solid Domain Deformation

Additionally, as it can be seen from presented deformation contour in Fig. 6.14, it is clear that the deformation in the mouth and nasal cavity is very small, and the most deformation can be seen at the end of the trachea, near the carina. The maximum deformation rate at 15 and 30 L/min flow rates is 6, which is 19 times greater than the 6 L/min flow rate, respectively. In other words, similar to Group **A**, with a marginal increase in flow rate, the deformation rate would be several times greater.

## Discussion

In order to get a more accurate answer, in a real model with DPM method and with the FSI boundary condition in the wall at the time of inhalation, the droplets were injected into the respiratory system from the entrance of the nose or mouth. Finally, a reliable model was developed, which, in spite of its complexity, has very reliable output responses and is consistent with the physiological behavior of the human body. Undoubtedly, tracking of the viral droplet effects on the respiratory tract can be helpful in understanding how to cope with, and treat the disease. When an infected person exhales, a great number of viral microdroplets are produced which can be suspended in the air and even move longer distances. Therefore, those who are in such an infected place inhale viral particles, and eventually the disease spread faster. The basic mode of comparisons for the flow rate was considered as 6 L/min; because, this number indicates the person's breathing rate in the rest position, and it is of great importance. It is more often that People in an indoor construction find themselves in such situation, in which the risk of virus transmission through micro-droplets increases with inappropriate ventilation. If a person starts moderate physical activity in the enclosed construction, depending on the level of activity, the results of the flow rate will be more practical at15 L/min and 30 L/min.

The presented results of this study are categorized in two groups: **A**. inhalation with nose (closed mouth), and **B**. inhalation with mouth (closed nose). In the both groups, the most deposition occurs in the nasal cavity, and in the mouth, respectively. The highest relaxation time occurs in the superior turbinate in the both groups; which occurs with a relatively high concentration in Group **A**, and with a very low concentration in Group **B**. Also according to Figs. 6.5 and 6.11, the larger stokes number lead to higher deposition efficiency in both groups. The coronavirus receptor is activated in the olfactory area. Olfactory nerve is the first pair among 12 pairs of cranial nerves which is a part of the odor system. On the other hand, it has a short path in the central nervous system. Olfactory receptor are located in the olfactory mucosa, which is a specific region of approximately 5 cm length in each nasal mucosa. Because of the viral droplet absorption in the superior turbinate, this region is a dangerous zone; which as shown in Fig. 6.15, the stroke occurrence probability, via the viral droplet absorption could be increased.

Other achievements of this study include the increasing of the deposition efficiency by the droplet diameter, density and flow rate rise (Figs. 6.6 and 6.12). Tables 6.1 and 6.2 summarize the deposition efficiency in the upper respiratory tract in Groups **A** and **B**, respectively. So that the last two columns of these tables present the percentage of total deposition and the percentage of output from the carina ring, and reached two lung bronchi. The droplet deposition percentage in the upper respiratory tract in Group **A** inhalation is always higher than that of Group **B**; in other words, the probability of a viral droplet deposition in Group **A** lungs is lower so that the values in the last column of Table 6.2 is always smaller than that of Table 6.1. Also, in Table 6.1, because the mouth is closed in the inhalation process, the amount of droplet deposition in the mouth is either zero or very low. Likewise, in Table 6.2, which illustrates the nasal inhalation process, the amount of droplet deposition in different areas of the nose is either zero or very low.

The case studied inhaled **12** times per minute in healthy condition. The number of normal breathes per minute for a healthy person older than 14 years, is 12 to 20

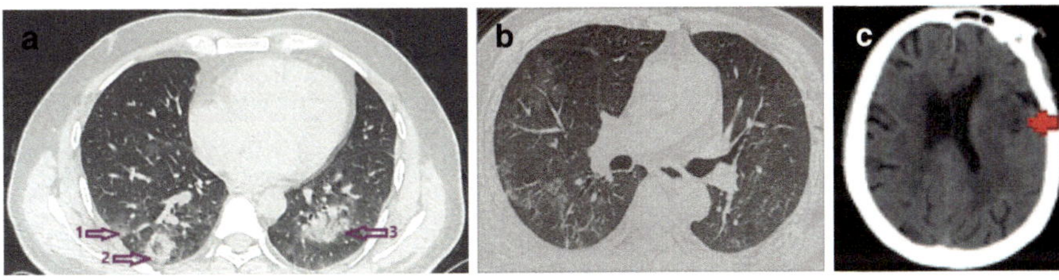


**Fig. 6.15** CT images of the chest and brain of COVID-19 male patients. (**a**) lesions to the patient lung have been identified in this study with a purple arrow. (**b**) CT images of the lung of a COVID-19 patient 1 day after stroke in another study [53]. (**c**) CT brain photo of the patient 1 day after a stroke [53]

**Table 6.1** Summary of the droplet deposition efficiency percentage with flow rate and droplet diameter changes in different areas of the upper respiratory system of Group **A**

| Condition | | Percent of droplet deposition efficiency in each zone | | | | | | | | | Total | |
|---|---|---|---|---|---|---|---|---|---|---|---|---|
| Capacity | Size | Oropharynx | Oral | Nasopharynx | Vestibule | Superior | Middle | Inferior | Larynx | Trachea | Deposited | Escaped |
| 6 L/min | 1 μm | 0.91 | 0 | 1.04 | 1.43 | 0.26 | 0.13 | 0.91 | 0 | 0.39 | 5.06 | 94.94 |
| | 5 μm | 0.65 | 0 | 0.91 | 1.43 | 0.26 | 1.82 | 2.08 | 0.13 | 0.65 | 7.92 | 92.08 |
| | 10 μm | 1.82 | 0.13 | 1.3 | 2.21 | 0.26 | 3.51 | 4.68 | 0.26 | 1.3 | 15.45 | 84.55 |
| 15 L/min | 1 μm | 1.43 | 0 | 2.34 | 2.21 | 0 | 1.17 | 1.04 | 0.65 | 0.78 | 9.61 | 90.39 |
| | 5 μm | 0.91 | 0 | 0.78 | 2.99 | 0.26 | 0.52 | 2.47 | 0.26 | 1.69 | 9.87 | 90.13 |
| | 10 μm | 4.03 | 0.13 | 2.60 | 3.38 | 0 | 0.91 | 3.25 | 1.69 | 1.69 | 17.66 | 82.34 |
| 30 L/min | 1 μm | 3.64 | 0.13 | 0.91 | 2.86 | 0.26 | 1.56 | 0.78 | 1.82 | 1.56 | 13.51 | 86.49 |
| | 5 μm | 11.30 | 0 | 1.30 | 3.51 | 0.39 | 2.34 | 3.64 | 4.29 | 4.81 | 31.56 | 68.44 |
| | 10 μm | 30.39 | 0 | 8.83 | 5.19 | 0.65 | 6.36 | 8.31 | 22.99 | 2.47 | 85.19 | 14.81 |

**Table 6.2** Summary of the droplet deposition efficiency percentage with flow rate and droplet diameter changes in different areas of the upper respiratory system of Group **B**

| Condition | | Percent of droplet deposition efficiency in each zone | | | | | | | | | Total | |
|---|---|---|---|---|---|---|---|---|---|---|---|---|
| Capacity | Size | Oropharynx | Oral | Nasopharynx | Vestibule | Superior | Middle | Inferior | Larynx | Trachea | Deposited | Escaped |
| 6 L/min | 1 µm | 1.64 | 4.23 | 0 | 0 | 0 | 0 | 0 | 0 | 0.70 | 6.57 | 93.43 |
| | 5 µm | 3.05 | 6.10 | 0 | 0 | 0.23 | 0.47 | 0.47 | 0 | 0.94 | 11.27 | 88.73 |
| | 10 µm | 3.29 | 6.34 | 0.47 | 0 | 0 | 0.23 | 0.47 | 0.47 | 3.29 | 14.55 | 85.45 |
| 15 L/min | 1 µm | 3.52 | 8.45 | 0.23 | 0.23 | 0 | 0 | 0 | 0.47 | 0.94 | 13.85 | 86.15 |
| | 5 µm | 4.46 | 13.15 | 0 | 0 | 0 | 0.47 | 0.23 | 0.23 | 1.88 | 20.42 | 79.58 |
| | 10 µm | 34.98 | 45.31 | 0 | 0 | 0 | 0 | 0 | 0 | 0.94 | 81.22 | 18.78 |
| 30 L/min | 1 µm | 4.69 | 11.97 | 0 | 0 | 0 | 0 | 0 | 0.23 | 0.23 | 17.14 | 82.86 |
| | 5 µm | 11.27 | 33.10 | 0 | 0 | 0 | 0 | 0 | 0.47 | 2.58 | 47.42 | 52.58 |
| | 10 µm | 1.64 | 97.18 | 0 | 0 | 0 | 0 | 0 | 0 | 0.23 | 99.06 | 0.94 |

**Table 6.3** The Maximum tracheal deformation at different flow rates

| | | Flow rate (L/min) | | |
|---|---|---|---|---|
| | Group type | 6 L/min | 15 L/min | 30 L/min |
| Max trachea deformation (mm) | **A** | 1.06 | 5.15 | 21.12 |
| | **B** | 0.24 | 1.42 | 4.69 |
| | Rati **A/B** | **4.42** | 3.63 | 4.50 |

times per minute [54]. However, after being infected with COVID-19 virus, the person's respiration rate increased to **20** times per minute. This increase is also seen in the Chen et al. study [55]. In other words, the patient's breathing rate increases at least $\frac{20}{12} = 1.67$ times per minute. Therefore, with respect to the increase in the number of inhalation per minute, the number of respiratory deformations and subsequently cyclic stresses in the tracheal wall and olfactory zone, also increase per minute compared to the healthy state. So, it comes with no surprise that according to the World Health Organization reports, one of the symptoms of the disease is pain/pressure in the chest and head.

It is noticeable that aspiration 6 liters of air per minute is equal to the amount of blood volume that the heart pumps per minute. Therefore, when due to COVID-19 infection, some parts of lungs are distorted, the lungs have to compensate this decrease by increasing the number of breaths per minute. Table 6.3 depicts the maximum deformations and the ratio between them, based on Figs. 6.8 and 6.14. According to this table, the most deformation of the trachea always occurs during nasal inhalation. Furthermore, the deformation changes rate is obtained 4.42 during breathing at rest through the nose with the closed mouth. Thus, according to Fig. 6.13, oral respiration not only minimizes viral infection in the nasal passages but also significantly reduces the rate of tracheal cyclic stresses per minute, and could cause less chest/head pain in patients.

Another important point in this FSI model is that in Group **A**, the most deformation can be seen in the carina zone, and the olfactory zone, respectively, while the least droplet deposition occurs in these areas. This is confirmed by the CT [32] images that the droplet deposition at the carina angle is smaller than the tracheal wall. Whereas in contrast, the result in unrealistic models is vice versa. Hence, the FSI method implementation in the analysis of droplet deposition in the upper human respiratory system is of great necessity to accurately detect viral-infected areas. For example, droplet deposition pattern contour is presented at the 1, 5, 10 μm diameters in the 30 L/min flow rate in Fig. 6.16.

When a person inhales through the mouth with closed nose, not only the droplet deposition in the nasal area is almost zero, but depositions in the mouth and throat can be transmitted to the stomach through drinking of fluids, and eventually the virus disappears in the stomach acid because COVID-19 virus receptor does not exist from the esophagus to the stomach. Only those droplets that reached the lungs could infect the person because along the respiratory tract from mouth to the lungs, the receptor of this virus just exists in the lungs; hence, the only way for the be virus to be transmitted to the body is through the lungs; and it is less probable to see

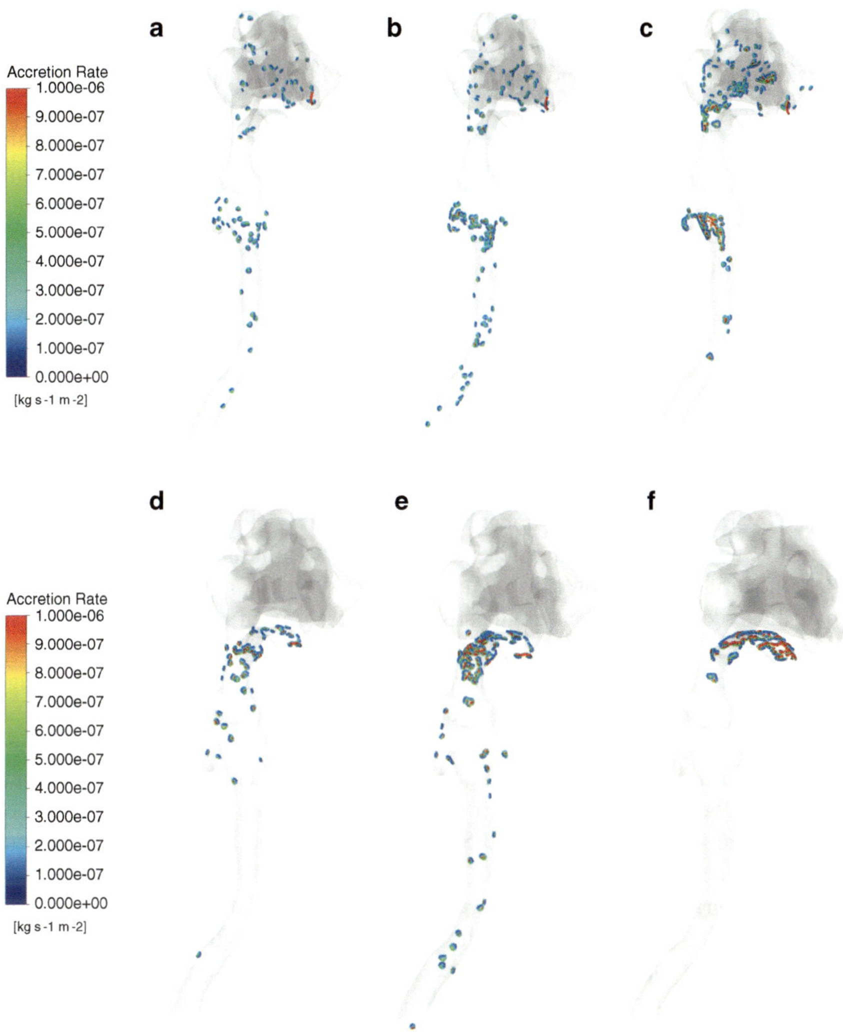


**Fig. 6.16** Droplet deposition with 1, 5, and 10 μm diameters at 30 L/min flow rate for Groups **A** and **B**. (**a**) Nostril inlet 1 μm droplet diameter, (**b**) Nostril inlet 5 μm droplet diameter, (**c**) Nostril inlet 10 μm droplet diameter, (**d**) Mouth inlet 1 μm droplet diameter, (**e**) Mouth inlet 5 μm droplet diameter, (**f**) Mouth inlet 10 μm droplet diameter

neurologic manifestations. Therefore, it is recommended to reduce the flow of the air entering through the nose with a special respiratory mask.

All the air that is inhaled does not carry the oxygen to the blood; in other words, the volume of the trachea and bronchi forms the anatomic dead space. Because in these spaces, the air does not get exposed to the blood in the respiratory capillaries. Usually this volume is about 150 $cm^3$ [51]. More details on the experimental tracking and numerical mapping of novel coronavirus microdroplet deposition through oral–nasal inhalation in the human respiratory system are mentioned in the Mortazavy et al. [56, 57] study and are not covered here for the sake of brevity. In the presented model, the available volume from carina to the mouth and nostril, regardless to the bronchus volume, is about 95 $cm^3$, which is part of the anatomic dead space, and is in contact with the air with the inner surface of 329 $cm^2$. This volume of air is returned to the lungs after an exhalation during the next inhalation. Therefore, if the anatomical dead space is contaminated with the virus, the droplet deposition relaxation time will increase significantly.

## Conclusion

Utilization of a realistic model with accurate and precise computational analysis can put an end to speculation about the deposition zone, accumulation, and the effects of the COVID-19 virus on the upper respiratory tract. On the other hand, recognizing of the virus-containing droplets' location can help in understanding the areas where the virus can first infect in the upper respiratory tract. In the meantime, mathematical models in different engineering fields have been pioneers in precise in vitro simulation [58–61].

The previous studies on particle deposition in the human respiratory system suggested that the results of each study depend on the biomechanical nature of the particles and the chosen realistic computational method. In this study, droplets containing the virus were examined using the FSI method, in a real geometry of human respiration. We believe that to reach the exact answer, the geometry of the model must be completely real, and the FSI condition must be applied for the human model. The actual model presented, demonstrates that the sense of smell of the studied person is disturbed due to the accumulation of viral droplet in the nasal cavity, and its high relaxation time in the superior turbinate. Therefore, it is recommended that the respirator masks should be made in such a way that the most air is inhaled through the mouth; so that in closed places where there is a high risk of virus contamination, the passage of air through the nose decreased.

Although oral inhalation also causes contamination in the olfactory area, however, the virus concentration is very low. Of course, this low concentration is trapped there due to the geometric structure of the upper area, and because of the high relaxation time in this area, a percentage of it is absorbed which is very small in comparison with nasal inhalation.

## References


1. Kahn JS, McIntosh K. History and recent advances in coronavirus discovery. Pediatr Infect Dis J. 2005;24(11 Suppl):S223–7, discussion S226.
2. Shiu EYC, Leung NHL, Cowling BJ. Controversy around airborne versus droplet transmission of respiratory viruses: implication for infection prevention. Curr Opin Infect Dis. 2019;32(4):372–9.
3. Gu J, Korteweg C. Pathology and pathogenesis of severe acute respiratory syndrome. Am J Pathol. 2007;170(4):1136–47.
4. Li YG, Chwang AT, Seto WH, Ho PL, Yuen PL. Understanding droplets produced by nebulisers and respiratory activities. Hong Kong Med J. 2008;14(Suppl 1):S29–32.
5. Chan TL, Lippmann M. Experimental measurements and empirical modelling of the regional deposition of inhaled particles in humans. Am Ind Hyg Assoc J. 1980;41:399.
6. Nowak N, Kakade PP, Annapragada AV. Computational fluid dynamics simulation of airflow and aerosol deposition in human lungs. Ann Biomed Eng. 2003;31(4):374–90.
7. Matida EA, et al. Improved numerical simulation of aerosol deposition in an idealized mouth–throat. J Aerosol Sci. 2004;35(1):1–19.
8. Heyder J. Deposition of inhaled particles in the human respiratory tract and consequences for regional targeting in respiratory drug delivery. Proc Am Thorac Soc. 2004;1(4):315–20.
9. Zhang Z, Kleinstreuer C. Airflow structures and nano-particle deposition in a human upper airway model. J Comput Phys. 2004;198(1):178–210.
10. Mahesh K, Constantinescu G, Moin P. A numerical method for large-eddy simulation in complex geometries. J Comput Phys. 2004;197(1):215–40.
11. Zhou Y, Cheng Y-S. Particle deposition in a cast of human tracheobronchial airways. Aerosol Sci Tech. 2005;39(6):492–500.
12. Jin HH, et al. Large eddy simulation of inhaled particle deposition within the human upper respiratory tract. J Aerosol Sci. 2007;38(3):257–68.
13. Farkas A, Balashazy I, Szocs K. Characterization of regional and local deposition of inhaled aerosol drugs in the respiratory system by computational fluid and particle dynamics methods. J Aerosol Med. 2006;19:329–43.
14. Xi J, Longest PW. Transport and deposition of micro-aerosols in realistic and simplified models of the oral airway. Ann Biomed Eng. 2007;35(4):560–81.
15. Shi H, Kleinstreuer C, Zhang Z. Modeling of inertial particle transport and deposition in human nasal cavities with wall roughness. J Aerosol Sci. 2007;38(4):398–419.
16. Li Z, Kleinstreuer C, Zhang Z. Simulation of airflow fields and microparticle deposition in realistic human lung airway models. Part II: particle transport and deposition. Eur J Mech B Fluids. 2007;26(5):650–68.
17. Lin CL, et al. Characteristics of the turbulent laryngeal jet and its effect on airflow in the human intra-thoracic airways. Respir Physiol Neurobiol. 2007;157(2–3):295–309.
18. Jayaraju ST, et al. Fluid flow and particle deposition analysis in a realistic extrathoracic airway model using unstructured grids. J Aerosol Sci. 2007;38(5):494–508.
19. Ma B, Lutchen KR. CFD simulation of aerosol deposition in an anatomically based human large-medium airway model. Ann Biomed Eng. 2009;37(2):271–85.
20. Mihaescu M, et al. Large Eddy simulation and Reynolds-averaged Navier-stokes modeling of flow in a realistic pharyngeal airway model: an investigation of obstructive sleep apnea. J Biomech. 2008;41(10):2279–88.
21. Shanley KT, et al. Numerical simulations investigating the regional and overall deposition efficiency of the human nasal cavity. Inhal Toxicol. 2008;20(12):1093–100.
22. Kleinstreuer C, Zhang Z. Airflow and particle transport in the human respiratory system. Annu Rev Fluid Mech. 2010;42(1):301–34.

23. Inthavong K, Zhang K, Tu J. Numerical modelling of nanoparticle deposition in the nasal cavity and the tracheobronchial airway. Comput Methods Biomech Biomed Engin. 2011;14(7):633–43.
24. Huang J, Zhang L. Numerical simulation of micro-particle deposition in a realistic human upper respiratory tract model during transient breathing cycle. Particuology. 2011;9(4):424–31.
25. Frank DO, et al. Effects of anatomy and particle size on nasal sprays and nebulizers. Otolaryngol Head Neck Surg. 2012;146(2):313–9.
26. Hopke PK, Wang Z. Particle deposition in the human respiratory tract. In: Fine particles in medicine and pharmacy; 2012. p. 223–40.
27. Li D, et al. Numerical simulation of particles deposition in a human upper airway. Adv Mech Eng. 2015;6.
28. Yousefi M, Inthavong K, Tu J. Microparticle transport and deposition in the human oral airway: toward the smart spacer. Aerosol Sci Tech. 2015;49(11):1109–20.
29. Varghese SK, Gangamma S. Particle deposition in human respiratory system: deposition of concentrated hygroscopic aerosols. Inhal Toxicol. 2009;21(7):619–30.
30. Basu S, Frank-Ito DO, Kimbell JS. On computational fluid dynamics models for sinonasal drug transport: relevance of nozzle subtraction and nasal vestibular dilation. Int J Numer Meth Biomed Eng. 2017;34(4):e2946.
31. Islam MS, et al. Euler–Lagrange approach to investigate respiratory anatomical shape effects on aerosol particle transport and deposition. Toxicol Res Appl. 2019;3:1–15.
32. Islam MS, et al. Euler-Lagrange prediction of diesel-exhaust polydisperse particle transport and deposition in lung: anatomy and turbulence effects. Sci Rep. 2019;9(1):12423.
33. Islam MS, et al. A review of respiratory anatomical development, air flow characterization and particle deposition. Int J Environ Res Public Health. 2020;17:380.
34. Ma B, et al. Potential effects of lingual fats on airway flow dynamics and particle deposition. Aerosol Sci Tech. 2019;54(3):321–31.
35. Keyhani K, Scherer PW, Mozell MM. Numerical simulation of airflow in the human nasal cavity. J Biomed Eng. 1995;117:429–41.
36. Hörschler I, Meinke M, Schröder W. Numerical simulation of the flow field in a model of the nasal cavity. Comput Fluids. 2003;32:39–45.
37. Grgic B, Finlay WH, Heenan AF. Regional aerosol deposition and flow measurements in an idealized mouth and throat. J Aerosol Sci. 2004;35(1):21–32.
38. Grgic B, et al. In vitro intersubject and intrasubject deposition measurements in realistic mouth–throat geometries. J Aerosol Sci. 2004;35(8):1025–40.
39. Heenan AF, et al. An investigation of the relationship between the flow field and regional deposition in realistic extra-thoracic airways. J Aerosol Sci. 2004;35(8):1013–23.
40. Shi H, Kleinstreuer C, Zhang Z. Laminar airflow and nanoparticle or vapor deposition in a human nasal cavity model. J Biomech Eng. 2006;128(5):697–706.
41. Xi J, Longest PW. Numerical predictions of submicrometer aerosol deposition in the nasal cavity using a novel drift flux approach. Int J Heat Mass Transf. 2008;51(23–24):5562–77.
42. Chen X, et al. Study on gas/solid flow in an obstructed pulmonary airway with transient flow based on CFD–DPM approach. Powder Technol. 2012;217:252–60.
43. Nicolaou L, Zaki TA. Direct numerical simulations of flow in realistic mouth–throat geometries. J Aerosol Sci. 2013;57:71–87.
44. Shinneeb AM, Pollard A. Investigation of the flow physics in the human pharynx/larynx region. Exp Fluids. 2012;53(4):989–1003.
45. Leung NHL, et al. Respiratory virus shedding in exhaled breath and efficacy of face masks. Nat Med. 2020;26(5):676–80.
46. Mortazavy Beni H, Hassani K, Khorramymehr S. In silico investigation of sneezing in a full real human upper airway using computational fluid dynamics method. Comput Methods Programs Biomed. 2019;177:203–9.

47. Mortazavy Beni H, Hassani K, Khorramymehr S. Study of the sneezing effects on the real human upper airway using fluid–structure interaction method. J Braz Soc Mech Sci Eng. 2019;41:1–3.
48. Decaro N. Betacoronavirus. In: Tidona C, Darai G, editors. The Springer index of viruses. New York, NY: Springer; 2011. p. 385–401.
49. Birch MJ, Srodon PD. Biomechanical properties of the human soft palate. Cleft Palate Craniofac J. 2009;46(3):268–74.
50. Cheng YS. Aerosol deposition in the extrathoracic region. Aerosol Sci Tech. 2003;37(8):659–71.
51. Cameron JR, Skofronick JG, Grant RM. Medical Physics: physics of the body. Madison, WI: Medical Physics Publishing Corporation; 1992.
52. Baig AM, et al. Evidence of the COVID-19 virus targeting the CNS: tissue distribution, host-virus interaction, and proposed neurotropic mechanisms. ACS Chem Nerosci. 2020;11(7):995–8.
53. Mao L, et al. Neurologic manifestations of hospitalized patients with coronavirus disease 2019 in Wuhan, China. JAMA Neurol. 2020;77(6):683–90.
54. Lu X, et al. SARS-CoV-2 infection in children. N Engl J Med. 2020;382(17):1663–5.
55. Chen T, et al. Clinical characteristics of 113 deceased patients with coronavirus disease 2019: retrospective study. BMJ. 2020;368:m1091.
56. Hamed M, Beni HM, Aghaei F, Sajadian H. SARS-CoV-2 droplet deposition path and its effects on the human upperairway in the oral inhalation. Comput Methods Programs Biomed. 2020;200:105843.
57. Mortazavy Beni H, Mortazavi H, Aghaei F, Kamalipour S. Experimental tracking and numerical mapping of novel coronavirus micro-droplet deposition through nasal inhalation in the human respiratory system. Biomech Model Mechanobiol. 2021;20(3):1087–100.
58. Beni HM, Mortazavi H, Tashvighi E, Islam MS. Investigation of the upper respiratory tract of a male smoker with laryngeal cancer by inhaling air associated with various physical activity levels. Atmosphere. 2022;13(5):717. https://doi.org/10.3390/atmos13050717.
59. Alaodolehei B, Jafarian K, Sheikhani A, Beni HM. Performance enhancement of an achalasia automatic detection system using ensemble empirical mode decomposition denoising method. J Med Biol Eng. 2020;40(2):179–88. https://doi.org/10.1007/s40846-019-00497-4.
60. Beni HM, Mortazavi H. Mathematical modeling of the solar regenerative heat exchanger under turbulent oscillating flow: applications of renewable and sustainable energy and artificial heart. Results Eng. 2022;13:100321. https://doi.org/10.1016/j.rineng.2021.100321.
61. Beni HM, Mortazavi H, Islam MS. Biomedical and biophysical limits to mathematical modeling of pulmonary system mechanics: a scoping review on aerosol and drug delivery. Biomech Model Mechanobiol. 2022;21(1):79–87. https://doi.org/10.1007/s10237-021-01531-8.

# Chapter 7
# SARS-CoV-2 Variants: Impact of Spike Mutations on Vaccine and Therapeutic Strategies

**Renuka Raman, Krishna J. Patel, and Kishu Ranjan**

## Introduction

The emergence of numerous severe acute respiratory syndrome coronavirus 2 (SARS-CoV-2) variants has raised global concern over early eradication of coronavirus disease 2019 (COVID-19), despite ongoing mass vaccination efforts across the globe. Most importantly, the mutated variants of SARS-CoV-2 are increasingly being transmitted across the population and are responsible for high mortality compared to earlier outbreaks caused by SARS viruses [1–4]. The SARS-CoV-2 virus is a positive single stranded RNA (ssRNA) virus (~ 30 kb genome size) flanked by 5′ and 3′ untranslated regions (UTRs), constituting 13–15 ORFs that encode proteins essential for viral assembly [5–7]. At the 5′ terminal, two large open reading frames (ORFs; ORF1a and ORF1b) encompassing more than two-thirds of the SARS-CoV-2 genome encode nonstructural proteins (NSPs) [7]. The 3′ terminal of the genome encodes four structural S (spike surface protein), E (envelope protein), M (membrane glycoprotein), and N (nucleocapsid phosphoprotein, RNA genome packaging) and nine accessory (3a, 3b, 6, 7a, 7b, 8b, 9a, 9b, and ORF10) proteins

Renuka Raman and Krishna J. Patel contributed equally with all other contributors.

R. Raman
Department of Medicine, Weill Cornell Medical College, New York, NY, USA
e-mail: rer2029@med.cornell.edu

K. J. Patel
Icahn School of Medicine at Mount Sinai, New York, NY, USA
e-mail: krishna.patel2@mssm.edu

K. Ranjan (✉)
School of Medicine, Yale University, New Haven, CT, USA
e-mail: kishu.ranjan@yale.edu


S. Adibi et al. (eds.), *Frontiers of COVID-19*,
https://doi.org/10.1007/978-3-031-08045-6_7

for viral assembly and establishment of infection in the host cell [6–9]. The SARS-CoV-2 trimeric S protein is composed of S1 [containing the N-terminal domain (NTD) and receptor binding domain (RBD) for viral attachment to host cell surface] and S2 (for membrane fusion and viral entry) subunits separated by a furin cleavage site [9–11]. Importantly, the S protein of coronaviruses are heavily glycosylated and are most susceptible to acquired mutations and shield epitopes from neutralizing antibodies [9, 12]. In the last several months, frequent mutations have been identified in the S protein leading to emergence of highly contagious variants causing the devastating rise of infection and mortality [13–17]. Mutations were also reported in ORF1ab, ORF8, NSP6, ORF3a, NSP4, and N regions with mild outcomes [18].

Like SARS virus, the SARS-CoV-2 preferers human angiotensin-converting enzyme 2 (hACE2) as a surface receptor for internalization across the cells [7, 19]. In addition, the activation of S protein through host proteases (furin, cathepsin L and TMPRSS2) is critical for viral infection and intracellular entry into the host [19–21]. After internalization, SARS-CoV-2 viral genome utilizes host transcriptional and translational machineries for synthesis and encapsulation of new viral progenies for further round of infections [16, 22, 23]. In most of the cases, individuals infected with SARS-CoV-2 start showing symptoms after 11–12 days of viral incubation, characterized by life-threatening respiratory pathologies and acute pneumonia-associated symptoms, such as dry cough, fever, muscle pain, and chills [5, 23]. It was found that some individuals remain asymptomatic post-SARS-CoV-2 infection; however, they serve as a carrier for transmission of viral infection in the vicinity [24, 25]. SARS-CoV-2 mutates more slowly than most RNA viruses due to proofreading function during replication, resulting in fewer mutations and higher accuracy in virus replication [15]. During replication in host cells, genomes of coronaviruses such as SARS-CoV-2, can alter their genome sequence referred to as mutations. A variant is a population of coronaviruses that inherits the same set of distinctive mutations. Most mutations have little to no impact on the virus' properties. Variants that confer a competitive advantage with respect to viral replication, viral transmission or escape from immunity are most likely to increase in frequency due to evolutionary pressure to survive and may create an opportunity for the emergence of new variants of moderate to severe pathogenicity [1, 2, 26]. Chance events, chronic infection in immunosuppressed individuals and host shifts could also increase the frequency of a particular strain. During early March 2020, the first SARS-CoV-2 variant carrying a single D614G mutation in the S glycoprotein was identified and remained predominant until June of 2020 [15, 17, 27]. Several fast-spreading SARS-CoV-2 variants with S protein mutation were also identified in the background [28], highlighting S protein as a potential target for designing COVID-19 vaccines [29]. Importantly, studies have shown that targeting S protein leads to robust humoral CD4+ T cell response [30]. In addition, vaccines targeting S protein significantly induce both humoral and cellular immune responses in clinical trials [31]. mRNA vaccine constructs, including BNT162b2 and mRNA-1273 have shown promising outcomes, with more than 95% protective efficacy against COVID-19 [32, 33]. However, these interventions were directed toward the initial SARS-CoV-2 virus that emerged in 2019. The emergence of novel SARS-CoV-2 variants is a global matter of concern since mutations accumulated by variants could potentially impact the structure of the protein, thereby modifying immune response or compromising the therapeutic efficacy of vaccines. Notably, an increased vaccination effort to general population will offer robust protection against hospitalization and severe disease.

The World Health Organization has classified variants as 'Variants of Interest' (VOI) and 'Variants of Concern' (VOC). As per the WHO (https://www.who.int/en/activities/tracking-SARS-CoV-2-variants/), a variant is classified as a VOC if one of the following criteria holds true.

1. Increase in transmissibility or detrimental change in COVID-19 epidemiology.
2. Increase in virulence or change in clinical disease presentation.
3. Decrease in effectiveness of public health and social measures or available diagnostics, vaccines, and therapeutics.

On the other hand, a variant is classified as a VOI if (1) the variant has genetic changes that are predicted or known to affect virus characteristics such as transmissibility, disease severity, immune escape, diagnostic or therapeutic escape; and (2) The variant has been identified to cause significant community transmission or multiple COVID-19 clusters, in multiple countries with increasing relative prevalence alongside increasing number of cases over time, or other apparent epidemiological impacts to suggest an emerging risk to global public health.

To provide an in-depth understanding regarding exacerbation of ongoing COVID-19 pandemic caused by SARS-CoV-2 variants, we have enlisted various SARS-CoV-2 variants based on the origin, mutational load, and pathogenicity. We have explored different vaccination platforms designed to effectively curb the propagation of variants. Additionally, we have systematically presented the efficacy of various vaccine candidates against identified variants. This comprehensive information will aid in informing health administrators, medical professionals, and the general population to understand how new variants could emerge in the future and may account for an epidemic rebound.

## Variants of Concern (VOC)

### *The B.1.1.7 Lineage (Alpha Variant)*

#### Origin

Alpha variant also known as B.1.1.7 variant or 20I/501Y.V1. B.1.1.7 was first detected in the UK in December 2020 and was named VOC 202012/01 since it quickly surged in other countries at an exponential rate [8]. The B.1.1.7 lineage has now been detected in over several countries, including the USA.

## Genetic Alterations, Impact on Protein Structure and Antigenicity

B.1.1.7 harbors several mutations in the S protein (Fig. 7.1), including two deletions, namely, H69/V70, and Y144/145, and six substitutions, including N501Y, A570D, P681H, T716I, S982A, and D1118H, which make the lineage 40–83% more infectious than the wild-type B1 strain (originally identified in Wuhan, China), resulting in higher nasopharyngeal viral loads and increased disease severity [34–36]. The N501Y substitution, H69/V70 deletion and P681H mutations are the key mutations in B.1.1.7 that are responsible for its increased transmissibility, disease severity and infection rate. Studies have demonstrated that the N501Y mutation in the RBD of the S protein helps the virus to increase binding to hACE2 receptors leading to increased rates of virus transmission and virulence in mouse and ferret models [37, 38]. The H69/V70 deletion modifies the immunodominant epitopes located at variable loops within NTD, conferring resistance to neutralization by sera from both convalescent patients and vaccinated individuals. Moreover, the H69/V70 deletion results in a twofold increase in S protein-mediated infectivity in vitro using pseudotyped lentivirus [39]. The Y144/145 deletion on the edge of the spike tip and is speculated to modify the binding of neutralizing antibodies to SARS-CoV-2 [40]. The P681 H mutation is another key mutation which is adjacent to the furin

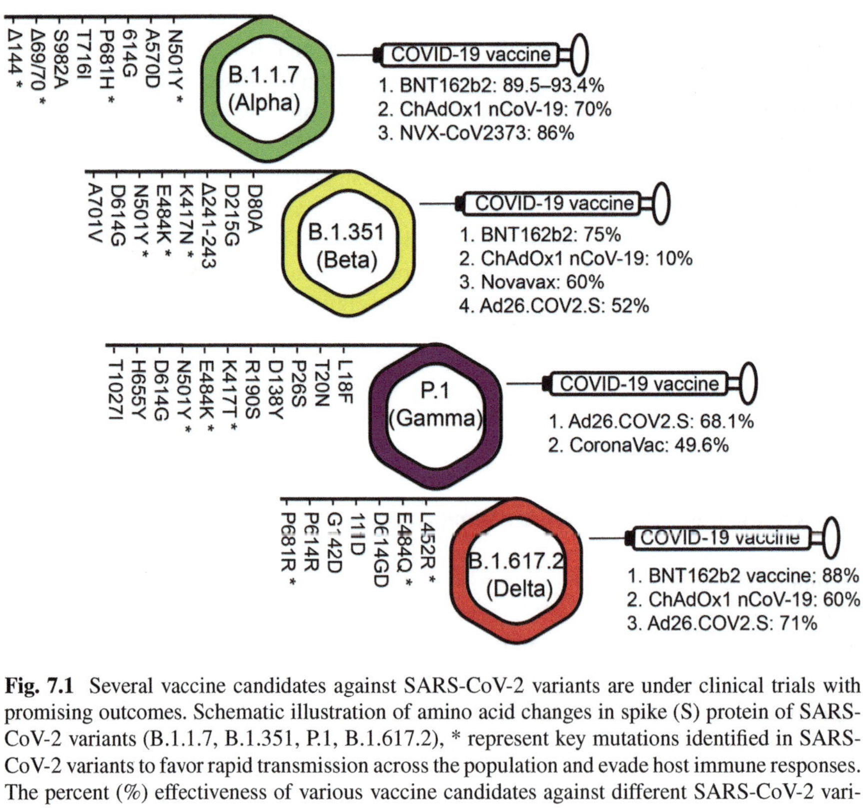


**Fig. 7.1** Several vaccine candidates against SARS-CoV-2 variants are under clinical trials with promising outcomes. Schematic illustration of amino acid changes in spike (S) protein of SARS-CoV-2 variants (B.1.1.7, B.1.351, P.1, B.1.617.2), * represent key mutations identified in SARS-CoV-2 variants to favor rapid transmission across the population and evade host immune responses. The percent (%) effectiveness of various vaccine candidates against different SARS-CoV-2 variants. https://www.who.int/en/activities/tracking-SARS-CoV-2-variants/

cleavage site that separates S1 and S2 subunits of the S protein and facilitates easier access of the human proteases to the furin cleavage site, thus increasing SARS-CoV-2 transmission and infection [10, 11].

## Effect on Convalescent and Vaccine Sera

Studies using pseudoviruses with the complete set of mutations described for B.1.1.7 variant have demonstrated reduced but, overall, largely preserved neutralizing antibody titers [41, 42]. Modest reductions in the neutralizing activity of both plasma from convalescent patients (2.7–3.8-fold) and sera from individuals that received mRNA vaccines (1.8–2-fold) have been observed [43, 44]. The protein-based vaccine (NVX-CoV2373) demonstrated an efficacy rate of 86.3% against mild, moderate, and severe COVID-19 caused by B.1.1.7 as compared to 96% efficacy seen in the wild-type B1 strain, whereas the viral vector—based Gam-COVID-Vac Sputnik V vaccine sera effectively neutralized B.1.1.7. viruses, albeit with highly variable titers [45, 46].

## Effect on Vaccine Efficacy

The overall efficacy of currently available vaccines is either similar or moderately lower against the B.1.1.7 variant (Fig. 7.1), although there are variations in study design (Table 7.1).

**Table 7.1** Percent effectiveness of vaccines on SARS-CoV-2 variants

| Vaccine | Alpha (B.1.1.7) | Beta (B.1.351) | Gamma (P.1) | Delta (B.1.617.2) |
|---|---|---|---|---|
| mRNA vaccine Pfizer (BNT162b2) | 89.5–93.4% [47, 48] | 75% [33, 49, 50] | Not reported | 88% [48] |
| Viral vector-based vaccine AstraZeneca (ChAdOx1 nCoV-19) | 70% [51] | 10% [52] | 82% effective against hospitalization or death 21 days after first dose [53] | 60% [48] |
| Viral vector-based vaccine Janssen (Ad26.COV2.S) | Not reported | 52% efficacy against moderate disease, 72% efficacy against severe disease [54] | 68.1% (against moderate to severe/critical disease), 87.6% (against severe/critical disease), where P1 was detected in 30.6% of sequences [55] | 71% effective against hospitalization, 85% effective against severe disease [56] |
| Protein-based vaccine Novovax (NVX-CoV2373) | 86% [57] | 60% [51] | Not reported | Not reported |

#### Effect on Antibody Therapy

The B.1.1.7 variant maintains high susceptibility to anti-SARS-CoV-2 monoclonal antibodies that are currently available through Emergency Use Authorization (EUA) [58] (Table 7.1).

### *The B.1.351 Lineage (Beta Variant)*

#### Origin

The Beta variant is also known as 20H/501Y.V2 and was first identified in South Africa in December 2020, with samples dating back to the beginning of October 2020 [59]. This variant is designated as a VOC since it demonstrates enhanced transmissibility and has been detected outside of South Africa, including in the USA.

#### Genetic Alterations and Impact on Protein Structure and Antigenicity

B.1.351 has two mutations in the RBD domain, namely, K417N and E484K that play a pivotal role in both the interaction with the receptor and immune evasion. B.1.351 also shares the N501Y mutation with B.1.1.7 in the RBD domain of the S protein (Fig. 7.1). The three mutations confer increased viral transmissibility and immune evasion to this variant. B.1.351 has 12 nonsynonymous mutations and one deletion as compared to the Wuhan reference strain (D614G). B.1.351 contains multiple mutations in the spike protein including L18F, D80A, D215G, 242–244 deletion, R246I, K417N, E484K, N501Y, D614G, and A701V, while the remaining ones are in ORF1a (K1655N), envelope (P71L), and N (T205I) viral proteins (Fig. 7.1). Out of these, the 242–244 deletion and R246I mutations are in the NTD, while K417N, E484K, and N501Y are in RBD, and A701V is located near the furin cleavage site [59]. Nelson et al. have demonstrated that the E484K mutation enhances spike RBD-ACE2 affinity and the combination of E484K, K417N, and N501Y mutations in the B.1.351 variant induce conformational changes greater than the N501Y mutant alone, resulting in an escape mutant [60].

#### Effect on Convalescent and Vaccine Sera

Compared to the D614G original isolate, pseudoviruses with spike containing K417N–E484K–N501Y–D614G and full B.1.351 mutations resulted in 2.7- and 6.4-fold geometric mean titer (GMT) reduction, respectively. Overall, vaccine sera show significantly reduced neutralization of B.1.351. Sera from individuals vaccinated with mRNA vaccines (Moderna and Pfizer-BioNTech) showed 12.4- and 10.3-fold decrease in viral load respectively [44]. On similar lines, sera from the Gam-COVID-Vac Sputnik V vaccine exhibited markedly reduced neutralization titers against the B.1.351 variant [45]. Serum samples obtained after the second dose of the inactivated vaccine based BBIBP-CorV vaccine (Sinopharm), or CoronaVac vaccine serum samples, also showed complete or partial loss of neutralization against B.1.351 [61].

#### Effect on Vaccine Efficacy

Mass immunization campaigns have revealed that the estimated effectiveness of the Pfizer-BioNTech vaccine against the B.1.351 variant was 75% at 14 or more days after the second dose, as compared to that of 89.5% against the B.1.1.7 variant [47]. Overall, the effectiveness of the BNT162b2 (Pfizer-BioNTech) vaccine against the B.1.351 variant was approximately 70%, which is lower than the effectiveness (> 90%) reported in the clinical trial [33] and in real-world conditions in Israel [49] and the USA [50] (Fig. 7.1; Table 7.1).

Clinical trials evaluating two dose regimens of AstraZeneca's vaccine (ChAdOx1 nCoV-19) in South Africa showed decreased protection against mild-to-moderate COVID-19 due to B.1.351 variant [52, 62]. On similar lines, randomized placebo-controlled trials reported by Novavax and Janssen companies in South Africa indicate significant reduction in the efficacy of their vaccines in places where the B.1.351 variant dominated [62, 63].

#### Effect on Antibody Therapy

One of the major concerns associated with the Beta variant is its resistance against a major group of potent monoclonal antibodies that target the RBD, including three authorized for emergency use [43, 64]. Studies suggest that combination of bamlanivimab plus etesevimab has markedly reduced activity against the B.1.351 variant. Similarly, Casirivimab activity is also significantly reduced, possibly due to the K417N and E484K mutation, although the combination of casirivimab and imdevimab appears to retain activity [58]. The US FDA revoked the EUA for bamlanivimab, because of an increasing number of reports of SARS-CoV-2 variants (having the E484K mutation) that are resistant to bamlanivimab alone, in addition to the Beta variant (Table 7.2).

**Table 7.2** Sensitivity of monoclonal antibodies (mAbs) targeted against SARS-CoV-2 variants

| mAbs | Alpha (B.1.1.7) | Beta (B.1.351) | Gamma (P.1) | Delta (B.1.617.2) |
|---|---|---|---|---|
| Eli Lilly (Bamlanivimab) | Susceptible [40] | Resistant | Resistant [40] | Resistant |
| Eli Lilly (Etesevimab) | Resistant [40] | Resistant [40] | Resistant [40] | Modest decrease in susceptibility to the combination of bamlanivimab and etesevimab, although the clinical implications of this finding are not fully known |
| Regeneron (REGN-COV2) (Casirivimab + Imdevimab) | Susceptible [40] | Activity of Casirivimab alone completely abolished, but combination retains activity [40] | Reduction in Casirivimab activity, although the combination retains activity [40] | Susceptible |

## *P.1 Variant (Gamma Variant)*

### Origin

The Gamma variant also known as P.1 or 20J/501Y.V3, is a branch of the B.1.1.28 lineage that was first detected in Brazil [65] and has become a dominant variant in Brazil [66].

### Genetic Alterations and Impact on Protein Structure and Antigenicity

The P.1 variant has accumulated 12 mutations in the spike protein, including the N501Y mutation, which is also present in B.1.1.7 and B.1.351, while L18F, K417T, E484K, and D614G mutations are shared with the B.1.351 variant (Fig. 7.1). P.1 contains several spike mutations in addition to D614G, including K417T, E484K, and N501Y in the RBD; L18F, T20N, P26S, D138Y, and R190S in the NTD; and H655Y near the furin cleavage site [65–67].

### Effect on Convalescent and Vaccine Sera

Neutralizing activity for the P.1 variant among vaccinated persons was lower by a factor of 6.7 for the BNT162b2 vaccine and by a factor of 4.5 for the mRNA-1273 vaccine [68]. A study using the CoronaVac vaccine showed that the immune plasma of COVID-19 convalescent blood donors had sixfold less neutralizing capacity against the P.1 variant than against the B-1 strain. Moreover, 5 months after booster immunization with CoronaVac, plasma from vaccinated individuals failed to efficiently neutralize P.1 lineage isolates [69]. However, real-world data demonstrates 49.6% effectiveness of the vaccine, which is similar to the vaccine's efficacy of 50.34% against symptomatic COVID-19 after both doses [70].

#### Effect on Vaccine Efficacy

The efficacy of the Oxford-AstraZeneca Ad26.COV2.S was seen to reduce to 68.1% against moderate to severe/critical disease and 87.6% against severe/critical disease, where P1 was detected in 30.6% of sequences [55] (Fig. 7.1) (Table 7.1).

#### Effect on Antibody Therapy

The P.1 variant is resistant to neutralization by several RBD-directed monoclonal antibodies including three having EUA including bamlanivimab, due to the presence of the E484K mutation which it shares with B.1.351 [42, 71, 72]. The combination of bamlanivimab plus etesevimab also has markedly reduced activity against the P.1 variant. Studies suggest that the K417T and E484 mutation, which are present in the P.1 variant, decrease casirivimab activity, although the combination of casirivimab and imdevimab appears to retain activity [58] (Table 7.2).

## *The B.1.617.2 (Delta Variant)*

### Origin

The *Delta variant*, known as the B.1.617 lineage, was first reported in October 2020 in Maharashtra, India and is also referred to as a "double mutation" variant. A detailed analysis of the genome and proteins of B.1.617 revealed it arose independently in India [56, 73]. Studies suggest that Delta is 40–60% more contagious than the Alpha (U.K./B.1.1.7) variant and may be the most transmissible variant the world has seen as of August 2021 [73]. On the 10th of May 2021, WHO designated B.1.617 and its sublineages, namely, B.1.617.1 (Kappa), B.1.617.2 (Delta), and B.1.617.3, as "VOC." The Delta variant has already spread to at least 135 countries as of 4th August 2021 (https://www.who.int/en/activities/tracking-SARS-CoV-2-variants/).

According to a report by Public Health England (PHE), an analysis of 38,805 sequenced cases in England unveiled that the Delta variant was associated with a 2.61 times higher risk of hospitalization within 14 days of infection than the Alpha variant. The Delta variant is more likely to spread among unvaccinated individuals since 73% of Delta cases are seen in unvaccinated people compared to only 3.7% Delta cases are in people who have had both doses [74].

## Genetic Alterations and Impact on Protein Structure and Antigenicity

B.1.617 harbors several mutations in the spike protein including D111D, G142D, L452R, E484Q, D614G, P614R, and P681R [16, 75] (Fig. 7.1). The Delta variant harbors the E484Q and L452R mutation in the spike protein that confer the variant with stronger binding potential to the hACE2 receptor, increased transmission, and infectivity as well as better ability to evade hosts' immune systems in comparison to other variants [38, 76].

The Delta variant led to a massive second wave of cases in India and replaced the Alpha variant in the UK. All three sublineages, namely, B.1.617.1 (Kappa), B.1.617.2 (Delta), and B.1.617.3, harbor the L452R and the P618R mutation. The P681R mutation in the furin cleavage site confers increased transmissibility to the Delta variant, enabling enhanced viral entry into lung cells. This enhanced entry can be accomplished due to more efficient membrane fusion of Delta with the host cell membrane [77]. However, Delta lacks mutations at amino acid positions 501 or 484 in its ACE2 receptor-binding domain, commonly associated with VOCs that escape from neutralizing antibodies (NAbs) [73, 75]. A new version of Delta known as "Delta plus" was first detected by PHE on June 11th, 2021. It has an additional K417N mutation which may contribute to immune escape [78]; however, the Delta plus variant is not more transmissible than the original Delta variant.

## Effect on Convalescent and Vaccine Sera

Wall et al. found that the neutralization antibody titers (NAbTs) were 5.8-fold reduced against B.1.617.2 relative to wild-type B1 strain in 250 participants after either one or two doses of the BNT162b2 vaccine. This reduction was similar to that observed against the B.1.351 variant [75]. B.1.617 partially evaded neutralization by the antibodies induced with the BNT162b2 and mRNA-1273 vaccine as well as through natural infection or immunization, while sera from individuals having received one dose of AstraZeneca/Oxford (ChAdOx1) vaccine barely inhibited B.1.617.2 [51, 79]. Convalescent sera from infected patients induced with the inactivated vaccine based BBV152 (Covaxin) were able to neutralize B.1.617 partially, but the effect was robust, as seen with mRNA vaccines [80]. Furthermore, heterologous boost with BNT162b2 following ChAdOx1 priming induces a more potent CD4+ and CD8+ T cell response as compared to homologous prime boost with ChAdOx1 [81].

## Effect on Vaccine Efficacy

Studies revealed that the effectiveness of BNT162b2 reduced from 93.4% with the Alpha variant to 87.9% with the Delta variant, while efficacy of Oxford-AstraZeneca vaccine ChAdOx1 reduced from 66.1% with Alpha to 59.8% with B.1.617.2 [68].

However, both vaccines were only 33% effective against symptomatic disease from Delta 3 weeks after the first dose [82]. PHE also found that Pfizer-BioNTech and the Oxford-AstraZeneca vaccine were 96% and 92% effective, respectively, at preventing hospitalization from the Delta variant [83] (Fig. 7.1). Recent studies have revealed a further drop in mRNA vaccine efficacy to ~ 50% [84].

#### Effect on Antibody Therapy

Recent studies have reported resistance of B.1.617.2 to neutralization by few anti-NTD and anti-RBD mAbs, including bamlanivimab and casirivimab, attributed to the L452R, E484Q, and E484K mutations [56] (Table 7.2). Thus, B.1.617.2 spread is associated with an escape to antibodies targeting epitopes on the S protein.

## Variants of Interest (VOI)

The WHO has described seven variants of interest (VOIs), namely, Epsilon (B.1.427 and B.1.429), Zeta (P.2), Eta (B.1.525), Theta (P.3), Iota (B.1.526), Kappa (B.1.617.1), and Lambda (C.37) (https://www.who.int/en/activities/tracking-SARS-CoV-2-variants/).

### *Epsilon (B.1.427 and B.1.429) Variants*

This variant discovered in California constitutes the B.1.427 and B.1.429 lineages and carries the L452R mutation, as seen in the lineage B.1.617 [76]. Molecular clock analysis suggest that the progenitor of both lineages emerged in May 2020 in the USA, diverging to give rise to the B.1.427 and B.1.429 independent lineages in June–July 2020 [85]. Epsilon is characterized by the S13I, W152C mutations in the NTD and by the L452R mutation in the RBD. The two lineages, B.1.427 and B.1.429, share the same spike protein mutations (S13I, W152C, and L452R), but harbor different mutations in other SARS-CoV-2 genes [86].

### *Zeta (P.2) Variant*

Zeta was first detected in Brazil in April 2020 and has key S protein mutations (L18F; T20N; P26S; F157L; E484K; D614G; S929I; and V1176F).

**Eta (B.1.525) and Iota (B.1.526) Variants**

The Eta and Iota variants were first identified in New York in November 2020. The reduction in neutralization by antibody treatments and vaccine sera is attributed to the mutation in these variants [231]. In addition to E484K, the Eta variant S protein mutations include A67V, Δ69/70, Δ144, D614G, Q677H, and F888L. Iota harbors L5F, T95I, D253G, S477N, D614G, and A701V, in addition to E484K [87].

## *Theta (P.3) Variant*

Theta is also called GR/1092K.V1 and was first detected in the Philippines and Japan in February 2021 and is classified as a VOI by the WHO. Theta harbors key S protein mutations 141–143 deletion E484K; N501Y; and P681H [88].

## *Kappa (B.1.617.1)*

Kappa was first detected in India in December 2021 and harbors key S protein mutations (T95I; G142D; E154K; L452R; E484Q; D614G; P681R; and Q1071H [88].

## *Lambda (C.37) Variant*

Lambda was first detected in Peru and has been designated as a VOI by the WHO in June 2021 due to an increased presence of this variant in the South American region.

## *Uganda Variant (A.23.1)*

A.23.1 has been detected in Uganda [89]. The S protein mutations in B.1.526 are L5F, T95I, D253G, and E484K or S477N, D614G, and A701V, while those in A.23.1 include R102I, F157L, V367F, Q613H, and P681R, respectively [88].

# Conclusion

Several variants of the SARS-CoV-2 virus have emerged over the past several months, leading to increased number of cases and mortality rate. An increased transmission of virus across the population further acquires genetic changes in the genome and develops a new strain of the virus. In this context, a comprehensive understanding of variants' genomic sequences associated with prolonged infections is important to explain the increased transmissibility. There is now emerging evidence of vaccine-induced immunity in protection against SARS-CoV-2 variants, which signifies that a collaborative effort to vaccinate global population may be the only way to fight the COVID-19 pandemic. Furthermore, extensive vaccination to the global population also requires bulk production of vaccines, rapid transport, large storage capacity, and uniform vaccine distribution. As of now, several vaccine projects are in the final stage of development, and almost ready to receive approval for general use by the end of 2021. Importantly, vaccines have retained their ability to prevent serious illness and death, in spite of the threat from VOCs including the Delta variant. According to Centers for Disease Control and Prevention (CDC, USA) the Delta variant has been detected in 8 in 10 samples in the USA. The rise in infection due to Delta variant reiterated the fact that variants exhibit antigenic variation and will further emerge and spread if a significant part of the population remains unvaccinated. Recently, developed nations approved to give booster vaccine shots (to protect against variants like Delta), which is limited to elderly and immunocompromised individuals; however, these efforts will largely remain ineffective if a significant portion of population remains unvaccinated. Altogether, a systematic global establishment is required to manage and track emerging variants and effective vaccine candidates against these variants for designing future strategies to control COVID-19 pandemic.

## References

1. Burki T. Understanding variants of SARS-CoV-2. Lancet. 2021;397(10273):298. https://doi.org/10.1016/s0140-6736(21)00298-1.
2. Gupta RK. Will SARS-CoV-2 variants of concern affect the promise of vaccines? Nat Rev Immunol. 2021;21(6):340–1. https://doi.org/10.1038/s41577-021-00556-5.
3. Peiris JS, Yuen KY, Osterhaus AD, Stohr K. The severe acute respiratory syndrome. N Engl J Med. 2003;349(25):2431–41. https://doi.org/10.1056/NEJMra032498.
4. Zhu N, Zhang D, Wang W, et al. A novel coronavirus from patients with pneumonia in China, 2019. N Engl J Med. 2020;382(8):727–33. https://doi.org/10.1056/NEJMoa2001017.
5. Lu R, Zhao X, Li J, et al. Genomic characterisation and epidemiology of 2019 novel coronavirus: implications for virus origins and receptor binding. Lancet. 2020;395(10224):565–74. https://doi.org/10.1016/S0140-6736(20)30251-8.
6. Wang Q, Wu J, Wang H, et al. Structural basis for RNA replication by the SARS-CoV-2 polymerase. Cell. 2020;182(2):417–28. https://doi.org/10.1016/j.cell.2020.05.034.
7. Yan R, Zhang Y, Li Y, et al. Structural basis for the recognition of SARS-CoV-2 by full-length human ACE2. Science. 2020;367(6485):1444–8. https://doi.org/10.1126/science.abb2762.
8. Chand GB, Banerjee A, Azad GK. Identification of novel mutations in RNA-dependent RNA polymerases of SARS-CoV-2 and their implications on its protein structure. PeerJ. 2020;8:e9492. https://doi.org/10.7717/peerj.9492.
9. Walls AC, Park YJ, Tortorici MA, et al. Structure, function, and antigenicity of the SARS-CoV-2 spike glycoprotein. Cell. 2020;181(2):281–92. https://doi.org/10.1016/j.cell.2020.02.058.

10. Hoffmann M, Kleine-Weber H, Pohlmann S. A multibasic cleavage site in the spike protein of SARS-CoV-2 is essential for infection of human lung cells. Mol Cell. 2020a;78(4):779–84. https://doi.org/10.1016/j.molcel.2020.04.022.
11. Peacock TP, Goldhill DH, Zhou J, et al. The furin cleavage site in the SARS-CoV-2 spike protein is required for transmission in ferrets. Nat Microbiol. 2021;6(7):899–909. https://doi.org/10.1038/s41564-021-00908-w.
12. Walls AC, Tortorici MA, Frenz B, et al. Glycan shield and epitope masking of a coronavirus spike protein observed by cryo-electron microscopy. Nat Struct Mol Biol. 2016;23(10):899–905. https://doi.org/10.1038/nsmb.3293.
13. Deng X, Garcia-Knight MA, Khalid MM, et al. Transmission, infectivity, and neutralization of a spike L452R SARS-CoV-2 variant. Cell. 2021;184(13):3426–37. https://doi.org/10.1016/j.cell.2021.04.025.
14. Edara VV, Norwood C, Floyd K, et al. Infection- and vaccine-induced antibody binding and neutralization of the B.1.351 SARS-CoV-2 variant. Cell Host Microbe. 2021;29(4):516–21. https://doi.org/10.1016/j.chom.2021.03.009.
15. Plante JA, Liu Y, Liu J, et al. Spike mutation D614G alters SARS-CoV-2 fitness. Nature. 2021;592(7852):116–21. https://doi.org/10.1038/s41586-020-2895-3.
16. Raman R, Patel KJ, Ranjan K. COVID-19: unmasking emerging SARS-CoV-2 variants, vaccines and therapeutic strategies. Biomolecules. 2021;11(7):993. https://doi.org/10.3390/biom11070993.
17. Zhou B, Thao TTN, Hoffmann D, et al. SARS-CoV-2 spike D614G change enhances replication and transmission. Nature. 2021;592(7852):122–7. https://doi.org/10.1038/s41586-021-03361-1.
18. Gordon DE, Jang GM, Bouhaddou M, et al. A SARS-CoV-2 protein interaction map reveals targets for drug repurposing. Nature. 2020;583(7816):459–68. https://doi.org/10.1038/s41586-020-2286-9.
19. Shang J, Wan Y, Luo C, et al. Cell entry mechanisms of SARS-CoV-2. Proc Natl Acad Sci USA. 2020;117(21):11727–34. https://doi.org/10.1073/pnas.2003138117.
20. Hoffmann M, Kleine-Weber H, Schroeder S, et al. SARS-CoV-2 cell entry depends on ACE2 and TMPRSS2 and is blocked by a clinically proven protease inhibitor. Cell. 2020b;181(2):271–80. https://doi.org/10.1016/j.cell.2020.02.052.
21. Matsuyama S, Nao N, Shirato K, et al. Enhanced isolation of SARS-CoV-2 by TMPRSS2-expressing cells. Proc Natl Acad Sci USA. 2020;117(13):7001–3. https://doi.org/10.1073/pnas.2002589117.
22. Tang T, Bidon M, Jaimes JA, et al. Coronavirus membrane fusion mechanism offers a potential target for antiviral development. Antivir Res. 2020;178:104792. https://doi.org/10.1016/j.antiviral.2020.104792.
23. V'Kovski P, Kratzel A, Steiner S, et al. Coronavirus biology and replication: implications for SARS-CoV-2. Nat Rev Microbiol. 2021;19(3):155–70. https://doi.org/10.1038/s41579-020-00468-6.
24. Bai Y, Yao L, Wei T, et al. Presumed asymptomatic carrier transmission of COVID-19. JAMA. 2020;323(14):1406–7. https://doi.org/10.1001/jama.2020.2565.
25. Rothe C, Schunk M, Sothmann P, et al. Transmission of 2019-nCoV infection from an asymptomatic contact in Germany. N Engl J Med. 2020;382(10):970–1. https://doi.org/10.1056/NEJMc2001468.
26. Garcia-Beltran WF, Lam EC, St Denis K, et al. Circulating SARS-CoV-2 variants escape neutralization by vaccine-induced humoral immunity. medRxiv. 2021;2021:704. https://doi.org/10.1101/2021.02.14.21251704.
27. Shahhosseini N, Babuadze GG, Wong G, Kobinger GP. Mutation signatures and in silico docking of novel SARS-CoV-2 variants of concern. Microorganisms. 2021;9(5):926. https://doi.org/10.3390/microorganisms9050926.

28. Korber B, Fischer WM, Gnanakaran S, et al. Tracking changes in SARS-CoV-2 spike: evidence that D614G increases infectivity of the COVID-19 virus. Cell. 2020;182(4):812–27. https://doi.org/10.1016/j.cell.2020.06.043.
29. Amanat F, Krammer F. SARS-CoV-2 vaccines: status report. Immunity. 2020;52(4):583–9. https://doi.org/10.1016/j.immuni.2020.03.007.
30. Grifoni A, Weiskopf D, Ramirez SI, et al. Targets of T cell responses to SARS-CoV-2 coronavirus in humans with COVID-19 disease and unexposed individuals. Cell. 2020;181(7):1489–501. https://doi.org/10.1016/j.cell.2020.05.015.
31. Bisht H, Roberts A, Vogel L, et al. Severe acute respiratory syndrome coronavirus spike protein expressed by attenuated vaccinia virus protectively immunizes mice. Proc Natl Acad Sci USA. 2004;101(17):6641–6. https://doi.org/10.1073/pnas.0401939101.
32. Anderson EJ, Rouphael NG, Widge AT, et al. Safety and immunogenicity of SARS-CoV-2 mRNA-1273 vaccine in older adults. N Engl J Med. 2020;383(25):2427–38. https://doi.org/10.1056/NEJMoa2028436.
33. Polack FP, Thomas SJ, Kitchin N, et al. Safety and efficacy of the BNT162b2 mRNA Covid-19 vaccine. N Engl J Med. 2020;383(27):2603–15. https://doi.org/10.1056/NEJMoa2034577.
34. Davies NG, Abbott S, Barnard RC, et al. Estimated transmissibility and impact of SARS-CoV-2 lineage B.1.1.7 in England. Science. 2021;372(6538):3055. https://doi.org/10.1126/science.abg3055.
35. Leung K, Shum MH, Leung GM, et al. Early transmissibility assessment of the N501Y mutant strains of SARS-CoV-2 in the United Kingdom, October to November 2020. Euro Surveill. 2021;26(1):2106. https://doi.org/10.2807/1560-7917.ES.2020.26.1.2002106.
36. Volz E, Mishra S, Chand M, et al. Assessing transmissibility of SARS-CoV-2 lineage B.1.1.7 in England. Nature. 2021;593(7858):266–9. https://doi.org/10.1038/s41586-021-03470-x.
37. Liu Y, Liu J, Plante KS, et al. The N501Y spike substitution enhances SARS-CoV-2 transmission. bioRxiv. 2021;2021:499. https://doi.org/10.1101/2021.03.08.434499.
38. Starr TN, Greaney AJ, Addetia A, et al. Prospective mapping of viral mutations that escape antibodies used to treat COVID-19. Science. 2021;371(6531):850–4. https://doi.org/10.1126/science.abf9302.
39. Kemp SA, Collier DA, Datir R, et al. Neutralising antibodies in spike mediated SARS-CoV-2 adaptation. medRxiv. 2020;2020:927. https://doi.org/10.1101/2020.12.05.20241927.
40. McCarthy KR, Rennick LJ, Nambulli S, et al. Recurrent deletions in the SARS-CoV-2 spike glycoprotein drive antibody escape. Science. 2021;371(6534):1139–42. https://doi.org/10.1126/science.abf6950.
41. Collier DA, De Marco A, Ferreira I, et al. Sensitivity of SARS-CoV-2 B.1.1.7 to mRNA vaccine-elicited antibodies. Nature. 2021;593(7857):136–41. https://doi.org/10.1038/s41586-021-03412-7.
42. Xie X, Liu Y, Liu J, et al. Neutralization of SARS-CoV-2 spike 69/70 deletion, E484K and N501Y variants by BNT162b2 vaccine-elicited sera. Nat Med. 2021;27(4):620–1. https://doi.org/10.1038/s41591-021-01270-4.
43. Wang P, Nair MS, Liu L, et al. Increased resistance of SARS-CoV-2 variants B.1.351 and B.1.1.7 to antibody neutralization. bioRxiv. 2021c;2021:428137. https://doi.org/10.1101/2021.01.25.428137.
44. Wu K, Werner AP, Moliva JI, et al. mRNA-1273 vaccine induces neutralizing antibodies against spike mutants from global SARS-CoV-2 variants. bioRxiv. 2021;2021:427948. https://doi.org/10.1101/2021.01.25.427948.
45. Ikegame S, Siddiquey M, Hung CT, et al. Neutralizing activity of Sputnik V vaccine sera against SARS-CoV-2 variants. Res Sq. 2021;2021:400230. https://doi.org/10.21203/rs.3.rs-400230/v1.
46. Novavax. Novavax confirms high levels of efficacy against original and variant COVID-19 strains in United Kingdom and South Africa trials. Gaithersburg: Novavax, Inc; 2021.

47. Abu-Raddad LJ, Chemaitelly H, Butt AA. National Study Group for C-V (2021) effectiveness of the BNT162b2 Covid-19 vaccine against the B.1.1.7 and B.1.351 variants. N Engl J Med. 2021;385(2):187–9. https://doi.org/10.1056/NEJMc2104974.
48. Lopez Bernal J, Andrews N, Gower C, et al. Effectiveness of Covid-19 vaccines against the B.1.617.2 (Delta) variant. N Engl J Med. 2021;385(7):585–94. https://doi.org/10.1056/NEJMoa2108891.
49. Dagan N, Barda N, Kepten E, et al. BNT162b2 mRNA Covid-19 vaccine in a Nationwide mass vaccination setting. N Engl J Med. 2021;384(15):1412–23. https://doi.org/10.1056/NEJMoa2101765.
50. Thompson MG, Burgess JL, Naleway AL, et al. Interim estimates of vaccine effectiveness of BNT162b2 and mRNA-1273 COVID-19 vaccines in preventing SARS-CoV-2 infection among health care personnel, first responders, and other essential and frontline workers—eight U.S. locations, December 2020–March 2021. MMWR Morb Mortal Wkly Rep. 2021;70(13):495–500. https://doi.org/10.15585/mmwr.mm7013e3.
51. Emary KRW, Golubchik T, Aley PK, et al. Efficacy of ChAdOx1 nCoV-19 (AZD1222) vaccine against SARS-CoV-2 variant of concern 202012/01 (B.1.1.7): an exploratory analysis of a randomised controlled trial. Lancet. 2021;397(10282):1351–62. https://doi.org/10.1016/S0140-6736(21)00628-0.
52. Madhi SA, Baillie V, Cutland CL, et al. Efficacy of the ChAdOx1 nCoV-19 Covid-19 vaccine against the B.1.351 variant. N Engl J Med. 2021;384(20):1885–98. https://doi.org/10.1056/NEJMoa2102214.
53. Nasreen S, Chung H, He S, et al. Effectiveness of COVID-19 vaccines against variants of concern in Ontario, Canada. medRxiv. 2021;2021:21259420. https://doi.org/10.1101/2021.06.28.21259420.
54. Janssen. Emergency use authorization (EUA) for an unapproved product review memorandum. Beerse: Janssen; 2021.
55. Sadoff J, Gray G, Vandebosch A, et al. Safety and efficacy of single-dose Ad26.COV2.S vaccine against Covid-19. N Engl J Med. 2021;384(23):2187–201. https://doi.org/10.1056/NEJMoa2101544.
56. Takuya T, Zhou H, View ORCID ProfileBelinda, Dcosta BM, Samanovic MI, Mulligan MJ, Landau NR, View ORCID, ProfileBelinda M. The spike proteins of SARS-CoV-2 B.1.617 and B.1.618 variants identified in India provide partial resistance to vaccine-elicited and therapeutic monoclonal antibodies. bioRxiv. 2021;2021:444076. https://doi.org/10.1101/2021.05.14.444076.
57. Mahase E. Covid-19: Novavax vaccine efficacy is 86% against UK variant and 60% against South African variant. BMJ. 2021a;372:n296. https://doi.org/10.1136/bmj.n296.
58. NIH. COVID-19 treatment guidelines panel. Coronavirus disease 2019 (COVID-19) treatment guidelines. National Institutes of Health; 2021. https://www.covid19treatmentguidelines.nih.gov/. Accessed 29 May 2021
59. Tegally H, Wilkinson E, Giovanetti M, et al. Detection of a SARS-CoV-2 variant of concern in South Africa. Nature. 2021;592(7854):438–43. https://doi.org/10.1038/s41586-021-03402-9.
60. Nelson G, Buzko O, Spilman P, Niazi K, Rabizadeh S, View ORCID ProfilePatrick Soon-Shiong. Molecular dynamic simulation reveals E484K mutation enhances spike RBD-ACE2 affinity and the combination of E484K, K417N and N501Y mutations (501Y.V2 variant) induces conformational change greater than N501Y mutant alone, potentially resulting in an escape mutant. bioRxiv. 2021;13:558. https://doi.org/10.1101/2021.01.13.426558.
61. Wang GL, Wang ZY, Duan LJ, et al. Susceptibility of circulating SARS-CoV-2 variants to neutralization. N Engl J Med. 2021a;384(24):2354–6. https://doi.org/10.1056/NEJMc2103022.
62. Callaway E. Mix-and-match COVID vaccines trigger potent immune response. Nature. 2021;593(7860):491. https://doi.org/10.1038/d41586-021-01359-3.
63. Shinde V, Bhikha S, Hoosain Z, et al. Efficacy of NVX-CoV2373 Covid-19 vaccine against the B.1.351 variant. N Engl J Med. 2021;384(20):1899–909. https://doi.org/10.1056/NEJMoa2103055.

64. Wibmer CK, Ayres F, Hermanus T, et al. SARS-CoV-2 501Y.V2 escapes neutralization by South African COVID-19 donor plasma. bioRxiv. 2021a;2021:427166. https://doi.org/10.1101/2021.01.18.427166.
65. Sabino EC, Buss LF, Carvalho MPS, et al. Resurgence of COVID-19 in Manaus, Brazil, despite high seroprevalence. Lancet. 2021;397(10273):452–5. https://doi.org/10.1016/S0140-6736(21)00183-5.
66. Faria NR, Mellan TA, Whittaker C, et al. Genomics and epidemiology of the P.1 SARS-CoV-2 lineage in Manaus, Brazil. Science. 2021;372(6544):815–21. https://doi.org/10.1126/science.abh2644.
67. Naveca FG, Nascimento V, de Souza VC, et al. COVID-19 in Amazonas, Brazil, was driven by the persistence of endemic lineages and P.1 emergence. Nat Med. 2021;27(7):1230–8. https://doi.org/10.1038/s41591-021-01378-7.
68. Abdool Karim SS, de Oliveira T. New SARS-CoV-2 variants- clinical, public health, and vaccine implications. N Engl J Med. 2021;384(19):1866–8. https://doi.org/10.1056/NEJMc2100362.
69. Souza WM, Amorim MR, Sesti-Costa R, et al. Neutralisation of SARS-CoV-2 lineage P.1 by antibodies elicited through natural SARS-CoV-2 infection or vaccination with an inactivated SARS-CoV-2 vaccine: an immunological study. Lancet Microbe. 2021;2(10):e527–35. https://doi.org/10.1016/S2666-5247(21)00129-4.
70. Moutinho S. Chinese COVID-19 vaccine maintains protection in variant-plagued Brazil. Science AAAS. 2021;2021:9414. https://doi.org/10.1126/science.abi9414.
71. Wang P, Nair MS, Liu L, et al. Antibody resistance of SARS-CoV-2 variants B.1.351 and B.1.1.7. Nature. 2021b;593(7857):130–5. https://doi.org/10.1038/s41586-021-03398-2.
72. Wibmer CK, Ayres F, Hermanus T, et al. SARS-CoV-2 501Y.V2 escapes neutralization by South African COVID-19 donor plasma. Nat Med. 2021b;27(4):622–5. https://doi.org/10.1038/s41591-021-01285-x.
73. Mahase E. Delta variant: what is happening with transmission, hospital admissions, and restrictions? BMJ. 2021b;373:n1513. https://doi.org/10.1136/bmj.n1513.
74. Subbaraman N. How do vaccinated people spread Delta? What the science says. Nature. 2021;596(7872):327–8. https://doi.org/10.1038/d41586-021-02187-1.
75. Wall EC, Wu M, Harvey R, et al. Neutralising antibody activity against SARS-CoV-2 VOCs B.1.617.2 and B.1.351 by BNT162b2 vaccination. Lancet. 2021;397(10292):2331–3. https://doi.org/10.1016/S0140-6736(21)01290-3.
76. Zhang W, Davis BD, Chen SS, et al. Emergence of a novel SARS-CoV-2 variant in Southern California. JAMA. 2021b;325(13):1324–6. https://doi.org/10.1001/jama.2021.1612.
77. Zhang J, Xiao T, Cai Y, et al. Membrane fusion and immune evasion by the spike protein of SARS-CoV-2 Delta variant. bioRxiv. 2021a;2021:456689. https://doi.org/10.1101/2021.08.17.456689.
78. Kannan SR, Spratt AN, Cohen AR, et al. Evolutionary analysis of the Delta and Delta plus variants of the SARS-CoV-2 viruses. J Autoimmun. 2021;124:102715. https://doi.org/10.1016/j.jaut.2021.102715.
79. Voysey M, Clemens SAC, Madhi SA, et al. Safety and efficacy of the ChAdOx1 nCoV-19 vaccine (AZD1222) against SARS-CoV-2: an interim analysis of four randomised controlled trials in Brazil, South Africa, and the UK. Lancet. 2021;397(10269):99–111. https://doi.org/10.1016/S0140-6736(20)32661-1.
80. Bharat Biotech. COVAXIN—India's first indigenous Covid-19 vaccine. Hyderabad: Bharat Biotech; 2021.
81. Barros-Martins J, Hammerschmidt SI, Cossmann A, et al. Immune responses against SARS-CoV-2 variants after heterologous and homologous ChAdOx1 nCoV-19/BNT162b2 vaccination. Nat Med. 2021;27(9):1525–9. https://doi.org/10.1038/s41591-021-01449-9.
82. Lacobucci G. Covid-19: single vaccine dose is 33% effective against variant from India, data show. BMJ. 2021;373:n1346.
83. Public Health England (PHE). Effectiveness of COVID-19 vaccines on hospitalisation disease with the Delta variant. 2021. https://www.gov.uk/government/news/vaccines-highly-effective-against-hospitalisation-from-delta-variant.

84. Puranik A, Lenehan PJ, Silvert E, et al. Comparison of two highly-effective mRNA vaccines for COVID-19 during periods of Alpha and Delta variant prevalence. medRxiv. 2021;2021:21261707. https://doi.org/10.1101/2021.08.06.21261707.
85. Cai Q, Yang M, Liu D, et al. Experimental treatment with Favipiravir for COVID-19: an open-label control study. Engineering (Beijing). 2020;6(10):1192–8. https://doi.org/10.1016/j.eng.2020.03.007.
86. McCallum M, Bassi J, De Marco A, et al. SARS-CoV-2 immune evasion by the B.1.427/B.1.429 variant of concern. Science. 2021;373(6555):648–54. https://doi.org/10.1126/science.abi7994.
87. Annavajhala MK, Mohri H, Zucker JE, et al. A novel SARS-CoV-2 variant of concern, B.1.526, identified in New York. medRxiv. 2021;2021:2259. https://doi.org/10.1101/2021.02.23.21252259.
88. Aleem A, Akbar Samad AB, Slenker AK. Emerging variants of SARS-CoV-2 and novel therapeutics against coronavirus (COVID-19). Treasure Island: StatPearls; 2021.
89. Bugembe DL, Kayiwa J, Phan MVT, et al. Main routes of entry and genomic diversity of SARS-CoV-2. Uganda Emerg Infect Dis. 2020;26(10):2411–5. https://doi.org/10.3201/eid2610.202575.

# Chapter 8
# Global Biologic Characteristics of Variants of Concern and Variants of Interest of SARS-CoV-2

**Jasdeep Singh, Nasreen Z. Ehtesham, Subhash Hira, Umid Kumar Shrestha, and Seyed E. Hasnain**

## Background

Coronaviruses (CoVs) are group of RNA viruses which primarily cause mild to lethal respiratory infections. In humans, the CoVs causing mild illness (common cold) include Rhinoviruses while lethal ones include the historical SARS-CoV (Severe Acute Respiratory Syndrome), MERS-CoV (Middle East Respiratory Syndrome), and the recently discovered SARS-CoV-2, responsible for COVID-19 pandemic which has claimed over 4.3 million lives globally between its outbreak in December 2019 and July 2021 [1–3]. The CoVs are enveloped viruses with single strand positive-sense RNA genome of size ranging from 26 to 32 Kb, flanked by untranslated regions at both 5′ and 3′ ends [2]. These regions contain cis-acting secondary RNA structures which are essential for synthesis of new RNA. About

J. Singh
Department of Biochemical Engineering and Biotechnology, Indian Institute of Technology-Delhi, New Delhi, Delhi, India

N. Z. Ehtesham
ICMR National Institute of Pathology, Safdarjung Hospital Campus, New Delhi, Delhi, India

S. Hira
Department of Global Health, University of Washington-Seattle, Seattle, WA, USA
e-mail: hiras2@uw.edu

U. K. Shrestha
Nepal Mediciti Hospital, Bhaisepati, Lalitpur, Nepal

S. E. Hasnain (✉)
Department of Biochemical Engineering and Biotechnology, Indian Institute of Technology-Delhi, New Delhi, Delhi, India

Department of Life Science, School of Basic Sciences and Research, Sharda University, Greater Noida, Uttar Pradesh, India
e-mail: seh@dbeb.iitd.ac.in


S. Adibi et al. (eds.), *Frontiers of COVID-19*,
https://doi.org/10.1007/978-3-031-08045-6_8

two-thirds of the genome from the 5′ end features two large open reading frames; ORF1a and 1b which encode non-structural proteins involved in various processes for maintaining the integrity of the genome. The other one-third of the genome encodes few viral accessory proteins and structural proteins, namely envelope (E), membrane (M), spike (S), and nucleocapsid (N) proteins. The accessory proteins are believed to modulate host responses to viral infection, acting as regulators of its pathogenicity. The E and M proteins form part of viral envelope to maintain its shape and size and the S protein which protrudes outside the envelope provides specificity for host cell receptors. The multifunctional N protein interacts with genomic RNA and plays crucial role in enhancing viral transcription and its assembly.

To establish host contact, human ACE2 (Angiotensin Converting Enzyme) acts as recognition receptors for S protein of SARS-CoV-2 [1, 4]. The host–virus interactions are mediated through receptor binding domain (RBD) of S protein and stabilized predominantly by polar interactions. Due to its crucial role, S protein is also the primary target in COVID-19 vaccines, neutralizing antibodies, and drug candidates. Consequently, during early phase of COVID-19 pandemic, a major thrust of scientific efforts was dedicated towards design of neutralizing antibodies and vaccine candidates targeting specifically the viral Spike (S) protein. However, with a modest mutation rate of $9.8 \times 10^{-4}$ substitutions per site per year [5], mutations in regions binding with antibodies (natural or vaccine induced) could pose a grave hurdle in the time to come. Till mid-2020, more than 0.1 million SARS-CoV-2 genome samples were sequenced indicating emergence of first globally dominant SARS-CoV-2 D614G variant over the ancestral strains. The D614G mutation of S protein was associated with enhanced infectivity, increased viral density, and increased replication in the human lung epithelial cells. The mutation also led to moderate reduction in vaccines elicited neutralization which initially paved way for universal COVID-19 vaccines [2, 6]. Despite a sluggish mutation rate, new emerging genetically distinct phylogenetic clusters of SARS-CoV-2 were reported all around world towards the end of 2020 (Fig. 8.1).

With possibilities of being more transmissible and infectious than previously dominant D614G variant, these new SARS-CoV-2 variants were designated as variants of interest (VOI)/variants under investigation (VUI) and later designated as variants of concern (VOC) by either WHO (World Health Organization), CDC-USA (Centers for Disease Control and Prevention), Public Health England or ECDC (European Centers for Disease Control and Prevention) public health organizations [7, 8]. As per their general recommendations, the VOCs are associated with either increased transmissibility or detrimental change in COVID-19 epidemiology, virulence or severity in presentation of clinical disease; or reduced effectiveness of public health, social measures or available therapeutics, vaccines, and diagnostics [4, 9, 10].

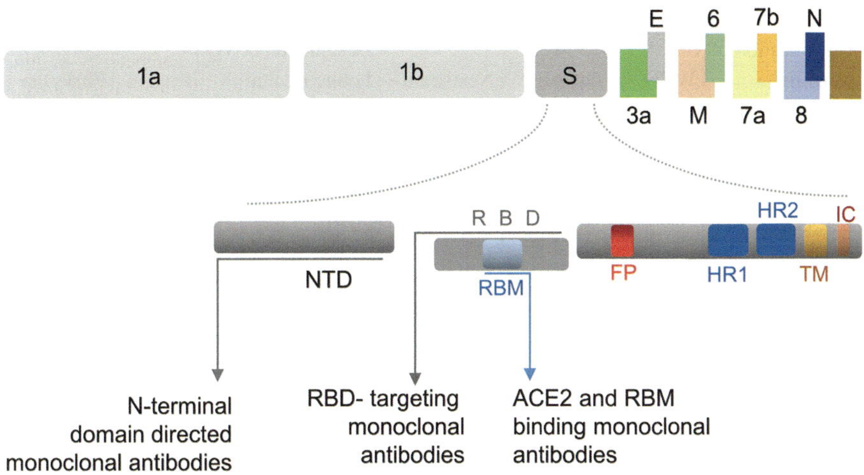


**Fig. 8.1** Organization of SARS-CoV-2 coding genome. The 5′ end features two large open reading frames; ORF1a and 1b. The 3′ end encodes viral structural proteins; envelope (E), membrane (M), spike (S), and nucleocapsid (N) and viral accessory proteins; 3a, 6, 7a, 7b, and ORF8. The SARS-CoV-2 Spike (S) protein can be further divided into S1 and S2 subunits. The S1 receptor binding subunit features the N-terminal (NTD) and receptor binding domain (RBD) which are targets for many monoclonal antibodies against S protein. The RBD consists of a receptor binding motif (RBM) which interacts with host ACE2 receptors and shares binding site with some RBD-targeting antibodies. The S2 acts as membrane fusion subunit which features fusion peptide, HR1 and 2 heptad regions, TM transmembrane domain and IC, intracellular tail. The initial host–viral contact is mediated via RBM-ACE2 interactions while entry through endocytosis occurs through S2 subunit

## SARS-CoV-2 Variants of Concerns and Their Characteristics

Till mid-2021, four SARS-CoV-2 genetic variants were classified by different names on various SARS-CoV-2 genome analysis platforms as Nextstrain, GISAID (Global Initiative On Sharing All Influenza Data,) WHO, and Pangolin (Phylogenetic Assignment of Named Global Outbreak) classifications. An overview of classifications of different VOCs along with geographic characteristics and key mutations in their S protein is outlined in Table 8.1.

Current SARS-CoV-2 VOCs; Alpha, Beta, Gamma, and Delta represent sub-lineage of B.1, characterized by co-occurring D614G and P323L mutations in S protein and ORF1ab, respectively. The single most-concerning mutation in the RBD region of S protein, frequent among Alpha, Beta, and Gamma variants is N501Y (Asparagine–Tyrosine). Other co-occurring mutations have been discussed extensively with each variant. Emergence of new SARS-CoV-2 variants are associated with four major concerns; increased transmissibility, disease severity, escape from

**Table 8.1** Classification and current designation of VOCs

| Classification of VOC | | | | Designation of VOC | | First identified |
|---|---|---|---|---|---|---|
| pangolin Lineage | WHO label | GISAID clade | Nextstrain clade | Public Health England | WHO | |
| B.1.1.7 | Alpha | GRY, 501Y.V1 | 20I (V1) | December 18, 2020 | December 18, 2020 | United Kingdom |
| B.1.351, B.1.351.2, B.1.351.3 | Beta | GH, 501Y.V2 | 20H (V2) | December 24, 2020 | December 18, 2020 | South Africa |
| B.1.1.28.1 (P.1), P.1.1, P.1.2 | Gamma | GR, 501Y. V3 | 20J (V3) | January 13, 2021 | January 11, 2021 | Brazil |
| B.1.617.2, AY.1, AY.2 | Delta | G/478K. V1 | 21A | May 6, 2021 | May 11, 2021 | India |

natural infection induced antibodies (reinfection potential), and escape from vaccination induced antibodies (vaccine breakthrough potential). In this chapter, we have discussed genomic characteristics and phenotypic manifestations of various VOCs and VOIs. The emergence of VOCs is compared with temporal variation in daily new cases, Ro (Reproduction number) and stringency index. Ro signifies how contagious is an infectious disease where Ro > 1 indicates that the virus will be transmitted across the population and Ro < 1 indicates existing infection will cause less than one new infection and thus disease will decline by itself. Stringency index refers to containment and closure policies or as lockdown policies based on Oxford COVID-19 government response tracker [11].

## *SARS-CoV-2 Alpha Variant*

During early December 2020, sequence analysis of genomic data from Kent, England revealed a phylogenetically distinct cluster from the rest of UK. This variant on detection of its high prevalence in Kent and North east London, was then designated as VUI-202012/01 (Variant Under Investigation with a year, month, and number) and later re-designated as VOC-202012/01 on December 18 2020.

The local prevalence (based on B.1.1.7 positive sequences) of Alpha in UK remained above 80% till April 2021 while globally it remained above 50% from late February to May 2021 (Fig. 8.2a). The rise in B.1.1.7 positive sequences was also accompanied by steep rise in daily COVID-19 cases in UK (Fig. 8.2b). However, owing to a national lockdown resulting in a stringency index above 80 could be accounted for lower Ro > 1.5 during high prevalence of Alpha variant (Fig. 8.2b). The Alpha (B.1.1.7) VOC is characterized by 13 non-synonymous and six synonymous mutations and four amino acid deletions. The non-synonymous mutations occur in ORF1ab, S, ORF8 (also contains stop codon), and N protein (Fig. 8.2c). More importantly, this variant accumulated large number of mutations in the S protein which extend multiple phenotypic advantages to the virus. The Alpha variant

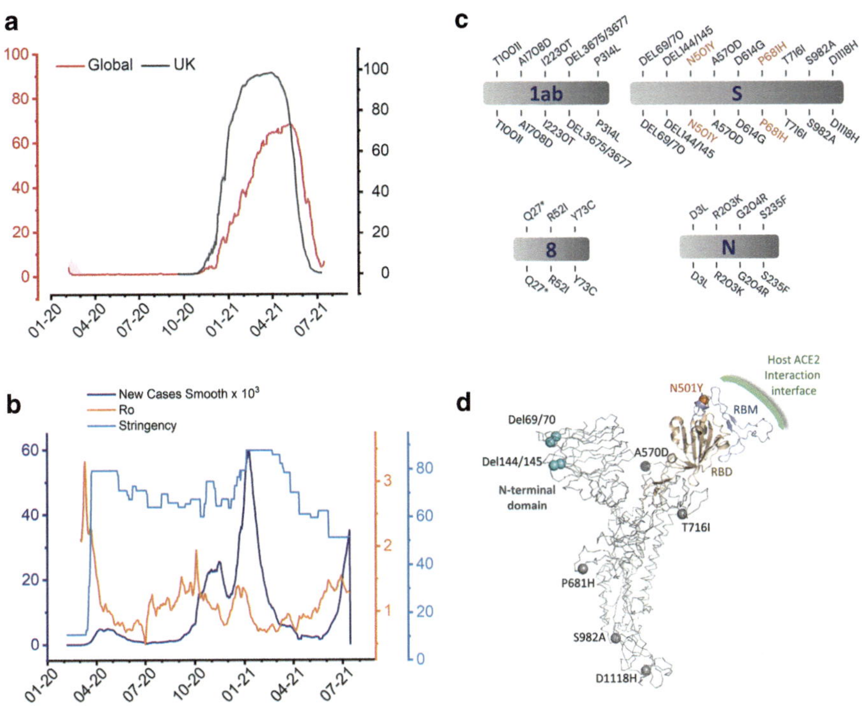


**Fig. 8.2** Characteristics of SARS-CoV-2 Alpha variant. (**a**) Temporal prevalence of Alpha variant globally (red) and in UK (dark gray) based on 7-day rolling average of percent of B.1.1.7-positive sequences. Shaded regions (light red and light gray) around the curves show 95% confidence intervals. (**b**) Temporal variations in daily new COVID-19 cases (navy blue), Ro (orange), and stringency index (light blue) in UK. Stringency index (0–100) is based on nine response indicators including school closures, workplace closures, and travel bans (100 is strictest). (**c**) ORF mutations in B.1.1.7 lineage with >75% prevalence. (**d**) Structural mapping of deletions and mutations (spheres) in the S protein monomer of Alpha variant. Cyan spheres indicate deletions. Orange spheres indicate mutations of concern occurring in RBD (gold) or RBM (pale blue) region. RBM–ACE2 interaction site is shown as green interface

carries only N501Y mutation in the RBD of its S protein (Fig. 8.2d). This mutation is associated with ~ two times higher affinity with host ACE2 receptors compared to ancestral D614G strain [12]. In accord with reports to characterize the spread of Alpha variant in United Kingdom [13], Davies NG et al. estimated a 43–90% increase in transmissibility over the predecessor lineage using combination of statistical and dynamic modeling approaches. Although the authors noted absence of its role in disease severity; the enhanced transmission may likely result in higher incidences and increase in hospital admitted patients [14]. In another report on analysis of ~two million positive SARS-CoV-2 community tests and 17,452 COVID-19 related deaths from November 2020 to February 2021, Davies NG et al. estimated 61% (95% CI 42–82%) higher risk of death with infection from Alpha variant in England indicating a more severe illness than infections from the pre-existing variants. However, in another cohort study of patients admitted to hospitals between November 9 and December 20, 2020 in London, Frampton D et al. albeit observed an increased viral load associated with Alpha variant but did not observe any association with disease severity [15]. As per early reports from Public Health England, a random effect model based on analysis of 1419 Alpha genomes and 33,972 non-Alpha genomes reported an additive effect of 0.74 (95% CI 0.44–1.29) to the reproduction number [16]. The other highly co-occurring P681H mutation (S protein) occurring in the vicinity of polybasic "RRAR" furin cleavage motif was also suspected to affect phenotypic characteristics of this strain [4].

Interestingly, the early detection of Alpha variants was a consequence of S gene target failures in a three-target diagnostic assay (N, ORF1ab, S) adopted in national testing system of United Kingdom [16]. Through molecular analysis of PCR amplicon products from diagnostic assays of S gene dropout samples, the S gene target failure was later ascribed to deletion of six nucleotides in Alpha variant leading to Δ69–70 deletion in the S protein. The deletions result in the failure of qPCR probes to bind target gene [17]. The enhanced transmission and diagnostic failures could be immediately addressed through appropriate COVID-19 behavior and upgradation of qPCR testing protocols [18]. However, notable concerns looming over accumulation of cluster of mutations in B.1.1.7 Alpha and other VOCs were their potential to escape neutralizing antibodies and at a time when vaccination programs were about to commence globally.

By December 2020, nearly 1.2 million people globally (~ 0.6 million in United Kingdom and ~ 0.5 million in USA) have received their single COVID-19 vaccine dose [8]. The modulation of efficacy of neutralization antibodies was suspected due to the N501Y mutation in the antigenic site of RBD. However, later follow-up studies indicated that the B.1.1.7 Alpha variant was only moderate in compromising neutralization potential by monoclonal antibodies and antibody responses by vaccination or natural infection; thus, less likely to be a major concern of reinfection or neutralization resistance. In a post-hoc analysis of the efficacy of Oxford-AstraZeneca (ChAdOx1/AZD1222) vaccine against B.1.1.7 variant, moderate reduction in clinical efficacy 70·4% (95% CI 43.6–84.5) was observed compared against non-B.1.1.7 lineages (clinical efficacy: 81.5%, CI 67.9–89.4) [19]. In another study, sera collected from 19 fully vaccinated individuals with Pfizer-Comirnaty messenger RNA (mRNA) vaccine were effectively potent against B.1.1.7 compared to D614G strain [20, 21]. While assessing mutational effects on monoclonal antibodies isolated from COVID-19 recovered individuals, decreased neutralization in N-terminal domain and receptor binding motif (part of RBD which interacts with host ACE2 receptors) directed antibodies was observed [21, 22]. Antibodies which bind outside the receptor binding motif were moderately affected by mutations in Alpha variant [22]. Another mRNA-based Moderna-mRNA-1273 vaccine was also equally effective with Pfizer-Comirnaty in preventing hospitalizations in the USA due to Alpha variant (vaccine efficacy, 97.3%; 95% CI 78.9–99.7%). The vaccine efficacy was reduced in patients with immunosuppression (59.2%; 95% CI 11.9–81.1%) than without immunosuppression (91.3%; 95% CI 85.5–94.7%) [23]. Similar results were obtained from testing vaccine effectiveness efficacy of Moderna-mRNA-1273 (double dose) against Alpha variant (100%; 95% CI 91.8–100.0%) prevalent in Qatar population [24]. The high vaccine efficacy observed against asymptomatic (92.5%; 95% CI 84.8–96.9%) and symptomatic infections (98.6%; 95% CI 92.0–100%) indicating the importance of a full vaccination protocol in viral neutralization. Emergence of Alpha variant only presented minimal threats to neutralization by convalescent and post-vaccination sera; the introduction of single E484K mutation to B.1.1.7 background resulted in higher neutralization resistance [25, 26] and disease severity [21].

## *SARS-CoV-2 Beta Variant*

The Beta variant or 501Y.V2 belongs to B.1.351 SARS-CoV-2 lineage and was first identified in South Africa in September 2020 and later designated as VOC in December 2020. By July 2021, the Beta lineage has spread over 100 nations with global prevalence of 1% and 63% in South Africa. While its global prevalence peaked near 2% during March 2021, it remained consistently high (>80%) from End-November 2020 till early May 2021 (Fig. 8.3a).

Emergence of Beta variant coincided with reduction in stringency index in South Africa, thus fueling its second COVID-19 infection wave in South Africa with Ro peaking above 1.5 (Fig. 8.3b). The third COVID-19 wave peaking around July 2021 could be attributed to introduction of Delta variants in South African population. Beta variant accumulated 23 mutations with 17 amino acid changes in ORF1ab, S, 3a, E, and N proteins (Fig. 8.3c). Besides N501Y, it carries two additional K417N and E484K mutations in the RBD and RBM, respectively (Fig. 8.3d). These mutations further enhance binding affinity of RBD with host ACE2 receptors by 2.32 and 4.62 times compared to that of Alpha variant and wild type SARS-CoV-2 [12]. The Beta variant was also estimated to be 50% more transmissible than pre-existing variants in South Africa [7]. Consequently, this variant's apparent cumulative prevalence was more than 80% in all sequenced samples in South Africa between December 2020 to early May 2021 and more than 1% globally from early January till June 2021 (Fig. 8.3a). Unlike Alpha variant, changes in disease severity or diagnostic test failures exclusively due to Beta variant could not be established. However, Jassat et al. in a cohort study from hospital admissions in South Africa established an increased risk of in-hospital mortality during the second infection wave [27].

The rapid expansion of B.1.351 lineage towards end of 2020 in South Africa was associated with increased transmissibility and immune evasive capabilities due to K417N, E484K, and N501Y key substitutions in the RBD of S protein. In earliest reports, the 501Y.V2 Beta variant was poorly cross neutralized from convalescent plasma of individuals recovered from first COVID-19 wave infections indicating the reinfection potential of the new variant and that previous infection might confer partial protection against this variant [28]. While the Alpha variant had moderate impacts on susceptibility to most of the monoclonal antibody treatments, the Beta showed significant susceptibility reduction to combination bamlanivimab and

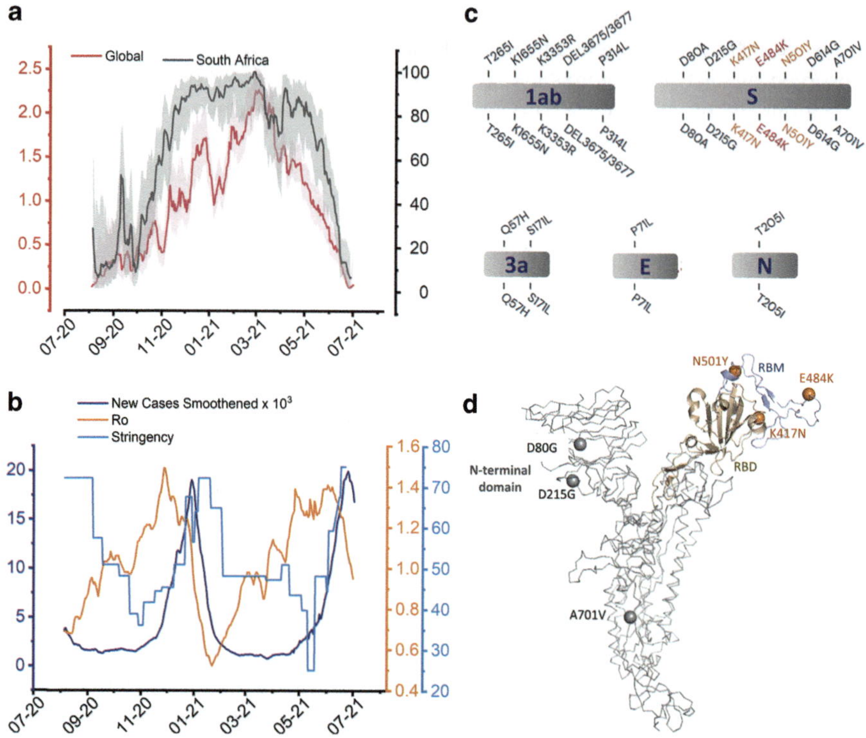


**Fig. 8.3** Characteristics of SARS-CoV-2 Beta variant. (**a**) Temporal prevalence of Beta variant globally (red) and in South Africa (dark gray) based on 7-day rolling average of percent of B.1.351-positive sequences. Shaded regions (light red and light gray) around the curves show 95% confidence intervals. (**b**) Temporal variations in daily new COVID-19 cases (navy blue), Ro (orange) and stringency index (light blue) in South Africa. (**c**) ORF mutations in B.1.351 lineage with >75% prevalence. (**d**) Structural mapping of deletions and mutations (spheres) in the S protein monomer of Beta variant. Cyan spheres indicate deletions. Orange spheres indicate mutations of concern occurring in RBD (gold) or RBM (pale blue) region

etesevimab monoclonal antibody treatments. With regard to vaccine induced immunity, multiple studies have indicated possibly reduced protection against symptomatic disease and infection while vaccine protection against severe COVID-19 by Beta variant is retained. The Janssen Ad26.COV2.S showed 81.7% and 64% efficacy against severe-critical and moderate to severe-critical COVID-19 infection, respectively indicating protection against symptomatic and asymptomatic COVID-19 infection and severe-critical disease that results in hospitalization and deaths [29]. The neutralizing antibody titers by Ad26.COV2.S were, however, reduced by fivefold compared to WA1/2020 SARS-CoV-2 strain while preserving complement deposition, cellular phagocytosis and natural killer cell activation responses against the B.1.351 variant [30]. The Pfizer-BioNTech mRNA vaccine has shown more than 90% efficacy against COVID-19 retained protection against severe disease. However, the effectiveness against Beta variant infection was moderately reduced to 75% (95% CI 70.5–78.9) but not translating to poor protection against severe-critical cases [31]. The Moderna-mRNA-1273 vaccine showed a 96.4% efficacy (95% CI 91.9–98.7%) in preventing infection (after double dose). Additionally, it showed high effectiveness against any severe-critical or fatal COVID-19 even at a single dose (81.6%, 95% CI 71.0–88.8%) and 95.7% (95% CI 73.4–99.9%) after second dose. In recent studies, the antibody neutralization titers against Beta variant were shown to be reduced by tenfold compared to Wuhan-related SARS-CoV-2 strain [32, 33]. The whole virion-inactivated BBV152 SARS-CoV-2 vaccine also showed threefold reduction in neutralization titers against Beta variant, although the vaccine showed an overall protective response against the VOC [34]. Among the in-use candidates, the AstraZeneca-Vaxzevria and Novavax-Covavax vaccine efficacies in preventing mild-moderate COVID-19 infections and neutralization against Beta variant were severely affected [35, 36]. The reduction in neutralization could be linked to loss of vaccine efficacy which could be further mediated by escape from T-cell immunity. However, this is less likely due to diversity of HLA alleles in the population [37]. Because the substitutions at E484 in the RBD were associated with largest decrease in neutralization, the Beta variant was highly refractory against polyclonal human plasma antibodies and to most of the in-use vaccines [38].

## *SARS-CoV-2 Gamma Variant*

The SARS-CoV-2 Gamma (501Y.V3) variant was first identified in Manaus, the capital city of Amazonas state in Brazil and was associated with second wave of COVID-19 infection. The Gamma or 501Y.V2 variant belongs to P.1 lineage which is a direct descendent of B.1.1.28, first detected in early March 2020 in Brazil [4, 7, 39]. The consecutive lineage replacements were predicted to be driven by emergence of P.1 along with variable levels of social distancing. Molecular clock analysis (used to estimate most recent common ancestor) using flexible nonparametric demographic tree indicated emergence of P.1 lineage around mid-November 2020. The local model also confirmed a higher evolutionary rate for branch ancestral to P.1 [39]. The global percentage of P.1-positive sequences remained above 3% from April to June 2021 while in Brazil it remained above 80% during the same time period (Fig. 8.1a). Since the beginning of pandemic, Brazil has recorded highest COVID-19 incidences besides India and USA. The stringency index has also remained below 50 since mid-2020 due to which multiple overlapping infections waves could be observed (Fig. 8.4b). The emergence of Gamma could be witnessed in terms of daily cases (average weekly) increasing beyond 60,000 per day. Contrastingly, the Ro fluctuated around 1.0 during this period.

The P.1 lineage also carried distinct set of mutations of concern (previously known to be of virological importance) in the RBD of S protein and other ORFs (Fig. 8.4c, d). The RBD harboring E484K, N501Y, and K417N mutations (Fig. 8.4d) showed two times higher binding affinity towards ACE2 compared to RBD from

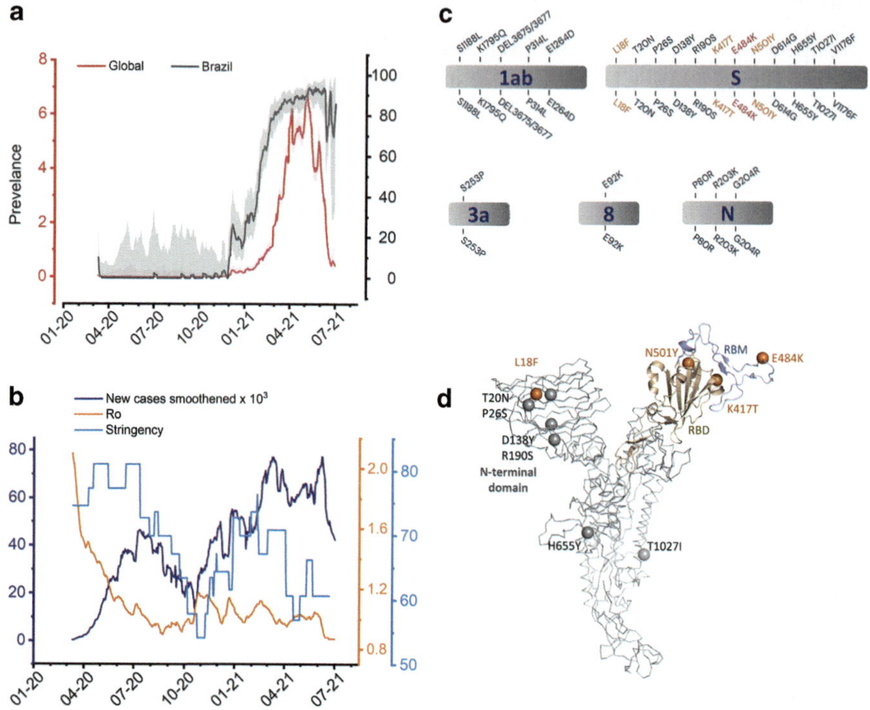


**Fig. 8.4** Characteristics of SARS-CoV-2 Gamma variant. (**a**) Temporal prevalence of Gamma variant globally (red) and in Brazil (dark gray) based on 7-day rolling average of percent of P.1-positive sequences. Shaded regions (light red and light gray) around the curves show 95% confidence intervals. (**b**) Temporal variations in daily new COVID-19 cases (navy blue), Ro (orange) and stringency index (light blue) in Brazil. (**c**) ORF mutations in P.1 lineage with >75% prevalence. (**d**) Structural mapping of deletions and mutations (spheres) in the S protein monomer of Gamma variant. Cyan spheres indicate deletions. Orange spheres indicate mutations of concern occurring in RBD (gold) or RBM (pale blue) region

wild type SARS-CoV-2 [40]. This was consistent with other in silico studies and epidemiological studies [4, 41, 42] which also estimated P.1 to be 1.7- to 2.4-fold more transmissible than non-P.1 variants in Brazil [39]. While the P.1 infected individuals had tenfold higher viral load than non-P.1 infected, the clear role of P.1 in causing higher disease severity has not been documented. Although recent studies indicate its role in possibly higher risk of hospitalization [25], this could be due to combination of rapid transmission of highly infectious P.1 and over-burdening of healthcare systems. The impact of P.1 on diagnostic failures has also not been reported.

As per latest epidemiological report from WHO (July 20, 2020), no evidence has been reported on modulation of vaccine protection against infection and severe disease by P.1 variant [43]. With regard to Sinovac-CoronaVac vaccine effectiveness against Gamma variant infecting in elderly population in Brazil, a reduction in symptomatic infection, hospitalizations, and deaths in adults (≥70 years) was observed but an age-dependent reduction in vaccine effectiveness was observed [44]. Another related study on health care workers ($\geq$18 years) in Manaus Brazil reported low estimated vaccine effectiveness against symptomatic infection, following a two-dose schedule [45]. The neutralizing activity in sera against P.1 was reduced by a factor of 6.7 and 4.5 for mRNA-based Pfizer-BNT162b2 and Moderna mRNA-1273 [7, 46] and 3·92 for CoronaVac vaccinated individuals [47]. In a recent study on assessment of Janssen Ad26.COV2.S vaccine against P.1, 2.7-fold lower median binding antibody titers were observed while T-cell responses and functional non-neutralizing antibody responses were largely preserved [30]. P.1 Gamma variant was also observed to be refractory to neutralization by convalescent plasma (3.4-fold) and combination of emergency-use approved antibodies; etesevimab, bamlanivimab, and casirivimab except imdevimab monoclonal antibody [48]. Interestingly, P.1 was observed to be profoundly refractory against NTD-directed antibodies; 2–17, 4–18, 4–19, and 5–7 [48] and sensitive to 5–24 and 4–8 (no neutralization activity against Beta variant) which were isolated from patients infected with SARS-CoV-2 with severe COVID-19 disease [49]. Despite harboring similar set of K417N/T, E484K, and N501Y mutations in RBD of S protein of Beta and Gamma variants, loss of neutralization by natural antibodies isolated from COVID-19 patients indicate crucial role of non-RBD regions in mediating viral neutralization.

## *SARS-CoV-2 Delta Variant*

The SARS-CoV-2 Delta (B.1.617.2) variant was associated with second COVID-19 infection wave in India from April to May 2021 [50]. As of August 2021, the Delta has been detected across more than 100 nations, including a notable increase in Delta cases in the United Kingdom and USA. It also comprises ~ 9% of total sequences (>2.4 million) submitted in GISAID (a global science initiative for rapid sharing of genomic, epidemiological, and clinical data from all human infecting viruses and coronaviruses). The apparent percentage of B.1.617.2-positive sequences remained above 50% globally and in India since mid-June and mid-April, respectively (Fig. 8.5a).

The Delta variant was responsible for fueling second COVID-19 infection in India despite relatively high stringency index (>60) (Fig. 8.5b). Consequently, Ro escalated beyond 1.5 indicating high penetration capacity of this variant. Compared to other VOCs, Delta harbors highest number of deletions and mutations in all ORFs (Fig. 8.5c). The variant carries two deletions and 27 non-synonymous mutations with key L452R–T468K–P681R mutations in the S protein (Fig. 8.5c, d). The key S protein mutations, distinct from Alpha, Beta, and Gamma were also associated with increased transmissibility and secondary attack rate [8, 43]. In a recent analysis using 1.72 million SARS-CoV-2 genome sequences, the Delta variant showed a statistically significant increase of 97% (95% CI 76–117%) in the pooled mean effective reproduction number compared to non-VOC/VOI strains [51]. The study

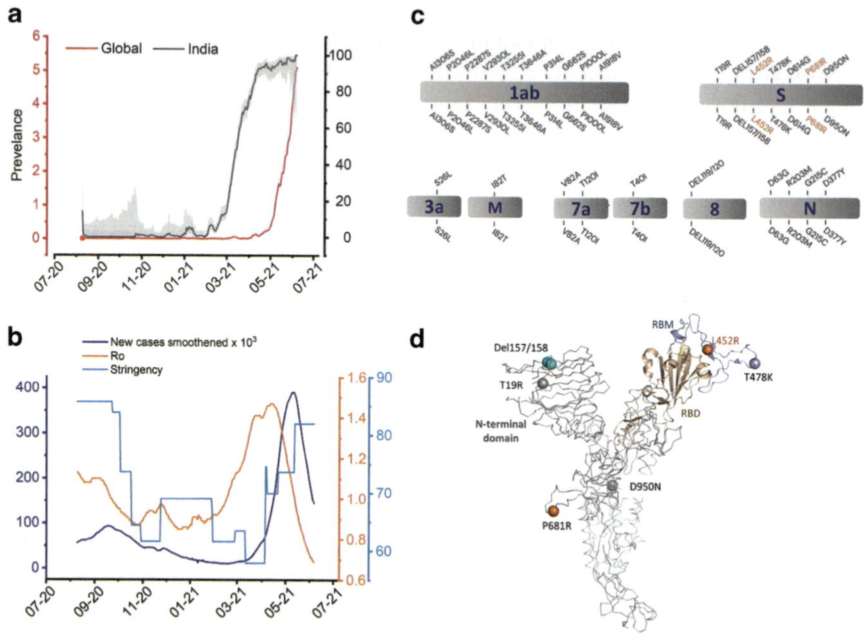


**Fig. 8.5** Characteristics of SARS-CoV-2 Delta variant. (**a**) Temporal prevalence of Delta variant globally (red) and in India (dark gray) based on 7-day rolling average of percent of B.1.617.2-positive sequences. Shaded regions (light red and light gray) around the curves show 95% confidence intervals. (**b**) Temporal variations in daily new COVID-19 cases (navy blue), Ro (orange) and stringency index (light blue) in India. (**c**) ORF mutations in P.1 lineage with >75% prevalence. (**d**) Structural mapping of deletions and mutations (spheres) in the S protein monomer of Delta variant. Cyan spheres indicate deletions. Orange spheres indicate mutations of concern occurring in RBD (gold) or RBM (pale blue) region

also suggested clear competitive advantage of B.1.617.2 Delta variant over other VOCs; Alpha, Beta, and Gamma with an estimated increase in effective reproduction number by 55% (95% CI 43–68%), 60% (95% CI 48–73%), and 34% (95% CI 26–43%) respectively. The mechanisms for increased transmissibility may be attributed to enhanced viral entry, altered host-mediated protease activity and host membrane fusion by B.1.617 lineage compared to D614G and B.1.1.7 variants [52]. From structural perspectives, an in silico study (preprint) indicates role of disruption of intra-molecular interactions within a hydrophobic patch in RBD (L452–L492–F490) which leads to slight increase in ACE2 affinity [53]. Another study hints at stabilization of RBD by Delta mutations which increase in the binding energy with ACE2 [54]. Delta variant was associated with higher risk of hospitalizations as viral loads in Delta affected patients in China were ~ 1000 times higher than non-VOCs [55]. In another study from Canada, the risk of hospitalization, intensive care unit admissions and deaths from Delta variant were increased by 120% (95% CI 93–153%), 287% (95% CI 198–399%), and 137% (95% CI 50–230%), respectively compared to non-VOCs [56]. The mutations in the Delta were however not observed to impact SARS-CoV-2 diagnostic tests [43].

Protection against severe disease by Delta variant is retained by most of current line vaccines while moderate reduction in protection against symptomatic disease, infection, and neutralization is reported. In one of the earliest reports on assessing efficacy of Pfizer-BioNTech and AstraZeneca-ChAdOx1 vaccines against Delta variant, high levels of protection against hospitalization with single or double doses of either vaccine was reported. Compared to Alpha variant, only modest differences in vaccine effectiveness against Delta was observed [57]. The Moderna mRNA-1273 vaccine also showed moderate (2.1-fold) reduction in neutralization of Delta compared to D614G (B.1) variant while it remained susceptible to vaccine elicited serum neutralization [58]. In two separate studies, the Delta variant was observed to be refractory against natural infection inflicted antibodies compared to other VOCs and D614G variant. The Sinovac-CoronaVac (inactivated vaccine) elicited neutralizing antibodies also showed moderate reduction (>twofold) in neutralizing antibody titers against Delta and B.1.617 parent lineage compared to natural and D614G infections [52, 59]. The whole-virion inactivated BBV152 SARS-CoV-2 vaccine also showed 2.7-fold reduction in neutralizing titers against Delta, although protective response against the VOC was maintained [34]. Interestingly, modest reduction (1.6-fold) in susceptibility to single dose Janssen Ad26.COV2.S vaccine elicited antibodies against Delta was reported [60]. The B.1.617 has also showed reduced neutralization sensitivity against five monoclonal antibodies (CQ012, CQ026, CQ038, CQ039, and CQ046) isolated from blood of COVID-19 convalescent patients by 3–4.5-fold compared to D614G variant [52]. Another study by Liu et al. assessed response of potent antibodies, isolated from COVID-19 recovered individuals to neutralize B.1.617.1 and B.1.617.2 Delta variants [61]. Compared to ancestral Victoria (SARS-CoV-2/human/AUS/VIC01/2020) strain, at least five antibodies showed fivefold reduction in neutralization of B.1.617.1 and Delta variants by virtue of L452R and E484Q mutations in the RBD of S protein. On assessment of sensitivity of RBD-targeting approved monoclonal antibodies for human use; Bamlanivimab was completely refractory while Etesevimab, Casirivimab, and Imdevimab retained their activity against Delta variant compared to D614G (B.1) [62]. B.1.617.2 Delta also contains T19R, G142D, del156–157, R158G, and A222V mutations in the NTD (S protein) which can potentially disrupt its antigenic supersite, target for many NTD-directed antibodies. Consequently, global loss of neutralization by some NTD-directed antibodies has also been reported [62]. In conclusions, the Delta variant may escape neutralization by some RBD or NTD-targeting antibodies.

Amid global concerns over phenotypic manifestations of Delta variant, the B.1.617.2 continues to evolve to two more VOCs; AY.1 and AY.2 (currently aggregated with Delta and provisionally called Delta plus). As of August 2021, the Delta plus: AY.1 and AY.2 is currently reported from 22 and 24 nations, respectively with cumulative prevalence of <0.5% globally.

The Delta plus variants carry an additional K417N mutation apart from L452R, T478K in the RBD of S protein. The mutation, however, did not confer any increase in infectivity with respect to Delta variant [63]. K417N alone or as co-occurring mutation was also associated with neutralization resistance [50]. On comparison to Delta, the AY.1 carries highly conserved W258L mutation in the unstructured (N5) loop region of NTD antigen supersite, previously described as binding region for NTD-directed high neutralization potency monoclonal antibodies [64, 65]. Interestingly, during assessment of recent vaccine breakthrough infections in USA, W258L was ~ 15.2-fold enriched in two B.1.427 VOI [66] indicating its role in NTD mediated antibody neutralization resistance. With respect to natural infection elicited antibodies, sera of individuals infected prior to the detection of VOCs showed modest (3.2–4.9-fold) decrease in neutralization against Delta or Delta plus variants. Antibodies from sera of 81 individuals vaccinated with Pfizer-BNT162b2 and Moderna-mRNA-1273 also showed modest 2.5–4.0-fold decrease in titer upon cross-reaction with the variants [63]. The Janssen Ad26.COV2.S vaccine which showed only modest decrease in neutralizing tires against Delta variant showed a more pronounced decrease (5.4-fold) against Delta plus compared to D614G (B.1) variant. The Delta plus variant was observed to be specifically refractory to casirivimab with ~ 93-fold decrease in neutralizing titer while modestly to imdevimab monoclonal antibodies due to K417N and L452R mutations, respectively [63]. As of August 2021, the Delta and Delta plus variants show positive transmission advantage compared to Alpha, Beta, and Gamma indicating their capability to outcompete other VOCs/VOIs.

Differences in current line vaccines against severe, symptomatic, infection and neutralization of SARS-CoV-2 are outlined in Table 8.2.

**Table 8.2** Summary of different types of COVID-19 vaccines against currently designated VOCs

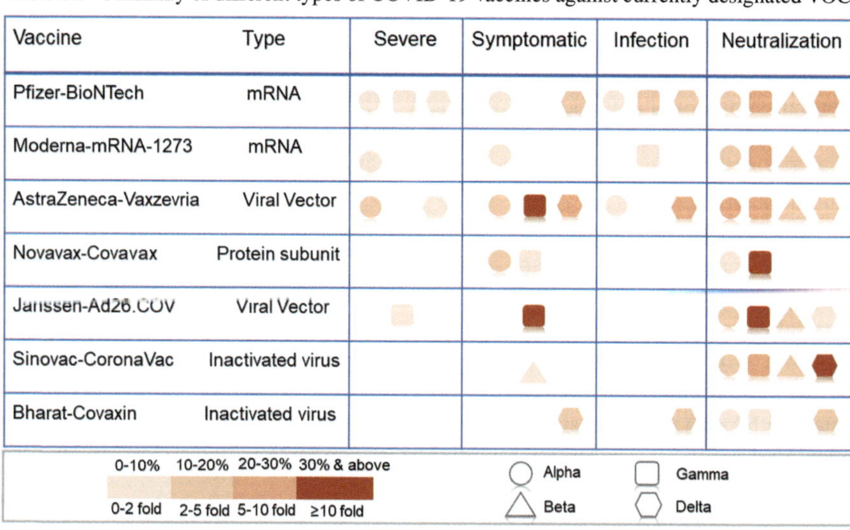

| Vaccine | Type | Severe | Symptomatic | Infection | Neutralization |
|---|---|---|---|---|---|
| Pfizer-BioNTech | mRNA | | | | |
| Moderna-mRNA-1273 | mRNA | | | | |
| AstraZeneca-Vaxzevria | Viral Vector | | | | |
| Novavax-Covavax | Protein subunit | | | | |
| Janssen-Ad26.COV | Viral Vector | | | | |
| Sinovac-CoronaVac | Inactivated virus | | | | |
| Bharat-Covaxin | Inactivated virus | | | | |



Adapted from WHO COVID-19 Weekly Epidemiological Update [43]

## SARS-CoV-2 Variants of Interest (VOI) and Their Characteristics

The SARS-CoV-2 VOIs are classified on the basis of specific genetic markers associated with possible increase in viral transmission or severity through modulation of host receptor binding, reduced neutralization by naturally or vaccine induced antibodies, potential diagnostic failures, or reduced therapeutic efficacies [43, 50]. As of August 2021, four major genetic variants have been classified as VOIs; B.1.525, B.1.526, B.1.617.1, and C.37 by WHO (Table 8.3).

The B.1.525 Eta variant was first identified in UK and Nigeria in early 2021. Till mid-July 2021, the global cumulative prevalence of Eta was <0.5% and ~47% in Nigeria till May 21 2021. This variant contains crucial E484K mutation (also present in Beta and Gamma VOCs), associated with escape from antibodies induced by natural infection or vaccines. The NTD del 69–70 and del144 (present in Alpha variant) are associated with antigenic escape and viral replication in immunocompromised patients. The CDC-USA has attributed potential reduction in neutralization by monoclonal antibodies, convalescent and post-vaccination sera based on E484K mutation of Eta variant [67]. However in a recent study, SARS-CoV-2 Alpha and theta authentic viruses were effectively neutralized by Pfizer-BNT162b2 vaccine elicited antibodies, followed by reduced neutralization of Beta and Gamma variants compared to B.1 lineage [68].

The B.1.526 Iota variant was first identified in the USA and later designated as VOI/VUI in March 2021. Since its last detection in mid-July 2021, cumulative prevalence of Iota was 2% while it accounted for 7% of total sequenced samples in USA. Among the total sequenced samples, D5F, T95I, D253G were most conserved mutations (>75% prevalence) and few (<20% of samples) harbored known mutations of concern; L452R, S477N, and E484K. Compared to D614G, Iota variants with S477N mutation were fully susceptible to sera and convalescent sera isolated from individuals vaccinated with the Moderna mRNA1273 and Pfizer-BNT162b2 vaccines and variants with E484K were neutralized with modest (3.5-fold) reduction [69].

**Table 8.3** Classification and current designation of VOIs

| Classification of VOC | | | | Designation of VOI | | |
|---|---|---|---|---|---|---|
| Pangolin lineage | WHO label | GISAID clade | Nextstrain clade | Public Health England | WHO | First identified |
| B.1.525 | Eta | G/484K.V3 | 21D | February 12, 2021 | March 17, 2021 | England, Nigeria |
| B.1.526 | Iota | GH/253G. V1 | 21F | March 10, 2021 | March 24, 2021 | USA |
| B.1.617.1 | Kappa | G/452R.V3 | 21B | April 1, 2021 | April 4, 2021 | India |
| C.37 | Lambda | GR/452Q. V1 | 21G | June 25, 2021 | June 14, 2021 | Peru |

The third B.1.617.1 Kappa VOI first detected in India (11% cumulative prevalence) has now been detected in 51 nations (<0.5% globally). In Kappa, L452R, E484Q occur as highly conserved mutations. These individual mutations associated with higher transmissibility were also suspected to confer synergistic effects in neutralization resistance. However, S protein bearing L452R or E484Q alone confers similar (to L452R–E484K co-occurring) and modestly reduced sensitivity to Pfizer-BNT162b2 vaccine elicited antibodies [70]. In another study, Kappa variant was observed to be 6.8-folds more resistant to neutralization by sera from Moderna mRNA1273 and Pfizer-BNT162b2 vaccinated individuals, although protective immunity by the mRNA vaccines were fully retained [71].

The fourth C.37 Lambda variant emerged in Peru and identified across American, European and Western pacific regions. While globally, Lambda encompasses 0.5% of sequenced samples, it has ~ 70% cumulative prevalence in Peru (July 2021). Lambda VOI is characterized by convergent deletion; del3675–3677in the ORF1a (also in Beta and Gamma VOCs) and notable mutations; L452Q and F490S in the RBD of S protein. The Lambda variant was observed to be associated with higher infectivity compared to D614G (B.1), Alpha and Gamma variants due to L45Q mutation [63]. Further compared to wild-type (lineage A), a modest 3.05-fold decrease in neutralization by CoronaVac vaccine elicited antibodies were observed followed by 2.03- and 2.33-fold decrease recorded for Alpha and Gamma variants, respectively [72]. More studies showed modest compromise in effectiveness of Moderna mRNA1273 and Pfizer-BNT162b2 mRNA vaccine against Lambda variant [63, 73], however, Janessen-Ad26.COV2.S vaccine elicited neutralizing antibodies showed pronounced decrease (five to sevenfold) in neutralizing titer indicating that its second immunization might increase protection against Lambda VOI. Additionally, no loss of titer was observed during neutralization of Lambda by the Regeneron therapeutic monoclonal antibody cocktail [73].

The SARS-CoV-2S protein has been the target of the most first-generation vaccines, almost exclusively using the D614 sequence, an early variant with an aspartic acid (D) to glycine (G) mutation at position 614, D614G. The recent fast-spreading variants-including B.1.1.7 (Alpha), B.1.351 (Beta), P.1 (Gamma), and B.1.617.2 (Delta) all contain the D614G substitution. Hence the vaccinations should be effective, at least to some extent, against these variants and will help to curtail the spread of infection and save fatalities to a great extent. However, the modified next generation of vaccines may be needed that would include the mutations E484K, N501Y, L452R and T478K in the RBD, and P681H/R mutation in the furin cleavage site as well as NTD deletions.

## Long-Term Manifestations of COVID-19

With emergence of VOCs and VOIs around the globe, we are witnessing immediate COVID-19 related complications as increase in disease incidence, disease burden, and severity, resistance against natural infection and vaccine induced antibodies stirring fears of reinfection. While we are still in the infancy of understanding these complications, researchers and medical practitioners are also anticipating long-term or long-haul effects of COVID-19. Prior to December 2020, there was absence of an agreed clinical definition of COVID-19 related long-term effects or of treatment pathway. In light of this, the Royal College of General Practitioners, National Institute for Health and Care Excellence and Scottish Intercollegiate Guidelines Network have jointly framed the rapid guideline for management of long-term complications of COVID-19 [74]. As per their guidelines, these complications can be defined as acute, ongoing-symptomatic and chronic or post-COVID-19. Acute infection covers presence of symptoms of COVID-19 up to 4 weeks, ongoing-symptomatic signs and symptoms extend beyond 4–12 weeks from initial onset of COVID-19 symptom, while chronic COVID-19 refers to symptoms extending beyond 12 weeks and are not related to alternative diagnosis. Ongoing or new symptoms; singularly or co-occurring, constant, transient, or fluctuating post-acute COVID-19 are listed in Table 8.4.

From standpoint of long-term health problems, cardiovascular, pulmonary, neurological, and behavioral manifestations could be major challenges for clinical researchers in near future. The pulmonary manifestations are immediately (after 12 weeks) observed following COVID-19, including fibrosis and interstitial thickening. Lower respiratory muscle strength and decreased carbon monoxide diffusion capacity occurred commonly among patients. Among the cardiovascular problems, myocarditis, cardiac arrhythmias and cardiomyopathy are increasingly being associated with COVID-19. A recent cardiac magnetic resonance imaging (performed at median of 70 days post COVID diagnosis) study revealed ongoing myocardial inflammation in 60% and cardiac involvement in 78% among hundred COVID-19 recovered patients [75]. Decline in pulmonary function compounded with cardiac manifestations could have severe cardiopulmonary consequences in already affected patients with either of diseases. Long-term neurological diseases are also anticipated considering diverse neurological conditions such as myopathy, seizures, strokes, cranial nerve palsies, encephalopathy and peripheral neuropathy with SARS-CoV-1 and MERS-CoV outbreaks in 2002 and 2012, respectively [76, 77].

**Table 8.4** Reported symptoms after acute COVID-19 infection (>4 weeks after the onset of acute symptoms)

| | |
|---|---|
| *Generalized*<br>Fatigue, fever, pain, skin hemorrhages, conjunctiva hemorrhages, uncontrolled hypertension >140/90 mmHg, uncontrolled diabetes mellitus | *Cardiovascular*<br>Palpitation, Chest pain |
| *Pulmonary*<br>Breathlessness, cough | *Psychological/psychiatric*<br>Depression, anxiety, aggression |
| *Neurological*<br>Cognitive impairment, sleep disturbance, peripheral neuropathy, delirium | *Gastrointestinal*<br>Abdominal pain, nausea, Diarrhea, anorexia, reduced appetite |
| *Musculoskeletal*<br>Joint and muscle pain | *Ear, nose, and throat*<br>Tinnitus, loss of smell/taste |

In this regard, "NeuroCovid" classification scheme has been proposed recently by Fotuhi et al., which integrates currently identified short-term challenges and the long-term sequalae of COVID-19 such as cognitive decline, compulsive obsessive disorder, accelerated aging, Alzheimer's or Parkinson's disease in the future [78].

## Conclusions

The current observations on emerging VOCs/VOIs indicate their high reinfection potential in individuals which were prior infected or have been fully vaccinated. In case of uncontrolled transmission and high breakthrough infections, the health policy makers ought to consider annual booster immunizations to prevent further loss of lives due to emerging variants. While most of vaccine candidates have shown potential to neutralize these variants, the public health apparatus in highly affected nations should primarily focus on large-scale full vaccinations and meticulous genome surveillance to check spread of new variants.

In addition to pulmonary complications arising out of initial COVID-19 illness, the true extent of extra-pulmonary cardiac-vascular, pancreatic, and neurological manifestations is yet to be determined. Given the psychological stress by the pandemic experienced by global population for more than a year, the recovered individuals are at greater risk of developing cardiopulmonary co-morbidities, anxiety, behavioral changes, depression and post-traumatic stress disorders. Long-COVID is adding chronic disease burden exponentially, with a cumulative differential towards mental health. With a pre-existing infection burden of more than 25,000 per million of world population and still escalating, the potential of non-COVID global health crisis should not be ignored either [79].

## References

1. Li Q, et al. The impact of mutations in SARS-CoV-2 spike on viral infectivity and antigenicity. Cell. 2020;182(5):1284–1294 e9.
2. Sheikh JA, et al. Emerging genetic diversity among clinical isolates of SARS-CoV-2: lessons for today. Infect Genet Evol. 2020;84:104330.
3. Sironi M, et al. SARS-CoV-2 and COVID-19: a genetic, epidemiological, and evolutionary perspective. Infect Genet Evol. 2020;81:104384.
4. Singh J, et al. Structure–function analyses of new SARS-CoV-2 variants B.1.1.7, B.1.351 and B.1.1.28.1: clinical, diagnostic, therapeutic and public health implications. Viruses. 2021;13(3):439.
5. van Dorp L, et al. No evidence for increased transmissibility from recurrent mutations in SARS-CoV-2. Nat Commun. 2020;11(1):5986.
6. Singh H, et al. Mapping the genomic landscape and diversity of COVID-19 based on >3950 clinical isolates of SARS-CoV-2: likely origin and transmission dynamics of isolates sequenced in India. Indian J Med Res. 2020;151(5):474–8.

7. Abdool Karim SS, de Oliveira T. New SARS-CoV-2 variants—clinical, public health, and vaccine implications. N Engl J Med. 2021;384(19):1866–8.
8. Julia LM, et al. outbreak.info. 2020. Accessed 18 Jul 2021.
9. Mukherjee A, et al. SARS-CoV-2 re-infection: development of an epidemiological definition from India. Epidemiol Infect. 2021;149:e82.
10. Sabino EC, et al. Resurgence of COVID-19 in Manaus, Brazil, despite high seroprevalence. Lancet. 2021;397(10273):452–5.
11. Hale T, et al. A global panel database of pandemic policies (Oxford COVID-19 Government Response Tracker). Nat Hum Behav. 2021;5(4):529–38.
12. Ramanathan M, et al. SARS-CoV-2 B.1.1.7 and B.1.351 spike variants bind human ACE2 with increased affinity. Lancet Infect Dis. 2021;21(8):1070.
13. Volz E, et al. Assessing transmissibility of SARS-CoV-2 lineage B.1.1.7 in England. Nature. 2021;593(7858):266–9.
14. Davies NG, et al. Estimated transmissibility and impact of SARS-CoV-2 lineage B.1.1.7 in England. Science. 2021;372(6538):305.
15. Frampton D, et al. Genomic characteristics and clinical effect of the emergent SARS-CoV-2 B.1.1.7 lineage in London, UK: a whole-genome sequencing and hospital-based cohort study. Lancet Infect Dis. 2021;21(9):1246–56.
16. Public Health England. Investigation of novel SARS-COV-2 variant of concern 202012/01. Public Health England, 2020. https://assets.publishing.service.gov.uk/government. Accessed 19 Jul 2021.
17. Brown KA, et al. S-gene target failure as a marker of variant B.1.1.7 among SARS-CoV-2 isolates in the greater Toronto area, December 2020 to March 2021. JAMA. 2021;325(20):2115–6.
18. Bal A, et al. Two-step strategy for the identification of SARS-CoV-2 variant of concern 202012/01 and other variants with spike deletion H69–V70, France, August to December 2020. Euro Surveill. 2021;26(3):2100008.
19. Emary KRW, et al. Efficacy of ChAdOx1 nCoV-19 (AZD1222) vaccine against SARS-CoV-2 variant of concern 202012/01 (B.1.1.7): an exploratory analysis of a randomised controlled trial. Lancet. 2021;397(10282):1351–62.
20. Planas D, et al. Sensitivity of infectious SARS-CoV-2 B.1.1.7 and B.1.351 variants to neutralizing antibodies. Nat Med. 2021;27(5):917–24.
21. Collier DA, et al. Sensitivity of SARS-CoV-2 B.1.1.7 to mRNA vaccine-elicited antibodies. Nature. 2021;593(7857):136–41.
22. Wang P, et al. Antibody resistance of SARS-CoV-2 variants B.1.351 and B.1.1.7. Nature. 2021;593(7857):130–5.
23. Tenforde MW, et al. Effectiveness of SARS-CoV-2 mRNA vaccines for preventing Covid-19 hospitalizations in the United States. medRxiv. 2021;2021:9776.
24. Chemaitelly H, et al. mRNA-1273 COVID-19 vaccine effectiveness against the B.1.1.7 and B.1.351 variants and severe COVID-19 disease in Qatar. Nat Med. 2021;27(9):1614–21.
25. Funk T, et al. Characteristics of SARS-CoV-2 variants of concern B.1.1.7, B.1.351 or P.1: data from seven EU/EEA countries, weeks 38/2020 to 10/2021. Eur Secur. 2021;26(16):2100348.
26. Jangra S, et al. SARS-CoV-2 spike E484K mutation reduces antibody neutralisation. Lancet Microbe. 2021;2(7):e283–4.
27. Jassat W, et al. Difference in mortality among individuals admitted to hospital with COVID-19 during the first and second waves in South Africa: a cohort study. Lancet Glob Health. 2021;9(9):e1216–25.
28. Cele S, et al. Escape of SARS-CoV-2 501Y.V2 from neutralization by convalescent plasma. Nature. 2021;593(7857):142–6.
29. Sadoff J, et al. Safety and efficacy of single-dose Ad26.COV2.S vaccine against Covid-19. N Engl J Med. 2021;384(23):2187–201.
30. Alter G, et al. Immunogenicity of Ad26.COV2.S vaccine against SARS-CoV-2 variants in humans. Nature. 2021;596(7871):268–72.

31. Abu-Raddad LJ, et al. Effectiveness of the BNT162b2 Covid-19 vaccine against the B.1.1.7 and B.1.351 variants. N Engl J Med. 2021;385(2):187–9.
32. Lustig Y, et al. Neutralising capacity against Delta (B.1.617.2) and other variants of concern following Comirnaty (BNT162b2, BioNTech/Pfizer) vaccination in health care workers, Israel. Eurosurveillance. 2021;26(26):2100557.
33. Liu Y, et al. BNT162b2-elicited neutralization against new SARS-CoV-2 spike variants. N Engl J Med. 2021;385(5):472–4.
34. Yadav PD, et al. Neutralization against B.1.351 and B.1.617.2 with sera of COVID-19 recovered cases and vaccinees of BBV152. bioRxiv. 2021;2021:177.
35. Shinde V, et al. Efficacy of NVX-CoV2373 Covid-19 vaccine against the B.1.351 variant. N Engl J Med. 2021;384(20):1899–909.
36. Madhi SA, et al. Efficacy of the ChAdOx1 nCoV-19 Covid-19 vaccine against the B.1.351 variant. N Engl J Med. 2021;384(20):1885–98.
37. Tarke A, et al. Comprehensive analysis of T cell immunodominance and immunoprevalence of SARS-CoV-2 epitopes in COVID-19 cases. Cell Rep Med. 2021;2(2):100204.
38. Greaney AJ, et al. Comprehensive mapping of mutations in the SARS-CoV-2 receptor-binding domain that affect recognition by polyclonal human plasma antibodies. Cell Host Microbe. 2021;29(3):463–76.
39. Faria NR, et al. Genomics and epidemiology of the P.1 SARS-CoV-2 lineage in Manaus, Brazil. Science. 2021;372(6544):815–21.
40. Vogel M, et al. SARS-CoV-2 variant with higher affinity to ACE2 shows reduced sera neutralization susceptibility. bioRxiv. 2021;2021:887.
41. Naveca FG, et al. COVID-19 in Amazonas, Brazil, was driven by the persistence of endemic lineages and P.1 emergence. Nat Med. 2021;27(7):1230–8.
42. Yang Y, et al. Key residues of the receptor binding domain in the spike protein of SARS-CoV-2 mediating the interactions with ACE2: a molecular dynamics study. Nanoscale. 2021;13(20):9364–70.
43. World Health Organization. COVID-19 weekly epidemiological update. 49th ed. Geneva: World Health Organization; 2021.
44. Ranzani OT, et al. Effectiveness of the CoronaVac vaccine in the elderly population during a Gamma variant-associated epidemic of COVID-19 in Brazil: a test-negative case-control study. medRxiv. 2021;2021:472.
45. Hitchings MDT, et al. Effectiveness of CoronaVac among healthcare workers in the setting of high SARS-CoV-2 Gamma variant transmission in Manaus, Brazil: a test-negative case–control study. medRxiv. 2021;2021:5081.
46. Liu J, et al. BNT162b2-elicited neutralization of B.1.617 and other SARS-CoV-2 variants. Nature. 2021;596(7871):273–5.
47. Chen Y, et al. Serum neutralising activity against SARS-CoV-2 variants elicited by CoronaVac. Lancet Infect Dis. 2021;21(8):1071–2.
48. Wang P, et al. Increased resistance of SARS-CoV-2 variant P.1 to antibody neutralization. Cell Host Microbe. 2021;29(5):747–751 e4.
49. Liu L, et al. Potent neutralizing antibodies against multiple epitopes on SARS-CoV-2 spike. Nature. 2020;584(7821):450–6.
50. Singh J, et al. SARS-CoV-2 variants of concern are emerging in India. Nat Med. 2021;27:1131–3.
51. Campbell F, et al. Increased transmissibility and global spread of SARS-CoV-2 variants of concern as at June 2021. Eur Secur. 2021;26(24):2100509.
52. Hu J, et al. Reduced neutralization of SARS-CoV-2 B.1.617 variant by inactivated and RBD-subunit vaccine. bioRxiv. 2021;2021:732.
53. Cherian S, et al. Convergent evolution of SARS-CoV-2 spike mutations, L452R, E484Q and P681R, in the second wave of COVID-19 in Maharashtra, India. bioRxiv. 2021;2021:932.
54. Kumar V, et al. Possible link between higher transmissibility of B.1.617 and B.1.1.7 variants of SARS-CoV-2 and increased structural stability of its spike protein and hACE2 affinity. bioRxiv. 2021;2021:933.

55. Li B, et al. Viral infection and transmission in a large well-traced outbreak caused by the Delta SARS-CoV-2 variant. medRxiv. 2021;2021:122.
56. Fisman DN, Tuite AR. Progressive increase in virulence of novel SARS-CoV-2 variants in Ontario, Canada. medRxiv. 2021;2021:050.
57. Lopez Bernal J, et al. Effectiveness of Covid-19 vaccines against the B.1.617.2 (Delta) variant. N Engl J Med. 2021;2021:8891. https://doi.org/10.1056/NEJMoa2108891.
58. Choi A, et al. Serum neutralizing activity of mRNA-1273 against SARS-CoV-2 variants. bioRxiv. 2021;2021:9914.
59. Vacharathit V, et al. SARS-CoV-2 variants of concern exhibit reduced sensitivity to live-virus neutralization in sera from CoronaVac vaccines and naturally infected COVID-19 patients. medRxiv. 2021;2021:232.
60. Jongeneelen M, et al. Ad26.COV2.S elicited neutralizing activity against Delta and other SARS-CoV-2 variants of concern. bioRxiv. 2021;2021:707.
61. Liu C, et al. Reduced neutralization of SARS-CoV-2 B.1.617 by vaccine and convalescent serum. Cell. 2021;184(16):4220–36.
62. Planas D, et al. Reduced sensitivity of SARS-CoV-2 variant Delta to antibody neutralization. Nature. 2021;596(7871):276–80. https://doi.org/10.1038/s41586-021-03777-9.
63. Tada T, et al. Comparison of neutralizing antibody titers elicited by mRNA and adenoviral vector vaccine against SARS-CoV-2 variants. bioRxiv. 2021;2021:2771.
64. Cerutti G, et al. Potent SARS-CoV-2 neutralizing antibodies directed against spike N-terminal domain target a single supersite. Cell Host Microbe. 2021;29(5):819–33.
65. Chi X, et al. A neutralizing human antibody binds to the N-terminal domain of the spike protein of SARS-CoV-2. Science. 2020;369(6504):650–5.
66. McEwen AE, et al. Variants of concern are overrepresented among post-vaccination breakthrough infections of SARS-CoV-2 in Washington State. medRxiv. 2021;2021:7679.
67. CDC-USA. SARS-CoV-2 variant classifications and definitions. Washington, DC: Centers for Disease Control and Prevention; 2021.
68. Zani A, et al. Serosurvey in BNT162b2 vaccine-elicited neutralizing antibodies against authentic B.1, B.1.1.7, B.1.351, B.1.525 and P.1 SARS-CoV-2 variants. Emerg Microbes Infect. 2021;10(1):1241–3.
69. Zhou H, et al. B.1.526 SARS-CoV-2 variants identified in New York City are neutralized by vaccine-elicited and therapeutic monoclonal antibodies. bioRxiv. 2021;2021:6620.
70. Ferreira I, et al. SARS-CoV-2 B.1.617 mutations L452 and E484Q are not synergistic for antibody evasion. J Infect Dis. 2021;224(6):989–94. https://doi.org/10.1093/infdis/jiab368.
71. Edara V-V, et al. Infection and vaccine-induced neutralizing antibody responses to the SARS-CoV-2 B.1.617.1 variant. bioRxiv. 2021;2021:3299.
72. Acevedo ML, et al. Infectivity and immune escape of the new SARS-CoV-2 variant of interest lambda. medRxiv. 2021;2021:9673.
73. Tada T, et al. SARS-CoV-2 lambda variant remains susceptible to neutralization by mRNA vaccine-elicited antibodies and convalescent serum. bioRxiv. 2021;2021:959.
74. Shah W, et al. Managing the long term effects of covid-19: summary of NICE, SIGN, and RCGP rapid guideline. BMJ. 2021;372:n136.
75. Puntmann VO, et al. Outcomes of cardiovascular magnetic resonance imaging in patients recently recovered from coronavirus disease 2019 (COVID-19). JAMA Cardiol. 2020;5(11):1265–73.
76. Wu Y, et al. Nervous system involvement after infection with COVID-19 and other coronaviruses. Brain Behav Immun. 2020;87:18–22.
77. Algahtani H, Subahi A, Shirah B. Neurological complications of Middle East respiratory syndrome coronavirus: a report of two cases and review of the literature. Case Rep Neurol Med. 2016;2016:3502683.
78. Fotuhi M, et al. Neurobiology of COVID-19. J Alzheimers Dis. 2020;76(1):3–19.
79. Singh J, Ehtesham NZ, Hasnain SE. Two parallel pandemics: the challenges faced by countries with COVID-19 and TB. Int J Tuberc Lung Dis. 2020;24(12):1319–20.

# Chapter 9
# Emergence of COVID-19 Variants and Its Global Impact

**Shekhar Kunal, Pranav Ish, Aditi, and Kashish Gupta**

## Introduction

Coronavirus disease 2019 (COVID-19), caused by a novel coronavirus, SARS-CoV-2 was first reported from Wuhan, China in December 2019 and subsequently declared as a pandemic by the World Health Organization (WHO) in March 2020 [1]. SARS-CoV-2, the third zoonotic-human coronavirus belongs to the *betacoronavirus* genera of the *Coronaviridae* family (subfamily *Coronavirinae*). SARS-CoV-2 is an enveloped RNA virus with a diameter of 50–200 nm. The basic structure of the virus includes a lipid envelope comprising spike glycoprotein (S), envelope protein (E), membrane glycoprotein (M) while the nucleocapsid protein (N) forms the core [2]. SARS-CoV-2 is a single stranded positive RNA virus and has one of the largest genomes (~29.9 kB in size) among all the RNA viruses which encodes for 29 proteins. The genetic constitution of SARS-CoV-2 comprises 14 open reading frames (ORFs) containing approximately 30,000 nucleotides. It has a 5′ untranslated region (UTR), replication complex (ORF1a and ORF1b), spike (S) gene, envelope (E) gene, membrane (M) gene, nucleocapsid (N) gene, 3′ UTR, several unidentified non-structural ORFs and a poly(A) tail. The S gene encodes the spike

S. Kunal (✉)
Department of Cardiology, Govind Ballabh Pant Institute of Postgraduate Medical Education and Research, New Delhi, Delhi, India

P. Ish
Department of Pulmonary, Critical Care and Sleep Medicine, Vardhman Mahavir Medical College and Safdarjung Hospital, New Delhi, Delhi, India

Aditi
Department of Pathology, Holy Family Hospital, New Delhi, Delhi, India

K. Gupta
Department of Medicine, SG Diabetes Center, New Delhi, Delhi, India


S. Adibi et al. (eds.), *Frontiers of COVID-19*,
https://doi.org/10.1007/978-3-031-08045-6_9

(S) glycoprotein which is a major contributor in the COVID-19 pathogenesis as well as evolution of various viral variants. The receptor binding domain (RBD; S1 subunit) of the S glycoprotein recognizes and binds to the human angiotensin-converting enzyme 2 (ACE2) receptor leading to infection with SARS-CoV-2 [2, 3].

Mutations are an integral component of viral replication especially among the RNA viruses. However, coronaviruses are known to have a stable genomic profile with lesser mutation rates as compared to other RNA viruses such as influenza [4]. Development of viral variants are often decided by the principle of natural selection wherein mutants having a competitive advantage in terms of viral replication, transmission, or immune escape becoming the dominant variant while those with reduced viral fitness tend to be removed from circulation. Epidemiological and genomic analysis of SARS-CoV-2 has documented the evolution of multiple viral variants worldwide with most of the mutations occurring in the RBD of the S-glycoprotein. An important distinction in terms of SARS CoV-2 has to be made regarding the usage of the terms such as mutation, variant, and strain which are often used interchangeably [5]. Mutation refers to the actual change in the genomic sequence of SARS-CoV-2. Variants refer to the viral genomes which actually differ in their sequence. A variant of SARS CoV-2 is termed as a strain when it has a distinct phenotype which can be in terms of its virulence, transmissibility or immune escape [5].

## Reasons for Emergence of SARS CoV-2 Variants

Viruses especially those having RNA as the genetic material are highly susceptible to mutations owing to the error prone RNA copying mechanisms. SARS CoV-2 being an RNA virus too is prone to genetic changes which can occur either due to (a) point mutations following single nucleotide polymorphisms (SNPs) as the RNA polymerase enzyme lacks a proofreading mechanism leading to copying errors and (b) recombination errors which leads to acquisition of new genetic material including those of the virus and the host [6]. Several factors have been thought to be the driving force behind viral evolution. These include the selective pressures by the host immune responses, longer replication period in immunocompromised hosts thereby acquiring greater number of mutations or nsp12 (viral RNA polymerase) mutations interfering with the virus's proofreading mechanism.

Random genetic changes leading to SNPs occur every time during viral replication with an intrinsic copy error rate of $1 \times 10^{-6}$ to $1 \times 10^{-7}$ mutations per nucleotide per genome replication for SARS-CoV-2. This leads to the development of one mutation for every 1–10 million nucleotides which are being replicated. Since, the SARS-CoV-2 genome comprises 30,000 nucleotides, there occurs one mutation for every 33–330 replications. However, in an infected individual, at peak of infection there are more than a 100 million viral genomes, hence a theoretical chance that every nucleotide of its genome can get mutated hundreds of time leading to emergence of multiple viral variants [7]. However, practically the risk for emergence of newer variants becomes less as most of these SNPs either lead to deleterious changes and a non-viable virus or do not lead to a change in the amino acid sequence. Occasionally, changes in the amino acid sequence due to SNPs can lead to alterations in the viral proteins giving a survival advantage for that particular variant [6]. In the presence of a selection pressure favoring that variant, it outstrips the growth rate of other variants and establishes itself to be the dominant variant. A classic example has been the emergence of variants with the D614G SNP in the spike glycoprotein in early March 2020. Population genetic and phylodynamic assessment showed that this change was associated with increased transmission as it enhances the ability of spike protein to bind to the ACE2 receptor [8, 9]. Another plausible method for emergence of viral variants include genetic recombination, a process leading to viruses swapping the genetic material producing new genetic sequences. This can either include deletion of parts of the genome or insertion of new sequences within the genome. These new sequences can either be acquired from other coronaviruses or from the host genome itself. An example of such would be the presence of a furin protease cleavage site at the S1/S2 junction in the S-glycoprotein gene in SARS-CoV-2 which occurred due to genetic recombination [10]. Certain portions of the SARS-CoV-2 genome especially the Spike protein gene is increasingly predisposed to such recombination's and have been termed as "hotspots." The key mutations in the SARS CoV-2 genome have been tabulated in Table 9.1.

**Table 9.1** Key mutations in the SARS-CoV2 genome

| Mutation | Type of mutation | Location of mutation | Variants | Mutation characteristic |
|---|---|---|---|---|
| D614G | Missense mutation—substitution of aspartic acid (D) to glycine (G) in amino acid position 614 of S protein | RBD of spike protein | Alpha or B.1.1.7<br>Beta or B.1.351<br>Delta or B.1.617.2<br>Gamma or P.1<br>Kappa or B.1.617.1<br>Iota or B.1.526<br>Eta or B.1.525<br>B.1.617.3 | • Higher infectivity—enhanced binding to hACE2<br>• In-vitro studies: increased replication in primary human bronchial and nasal airway epithelial cultures<br>• Markedly increased replication and transmissibility |

(continued)

**Table 9.1** (continued)

| Mutation | Type of mutation | Location of mutation | Variants | Mutation characteristic |
|---|---|---|---|---|
| N501Y | Missense mutation—substitution of asparagine (N) to tyrosine (Y) in amino acid position 501 | RBD of spike protein | Alpha or B.1.1.7<br>Beta or B.1.351<br>Gamma or P.1 | • Increased ACE2 binding affinity-greater time spent in the 'open' conformation<br>• Stronger hydrophobic interactions of RBD-ACE2<br>• N501Y—highest binding affinity in VOC RBD to hACE2<br>• Risk of a possible persistent reservoir in wild rodents/mustelids<br>• Small but significant reduction in neutralization of Pfizer-BioNTech and Moderna vaccinated individuals |
| E484K | Missense mutation—glutamic acid (E) is replaced by lysine (K) at amino acid position 484 | RBD of spike protein | Beta or B.1.351<br>Gamma or P.1 | • Reduced convalescent serum neutralization<br>• Immune escape and re-infection<br>• Increased hACE2 receptor binding—greater infectivity<br>• Increased binding affinity by altering electrostatic interactions<br>• Reduce neutralizing ability of a combination of mAbs (REGN10989 and REGN10934) |
| K417N/T | Missense mutation—lysine replaced by either asparagine (N) or threonine (T) at amino acid position 417 | RBD of spike protein | Beta or B.1.351<br>Gamma or P.1<br>Delta Plus | • Enhanced immune evasion<br>• Increased S1 RBD binding to hACE2<br>• Synergistic effect in conjugation with mutation L452R |
| L452R | Missense mutation—leucine (L) is replaced by arginine (R) at amino acid position 452 | RBD of spike protein | Delta or B.1.617.2<br>Kappa or B.1.617.1<br>Epsilon or B.1.427 | • Enhanced hACE2 receptor binding ability<br>• Reduce vaccine-stimulated antibodies from attaching to altered spike protein<br>• Resistant to T cell response<br>• Decreased binding ability of REGN10933 and P2B-2F6 antibodies<br>• Escape from human leukocyte antigen (HLA) 24-restricted cellular immunity |

**Table 9.1** (continued)

| Mutation | Type of mutation | Location of mutation | Variants | Mutation characteristic |
|---|---|---|---|---|
| Q677P/H | Missense mutation—glutamine replaced by either proline (P) or histidine (H) at amino acid position 677 | S1–S2 furin cleavage site | 20G (20C-US clade) | • Influences S1/S2 cleavage—promotes more efficient viral entry |
| E484Q | Missense mutation—glutamic acid (E) is replaced by glutamine (Q) at position 484 | RBD of spike protein | Kappa or B.1.617.1 | • Reduced convalescent serum neutralization<br>• Increased ACE2 receptor binding—greater infectivity<br>• Decrease the binding ability of REGN10933 and P2B-2F6 antibodies to the variant strains |
| Δ69/70 | 6-nucleotide deletion (21765–21770) of S gene: deletion of two amino acids at sites 69 (histidine) and (70 valine) in spike protein | N-terminal domain of spike S1 fragment | Alpha or B.1.1.7<br>Eta or B.1.525<br>B.1.258<br>B.1.1.298<br>B.1.160<br>B.1.177<br>B.1.375 | • Conformational change in the spike protein<br>• S gene "drop out" in RT-PCR assays<br>• Increased infectivity<br>• Evasion of the immune response |
| P681R | Missense mutation—proline (P) is replaced by arginine (R) at amino acid position 681 | S1–S2 furin cleavage site | Kappa or B.1.617.1<br>Delta or B.1.617.2 | • Increased rate of membrane fusion, internalization—better transmissibility |

*hACE2* human angiotensin-converting enzyme 2, *RBD* receptor binding domain, *S protein* spike protein, *VOC* variant of concern

## Nomenclature of the SARS CoV-2 Variants

COVID-19 variants are classified based on the variant classification scheme jointly developed by the Centers for Disease Control and Prevention (CDC) [11] and the WHO [12]. As per this scheme, there are three classes of SARS-CoV-2 variants including (a) Variant of Interest (VOI), (b) Variant of Concern (VOC), and (c) Variant of High Consequence. COVID-19 variants are designated as VOI when they are associated with changes in the receptor binding, potential diagnostic impact, decreased neutralization by antibodies generated through natural infection/vaccination, reduced treatment efficacy or leading to increase in the disease transmissibility or severity. WHO defines VOI [13] as "A SARS-CoV-2 isolate is a VOI if it is phenotypically changed (changes in the epidemiology, antigenicity, or virulence or changes that have or potentially have a negative impact on available diagnostics, or public health and social measure) compared to a reference isolate or has a genome with mutations that lead to amino acid changes associated with established or suspected phenotypic implications AND has been identified to cause community transmission/multiple COVID-19 cases/clusters, or has been detected in multiple countries OR is otherwise assessed to be a VOI by WHO in consultation with the WHO SARS-CoV-2 Virus Evolution Working Group." VOI are often associated with increased proportion of cases or new outbreaks in clusters. This often requires appropriate public health action including genomic surveillance, epidemiological surveys in order to ascertain specific characteristics leading to disease spread and immune escape. Currently, WHO has designated five SARS CoV-2 variants as VOI [12].

COVID-19 VOIs are designated as VOC when there is a definite evidence for that VOI to have increased transmissibility, causing more severe disease leading to greater number of hospitalizations or deaths along with significant reduction in neutralization by antibodies generated through natural infection/vaccination, diagnostic detection failures and reduced effectiveness of current therapies or vaccination failure. WHO defines VOCs [13] as "A VOI is a VOC if through a comparative assessment it has been demonstrated to be associated with increase in transmissibility or detrimental change in COVID-19 epidemiology, increase in virulence or change in clinical disease presentation, or decrease in effectiveness of public health and social measures or available diagnostics, vaccines, therapeutics OR assessed to be a VOC by WHO in consultation with the WHO SARS-CoV-2 Virus Evolution Working Group." Currently, WHO has designated four SARS CoV-2 variants as VOCs [12]. A VOC is labelled as a Variant of High Consequence when there is ample evidence that "prevention measures or medical countermeasures (MCMs) have significantly reduced effectiveness relative to previously circulating variants." Variant of High Consequence have a definite impact on the MCMs along with failure of diagnostic tests to detect these variants culminating in a far more severe form disease with increased hospitalizations, deaths, and significantly reduced vaccine effectiveness with higher vaccine breakthrough cases. Variant of High Consequence requires notification to the WHO and CDC along with the need for strategies to prevent transmission and treatment modalities. Currently, there are no SARS-CoV-2 variants that can be labelled as high consequence [12].

According to the WHO, a previously designated VOI/VOC which has been demonstrated to not pose a major added risk to global public health in approaching times compared to other circulating SARS-CoV-2 variants, can be reclassified through a critical expert assessment of several criteria, such as ongoing impact on control measures, observed incidence or prevalence of variant between geographical locations and the presence of other risk factors.

WHO also defines "*variants under monitoring*" as a "SARS-CoV-2 variant with genetic changes that are suspected to affect virus characteristics with some indication that it may pose a future risk, but evidence of phenotypic or epidemiological impact is currently unclear, requiring enhanced monitoring and repeat assessment pending new evidence."

The major variants of concern, variants of interest and variants under monitoring for COVID-19 are listed in Table 9.2.

**Table 9.2** Major variants of concern, variants of interest and variants under monitoring for COVID-19

| Variants of concern (VOC) | Variants of interest (VOI) | Variants under monitoring |
|---|---|---|
| Alpha or B.1.1.7<br>Earliest documented in UK in Sept 2020 and designated VOC on 18-12-2020 | Eta or B.1.525<br>Earliest documented in many countries in Dec 2020 and designated VOI on 17-3-2021 | B.1.427<br>B.1.429<br>Earliest documented samples from USA in Mar 2020 |
| Beta or B.1.351<br>Earliest documented in SA in May 2020 and designated VOC on 18-12-2020 | Iota or B.1.526<br>Earliest documented in USA in Nov 2020 and designated VOI on 24-3-2021 | R.1<br>B.1.1.318<br>B.1.1.519<br>Earliest documented samples from multiple countries |
| Gamma or P.1<br>Earliest documented in Brazil in Nov 2021 in May 2020 and designated VOC on 11-1-2021 | Kappa or B.1.617.1<br>Earliest documented in India in Oct 2020 and designated VOI on 4-4-2021 | B.1.466.2<br>Earliest documented samples from Indonesia in Nov 2020 |
| Delta or B.1.617.2<br>Earliest documented in India in OCT 2020 in May 2020 and designated VOC on 11-5-2021 | Lambda or C.37<br>Earliest documented in Peru in Dec 2020 and designated VOI on 14-6-2021 | C.36.3<br>B.1.214.2<br>B.1.1.523<br>B.1.619<br>B.1.620<br>Earliest documented samples from multiple countries |
| | Mu or B.1.621<br>Earliest documented in Colombia in Jan 2021 and designated VOI on 30-8-2021 | C.1.2<br>Earliest documented samples from SA in May 2021 |

*UK* United Kingdom, *SA* South Africa, *USA* United States of America

## Major COVID-19 Variants

The WHO Virus Evolution Working Group in collaboration with scientists from the WHO COVID-19 reference laboratory network, GISAID, Pango and Nextstrain proposed a simplified nomenclature scheme for the VOI and VOC of COVID-19 which are easy-to-pronounce and non-stigmatizing [12]. This expert group suggested the use of Greek alphabets such as alpha, beta, gamma, and delta for naming of various COVID-19 variants [14]. Major variants of concern and their global prevalence have been depicted in Figs. 9.1 and 9.2.

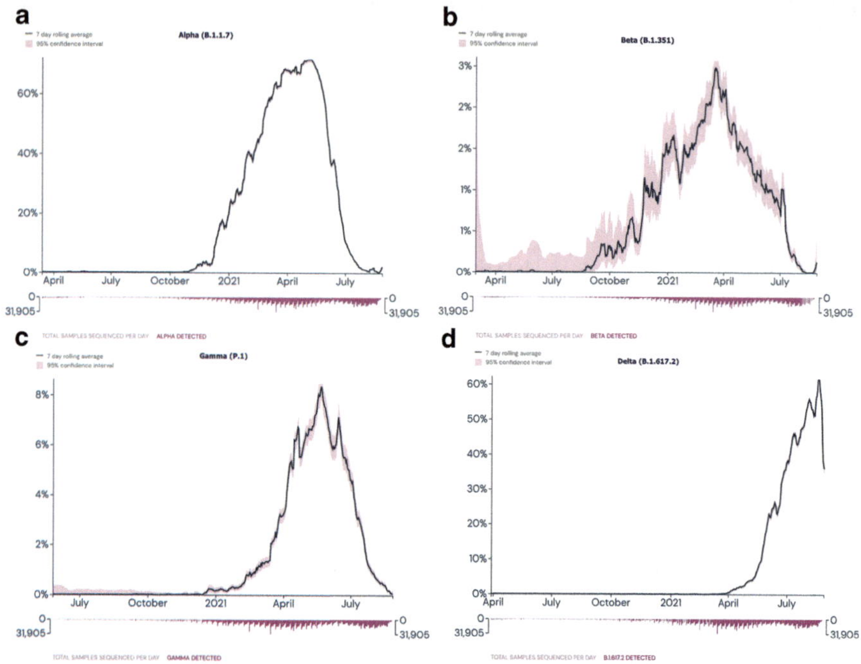


**Fig. 9.1** (**a**) Line graph depicting the average daily of Alpha (B.1.1.7) variant prevalence globally. (**b**) Line graph depicting the average daily of Beta (B.1.351) variant prevalence globally. (**c**) Line graph depicting the average daily of Gamma (P.1) variant prevalence globally. (**d**) Line graph depicting the average daily of Delta (B.1.617.2) variant prevalence globally. (**a–d**) Source: Outbreak.info; Available online: https://outbreak.info/ [57]

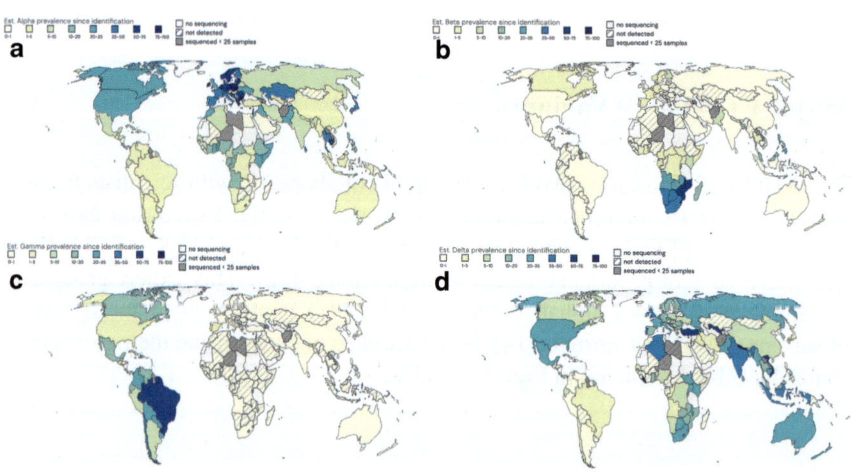


**Fig. 9.2** (**a**) World map depicting the cumulative prevalence of Alpha (B.1.1.7) variant globally. (**b**) World map depicting the cumulative prevalence of Beta (B.1.351) variant globally. (**c**) World map depicting the cumulative prevalence of Gamma (P.1) variant globally. (**d**) World map depicting the cumulative prevalence of Delta (B.1.617.2) variant globally. (**a–d**) Source: Outbreak.info; Available online: https://outbreak.info/ [57]

## *Variants of Concern*

### B.1.1.7 or the Alpha Variant

The B.1.1.7 variant, also known as VOC 202012/01 or 20B/501Y.V1 (Alpha variant), was first identified in Southern England in December 2020 [15]. It has become the dominant variant in the United Kingdom (UK) having fueled the second wave of COVID-19 in Europe and has been documented in more than 114 countries worldwide (Figs. 9.1a and 9.2a). As compared to its ancestral SARS-CoV-2 virus variant containing the D614G mutation, this particular variant had 17 novel mutations with eight of them being in the S protein. Three characteristic mutations in this particular variant are (a) N501Y mutation at position 501 in the RBD of S protein leading to increased affinity for the human ACE2 and greater transmission, (b) P681H mutation augmenting infectivity and disease transmissibility, and (c) ΔH69/ΔV70 deletion in the S region leading to immune escape and greater infectivity. This particular deletion in the S protein was also responsible for the failure of certain commercial testing kits to detect the S gene leading to "S gene target failure" [16].

Data from the COG-UK dataset revealed that the relative population growth rate of the alpha variant in the first 30 days after its detection was higher than that of all the other 307 other lineages [17]. Multiple hypothesis were proposed for increased infectivity of alpha variant and includes: (a) higher viral load as reflected by a lower cycle threshold (*Ct*) values suggesting this variant to be more transmissible per contact with an index case than preexisting variants, (b) longer duration of viral shedding and hence greater infectiousness, (c) immune escape attributed to the ΔH69/ΔV70 deletion leading to breakthrough infections in individuals with natural immunity or post vaccination, (d) shorter generation time than previously circulating variants leading to increased growth rates [17]. The higher infectivity of this variant was reflected in a community-based cohort study involving 54,906 low risk individuals wherein the mortality hazard ratio associated with infection with alpha variant was 1.64 (95% CI 1.32–2.04) as compared to those infected with previously circulating variants. This translated into a 32–104% increased risk of death with the novel variant [18].

### B.1.351 or the Beta Variant

The B.1.351 variant also known as the 20H/501Y.V2 or Beta variant was first identified in South Africa in October 2020 and has been widely in circulation since then (Figs. 9.1b and 9.2b) [19]. This particular variant has 23 mutations with the notable ones being the K417N, E484K, and N501Y in the RBD of the S protein. Of these, the E484K mutation is responsible for increased affinity with the ACE2 receptor as well as immune escape leading to reduced sensitivity to the vaccines [20]. This variant was identified to be nearly 50% more transmissible than the preexisting variants in South Africa [20]. As compared to the D614G reference SARS-CoV-2 virus strain, both the Pfizer Comirnaty (also termed BNT162b2) and the Moderna mRNA-1273 vaccine had lower protective efficacy against the B.1.351 variant [21].

## P.1 or the Gamma Variant

The gamma variant also known as 20J/501Y.V3 was first identified in Japan among four travellers returning to Japan from the city of Manaus in the Amazonas state, Brazil in December 2020 (Figs. 9.1c and 9.2c). Soon, this variant became an emergent lineage in Manaus and fueled the second wave of the pandemic in January 2021 despite a sero-survey in October 2020 reporting that 78% of its population were sero-positive for COVID-19 [22]. Overall, it has 35 mutations with the notable ones being the K417T, E484K, and N501Y in the RBD of the S-protein. The E484K and N501Y mutation is seen in other lineages of the SARS-CoV-2 virus including the beta variant strains. The presence of both the K417T and N501Y mutation tends to influence host cell entry and virus transmission increase the transmissibility of the variant by enabling greater affinity for ACE2 receptors in human cells [23, 24]. In a study by Naveca et al. [25], it was found that this variant is 2.2 times higher transmissible that led to a few cases of reinfection who recovered from COVID-19, and almost has a similar rate infection in the younger (18–59 years old) and older (>60 years old) patients. In terms of its impact on the vaccine efficacy, this particular variant had a modest loss of neutralization efficacy (3.8–4.8-fold) by convalescent plasma and vaccinee sera following Moderna or Pfizer vaccination. Similarly, a recent study also demonstrated marked/complete loss of neutralizing activities of various monoclonal antibodies such as REGN10933 (casirivimab), LY-CoV555 (bamlanivimab), and CB6 (etesevimab). However, the monoclonal antibody REGN10987 (Imdevimab) did retain its neutralization activity against this particular variant [26].

## B.1.617.2 or the Delta Variant

The Delta variant also known as 21A/S:478K was first reported from the state of Maharashtra, India in October 2020 and has been largely responsible for the devastating second wave of COVID-19 pandemic in India (Figs. 9.1d and 9.2d) [12]. This belongs to the Lineage B.1.617 which has three sub-lineages (B.1.617.1: Kappa variant, B.1.617.2: Delta variant, and B.1.617.3). This variant has now spread to 163 countries across the globe and soon can become the dominant strain globally [27]. It has 13 mutations with the notable ones being D614G, T478K, L452R, and P681R in the RBD of the Spike protein. The L452R mutation previously reported in the California variants (B.1.427 and B.1.429) is known to increase affinity of spike proteins to ACE2 receptors making it more transmissible [28]. Additionally, it has also been known to mediate immune escape. The P681R mutation is located near the cleavage site between S1 and S2 and has been shown to increase cellular infectivity by facilitating cleavage of the precursor S protein to the S1/S2 active configuration [29]. Delta variant has been reported to be 40–60% more transmissible than Alpha variant [30]. A recent study by the Guangdong Provincial Center for Disease Control and Prevention reported that viral load with the Delta variant to be around 1000 times higher than with the Wuhan strain [31]. Epidemiologists from the

University of Toronto reported that the Delta variant had a 120% greater risk of hospitalization, 287% greater risk of ICU admission, and 137% greater risk of death as compared to the non-VOC strains of SARS-COV-2 [32]. The Delta variant has given rise to various sub-lineages which have been labelled as AY.1 to AY.22 which have been termed as "Delta Plus variant." It refers to the presence of Delta variant with an additional K417N mutation [30]. Of the various sub-lineages of the Delta variant, the AY.12 has recently gained importance and is currently been thought to be the reason behind the recent surge in COVID-19 cases in Israel despite nearly 60% of the population being fully vaccinated [33].

## *Variants of Interest*

Currently, WHO has declared five variants as VOI which includes Eta (B.1.525), Iota (B.1.526), Kappa (B.1.617.1), Lambda (C.37), and Mu (B.1.621) [12]. The Eta variant was first identified in United Kingdom and Nigeria in December 2020 and has E484K, D614G, and ΔH69/ΔV70 deletion as important mutations. This variant was shown to have reduction in neutralization by monoclonal antibody treatments and by convalescent and post-vaccination sera [34]. The Iota variant was first reported from United States (New York) in November 2020 and has L452R, E484K, and D614G as notable mutations. This variant has been shown to have reduced neutralization by convalescent and post-vaccination sera [35]. The Kappa variant was identified in India in December 2020 and has a host of mutations including E154K, L452R, E484Q, D614G, and P681R. This variant too has an impact on the efficacy of vaccines and monoclonal antibodies [36]. The Lambda variant, first identified in Peru in October 2020, has now been reported in more than 25 countries across the globe. It is believed to be the dominant strain in various South American countries such as Peru, Chile, Ecuador, and Argentina. Lambda variant has been shown to have a greater infectivity than the Alpha and Gamma variants [37]. Additionally, studies have shown decreased effectiveness of the Chinese Sinovac vaccine (CoronaVac) against the Lambda variant [38]. Recently in August 2021, the WHO added Mu (B.1.621) as a variant of interest. This variant was first detected in Colombia in January 2021 and has been reported from 39 countries. It has R346K, E484K, N501Y, D614G, and P681H as some of the notable mutations. Preliminary estimates for this variant indicate potential properties of immune escape along with reduction in neutralization capacity of convalescent and vaccinee sera [39].

## *Other Notable Variants*

The other notable variants include previously designated VOIs such as Epsilon (lineages B.1.429, B.1.427, CAL.20C), Zeta (lineage P.2), Theta (lineage P.3) as well as the Lineage B.1.1.207 and Lineage C.1.2 [12]. Epsilon variant or lineage B.1.429

had five distinct mutations of which the L452R was of major concern. This variant was first detected in July 2020 in California and soon spread to other US states. However, this variant was soon outcompeted by the Delta variant and is no longer a VOI. Zeta variant (P.2) is a sub-lineage of B.1.1.28 and was first detected in Rio de Janeiro, Brazil. It differs from P1 as it does not harbor N501Y and K417T mutations. Though initially listed as a VOI, WHO as of July 2021, no longer considers it a VOI. Lineage B.1.1.207 was first reported from Nigeria in August 2020 and has been labelled as an emerging variant by the CDC [40]. Lineage C.1.2 is one of the notable variants to have been emerged off late and was first identified in May 2021 in South Africa. It has a host of mutations including multiple substitutions such as R190S, D215G, N484K, N501Y, H655Y, and T859N and deletions such as Y144del, L242-A243del within the S protein. These mutations are associated with greater transmissibility and reduced neutralization sensitivity. However, one of the major concerns is the presence of additional mutations such as C136F, Y449H, and N679K which can have an impact neutralization sensitivity or furin cleavage [41].

## *Impact of Viral Variants*

Emergence of viral variants are associated with a host of issues including its impact on diagnostic tests, vaccine efficacy as well as varied clinical presentation and disease severity. There are multiple challenges associated with novel viral variants including immune escape, breakthrough viral infections despite prior infection/vaccination and greater virulence [42]. The following are the impact of various viral variants.

## *Impact on Disease Spread, Virulence, and Therapeutics*

An important challenge currently being faced following emergence of newer variants is its ability to spread rapidly among different population groups. Most of the variants have a mutation in the RBD of the S-protein which leads to increased affinity for binding to the ACE2 receptor thereby leading to greater transmissibility. Variants such as B1.1.7 or 20I/501Y.V1 were found to be 30–80% more transmissible with higher nasopharyngeal viral loads and a 30% increase in mortality risk as compared to the original SARS-CoV-2 strain [43]. Similarly, the Delta variant was found to have 40–60% higher transmissibility as well as greater hospital admission rates as compared with the alpha variant [30]. The greater transmissibility of the novel variants translates into increased infection rates and higher levels of hospitalizations thereby increasing the pressure on the already overburdened healthcare system. The CDC guidelines recommended against the use of bamlanivimab plus etesevimab combination therapy as the Gamma (P.1) and Beta (B.1.351) VOCs have reduced susceptibility to both the agents [44].

## *Impact on Diagnostic Tests*

Routine testing for SARS-CoV-2 is based on molecular methods using nucleic acid amplification tests (NAATs) including those based on PCR. This involves detection of specific portion of the viral genome using primers which are short DNA sequences which bind and detect specific virus RNA target sequences. Mutations within these primer specific target sequences would lead to a false negative test result and failure of the NAATs to detect SARS CoV-2. As a result, viral mutations do have the potential to reduce the diagnostic accuracy of NAATs. However, in clinical practice, most of the NAATs have multiple genetic targets rather than one hence the chances of false negative due to a viral variant gets minimized [42]. Additionally, mutations can also affect the diagnostic performance of the antigen and antibody tests by causing an alteration to the protein or physical structure of the viral antigen targeted by the test. Such had been the impact with the B.1.1.7 variant where deletions at amino acid positions 69 and 70 in the S-gene led to false negative results with the Taq-Path COVID-19 Combo Kit and the Linea COVID-19 Assay Kit. This calls for periodic assessment of diagnostic performance of various molecular tests based upon the local circulating variants as was highlighted in a recent US food and drug administration (FDA) guidance statement [45].

Herd immunity or protective seroprevalence becomes a questionable concept with the emergence of newer variants as immunity gained either through natural infection or following vaccination may not be protective. COVID-19 variants can lead to immune escape and breakthrough/reinfection in previously infected individuals thereby hampering disease control. Vaccine resistance and immune escape have become a major challenge both in developing and developed countries worldwide with newer emerging variants [42]. This was highlighted in a recent case report wherein two fully vaccinated individuals having received BNT162b2 (Pfizer-BioNTech) and mRNA-1273(Moderna), respectively, developed breakthrough infection with novel variants 19 and 36 days following the second dose. This novel COVID-19 variant had marked similarity with the B.1.1.7 and B.1.526 variants [46]. Most of the vaccines available currently utilize the S-protein of SARS-CoV-2 as a target antigen against which antibodies develop. Since a majority of the variants have a mutation within the RBD of the S-protein, there is always a doubt regarding the efficacy of various vaccines [42]. In vitro studies have reported that plasma from vaccinated individuals were less effective in neutralizing variants with the E484K, N501Y, or K417N/E484K/N501 mutations within the RBD of S-protein [47, 48]. In a multicentric, randomized double blind study, Madhi et al. [49] reported that the two dose regimen of the ChAdOx1 nCoV-19 vaccine (AZD1222) failed to provide protection from mild to moderate COVID-19 disease caused by the B1.351 variant which was widespread in South Africa. This study presented ample evidence that the B.1.351 variant possesses mutations which enables it to escape the host immune response in previously vaccinated individuals and forced the South African authorities to halt the roll out of the Astra Zeneca's ChAdOx1 nCoV-19 vaccine [50]. However, for the B.1.1.7 variant, the efficacy of the ChAdOx1 nCoV-19 vaccine in preventing symptomatic infection was 70.4% as compared to the non-B.1.1.7

lineages where it was reported to be 81.5% [51]. In an another study to evaluate the real world effectiveness of the mRNA-1273 (Moderna) vaccine against SARS-CoV-2 variants of concern [B.1.1.7 (Alpha) and B.1.351 (Beta)] in Qatar, the authors reported effectiveness for the B.1.1.7 infection was 88.1% following the first dose and 100% after the second dose. Similarly, for the B.1.351 infection the effectiveness was 61.3% following first dose and 96.4% post the second dose [52]. Data regarding the efficacy of vaccines for the Delta variant is limited. Bernal and colleagues [53] from the Public Health England (PHE) in a non-randomized study reported the effectiveness of BNT162b2 and ChAdOx1 vaccines against the two variants: alpha (B.1.1.7) and the delta (B.1.617.2) following one or two doses. A recent study from Canada evaluated the effectiveness of BNT162b2, mRNA-1273, and ChAdOx1vaccines against symptomatic SARS-CoV-2 infection and outcomes caused by the Alpha (B.1.1.7), Beta (B.1.351), Gamma (P.1), and Delta (B.1.617.2) variants of COVID-19. The study reported that for infections caused by the Alpha variant, effectiveness of partial vaccination (≥ 14 days post first dose) was higher for mRNA-1273 (83%) than BNT162b2 (66%) and ChAdOx1(64%). The protection against infection caused by Beta/Gamma variant was lower with partial vaccination for ChAdOx1 (48%) than mRNA-1273 (77%). In terms of protection against Delta variant, vaccine effectiveness following partial vaccination was lower than that against Alpha for BNT162b2 (56% vs. 66%) and mRNA-1273 (72% vs. 83%) however, was similar to Alpha for ChAdOx1 (67% vs. 64%). A full vaccination with BNT162b2 increased protection against Delta variant (87%) to comparable levels with Alpha (89%) and Beta/Gamma (84%) [54].

## *Strategies to Prevent Emergence of Newer Variants*

Multiple strategies need to be devised to tackle the ever-growing menace of the COVID-19 variants. This would include genomic surveillance, data sharing, and global cooperation as well as adopting a rapid rate of immunization against COVID-19 worldwide.

Genomic surveillance has been on the forefront in this fight against COVID-19 infection and bringing the pandemic under control. Genomic surveillance using whole genomic sequencing remains a key in the identification of novel COVID-19 variants evolving over a period of time. WHO advocates for genomic surveillance as a worldwide priority and has previously achieved success with Ebola virus disease and influenza virus [55]. Genomic surveillance would not only monitor for the emergence of the variants but would also help in the rapid assessment of their affects. It has been well documented that variants such as B.1.1.7 and B.1.617 with a high transmissibility can lead to new waves of infection and collapse of the healthcare system as had been evident in the deadly second wave of COVID-19 in UK and India [42]. This calls in for setting up and strengthening the genomic surveillance network. Emergence of the alpha variant of COVID-19 led to the establishment of the Indian SARS-CoV2 Genomic Consortia (INSACOG) under the Ministry of Health and Family Welfare, Government of India in December 2020.This consortium comprising a of ten national laboratories is responsible for monitoring the genetic variations and genomic surveillance across India. Additionally, it shares it data with international databases such as GISAID which further strengthens the global cooperation for genomic surveillance [42, 56]. The genomic surveillance program must be fast with the data made available publicly in a short period of time to allow for timely decision-making by public health agencies and vaccine manufacturers. However, there seems to be a disparity in the genomic surveillance data from the developed as well developing countries. Countries with poor infrastructure lacks behind in the genomic surveillance and such novel COVID-19 variants can get unrecognized and spread globally [42]. Data from the GISAID database reflects that countries such as India trail behind a lot many countries in terms of genomic sampling of SARS-CoV-2 with just 44,705 (0.136%) of the 32,768,880 cases sequenced. This is in stark contrast to the data from the developed nations such as Australia, Denmark, UK, and the USA with sequencing rates of 48.6%, 45.2%, 11.2%, and 2.2%, respectively (Fig. 9.3) [57, 58]. There is a need to set-up newer laboratories

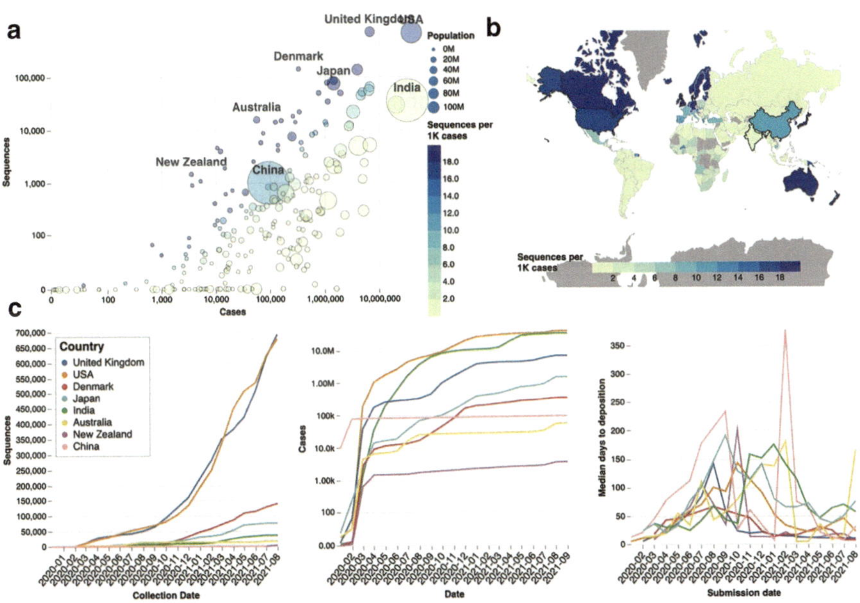


**Fig. 9.3** (**a**) Bubble plot comparing the population, actual number of COVID-19 cases and the genome sequencing data (per 1000 cases) deposited in the GISAID database for major countries globally. (**b**) Map comparing the genome sequencing data (per 1000 cases) deposited in GISAID database across the globe. Developed countries such as the USA, United Kingdom, and Australia (marked in purple) have the maximum contribution to genomic surveillance while developing nations in Asia and Africa lag well behind (marked in light green). (**c**) Plot showing the relative contribution of various countries to genomic surveillance, prevalence of disease and the median days to deposition to the GISAID data-base. India (green line) is in the lower part of the curve in terms of genomic sequencing reflecting poor genomic surveillance, however, is ranked second just behind the US (orange line) in terms of absolute number of cases. [**a–c** Source: COVID CoV Genomics (CG); Available at: covidcg.org] [58]

for genomic sequencing along with addressing issues such as lack of technical expertise or limited availability of reagents and raw materials. All of these call for capacity building with a better coordination among the network labs and involvement of the public and private sector enterprises. Apart from genomic surveillance, preventing spread of disease either through social distancing measures or vaccination remains a key in preventing emergence of variants. This calls for large scale immunization activities globally involving an equitable distribution of vaccines in the both developing as well as developed nations.

Apart from that following emergence of variants, there is a need to change the vaccine administration regimen. This would include an additional booster dose or optimizing the vaccine as per the variant (e.g. developing new version of the vaccines with an updated spike protein as per the genetic variation) or combining two different vaccine platforms in a "mix and match" strategy to ensure a stronger immune response [59].

## Conclusion

COVID-19 continues to remain a major public health issue worldwide with multiple waves of infection sweeping across different parts of the globe. Emergence of novel COVID-19 variants has left a major challenge for the healthcare providers in view of an increased transmissibility, greater disease severity, and immune escape. Though genomic surveillance for SARS-CoV-2 has increased our ability to detect and track evolution of these variants, there is a need to maintain a constant vigil along with large scale vaccination drives to curb the ever-rising tide of COVID-19 infection.

## References

1. Kunal S, Gupta K, Sharma SM, Pathak V, Mittal S, Tarke C. Cardiovascular system and COVID-19: perspectives from a developing country. Monaldi Arch Chest Dis. 2020;90(2):1305. https://doi.org/10.4081/monaldi.2020.1305.
2. Kim D, Lee JY, Yang JS, Kim JW, Kim VN, Chang H. The architecture of SARS-CoV-2 transcriptome. Cell. 2020;181:914–21. https://doi.org/10.1016/j.cell.2020.04.011.
3. Naqvi AAT, Fatima K, Mohammad T, Fatima U, Singh IK, Singh A, et al. Insights into SARS-CoV-2 genome, structure, evolution, pathogenesis and therapies: structural genomics approach. Biochim Biophys Acta Mol Basis Dis. 2020;1866:165878. https://doi.org/10.1016/j.bbadis.2020.165878.
4. Abdelrahman Z, Li M, Wang X. Comparative review of SARS-CoV-2, SARS-CoV, MERS-CoV, and influenza a respiratory viruses. Front Immunol. 2020;11(11):552909. https://doi.org/10.3389/fimmu.2020.552909.
5. Lauring AS, Hodcroft EB. Genetic variants of SARS-CoV-2-what do they mean? JAMA. 2021;325:529–31. https://doi.org/10.1001/jama.2020.27124.

6. Pachetti M, Marini B, Benedetti F, Giudici F, Mauro E, Storici P, et al. Emerging SARS-CoV-2 mutation hot spots include a novel RNA-dependent-RNA polymerase variant. J Transl Med. 2020;18:179. https://doi.org/10.1186/s12967-020-02344-6.
7. Tomaszewski T, DeVries RS, Dong M, Bhatia G, Norsworthy MD, Zheng X, et al. New pathways of mutational change in SARS-CoV-2 proteomes involve regions of intrinsic disorder important for virus replication and release. Evol Bioinform Online. 2020;16:1176934320965149. https://doi.org/10.1177/1176934320965149.
8. Korber B, Fischer WM, Gnanakaran S, Yoon H, Theiler J, Abfalterer W, et al. Tracking changes in SARS-CoV-2 spike: evidence that D614G increases infectivity of the COVID-19 virus. Cell. 2020;182:812–27. https://doi.org/10.1016/j.cell.2020.06.043.
9. Volz E, Hill V, McCrone JT, Price A, Jorgensen D, O'Toole Á, COG-UK Consortium, et al. Evaluating the effects of SARS-CoV-2 spike mutation D614G on transmissibility and pathogenicity. Cell. 2021;184:64–75. https://doi.org/10.1016/j.cell.2020.11.020.
10. Andersen KG, Rambaut A, Lipkin WI, Holmes EC, Garry RF. The proximal origin of SARS-CoV-2. Nat Med. 2020;26:450–2. https://doi.org/10.1038/s41591-020-0820-9.
11. CDC. SARS-CoV-2 variant classifications and definitions. https://www.cdc.gov/coronavirus/2019-ncov/variants/variant-info.html. Accessed 22 Aug 2021.
12. WHO. Tracking SARS-CoV-2 variants. https://www.who.int/en/activities/tracking-SARS-CoV-2-variants. Accessed 22 Aug 2021.
13. WHO. Weekly epidemiological update. Published on 25 February 2021. https://www.who.int/publications/m/item/covid-19-weekly-epidemiological-update. Accessed 22 Aug 2021.
14. WHO announces simple, easy-to-say labels for SARS-CoV-2 variants of interest and concern. Published on 31 May 2021. https://www.who.int/news/item/31-05-2021-who-announces-simple-easy-to-say-labels-for-sars-cov-2-variants-of-interest-and-concern. Accessed 22 Aug 2021.
15. Public Health England. Investigation of novel SARS-CoV-2 variant: variant of concern 202012/01, technical briefing 3. London: Public Health England; 2020. https://assets.publishing.service.gov.uk/government/uploads/system/uploads/attachment_data/file/950823/Variant_of_Concern_VOC_202012_01_Technical_Briefing_3_-_England.pdf. Accessed 22 Aug 2021.
16. Galloway SE, Paul P, MacCannell DR, Johansson MA, Brooks JT, MacNeil A, et al. Emergence of SARS-CoV-2 B.1.1.7 lineage—United States, December 29, 2020–January 12, 2021. MMWR Morb Mortal Wkly Rep. 2021;70:95–9. https://doi.org/10.15585/mmwr.mm7003e2.
17. Davies NG, Abbott S, Barnard RC, Jarvis CI, Kucharski AJ, Munday JD, CMMID COVID-19 Working Group; COVID-19 Genomics UK (COG-UK) Consortium, et al. Estimated transmissibility and impact of SARS-CoV-2 lineage B.1.1.7 in England. Science. 2021;372:eabg3055. https://doi.org/10.1126/science.abg3055.
18. Challen R, Brooks-Pollock E, Read JM, Dyson L, Tsaneva-Atanasova K, Danon L. Risk of mortality in patients infected with SARS-CoV-2 variant of concern 202012/1: matched cohort study. BMJ. 2021;9(372):n579. https://doi.org/10.1136/bmj.n579.
19. Tegally H, Wilkinson E, Giovanetti M, Iranzadeh A, Fonseca V, Giandhari J, et al. Detection of a SARS-CoV-2 variant of concern in South Africa. Nature. 2021;592:438–43. https://doi.org/10.1038/s41586-021-03402-9.
20. Pearson CAB, Russell TW, Davies N, et al. Estimates of severity and transmissibility of novel SARS-CoV-2 variant 501Y.V2 in South Africa. London: CMMID Repository. 2021. https://cmmid.github.io/topics/covid19/sa-novel-variant.html. Accessed 29 Aug 2021.
21. Abdool Karim SS, de Oliveira T. New SARS-CoV-2 variants—clinical, public health, and vaccine implications. N Engl J Med. 2021;384:1866–8. https://doi.org/10.1056/NEJMc2100362.
22. Buss LF, Prete CA Jr, Abrahim CMM, Mendrone A Jr, Salomon T, de Almeida-Neto C, et al. Three-quarters attack rate of SARS-CoV-2 in the Brazilian Amazon during a largely unmitigated epidemic. Science. 2021;371:288–92. https://doi.org/10.1126/science.abe9728.
23. Faria NR, Mellan TA, Whittaker C, Claro IM, Candido DDS, Mishra S, et al. Genomics and epidemiology of the P.1 SARS-CoV-2 lineage in Manaus, Brazil. Science. 2021;372:815–21. https://doi.org/10.1126/science.abh2644.

24. Gómez CE, Perdiguero B, Esteban M. Emerging SARS-CoV-2 variants and impact in global vaccination programs against SARS-CoV-2/COVID-19. Vaccines (Basel). 2021;9:243. https://doi.org/10.3390/vaccines9030243.
25. Naveca FG, Nascimento V, de Souza VC, Corado AL, Nascimento F, Silva G, et al. COVID-19 in Amazonas, Brazil, was driven by the persistence of endemic lineages and P.1 emergence. Nat Med. 2021;27:1230–8. https://doi.org/10.1038/s41591-021-01378-7.
26. Wang P, Casner RG, Nair MS, Wang M, Yu J, Cerutti G, et al. Increased resistance of SARS-CoV-2 variant P.1 to antibody neutralization. Cell Host Microbe. 2021;29:747–51. https://doi.org/10.1016/j.chom.2021.04.007.
27. Kirola L. Genetic emergence of B.1.617.2 in COVID-19. New Microbes New Infect. 2021;43:100929. https://doi.org/10.1016/j.nmni.2021.100929.
28. Harvey WT, Carabelli AM, Jackson B, Gupta RK, Thomson EC, Harrison EM, et al. SARS-CoV-2 variants, spike mutations and immune escape. Nat Rev Microbiol. 2021;19:409–24. https://doi.org/10.1038/s41579-021-00573-0.
29. Cherian S, Potdar V, Jadhav S, Yadav P, Gupta N, Das M, COVID-19 Genomics UK (COG-UK) Consortium, et al. SARS-CoV-2 spike mutations, L452R, T478K, E484Q and P681R, in the second wave of COVID-19 in Maharashtra, India. Microorganisms. 2021;9:1542. https://doi.org/10.3390/microorganisms9071542.
30. Ministry of Health and Family Welfare, Government of India. B.1.617.2, known as the Delta variant, is around 40–60% more transmissible than Alpha Variant. 2021. https://pib.gov.in/PressReleasePage.aspx?PRID=1736665. Accessed 22 Aug 2021.
31. Li B, Deng A, Li K, Hu Y, Li Z, Xiong Q, et al. Viral infection and transmission in a large well-traced outbreak caused by the Delta SARS-CoV-2 variant. medRxiv. 2021;2021:122. https://doi.org/10.1101/2021.07.07.21260122.
32. Fisman DN, Tuite AR. Progressive increase in virulence of novel SARS-CoV-2 variants in Ontario, Canada. medRxiv. 2021;2021:21260050. https://doi.org/10.1101/2021.07.05.21260050.
33. INSACOG Weekly Bulletin. 2021. https://dbtindia.gov.in/insacog. Accessed 29 Aug 2021.
34. Vasireddy D, Vanaparthy R, Mohan G, Malayala SV, Atluri P. Review of COVID-19 variants and COVID-19 vaccine efficacy: what the clinician should know? J Clin Med Res. 2021;13:317–25. https://doi.org/10.14740/jocmr4518.
35. Annavajhala MK, Mohri H, Wang P, Nair M, Zucker JE, Sheng Z, et al. A novel and expanding SARS-CoV-2 variant, B.1.526, identified in New York. medRxiv. 2021;2021:21252259. https://doi.org/10.1101/2021.02.23.21252259.
36. World Health Organization. Weekly epidemiological update on COVID-19. 2021. https://www.who.int/publications/m/item/weekly-epidemiological-update-on-covid-19%2D%2D-27-april-2021. Accessed 29 Aug 2021.
37. Liu H, Wei P, Zhang Q, Aviszus K, Linderberger J, Yang J, et al. The Lambda variant of SARS-CoV-2 has a better chance than the Delta variant to escape vaccines. bioRxiv. 2021;2021:457692. https://doi.org/10.1101/2021.08.25.457692.
38. Acevedo ML, Alonso-Palomares L, Bustamante A, Gaggero A, Paredes F, Cortés CP, et al. Infectivity and immune escape of the new SARS-CoV-2 variant of interest Lambda. medRxiv. 2021;2021:21259673. https://doi.org/10.1101/2021.06.28.21259673.
39. World Health Organization. Weekly epidemiological update on COVID-19. 2021. https://www.who.int/publications/m/item/weekly-epidemiological-update-on-covid-19%2D%2D-31-august-2021. Accessed 1 Sept 2021.
40. Sanyaolu A, Okorie C, Marinkovic A, Haider N, Abbasi AF, Jaferi U, et al. The emerging SARS-CoV-2 variants of concern. Ther Adv Infect Dis. 2021;8:20499361211024372. https://doi.org/10.1177/20499361211024372.
41. Scheepers C, Everatt J, Amoako DG, Mnguni A, Ismail A, Mahlangu B, et al. The continuous evolution of SARS-CoV-2 in South Africa: a new lineage with rapid accumulation of mutations of concern and global detection. medRxiv. 2021;2021:21262342. https://doi.org/10.1101/2021.08.20.21262342.
42. Kunal S, Aditi GK, Ish P. COVID-19 variants in India: potential role in second wave and impact on vaccination. Heart Lung. 2021;50:784–7. https://doi.org/10.1016/j.hrtlng.2021.05.008.

43. Twohig KA, Nyberg T, Zaidi A, Thelwall S, Sinnathamby MA, Aliabadi S, COVID-19 Genomics UK (COG-UK) Consortium, et al. Hospital admission and emergency care attendance risk for SARS-CoV-2 delta (B.1.617.2) compared with alpha (B.1.1.7) variants of concern: a cohort study. Lancet Infect Dis. 2021;21(1):35–42. https://doi.org/10.1016/S1473-3099(21)00475-8.
44. COVID-19 Treatment Guidelines Panel. Coronavirus Disease 2019 (COVID-19) treatment guidelines. Bethesda: National Institutes of Health. https://www.covid19treatmentguidelines.nih.gov/. Accessed 22 Aug 2021.
45. Policy for Evaluating Impact of Viral Mutations on COVID-19 Tests. https://www.fda.gov/regulatory-information/search-fda-guidance-documents/policy-evaluating-impact-viral-mutations-covid-19-tests. Accessed 22 Aug 2021.
46. Hacisuleyman E, Hale C, Saito Y, Blachere NE, Bergh M, Conlon EG, et al. Vaccine breakthrough infections with SARS-CoV-2 variants. N Engl J Med. 2021;384:2212–8. https://doi.org/10.1056/NEJMoa2105000.
47. Wang Z, Schmidt F, Weisblum Y, Muecksch F, Barnes CO, Finkin S, et al. mRNA vaccine-elicited antibodies to SARS-CoV-2 and circulating variants. Nature. 2021;592:616–22. https://doi.org/10.1038/s41586-021-03324-6.
48. Collier DA, De Marco A, Ferreira IATM, Meng B, Datir RP, Walls AC, CITIID-NIHR BioResource COVID-19 Collaboration; COVID-19 Genomics UK (COG-UK) Consortium, et al. Sensitivity of SARS-CoV-2 B.1.1.7 to mRNA vaccine-elicited antibodies. Nature. 2021;593:136–41. https://doi.org/10.1038/s41586-021-03412-7.
49. Madhi SA, Baillie V, Cutland CL, Voysey M, Koen AL, Fairlie L, NGS-SA Group; Wits-VIDA COVID Group, et al. Efficacy of the ChAdOx1 nCoV-19 Covid-19 vaccine against the B.1.351 variant. N Engl J Med. 2021;384:1885–98. https://doi.org/10.1056/NEJMoa2102214.
50. BBC. Covid: South Africa halts AstraZeneca vaccine rollout over new variant. 2021. https://www.bbc.co.uk/news/world-africa-55975052. Accessed 22 Aug 2021.
51. Emary KRW, Golubchik T, Aley PK, Ariani CV, Angus B, Bibi S, COVID-19 Genomics UK Consortium; AMPHEUS Project; Oxford COVID-19 Vaccine Trial Group, et al. Efficacy of ChAdOx1 nCoV-19 (AZD1222) vaccine against SARS-CoV-2 variant of concern 202012/01 (B.1.1.7): an exploratory analysis of a randomised controlled trial. Lancet. 2021;397:1351–62. https://doi.org/10.1016/S0140-6736(21)00628-0.
52. Chemaitelly H, Yassine HM, Benslimane FM, Al Khatib HA, Tang P, Hasan MR, et al. mRNA-1273 COVID-19 vaccine effectiveness against the B.1.1.7 and B.1.351 variants and severe COVID-19 disease in Qatar. Nat Med. 2021;27(9):1614–21. https://doi.org/10.1038/s41591-021-01446-y.
53. Lopez Bernal J, Andrews N, Gower C, Gallagher E, Simmons R, Thelwall S, et al. Effectiveness of Covid-19 vaccines against the B.1.617.2 (Delta) variant. N Engl J Med. 2021;385:585–94. https://doi.org/10.1056/NEJMoa2108891.
54. Nasreen S, He S, Chung H, Brown KA, Gubbay JB, Buchan SA, et al. Effectiveness of COVID-19 vaccines against variants of concern. medRxiv. 2021;2021:21259420. https://doi.org/10.1101/2021.06.28.21259420.
55. World Health Organization. COVID-19 new variants: knowledge gaps and research. 2021. https://www.who.int/publications/m/item/covid-19-new-variants-knowledge-gaps-and-research. Accessed 22 Aug 2021.
56. Shu Y, McCauley YJ. GISAID: Global initiative on sharing all influenza data from vision to reality. Euro Surveill. 2017;22:30494.
57. Mullen JL, Tsueng G, Latif AA, et al. The Center for Viral Systems Biology. https://outbreak.info/. 2020. Accessed 1 Sept 2021.
58. Chen AT, Altschuler K, Zhan SH, et al. COVID-19 CG enables SARS-CoV-2 mutation and lineage tracking by locations and dates of interest. elife. 2021;10:e63409.
59. Kunal S, Sakthivel P, Gupta N, Ish P. Mix and match COVID-19 vaccines: potential benefit and perspective from India. Postgrad Med J. 2021;98(e2):140648. https://doi.org/10.1136/postgradmedj-2021-140648.

# Part II
# Clinical Observations

# Chapter 10
# Psychological Impacts of the COVID-19 Pandemic

**Samuel K. Powell, Alexandra Saali, Randal A. Serafini, Callan P. O'Shea, Justin J. Frere, and Craig L. Katz**

## Introduction

The burden of infectious disease and consequent mortality brought on by the COVID-19 pandemic is paralleled only by the pervasive effects the pandemic has had on global mental health. For too many reasons, there have and will continue to be adverse psychological and psychiatric effects of the pandemic. With each of the approximately five million deaths that have occurred globally thus far, there are the

S. K. Powell (✉) · C. P. O'Shea
Department of Psychiatry, Icahn School of Medicine at Mount Sinai, New York, NY, USA

Department of Neuroscience, Icahn School of Medicine at Mount Sinai, New York, NY, USA

Department of Genetics and Genomic Sciences, Icahn School of Medicine at Mount Sinai, New York, NY, USA
e-mail: Samuel.powell@icahn.mssm.edu

A. Saali
Department of Medical Education, Icahn School of Medicine at Mount Sinai, New York, NY, USA
e-mail: Alexandra.saali@icahn.mssm.edu

R. A. Serafini
Department of Neuroscience, Friedman Brain Institute, Icahn School of Medicine at Mount Sinai, New York, NY, USA
e-mail: Alex.serafini@icahn.mssm.edu

J. J. Frere
Department of Microbiology, Icahn School of Medicine at Mount Sinai, New York, NY, USA
e-mail: Justin.frere@icahn.mssm.edu

C. L. Katz
Departments of Psychiatry, Global Health & System Design, and Medical Education, Icahn School of Medicine at Mount Sinai, New York, NY, USA
e-mail: Craig.katz@mssm.edu


S. Adibi et al. (eds.), *Frontiers of COVID-19*,
https://doi.org/10.1007/978-3-031-08045-6_10

family and loved ones left behind to grieve. For those who survive COVID-19, the trauma can have lasting impacts. And for individuals throughout the world, all are forced to continue adapting to uncertain and often highly dangerous circumstances.

This chapter focuses on the psychological impacts of the COVID-19 pandemic. We begin with the acute effects of the pandemic in substantially increasing rates of psychological distress and symptoms of psychiatric disorders. Throughout, we highlight broad findings from the general population as well as sub-group-specific impacts on those of different ages, genders, races and ethnicities, familial roles, and occupations, among others. We next explore both risk and protective factors for psychological distress and psychopathology during the pandemic. We also provide an overview the psychiatric manifestations and sequelae of COVID-19 itself, exploring potential psychological and pathophysiological mechanisms. We conclude with promising coping and psychological adaptation strategies, drawing from evidence reported during prior pandemics as well as early data reported during the ongoing pandemic. It is hoped that lessons learned from history and our collective current struggle can inform approaches to not only cope with the pandemic but emerge more resilient than before it.

## Psychological and Psychiatric Impacts of the COVID-19 Pandemic

The initial onset of the COVID-19 pandemic precipitated fear and psychological distress worldwide. This section describes results from numerous countries documenting heightened psychiatric symptoms and psychological distress beginning with large, nationally and regionally representative prevalence rates. We then highlight adverse psychological and psychiatric effects on specific subgroups of people defined by sociodemographic, familial, and occupational characteristics. Subsequently, we cover the complexities of whether the pandemic has affected suicide, distinguishing between suicidal ideation, self-injurious behavior, and completed suicides. Having provided snapshot estimates, we finally overview important evidence that changes in mental health have been heterogenous within overall populations, showing several patterns of change—or lack thereof—that vary over time.

### *General Population-Based Estimates of COVID-19-Related Psychiatric Symptoms and Psychological Distress*

In one of the first nationally representative surveys out of China, almost 35% of individuals reported psychological distress with the onset of the COVID-19 pandemic [1]. This finding was consistent with sentiment analyses of posts on the social media platform Weibo, which found psychological indices of depression, anxiety, indignation, and sensitivity to social risks increased while indices of happiness and life satisfaction decreased [2]. During the initial outbreak in Wuhan, the prevalence of depression was 48% and anxiety was 22.6%, and 19% had both depression and anxiety [3]. Furthermore, an estimated 7% of Wuhan adults had significant symptoms of post-traumatic stress [4]. Over half of residents in the Liaoning Providence reported feeling apprehensive and horrified due to the pandemic [5]. In Hong Kong, 19% and 14% of adults met threshold criteria for depression and anxiety, respectively, and approximately 25% reported that their mental health had deteriorated since the onset of the pandemic [6]. These data demonstrated clearly the adverse effects on mental health that had arisen in the acute onset of the pandemic and served as indicators of what was to come in other parts of the world.

Studies from the USA emerged soon after the first case of COVID-19 was reported in January of 2020. As in China, nationwide social media content reflected significant distress with the onset of the pandemic. A sentiment analysis database of U.S. Twitter posts termed the "Hedonometer" [7] showed that overall indicators of happiness dropped precipitously, with the lowest period from May 26th to June 9th [8]. In parallel, estimates of depression prevalence rates were threefold higher among U.S. adults during the beginning of the pandemic compared to pre-pandemic periods [9]. Data from the Center for Disease Control and Prevention (CDC) indicated that, beginning in April and persisting through July of 2020, about 30% of adults nationwide reported symptoms of anxiety and 25% reported symptoms of depression [10]. These estimates are markedly higher than those reported by the CDC in 2019, when 8.1% and 6.5% of adults had symptoms of anxiety and depression, respectively [11]. In June of 2020, an estimated 26% of adults were experiencing symptoms of stress- and trauma-related disorders due to the pandemic, and just over 13% of adults reported either starting or increasing their use of substances in order to cope with stress and difficult emotions related to the pandemic [12].

In the United Kingdom, rates of anxiety nearly doubled, increasing from 13% pre-pandemic to 24%, while estimates of depression remained constant [13]. 21% and 19%, respectively, of Austrian citizens met or exceeded threshold criteria for depression and anxiety, and 16% reported experiencing clinical insomnia [14]. During the first week of the government-mandated shutdown from March 13th to 18th, 35.6% of Italian adults had clinically significant levels of distress, with 29% experiencing symptoms of post-traumatic stress; symptoms of depression and anxiety were reported by 37.8% and 51.1%, respectively [15]. A nationally representative study found that 64% and 53% of adults in Cyprus reported above-minimal symptoms of anxiety and depression, respectively, and that two-thirds felt they had experienced a decreased quality of life due to the pandemic [16]. Data from Jordan indicated that, in March of 2020, 23% of the population had depression and 13% had anxiety [17]. Overall, a comprehensive meta-analysis of all studies ascertaining prevalence rates of depression and anxiety throughout the world in 2020 found that the pandemic contributed to an additional 53.2 million cases of major depressive disorder and 76.2 million additional cases of anxiety disorders globally, representing increases of 27.6% and 25.6%, respectively [18]. In sum, these findings indicate clearly that the COVID-19 pandemic has led to markedly high rates of psychological distress and psychopathology globally.

## *Distress and Psychiatric Symptoms Among Specific Sociodemographic Groups*

The COVID-19 pandemic has exacted differential impacts on various groups based on sociodemographic, familial, and occupational factors. In this section, we provide an overview of results documenting rates of psychological distress and psychopathology among subgroups of individuals defined by age, gender, education, occupational status, and racial/ethnic minority group. Here, our aim is to provide only descriptive results among these various subgroups; evidence for potential demographic, occupational, and clinical *risk factors* for COVID-19-related distress and psychiatric symptoms is covered in section "Risk and Protective Factors for Psychological Distress and Psychiatric Illness During the COVID-19 Pandemic".

### Children and Adolescents

Substantial concerns have been raised about the potential impact of the pandemic on children and adolescents due to the limitations in social interaction, reduced access to school and educational resources, and intrafamilial discord [19, 20, 25, 36, 37]. In tandem, the tragic deaths of parents and other caregivers have caused unimaginable devastation to children throughout the world, as more than 1.5 million have lost primary or secondary caregivers globally [21]. Lockdown orders and school closures have left children in a mentally vulnerable position, as elevated rates of depression and anxiety have been noted in children as young as 6 years old [40]. In adolescents, pandemic-era rates of anxiety and depression were reported to be approximately 12% and 19%, respectively [22]. As of March 2021, estimates of the global prevalence rates of depression and anxiety among children and adolescents were 25.2% (depression) and 20.5% (anxiety) [37], increased from earlier estimated rates of ~10–15% (e.g., [24]).

Disruption in daily routines, social interaction, and education have contributed significantly to the increased burden of distress and psychiatric conditions among youths. Digital education was found to be exhausting for many children, potentially impacting future scholarly performance [24]. Evidence exists showing disruptions in sleep-wakefulness patterns among children overall, with potentially greater impact on children with neurodevelopmental conditions [29]. Distance learning may be particularly challenging for children with ADHD [26, 27]. Of note, children with attention-deficit/hyperactivity disorder or poor emotion regulation before COVID-19 appear to suffer from greater exacerbations on mental health during the pandemic [36].

For both children and adolescents, it is still unclear what the long-lasting effects of the drastic reduction in physical activities on mental and physical health will be [32]. Early data show clearly negative effects: a large cross-sectional survey of children (ages 6–10 years) and adolescents (ages 11–17 years) found associations between lower physical activity, higher screen time, and greater mental health symptoms [33]. The heightened adverse effects on the mental health of children and adolescents with ADHD varies strongly by whether or not ADHD children participate in sports [211], suggesting particularly negative impacts of stay-at-home/shelter-in-place orders on children with ADHD.

Familial discord due to stay-at-home orders, pandemic-related stress, and increased demands of online education have also contributed directly to distress among youth. Studies have found that increased familial quarrels have led to increased psychological distress in adolescents during COVID-19 [30, 31]. A direct, positive relationship has been documented between children's COVID-19-related fear and levels of parental anxiety, suggesting the possibility of self-reinforcing patterns of distress in the parent-child relationship [28]. Of particularly grave concern is the risk of increased child abuse in the context of these stressors, coupled with decreased contacts with mandated reporters. In the USA, the CDC reported that the proportion of emergency department (ED) visits related to child neglect and abuse that results in hospitalization increased despite an overall decrease in the number of such ED visits [35]. These data suggest that the severity of child abuse has worsened and/or that only the most severe cases are brought to medical attention. An independent study found that ED visits for suspected child abuse or neglect increased from March to October of 2020 compared to rates from the same period of time in 2019 [81]. Overall rates child and adolescent discharge from the ED for assault and maltreatment were lower in Ontario than pre-pandemic levels, but it is unclear if there were changes in the severity of injuries documented [34]. Alarmingly, the rates of children ages 0–5 years admitted to the hospital for physical abuse increased substantially in a French study [35]. For these reasons, it appears that children may be at increased risk of harm and mistreatment during the pandemic, although much further study and monitoring is warranted considering the severe negative consequences that abuse and neglect have on children's mental health.

## Students and Young Adults

Numerous studies have examined the psychological impacts of the pandemic on students and young adults. In the U.S., available evidence indicates high levels of psychopathology, with 43.3% of young adults having depression, 45.4% having anxiety, and 31.8% having PTSD symptoms; furthermore, 61.5% reported feelings of loneliness [38]. These findings are aligned with results from studies of students in undergraduate, graduate, and professional school settings. Estimates of anxiety and depression among college students in the Guangdong Providence of China were 26.60% and 21.16%, respectively [42]. Among Chinese college students quarantined at home, prevalence rates of PTSD and depression were found to be 2.7% and 9.0%, respectively. Data from Ukraine indicated that 24% of college students met criteria for generalized anxiety disorder (GAD) and 32% met criteria for depression [43]. A longitudinal study of U.K. college psychology students found that one-third could be classified as having clinical depression at the time of lockdown compared to 15% at baseline and that this rise in depression strongly correlated with worsened sleep quality and a shift toward a later sleep and wake time [41]. Increased consumption of alcohol and other drugs may contribute to these findings, as a study of US college students found that, compared to pre-lockdown levels, rates of alcohol and cannabis use increased by 13% and 24%, respectively [39]. Furthermore, a smartphone-based study found increased levels of sedentary behavior, anxiety, and depression among college students compared to previous term periods in a manner that correlated positively with COVID-19-related media consumption [40]. Across 40 U.S. medical schools, 24.3% of students were depressed and 30.6% had anxiety [44]. Comparable estimates were found among nursing students, with 38.8% and 37.4% had anxiety and depression, respectively [45]. Overall, the pandemic has had sweeping negative impacts on young adult students, in part due to the heightened vulnerability of younger individuals to COVID-19-related distress and psychiatric conditions (discussed below).

## Frontline Healthcare Workers

The pandemic has placed a burden on frontline healthcare workers that is unprecedented in recent history. Early in the course of the pandemic, several reports documented increased symptoms of depression, anxiety, insomnia, and stress among those working in medical occupations. More than half of healthcare workers in Wuhan self-reported severe levels of perceived stress during the first few months of the pandemic [47] and greater than 50% in Chinese hospitals overall reported symptoms of depression and distress [48]. Medical workers, compared to non-medical workers, had higher rates of insomnia, depression, anxiety, somatization, and OCD symptoms in the early stages of the pandemic [49]. Estimates of more clinically severe depression, anxiety, stress, and psychological distress were 5.3%, 8.7%, 2.2%, and 3.8%, respectively [50]. Nurses in Hubei, China, were found to have a 16.83% incidence of PTSD in the context of the pandemic 16.83% [51]. In parallel, there has been a precipitous decline in workplace satisfaction among essential healthcare workers; one study reported that the proportion of those working in an obstetric hospital who were at least somewhat satisfied with their job declined from 93% pre-pandemic to 62% after it began and that the rates of anxiety related to their responsibilities increased substantially [52]. Overall, meta-analytic results suggest that the estimated rates of depression and anxiety among healthcare workers to be ~20% [53], indicating a substantial burden of psychopathology.

## Other Essential Workers

Essential workers in occupations such as maintenance, retail, grocery, cleaning, and law enforcement, among others, were largely exempted from social distancing measures that required most others to work from home. Not surprisingly, the comparatively higher levels of potential exposure to SARS-CoV-2 infection and increased workplace demands have negatively impacted the mental health of these individuals. Fear of contracting and spreading the virus have significantly increased worker's overall stress during the pandemic [12]. Surveys taken during the pandemic discovered that essential workers are more likely to report symptoms of anxiety or depressive disorders (42% vs. 30%), starting or increasing substance use (25% vs. 11%), and suicidal thoughts (22% vs. 8%) than non-essential workers [54]. The American Psychological Association's ongoing *Stress in America* research revealed that 29% of essential workers in 2020 reported that their mental health had deteriorated since the pandemic and that more than half have been relying on self-reported unhealthy habits to get through the pandemic, including 39% of workers who reported drinking more alcohol [55]. This same report also found that essential workers were more than twice as likely to have been diagnosed with a psychiatric condition since the pandemic began compared to those who were not essential workers (25% vs. 9%) [55]. Consistent with these findings are those from an online survey-based study of essential workers in Brazil and Spain which found that 27.4% had both anxiety and depression, 8.3% had depression alone, and 11.6% had anxiety alone [56]. Data from Australia indicated that non-medical essential workers had higher rates of depression, anxiety, and stress and lower quality of life than both the general population and essential workers in healthcare [57]. Among retail grocery store workers during the pandemic, the point prevalence of anxiety and depression were estimated to be 24% and 8%, respectively [58]. Without a doubt, the societal burdens placed on those working in these occupations has come at the cost of significant psychiatric morbidity and distress.

## Parents

Parents and primary caregivers of children face additional disruption and daily stressors due to the sudden and massive shift to online learning platforms as education systems worldwide enforced social distancing measures. Thus far, data on parental perceptions of online education indicate general dissatisfaction and increased stress as well as a perception that teachers were expecting too much from them [59]. Furthermore, childcare has been cited as a leading cause for concern among parents in the USA [60]. These findings parallel survey-based research showing that an overwhelming majority of parents agreed that the COVID-19 pandemic made the 2019–2020 school year extremely stressful for them, especially among those with children ages 8–12 [61]. The challenges with childhood online education have been accompanied by increased symptoms of mood and anxiety disorders among parents, as 47% of mothers and 30% of fathers who had children at home for remote education said that their mental health had worsened [62]. In parallel, half of all U.S. parents reported increased levels of stress compared to their pre-pandemic levels; this figure rose to 62% for parents with children at home engaged in remote learning [61]. Following the closure of schools, almost a quarter of caregivers reported anger and agitation, with over a third also noting anxiety stress and loneliness, suggesting up to a fourfold increase in psychiatric symptoms [63]. Similarly, Czeisler et al. identified more substance use (32.9%) and suicidal ideation (30.7%) among primary caregivers [12]. A longitudinal study of Canadian mothers found that within-subjects depression and anxiety scores increased by a mean of 2.3 and 1.04 points, respectively, and that one-third experienced clinically significant levels of depression and anxiety at the COVID-19 time point; these rates were higher than those observed at previous time points in the 8-year study period [64]. Parental stress associated with the COVID-19 pandemic may be even higher among caregivers of children with neurodevelopmental disorders and disabilities [65], a phenomenon that may vary with the mental health status of caregivers themselves, with low-mental-health caregivers experiencing even higher rates of increased psychological distress [66]. In a study of over 500 Portuguese mothers who gave birth to infants aged 0–12 months either before or during the pandemic, 27.5% of mothers overall had clinically significant symptoms of depression and anxiety; furthermore, mothers who gave birth during the pandemic were found to have signs of decreased emotional awareness of their children and more impaired infant-mother bonding [67]. Although not surprising, these findings highlight the tremendous impact the pandemic has had on parents throughout the world.

## Pregnant Individuals

Pregnant individuals have had to confront heightened uncertainty during the pandemic due to worries about their health and that of their pregnancies, combined with restrictions to healthcare access resulting from social-distancing measures [68]. High rates of post-traumatic stress, anxiety, and depression have been documented in pregnant mothers during the pandemic, with worries associated with their pregnancies, delivery plans, family presence during and after the birthing process, and exposure of the fetus to COVID-19 cited as the top concerns [69]. Additional studies have found that about one-third of pregnant women reported elevated symptoms of depression [70] and that expected mothers had higher increases in depression, anxiety, and negative affect than non-pregnant women [71]. In contrast, however, a study in China found that pregnant women had lower overall rates of depression, anxiety, insomnia, and PTSD than non-pregnant women [72]. A study of routine, prenatal urinalysis screens in a large Californian healthcare-delivery system found a 25% increase in the proportion of expectant mothers using cannabis during their pregnancies [73]. Perhaps not surprisingly, a large, representative survey-based study of mothers in New York City found that about half of mothers who had been trying to become pregnant before the pandemic ceased trying with the pandemic's onset; importantly, ~43% of those who stopped trying to become pregnant reported that they would not resume after the pandemic, suggestive of potential negative perceptions of longer-term futures families in general and mothers and their children in particular [74]. Thus, the preponderance of existing data shows high rates of distress and psychiatric symptoms among pregnant women during the COVID-19 pandemic.

#### Members of Racial and Ethnic Minority Groups

Individuals belonging to racial and ethnic minority groups have seen disproportionately higher adverse mental health consequences during the COVID-19 pandemic. In 2021, non-Hispanic Black adults (48%) and Hispanic or Latino adults (46%) were more likely to report symptoms of anxiety and/or depressive disorders than Non-Hispanic White adults (41%) [12]. Similarly, Hispanic individuals have reported higher prevalence of COVID-19–related trauma symptoms, increased substance use, and suicidal ideation than non-Hispanic Whites or non-Hispanic Asian individuals. Those identifying as Black reported increased substance use and serious consideration of suicide in the previous 30 days more commonly than White and Asian respondents [12]. In 2020, Hispanic Americans had the highest levels of self-reported disruptions in sleep, and Black Americans were the most likely to report concerns about the future. Black and Hispanic children were found to be more likely to suffer adverse mental health effects of remove versus in-person learning [77]. As discussed below, rates of suicide have increased among Black residents in some states [76, 77]. In the U.S. overall, rates of overdose-related cardiac arrest events recorded by emergency medical services increased by ~40% in the initial months of the pandemic, but the highest increases were found among Latinx (49.7%) and Black or African American (50.3%) individuals [79]. Worse still, people of color have historically faced challenges accessing mental health care, and such barriers have likely only increased during the pandemic [76]. For these reasons, expanded access to mental healthcare resources and community-driven research efforts to evaluate potential approaches to reducing these disparities are sorely needed.

We turn now to a critical evaluation of the potential impact of the COVID-19 pandemic on levels of suicide throughout the world.

### *Suicidality*

With the enormous increase in depression, anxiety, trauma, and distress globally, there remains much concern about a parallel increase in suicide. Although the number of individuals with suicidal ideation and passive death wishes has clearly grown, it is unclear if rates of completed suicide have increased in the population overall. Instead, where changes have been reported, they seem specific to certain sub-groups of people and also vary in the direction of change. Here, we discuss the current state of the evidence, making the important distinction between suicidal ideation, self-injurious behaviors and suicide attempts, and completed suicides.

Many studies have estimated rates of suicidal ideation from several countries during the COVID-19 pandemic. Assessment of trends in Google searches using terms indicative of users searching for suicide techniques found evidence that these searches were in fact lower than expected during the first month of the pandemic, even though there was an increase in searches related to help-seeking behavior and mental health problems such as depression, anxiety, and loneliness [82]. In the USA, a nationally representative study found that 10.7% of adults reported seriously considering suicide in 2020, more than double a previous estimate from 2018 [80], with greater increases among Hispanic and Black Americans, essential workers, and unpaid caregivers for adults [83]. Similarly, a Canadian study found that there was an increase in passive suicidal ideation among the general population and especially among participants who were young, Indigenous, unemployed, single, and with pre-existing psychiatric conditions [84]. In contrast, a prospective cohort study of U.S. military veterans found a decrease in rates of suicidal ideation rates from November 2019 to December 2020 [85]. With the widespread surge in depression overall, it is generally not surprising that rates of suicidal ideation have increased, as it is a core symptom of the disorder.

In the case of self-harming behavior and suicide attempts, the picture appears more complicated. Data from over 1600 primary care clinic electronic health record systems indicated substantial decreases in the number of recorded instances of self-harm during the first several months of the pandemic; this may have been due to limited availability of on-site primary care, as this difference normalized by September of 2020 [86]. Among youths aged 13–17, there was an initial decrease in the incidence rates of suicide-related ED visits in the first 3 months of the pandemic, potentially due to stay-at-home orders and shifting needs in healthcare utilization [87]. After May, however, the overall rates returned to pre-pandemic levels observed during the summer months, and female youths had higher rates from June to December of 2020 compared to the same periods of time in 2019 [87]. Analysis of about 190 million US ED encounters found increased visit rates for suicide attempts as well as drug overdoses in March to October of 2020 compared to the same months in the year prior [36]. In contrast, a large study of Sri Lankan individuals found a 32% decrease in hospital presentations for intentional self-poisonings [88] in data analyzed from January 1st, 2019 to August 31st, 2020.

Finally, any changes in the levels of completed suicide appear to be specific to certain demographic groups and locations. An interrupted time-series analysis of data from an Australian register did not find evidence that rates of suicide increased during the first 7 months after Queensland proclaimed a public health emergency due to the pandemic compared to pre-pandemic estimates [93]. A similar analytic approach was used in a study that found no increase in rates of suicide across 21 middle- and upper-income countries from April to July of 2020; in fact, expected rates were lower than expected in some areas examined [94]. Data from Massachusetts did not find increased suicides during the initial stay-at-home orders from March to May of 2020 [89]. However, results from a Maryland study indicated an increase in suicide among Black residents during the first few months of the pandemic, while the rate among White residents decreased in the same period of time [90]. Similar results were found in a study comparing suicide rates among White and non-White residents of Connecticut [91]. Importantly, this took place in the context of already increasing suicide rates among Black and Asian or Pacific Islander Americans beginning in 2014 and continuing to 2019, with rates increasing by 30% for Black Americans and 16% for Asian or Pacific Islander Americans during that time period [92]. A comprehensive study of monthly suicide rates in Japan found that while suicide slightly decreased in the first 5 months of the pandemic, there was a sharp increase during the second outbreak from July to October of 2020, particularly among females, children, and adolescents [95]. These findings were corroborated by a separate study reporting that monthly suicide rates in 2020 compared to the same months in years prior did not increase until July (and including every month through November) for women and October (and through November) for men [93]. These important results indicate clearly that the mental health effects of the pandemic change over time with increasing durations of isolation, lock-down and social distancing-measures, and outbreaks.

## *Heterogeneity and Temporal Variability of Adverse Psychiatric Effects Associated with the COVID-19 Pandemic*

As suggested from above discussion on suicidality, new and exacerbated psychiatric symptoms and disorders have varied through time and affect subgroups of individuals within populations in a heterogenous manner. The most convincing evidence comes from a large longitudinal study in the U.K. that identified different trajectories of mental health-related symptoms during the pandemic over time [100]. Using latent class analysis, investigators uncovered five broad patterns of temporal change in psychological health and symptoms which varied by baseline level of psychopathology at the onset of the pandemic, the direction of change in symptoms (increase or decrease), and the stability of symptoms over time. These findings have been generally consistent with those from other studies as well [96–98], further demonstrating that the psychological wellbeing of individuals has not been uniformly impacted by the pandemic. Instead, there appear to be those who are resilient to adverse psychological effects, those whose level of symptoms remained constant, and even some who appeared to improve during the pandemic. These data have yielded crucial insights into risk and protective factors for distress and psychopathology during the pandemic, as explored in the section that follows.

## Risk and Protective Factors for Psychological Distress and Psychiatric Illness During the COVID-19 Pandemic

The previous section provided a description of the pandemic's adverse effects on the mental health of the general population and specific subgroups of people. We now review existing evidence of differential psychological and psychiatric impacts of the pandemic that may reflect risk or protective factors.

### *Potential Risk Factors for Increased Distress and Psychopathology in the COVID-19 Pandemic*

#### Younger Age

Numerous studies have documented associations between younger age and increased risk of psychopathology and general distress during the COVID-19 pandemic. The longitudinal UK study mentioned immediately above found that although psychiatric symptoms increased above pre-pandemic levels across the entire population, this spike was the most pronounced in those ages 16–24; furthermore, those in one trajectory characterized by consistently good mental health were more likely to be 45 years or older, while those in another trajectory characterized by deteriorating mental health were more likely to be ages 16–35 [100]. Higher rates of depression and anxiety among younger adults were also reported in an additional longitudinal study in the U.K. [13]. Increased psychological distress was documented among younger Chinese individuals during the early months of the pandemic [101, 102], and student status was associated with higher levels of stress, depression, and anxiety during the initial outbreak in China [104]. These findings are consistent with nationally representative data from Cyprus finding that young adults aged 18–29 reported higher levels of depression and anxiety than did those in other age groups [16]. During the initial lockdown period in Italy, older age was found to be associated with lower risk of PTSD [15].

In the USA, individuals aged 18–23 had the highest average level of self-reported stress in 2020, followed by those ages 24–41, and those in this age range had the greatest overall increases in stress from years prior [61]. In 2021, people ages 18–23 were the most likely to state that their mental health had worsened due to the COVID-19 pandemic [62], and compared to all adults, young adults were more likely to report substance use (25% vs. 13%) and suicidal thoughts (26% vs. 11%) [103]. Younger individuals in the USA experienced higher rates of anxiety and depression in the first few months of the pandemic compared to older individuals [106]. College students, in particular, may be heavily impacted, as about half of students self-reported enhanced psychologic distress is a study from a large Northeastern U.S. university [105]. A Japanese study found that rates of internet gaming disorder increased overall during the pandemic but that individuals younger than 30 years old were at heightened risk [107]. Although robust statistical models of the impacts social distancing and lock-down measures demonstrate clear benefit of these interventions on reducing risk of Sars-CoV-2 infection and COVID-19-related hospitalization and mortality (e.g., [108]), these measures have unintended adverse impacts on mental health: analyses from a nationally representative sample found that the mental health of U.S. young adults (ages 18–34) was more negatively impacted by social distancing, lockdowns, and quarantine measures [109].

Importantly, however, not all studies report a simple, linear relationship between age and adverse psychological impacts. For example, during the onset of the pandemic, Chinese individuals younger than 18 experienced the lowest levels of distress while those between ages 18 and 30 or above 60 years of age had the highest distress levels [1]. Additionally, it appears that older healthcare providers were more likely than younger ones to experience symptoms of stress, anxiety, and depression [50]. Overall, however, a meta-analysis of studies throughout the world found that younger age was indeed associated with greater increases in the prevalence of depression and anxiety disorders [18]. Undoubtedly, understanding of the additional factors mediating relationships between age and pandemic-associated distress and psychopathology remain incomplete and are a target of active investigation.

## Female Sex/Gender

Both in the general population and among particular subgroups, several studies have documented elevated levels of distress in females [110–112], albeit with conflicting results and a lack of clarity about whether sex or gender was the variable under study. In one of the earliest nationwide reports, Chinese females had higher levels of distress than males ([1], although this was not found in a separate study [101]). Another group reported that males, rather than females, had higher overall scores on the stress, depression, and anxiety subscales of the depression, anxiety, and stress scale [104]. Female gender was also found to be the leading risk factor for symptoms of depression and anxiety among Chinese high school students [46]. For symptoms of post-traumatic stress, women reported greater symptoms than did men 1 month after the onset of the pandemic in China [4]. Among those who had been hospitalized for COVID-19 in Wuhan, China, female sex was associated with higher risk of prolonged fatigue 1 year after discharge [113]. In the Jordanian population, females were at the highest risk of depression and anxiety [17]. Similarly, Italian females were more likely to meet criteria for PTSD during the initial lockdown [15]. An Israeli study also found that women experienced higher rates of emotional distress during the pandemic than did men [114].

Female individuals from a longitudinal study in the U.K. were less likely to have a mental health trajectory characterized by consistently good mental health both before and during the COVID-19 pandemic and more likely to follow trajectories of deteriorating mental health throughout the pandemic or consistently poor before and after it [100]. Of note, the same study found a greater proportion of females in a trajectory characterized by an initial decline in mental health followed by a recovery as the pandemic progressed [94]. In the USA, while men are more likely to report COVID-19 related substance use disorder and insomnia, women had higher rates of anxiety and depression [103] From a peak in April of 2020, rates of depression and anxiety declined overall, but began and remained elevated among female participants in a large US study [106]. Female sex was a leading risk factor for increased rates of positive depression and suicide screens among adolescents in a primary care setting, with a 34% increase in the proportion of female adolescents reporting suicide thoughts in the latter half of 2020 compared to the same time period in the year prior [23].

Higher rates of psychological distress were reported among female college students compared to male college students [105]. Female gender was associated with higher rates of depression and anxiety in both medical [44] and nursing [45] schools. In the medical profession, female healthcare workers had higher rates of depression, anxiety, OCD, somatic symptoms, and insomnia than did their male counterparts [49]. Compared to male nurses, female nurses were reported to be at greater risk of PTSD [51], and this is consistent with findings from a meta-analysis of psychological risk factors among healthcare workers during the COVID-19 pandemic [53].

Socioeconomic impacts of the pandemic, cultural factors, and the responsibilities of raising children have likely influenced these disparities. Many early-career women were responsible for both consistent job performance and childcare [116, 117]. As discussed previously, pregnant women faced additional stressors, such as concerns over prenatal care, fetal health, and quality of delivery procedures in a limited hospital environment [68]. Internationally, high levels of post-traumatic stress, depression, and anxiety have been documented among pregnant women [69]. Compared to men with children, women with children (49%) are more likely to report symptoms of anxiety and/or depressive disorder than men with children (40%) [28]. Additionally, women were exposed to an elevated risk of domestic violence due to forced co-habitation with their partners during stay-at-home orders [118, 119].

Overall, a global meta-analysis found a much greater increase in the prevalence of depression and anxiety disorders among females than in males [18]. Among children and adolescents, global estimates of depression and anxiety were also found to be higher in girls than in boys [45]. Moving beyond broad point estimates, however, shows a complex pattern of associations between sex/gender and risk of psychological distress and psychopathology that is likely influenced by familial and occupational roles, clinical factors, and pre-existing socioeconomic challenges.

## Pre-existing Psychiatric Conditions

Cross-culturally, the mental health of individuals with psychiatric conditions has been negatively affected by the pandemic, and emerging data suggest that pre-existing psychopathology may be independently associated with additional psychopathology. During the peak of pandemic-related lockdown measures in China, those with a pre-existing psychiatric disorder experienced the pandemic as more stressful overall and had a higher magnitude of depressive and anxious symptoms than those without psychiatric conditions; of note, more than one-third of those with a mental health disorder were estimated to meet full criteria for PTSD [120]. In the early months of the pandemic, substance use was associated with higher risk of both depression and anxiety among Chinese adults [102]. Indeed, individuals with pre-existing anxiety disorders reported higher COVID-related stress and self-isolation distress than those without prior mental health diagnoses [121]. Not surprisingly, those with mood and anxiety disorders had much higher rates of anxious and depressive symptoms, and this remained throughout the first 10 weeks of the pandemic beginning in early April of 2020, despite a general decline from peak levels overall [106].

Of note, patients with affective disorders fared worse than those with psychotic disorders due to increases in perceived loneliness/social restrictions [122]. Within inpatient psychiatry patient populations, those with affective disorders, as opposed to those suffering from substance use disorder or schizophrenia, also demonstrated substantially elevated stress [124]. The pandemic has also been associated with reduced inpatient admissions to psychiatric wards, as well as increased suicidality—two observations that may very well be related [125, 126]. Among those with schizophrenia, social anxiety is associated with even higher rates of COVID-19-related psychological distress and sleep disturbance [117]. In a study of Spanish psychiatric patients, depressive and negative psychotic-like symptom domains were specifically associated with greater risk of moderate to severe neurocognitive impairment [130]. Our group also found further elevations in stress and psychiatric symptoms in an underserved minority patient population at an outpatient psychiatry clinic [123].

Most convincingly, those with a pre-existing mental illness were more likely to follow a trajectory of deteriorating mental health in a longitudinal study during the COVID-19 pandemic [100]. An analysis of 12 longitudinal studies from the U.K. found that those with higher levels of psychological distress before the pandemic were at greater risk of significant life disruptions in housing, employment, and access to healthcare [128], directly supporting the hypothesis that those with pre-existing psychological struggles were more likely to experience major negative impacts of the pandemic, all of which are contributors to further exacerbations in psychological distress.

There is now robust evidence that pre-existing psychiatric conditions also place individuals at higher risk for negative outcomes from COVID-19; as discussed below, the psychiatric sequelae of COVID-19 may in turn exacerbate existing mental health disorders and precipitate new ones. Psychiatric conditions overall, especially severe mental illnesses, are associated with increased risk for mortality from COVID-19 [206]. Those with Autism Spectrum Disorders and intellectual disabilities were found to be at greater risk for SARS-CoV-2 infection and complications from COVID-19 [207]. Compared to those without a mood disorder, those with a mood disorder are at increased risk of COVID-19-related hospitalization (OR = 1.31) and death (OR = 1.51) but not for COVID-19 susceptibility nor severe events [208]. Those with tobacco use disorder, cannabis use disorder, and cocaine use disorder appear to be at higher risk of breakthrough infections after full vaccination; even when matching for lifetime comorbidities and indicates of socioeconomic disadvantage, those with cannabis use disorder remained at higher risk of breakthrough infection [209]. An independent study based upon retrospective chart-review of electronic health records for over 73 million patients found that those diagnosed with a substance use disorder in the past year were at elevated risk for COVID-19, especially among those with opioid use disorder followed by tobacco use disorder [135]. In sum, these factors may interact synergistically to have disproportionately adverse impacts on those with mental health disorders.

### Socioeconomic Disadvantage

The association between low socioeconomic status and mental health conditions has been long documented and has persisted during the COVID-19 pandemic. Even with adjusting for pre-pandemic levels, those facing socioeconomic adversity in the U.K. had elevated rates of depression and anxiety compared to those who did not [13]. Importantly, financial difficulties were associated with a trajectory of deteriorating mental health in the largest longitudinal study in the U.K. [100]. Overall, having lower income and/or less than $5000 in savings has been closely linked to increased depressive symptoms during COVID-19 [9]. Low household income was identified as a key driver of elevated depressive symptoms throughout the first year of the COVID-19 pandemic [138]. A longitudinal study found that decreasing levels of household income corresponded directly to increased levels of depression and anxiety throughout several early months of the pandemic [106]. Income disruption independently predicted greater increases in anxiety symptoms among mothers during the pandemic [64]. Children from lower income households were more likely to suffer adverse mental health effects associated with school closures [77]. A nationally representative survey-based study found that 46% of U.S. adults reported moderate or severe psychological distress, and that those with housing insecurity had a higher likelihood of distress [136]. Unemployment is also associated with higher risk of depression and anxiety [16], and living in deprived neighborhoods predicted a consistently poor trajectory of mental health throughout the pandemic [100]. In the USA, living in impoverished neighborhoods was a risk factor for increased rates of overdose-related cardiac arrest events recorded by emergency medical services [79]. As is often the case in public health crises, those who are most negatively affected are those who were already struggling the most.

### Racism

The relationships between experiences of racism and adverse mental health effects have been previously documented [139], and the COVID-19 pandemic has led to a rise in racism and racial discrimination against Asian Americans [140]. Sentiment analysis of over 3,300,000 tweets from November 2019 to March 2020 found a substantial increase (from 9.79% to 16.49%, an increase of 68.4%) in negative tweets referencing Asian individuals, while there was little change in the number of negative tweets about other racial/ethnic minority groups [143]. A study of Asian

American families found that over 75% of both parents and children had experienced at least one instance of vicarious racism in person or online since the onset of the pandemic and that perceived racism and racial discrimination were associated with poorer mental health [141]. An online survey study found that about 1/3 of participants reported that they had experienced COVID-19-related racial discrimination and that this was positively associated with depressive symptoms [142]. Of note, Asian individuals in the U.K. were more likely experience longitudinal deterioration in mental health during the pandemic [100]. In these ways, a pandemic that is already taxing heavily the mental well-being of all has been associated with further determinants to psychological health for some due to new and exacerbated racism.

## *Possible Protective Factors Against Psychopathology During the COVID-19 Pandemic*

Unfortunately, the evidence available on factors that may protect against or lessen distress and psychiatric conditions during the COVID-19 pandemic is more limited. Largely, these factors appear to be related to knowledge about the pandemic itself, behavioral adaptations aimed at decreasing risk of infection, coping styles, and higher age.

### Increased Age

Demographically, some data suggests that higher age may be a protective factor, as older age was associated with lower anxious and depressive symptoms in nationally representative Italian sample [144]. As discussed previously, the mental health profiles of individuals aged 45 and older were more likely to follow a trajectory characterized by consistently good mental health both before and during the COVID-19 pandemic [100]. Overall, however, the extent to which higher age protects against pandemic-related psychopathology remains unknown.

### Healthcare Knowledge and Adoption of Precautionary Measures

Recent evidence indicates that having appropriate healthcare knowledge and the adoption of safety behaviors may protect against psychological distress. In China, scores for COVID-19 knowledge, prevention and control measures, and trend projections were higher among high school students without depressive and anxiety symptoms than in students with depressive and anxiety symptoms [46]. In the overall population, receiving quality health information that was specific and up-to-date as well as adoption of appropriate precautionary measures such as wearing a mask and hand-washing were associated with lower levels of anxiety, depression, and stress [104]. A 10-week longitudinal study of rates of depression and anxiety found a negative correlation between levels of informedness and magnitude of depressive symptoms overtime but a positive relationship between social media use and anxiety [106]. Others studies have also found that a lack of understanding of the pandemic and increased use of social technologies (smartphones, social media, and gaming) led to increased psychological distress in adolescents during COVID-19 [30, 31]. Among Canadian mothers, those who work in healthcare had smaller increases in depressive symptoms compared to mothers who did not work in healthcare [64]. In general, these findings are highly consistent with the notion that adequate, timely knowledge about COVID-19 and precautionary measures may help reduce uncertainty and ameliorate distress during the pandemic.

### Psychological Traits and Behaviors

Finally, certain psychological traits and behaviors are associated with lower risk of distress and psychiatric symptoms. Not surprisingly, those who spend more time with close friends and family reported lower levels of distress [5]. Those with higher overall defensive functioning were less likely to develop PTSD during the first month of the pandemic-related lockdown [144]. Negative coping styles predicted higher psychological distress in the early stages of the pandemic among a large convenience sample of Chinese individuals [97], as well as increased risk of PTSD symptoms in Chinese young adults [135]. Other studies have found that coping strategies associated with better mental health include positive reframing, acceptance, humor, mediation, work distractions, and COVID-19 preventative education [177, 178]. In contrast, avoidant coping style predicted higher psychiatric symptoms among third-year medical students during the pandemic [143]. A separate report found that both secure and avoidant attachment styles appear to be protective against moderate-to-severe levels of psychological distress [136]. In parallel, there was a negative correlation between attachment anxiety and the quality of romantic relationships among couples during periods of lockdown [137].

While these preliminary findings are promising, much additional research is needed to better understand protective factors in order to adequately inform potential interventions that may be of benefit to those at risk for psychopathology during the COVID-19 pandemic.

## Psychiatric Manifestations of COVID-19 and Its Aftermath

There is an increasing recognition that COVID-19 is often accompanied by neuropsychiatric symptoms. Furthermore, the emerging phenomenon of "Long COVID-19" is frequently marked by subtle psychological and neurocognitive complaints. Orthogonal lines of evidence show substantial levels of psychiatric sequelae among those who survive and even completely recover, likely due to experiencing illness-related trauma. In this section, we review each of these important topics, beginning first with psychiatric manifestations of COVID-19 and Long

COVID-19, briefly focusing on potential pathophysiologic mechanisms, and then covering research on the trauma-related sequelae documented among survivors of COVID-19.

## *Neuropsychiatric Manifestations of COVID-19 and Putative Pathophysiologic Mechanisms*

Although the respiratory tract is presently seen as the primary replication site of the virus, SARS-CoV-2 is also able to infect neurons [139]. Postmortem biopsy studies of COVID-19 patients have confirmed the presence of SARS-CoV-2 in endothelial cells of blood vessels supporting brain parenchyma [140]. It is therefore unsurprising that COVID-19 patients have reported a multiplicity of neuropsychiatric symptoms associated with their disease. Psychiatric complaints have been noted in almost 60% of hospitalized COVID-19 patients [141]. These findings were corroborated by additional data showing that up to one-third of COVID-19 patients present with acute changes in behavior, personality, cognition, and level of consciousness [142]. Numerous sources have documented an expansive array of psychiatric symptomatology in patients with ongoing COVID-19 that has included agitation [143], mania [144], anxious and depressive symptoms [145], delirium [146], confusion [140], dysexecutive syndrome [147], and psychosis [142].

The pathophysiology driving psychiatric symptoms in COVID-19 remains uncertain; while precise mechanisms have not been established, a growing consensus focuses on the immunological effects of the disease on brain tissue [158]. Some have suggested that direct neural infiltration by the virus could result in the aforementioned symptoms [147], while others posit that these symptoms could be due to overabundant cytokine production [148]. This latter hypothesis is consistent with findings of a positive correlation between the magnitude of inflammatory markers in the blood of patients hospitalized with COVID-19 and the severity of depressive symptoms [145]. The inflammatory hypothesis is further corroborated by an evergrowing line of research supporting the potential role of heightened inflammation in the development and progression of psychiatric diseases [149], including psychoses [150], mood disorders [151], and anxiety disorders [152]. The extent to which neuropsychiatric manifestations of COVID-19 are driven by non-specific inflammatory processes versus pathways unique to SARS-CoV-2 infection is presently under exploration by several investigative groups.

## *"Long COVID-19," Its Neuropsychiatric Symptoms, and Potential Mechanisms*

A period of prolonged symptoms following acute COVID-19 disease, often extending many months after clearance of the SARS-CoV-2 virus, has been named "Long COVID-19" or "Post-Acute Sequelae of SARS-CoV-2 Infection" (PASC) [153,

154]. Although cardiovascular and pulmonary symptoms are the primary complaints of those experiencing PASC, a significant body of work has shown that neuropsychiatric symptoms are extremely common [155]. COVID "long-haulers" have been noted to suffer from headache, anhedonia, fatigue, and impaired memory and concentration [155, 156]. A large cohort study of individuals who had been hospitalized for COVID-19 in Wuhan, China found that fatigue and anxiety were among the most common symptoms reported at one-year follow-up after discharge [108]. One study found that more than half of patients hospitalized with COVID-19 experienced clinically significant cognitive impairment 3–4 months following discharge and that the magnitude of impairment was associated with d-dimer levels during acute illness as well as the degree of residual pulmonary impairment [157]. Although milder COVID-19 infection does not appear to be associated with cognitive impairment, symptoms of anxiety and depression were elevated at follow-up compared to those individuals unaffected by PASC [158].

The pathophysiology of PASC remains unclear, although multiple hypotheses have been proposed in an attempt to account for the high prevalence of psychiatric symptomatology. One hypothesis suggests that the virus itself induces permanent systemic changes, including potential scarring and/or induction of autoimmune reactions, that, in turn, disrupt healthy neural functioning [154]. Others have proposed that persistent viral reservoirs of SARS-CoV-2 cause chronic inflammation that brings about the myriad reported symptoms [159]. At the time of this writing, however, the causes and pathophysiological mechanisms of Long-COVID-19 are speculative, and it remains diagnostically challenging, if not impossible, to completely distinguish psychiatric *symptoms* of PASC from psychiatric *consequences* of the stressful and sometimes traumatic experience of COVID-19 itself, discussed next.

## *Psychiatric Sequelae of COVID-19*

Survivors of COVID-19 are at heightened risk of psychiatric sequelae. Several research groups have observed a positive association between mild infection cases and lasting psychiatric conditions, including stress, anxiety, and depression [160, 161]. A follow-up study that took place 1 month after hospital discharge found that 31% of patients reported depression, 28% reported PTSD, 42% reported anxiety, 40% reported insomnia, and 20% reported symptoms of OCD [171]. 23% of patients discharged from a hospital in Wuhan, China, had anxiety or depression at 6 months follow-up [162]; strikingly, the same group found that this increased to 26% at 12 months follow-up [163]. A meta-analysis found that fatigue (58%) and attentional disorder (27%) were among the top-five most commonly experienced symptoms among those who had recovered from SARS-CoV-2 infection [169]. Whether these symptoms are due to PASC or secondary psychological consequences of COVID-19, or both, is unclear. Of note, however, is that rates of psychopathology due to COVID-19 are higher than those observed among patients admitted for influenza or other respiratory tract infections [164]. A large retrospective cohort study found that those without psychiatric histories had increased incidences of first psychiatric diagnosis at 14–90 days compared to those who had experienced six other health conditions [165], indicating that not just symptoms but also full psychiatric disorders can occur after the disease.

COVID-19 has also been linked with higher incidence of PTSD due to trauma induced by infection itself, as well as pandemic-associated stress, loss, and restrictive measures. About 13% of Chinese young adults had symptoms of PTSD in the first month of the pandemic [135]. One study found that almost 30% of the Italian population had PTSD symptomatology during the onset of the pandemic [170]. Almost 30% of individuals who had presented for emergency care with COVID-19 met *DSM-5* criteria for PTSD 30–120 days later [172], although these rates have varied by the duration of follow-up [173]. Undoubtedly, the pandemic has precipitated vast amounts of psychiatric illness and will likely continue to do so, thus necessitating the need for robust clinical monitoring and treatment interventions.

## Psychological and Behavior Adaptation Strategies

We have thus far described the substantial body of work showing adverse psychological impacts of the COVID-19 pandemic and those factors that may place individuals at increased risk of such effects. In the section that follows, we utilize empirical data to propose potential strategies for reducing negative psychological and psychiatric consequences of the COVID-19 pandemic as well as adaptive approaches to decrease the likelihood of additional worsening of mental health overall. Importantly, effective psychotherapeutic and psychopharmacologic treatments are still the mainstay of treatment for new psychiatric conditions. At the same time, interventions developed specifically for the COVID-19 pandemic have shown early evidence of efficacy, and the delivery of mental health services through virtual approaches has expanded dramatically to meet individual needs during times of social distancing and quarantine measures.

While several factors inherently contribute to the risk of lasting psychological symptoms due to COVID-19, research during the pandemic has highlighted successful methods of overcoming distress. From a cognitive perspective, mindfulness, optimism, and a sense of trust have been considered protective, as measured by tools such as the Mindfulness Attention Awareness Scale and the Life Orientation Test [39, 176]. An impressive clinical trial consisting of over 20,000 participants across 87 countries found that a brief intervention utilizing cognitive reappraisal, an emotion-regulation technique, was effective in both reducing negative emotions and increasing positive emotions [175]. Additionally, interventions to target uncertainty tolerance among children have been specifically suggested [214].

Many groups have called for improvement of remote psychiatric infrastructure in order to provide patients with the social support and mental health services they need during the pandemic [179–181]. Importantly, evidence-based guidelines on the appropriate and effective use of telepsychiatry-based mental health services have been developed and continue to evolve as more data emerge [192]. Intriguingly, there may be adherence and attendance advantages to remote versus in-person psychological service appointments for those with dementia [193] and adults receiving CBT for major depressive disorder [187], among others. Several successful remote clinical psychiatry efforts, which included the delivery of CBT, psychopharmaceutical management, and eye movement desensitization and reprocessing, improved symptoms and functioning for individuals of diverse backgrounds, including front-line healthcare workers and those with an existing psychiatric disorder [118, 182–186]. During the 6 months of lockdown in Wuhan, China, there was increased usage of a publicly available computerized CBT training program that was found to be effective in reducing the severity of both depression and anxiety [174]. Pilot data from a telecare-based model of case-management for home-bound elderly persons in China did not find evidence of benefit for overall self-efficacy and self-care behaviors; however, higher medication adherence and better quality of life were associated with the telecare intervention [210]. A small study found that patients with PTSD preferred face-to-face visits compared with telepsychiatry sessions, but most reported that they would continue treatment via virtual platforms [205].

Additional lifestyle factors and intervention programs aimed at relaxation training are of benefit to those both with and without psychopathology during COVID-19. Exercise was shown to deter psychological symptoms, while reliance on digital entertainment and the news actually increased the risk of depression and anxiety [38, 198–200]. Outdoor exercise has also been effective at counteracting perceived reductions in mental health during the pandemic, particularly in the context of increased time with several types of screens [201]. Alternative physical relaxation strategies that provided mental health benefits include yoga and progressive muscle relaxation [202]. Furthermore, progressive muscle relaxation showed benefit in reducing anxiety and improving sleep in a small study of patients hospitalized with COVID-19 [203]. A self-help relaxation and mindfulness training program may also be beneficial to those with COVID-19 and mild-to-moderate anxiety or depression [204]. Brief crisis intervention focused on psychological support led to improved quality of life and reduced stress, depression, and anxiety among those with COVID-19 [205].

The ability of individuals to have support networks, either in-person or digitally, during lockdowns was also highly protective against mental health deterioration [187–189]. However, lockdowns with other individuals have also been cited as a source of distress or even physical harm [190, 191]. For this reason, we believe that additional emphasis should be placed on remote couples or family therapy for the ongoing pandemic and future lockdowns, as strong bonds can be therapeutic. Information on interesting activities to do as a group should also be regularly disseminated. Policy suggestions have been developed to further support and address new challenges faced by informal (unpaid) caregivers, such as parents, including assistance in helping families form "closed support bubbles," consisting of small groups of families providing mutual support, companionship, and assistance to members in need [203]. Others [204] have developed perinatal planning guides in light of the unique burden the pandemic has placed upon perinatal women. These guides are designed to help decrease the chances of and impacts from perinatal mood and anxiety disorders, and they consist of both concrete steps to prevent or alleviate future challenges that could be expected and information on available evidence-based treatments for women during this time [204].

Lockdown orders and school closures have also left children in a mentally vulnerable position, as elevated rates of depression and anxiety have been noted in kids as young as 6 years old [41]. This consideration is important from both the perspective of impaired social interaction skills and inability to access mental health attention, which is often provided in the school setting [194]. During this pandemic there was a dearth of information for guiding parents on child-raising during a lockdown and preventing a trajectory towards psychological distress. Based on cited risk factors, potential strategies include limiting screen time, regularly providing interactive activities and parent-child discussions, promoting digital interaction with other children, and ensuring access to pediatric care [212–214]. Without sufficient additional supports to parents, especially those among low-income and disadvantaged groups, gaps in educational achievement and mental health are likely to become further exacerbated by the ongoing pandemic [127].

The well-being of healthcare workers similarly deserves special attention, and a small number of studies have reported on promising interventions aimed at increasing coping skills and treating psychological distress. The Toolkit for Emotional Coping for Healthcare Staff (TECHS) is an online resource to help screen for traumatic stress reactions among healthcare workers that also has demonstrated efficacy in helping them develop coping skills based upon principles of family therapy and cognitive-behavior therapy [215]. Additionally, mindfulness-based stress reduction demonstrated efficacy in improving quality of sleep among nurses working COVID-19 hospital treatment units [216]. Finally, cannabidiol was found to further decrease symptoms of emotional distress and burnout among frontline healthcare workers caring for those COVID-19 when added to standard care [217]. It is our hope that continued research provides a robust foundation for evidence-based treatment approaches for the prevention and treatment of psychological distress and psychiatric conditions associated with the COVID-19 pandemic.

## Conclusion

The adverse psychological and psychiatric impacts of the COVID-19 pandemic have been paralleled only by the devastating loss of life and physical illness affecting individuals, families, and communities worldwide. Unprecedented in the resulting chronic social isolation, sweeping unemployment, and constant uncertainty, the pandemic has and will likely continue to negatively impact the mental health of the global population.

While there has been a broad and global increase in distress, psychiatric symptoms, and mental health disorders, investigators have identified heterogeneity in patterns of psychopathology over time and groups of individuals defined by several sociodemographic, occupational, and familial factors. Young people, women, those with pre-existing psychiatric conditions, the poor, and members of racial and ethnic minorities have suffered disproportionately higher degrees of adverse psychological consequences of the pandemic. Increasing substance abuse, drug overdose, and suicidal ideation pose active threats of elevated rates of suicide. Particularly troubling phenomena are already increased rates of suicide among people of color in the USA and suggestive evidence from multiple countries of worsening child abuse and neglect.

With a continually improved understanding of the negative psychological effects of the pandemic and the risk and protective factors for those effects, evidence-based treatment and prevention efforts may be implemented successfully to reduce the overall burden of mental illness; indeed, nascent research reviewed herein is cause for cautious optimism. Ongoing investigative efforts should continue to unveil ways in which individuals and societies can best adapt to a new world in which COVID-19 is an inevitable fact of life.

## Further Readings

1. Qiu J, Shen B, Zhao M, Wang Z, Xie B, Xu Y. A nationwide survey of psychological distress among Chinese people in the COVID-19 epidemic: implications and policy recommendations. Gen Psychiatr. 2020;33(2):e100213.
2. Li S, Wang Y, Xue J, Zhao N, Zhu T. The impact of covid-19 epidemic declaration on psychological consequences: a study on active weibo users. Int J Environ Res Public Health. 2020;17(6):2032.
3. Gao J, Zheng P, Jia Y, Chen H, Mao Y, Chen S, et al. Mental health problems and social media exposure during COVID-19 outbreak. PLoS One. 2020;15(4):e0231924.
4. Liu N, Zhang F, Wei C, Jia Y, Shang Z, Sun L, et al. Prevalence and predictors of PTSS during COVID-19 outbreak in China hardest-hit areas: gender differences matter. Psychiatry Res. 2020;287:112921.
5. Zhang Y, Ma ZF. Impact of the COVID-19 pandemic on mental health and quality of life among local residents in Liaoning Province, China: a cross-sectional study. Int J Environ Res Public Health. 2020;17:2381.
6. Choi EPH, Hui BPH, Wan EYF. Depression and anxiety in Hong Kong during covid-19. Int J Environ Res Public Health. 2020;17:3740.
7. Dodds PS, Harris KD, Kloumann IM, Bliss CA, Danforth CM. Temporal patterns of happiness and information in a global social network: Hedonometrics and Twitter. PLoS One. 2011;6:26752.
8. Viglione G. Has Twitter just had its saddest fortnight ever? Nature. 2020.
9. Ettman CK, Abdalla SM, Cohen GH, Sampson L, Vivier PM, Galea S. Prevalence of depression symptoms in US adults before and during the COVID-19 pandemic key points + invited commentary. JAMA. 2020;3:e2019686.
10. CDC National Center for Health Statistics. Indicators of anxiety or depression based on reported frequency of symptoms during the last 7 days. Household Pulse Survey. Atlanta: CDC National Center for Health Statistics; 2020. [cited 2021 Jun 30]. Available from: https://www.cdc.gov/nchs/covid19/pulse/mental-health.htm.
11. CDC National Center for Health Statistics. Early release of selected mental health estimates based on data from the January–June 2019 National Health interview survey. Atlanta: CDC

National Center for Health Statistics; 2019. Available from: https://www.cdc.gov/nchs/covid19/pulse/mental-health.htm.

12. Czeisler MÉ, Lane RI, Petrosky E, Wiley JF, Christensen A, Njai R, et al. Mental health, substance use, and suicidal ideation during the COVID-19 pandemic—United States, June 24–30, 2020. Morb Mortal Wkly Rep. 2020;69:1049–57.
13. Kwong ASF, Pearson RM, Adams MJ, Northstone K, Tilling K, Smith D, et al. Mental health before and during the COVID-19 pandemic in two longitudinal UK population cohorts. Br J Psychiatry. 2021;218:334–43.
14. Pieh C, Budimir S, Probst T. The effect of age, gender, income, work, and physical activity on mental health during coronavirus disease (COVID-19) lockdown in Austria. J Psychosom Res. 2020;136:110186.
15. di Giuseppe M, Zilcha-Mano S, Prout TA, Perry JC, Orrù G, Conversano C. Psychological impact of coronavirus disease 2019 among Italians during the first week of lockdown. Front Psych. 2020;11:1.
16. Solomou I, Constantinidou F. Prevalence and predictors of anxiety and depression symptoms during the COVID-19 pandemic and compliance with precautionary measures: age and sex matter. Int J Environ Res Public Health. 2020;17:1–19.
17. Naser AY, Dahmash EZ, Al-Rousan R, Alwafi H, Alrawashdeh HM, Ghoul I, et al. Mental health status of the general population, healthcare professionals, and university students during 2019 coronavirus disease outbreak in Jordan: a cross-sectional study. Brain Behav. 2020;10:e01730.
18. Santomauro DF, Herrera AMM, Shadid J, Zheng P, Ashbaugh C, Pigott DM, et al. Global prevalence and burden of depressive and anxiety disorders in 204 countries and territories in 2020 due to the COVID-19 pandemic. Lancet. 2021;398(10312):1700–12.
19. Guessoum SB, Lachal J, Radjack R, Carretier E, Minassian S, Benoit L, et al. Adolescent psychiatric disorders during the COVID-19 pandemic and lockdown. Psychiatry Res. 2020;291:113264.
20. Racine N, Cooke JE, Eirich R, Korczak DJ, McArthur BA, Madigan S. Child and adolescent mental illness during COVID-19: a rapid review. Psychiatry Res. 2020;292:113307.
21. Hillis SD, Unwin HJT, Chen Y, Cluver L, Sherr L, Goldman PS, et al. Global minimum estimates of children affected by COVID-19-associated orphanhood and deaths of caregivers: a modelling study. Lancet. 2021;398:391–402.
22. Chen F, Zheng D, Liu J, Gong Y, Guan Z, Lou D. Depression and anxiety among adolescents during COVID-19: a cross-sectional study. Brain Behav Immun. 2020;88:36–8.
23. Racine N, McArthur BA, Cooke JE, Eirich R, Zhu J, Madigan S. Global prevalence of depressive and anxiety symptoms in children and adolescents during COVID-19: a meta-analysis. JAMA Pediatr. 2021;175(11):1142–50.
24. Lu W. Adolescent depression: national trends, risk factors, and healthcare disparities. Am J Health Behav. 2019;43:181–94.
25. Ravens-Sieberer U, Kaman A, Otto C, Adedeji A, Devine J, Erhart M, et al. Mental health and quality of life in children and adolescents during the COVID-19 pandemic—results of the copsy study. Dtsch Arztebl Int. 2020;117(48):828–9.
26. Bruni O, Breda M, Ferri R, Melegari MG. Changes in sleep patterns and disorders in children and adolescents with attention deficit hyperactivity disorders and autism spectrum disorders during the COVID-19 lockdown. Brain Sci. 2021;11(9):1139. https://doi.org/10.3390/brainsci11091139.
27. Tessarollo V, Scarpellini F, Costantino I, Cartabia M, Canevini MP, Bonati M. Distance learning in children with and without ADHD: a case-control study during the COVID-19 pandemic. J Atten Disord. 2022;26(6):902–14.
28. Breaux R, Dvorsky MR, Marsh NP, Green CD, Cash AR, Shroff DM, et al. Prospective impact of COVID-19 on mental health functioning in adolescents with and without ADHD: protective role of emotion regulation abilities. J Child Psychol Psychiatry Allied Discip. 2021;62(9):1132–9.

29. Xiang M, Zhang Z, Kuwahara K. Impact of COVID-19 pandemic on children and adolescents' lifestyle behavior larger than expected. Prog Cardiovasc Dis. 2020;63:531–2.
30. Tandon PS, Zhou C, Johnson AM, Schoenfelder Gonzalez E, Kroshus E. Association of children's physical activity and screen time with mental health during the COVID-19 pandemic. JAMA Netw Open. 2021;4(10):e2127892.
31. Karci CK, Gurbuz AA. Challenges of children and adolescents with attention-deficit/hyperactivity disorder during the COVID-19 pandemic. Nord J Psychiatry. 2021. Available from: https://www.tandfonline.com/action/journalInformation?journalCode=ipsc20.
32. Chen IH, Chen CY, Pakpour AH, Griffiths MD, Lin CY. Internet-related behaviors and psychological distress among schoolchildren during COVID-19 school suspension. J Am Acad Child Adolesc Psychiatry. 2020;59:1099–1102.e1.
33. Sharma V, Reina Ortiz M, Sharma N. Risk and protective factors for adolescent and young adult mental health within the context of COVID-19: a perspective from Nepal. J Adolesc Health. 2020;67:135–7.
34. Suffren S, Dubois-Comtois K, Lemelin J-P, St-Laurent D, Milot T. Relations between child and parent fears and changes in family functioning related to COVID-19. Int J Environ Res Public Health. 2021;18:1786. https://doi.org/10.3390/ijerph18041786.
35. Swedo E. Trends in U.S. Emergency Department visits related to suspected or confirmed child abuse and neglect among children and adolescents aged 18 years before and during the COVID-19 pandemic—United States, January 2019–September 2020. Morb Mortal Wkly Rep. 2020;69:1841–7.
36. Holland KM, Jones C, Vivolo-Kantor AM, Idaikkadar N, Zwald M, Hoots B, et al. Trends in US Emergency Department visits for mental health, overdose, and violence outcomes before and during the COVID-19 pandemic. JAMA Psychiat. 2021;78(4):372–9.
37. Saunders N, Plumptre L, Diong C, Gandhi S, Schull M, Guttmann A, et al. Acute care visits for assault and maltreatment before vs during the COVID-19 pandemic in Ontario, Canada. JAMA Health Forum. 2021;2:e211983.
38. Loiseau M, Cottenet J, Bechraoui-Quantin S, Gilard-Pioc S, Mikaeloff Y, Jollant F, et al. Physical abuse of young children during the COVID-19 pandemic: alarming increase in the relative frequency of hospitalizations during the lockdown period. Child Abuse Negl. 2021;122:105299.
39. Liu CH, Zhang E, Wong GTF, Hyun S, Chris HH. Factors associated with depression, anxiety, and PTSD symptomatology during the COVID-19 pandemic: clinical implications for U.S. young adult mental health. Psychiatry Res. 2020;290:113172. https://doi.org/10.1016/j.psychres.2020.113172.
40. Chang J, Yuan Y, Wang D. Mental health status and its influencing factors among college students during the epidemic of COVID-19. Nan Fang Yi Ke Da Xue Xue Bao. 2020;40:171–6.
41. Rogowska AM, Pavlova I, Kuśnierz C, Ochnik D, Bodnar I, Petrytsa P. Does physical activity matter for the mental health of university students during the COVID-19 pandemic? J Clin Med. 2020;9:3494.
42. Evans S, Alkan E, Bhangoo JK, Tenenbaum H, Ng-Knight T. Effects of the COVID-19 lockdown on mental health, wellbeing, sleep, and alcohol use in a UK student sample. Psychiatry Res. 2021;298:113819.
43. Schepis TS, de Nadai AS, Bravo AJ, Looby A, Villarosa-Hurlocker MC, Earleywine M. Alcohol use, cannabis use, and psychopathology symptoms among college students before and after COVID-19. J Psychiatr Res. 2021;142:73–9.
44. Huckins JF, da Silva AW, Wang W, Hedlund E, Rogers C, Nepal SK, et al. Mental health and behavior of college students during the early phases of the COVID-19 pandemic: longitudinal smartphone and ecological momentary assessment study. J Med Internet Res. 2020;22(6):e20185.
45. Halperin SJ, Henderson MN, Prenner S, Grauer JN. Prevalence of anxiety and depression among medical students during the Covid-19 pandemic: a cross-sectional study. J Med Educ Curric Dev. 2021;8:238212052199115.

46. Pouralizadeh M, Bostani Z, Maroufizadeh S, Ghanbari A, Khoshbakht M, Alavi SA, et al. Anxiety and depression and the related factors in nurses of Guilan University of Medical Sciences hospitals during COVID-19: a web-based cross-sectional study. Int J Afr Nurs Sci. 2020;13:100233.
47. Du J, Dong L, Wang T, Yuan C, Fu R, Zhang L, et al. Psychological symptoms among frontline healthcare workers during COVID-19 outbreak in Wuhan. Gen Hosp Psychiatry. 2020;65:144–5.
48. Lai J, Ma S, Wang Y, Cai Z, Hu J, Wei N, et al. Factors associated with mental health outcomes among health care workers exposed to coronavirus disease 2019. JAMA Netw Open. 2020;3:203976.
49. Zhang W, Wang K, Yin L, Zhao W, Xue Q, Peng M, et al. Mental health and psychosocial problems of medical health workers during the COVID-19 epidemic in China. Psychother Psychosom. 2020;89:242–50.
50. Chew NWS, Lee GKH, Tan BYQ, Jing M, Goh Y, Ngiam NJH, et al. A multinational, multicentre study on the psychological outcomes and associated physical symptoms amongst healthcare workers during COVID-19 outbreak. Brain Behav Immun. 2020;88:559–65.
51. Wang YX, Guo HT, Du XW, Song W, Lu C, Hao WN. Factors associated with post-traumatic stress disorder of nurses exposed to corona virus disease 2019 in China. Medicine. 2020;99:e20965.
52. Bender WR, Srinivas S, Coutifaris P, Acker A, Hirshberg A. The psychological experience of obstetric patients and health care workers after implementation of universal SARS-CoV-2 testing. Am J Perinatol. 2020;37:1271–9.
53. Pappa S, Ntella V, Giannakas T, Giannakoulis VG, Papoutsi E, Katsaounou P. Prevalence of depression, anxiety, and insomnia among healthcare workers during the COVID-19 pandemic: a systematic review and meta-analysis. Brain Behav Immun. 2020;88:901–7.
54. Kamal R, Panchal N, Garfield R. Both remote and on-site workers are grappling with serious mental health consequences of COVID-19. KFF. 2020. [cited 2021 Jun 30]. Available from: https://www.kff.org/policy-watch/both-remote-and-on-site-workers-are-grappling-with-serious-mental-health-consequences-of-covid-19/.
55. Essential workers more likely to be diagnosed with a mental health disorder during pandemic. [cited 2021 June 30]. Available from: https://www.apa.org/news/press/releases/stress/2021/one-year-pandemic-stress-essential.
56. de Boni RB, Balanzá-Martínez V, Mota JC, de Azevedo CT, Ballester P, Atienza-Carbonell B, et al. Depression, anxiety, and lifestyle among essential workers: a web survey from Brazil and Spain during the COVID-19 pandemic. J Med Internet Res. 2020;22(10):e22835.
57. Toh WL, Meyer D, Phillipou A, Tan EJ, van Rheenen TE, Neill E, et al. Mental health status of healthcare versus other essential workers in Australia amidst the COVID-19 pandemic: initial results from the collate project. Psychiatry Res. 2021;298:113822.
58. Lan FY, Suharlim C, Kales SN, Yang J. Association between SARS-CoV-2 infection, exposure risk and mental health among a cohort of essential retail workers in the USA. Occup Environ Med. 2021;78:237–43.
59. Fontenelle-Tereshchuk D. 'Homeschooling' and the COVID-19 crisis: the insights of parents on curriculum and remote learning. Interchange. 2021;52:167–91.
60. Nelson LM, Simard JF, Oluyomi A, Nava V, Rosas LG, Bondy M, et al. US public concerns about the COVID-19 pandemic from results of a survey given via social media. JAMA Intern Med. 2020;180:1020–2.
61. American Psychological Association. Stress in America™ 2020: a national mental health crisis. American Psychological Association; 2020. [cited 2021 Jun 30]. Available from: https://www.apa.org/news/press/releases/stress/2020/report-october.
62. American Psychological Association. Stress in America: one year later, a new wave of pandemic health concerns. American Psychological Association; 2021; Available from: https://www.apa.org/news/press/releases/stress/2013/stress-report.pdf.

63. Raviv T, Warren CM, Washburn JJ, Kanaley MK, Eihentale L, Goldenthal HJ, et al. Caregiver perceptions of children's psychological well-being during the COVID-19 pandemic. JAMA Netw Open. 2021;4:e2111103.
64. Racine N, Hetherington E, McArthur BA, McDonald S, Edwards S, Tough S, et al. Maternal depressive and anxiety symptoms before and during the COVID-19 pandemic in Canada: a longitudinal analysis. Lancet Psychiatry. 2021;8:405–15.
65. Siracusano M, Riccioni A, Gialloreti LE, Segatori E, Arturi L, Vasta M, et al. Parental stress and disability in offspring: a snapshot during the COVID-19 pandemic. Brain Sci. 2021;11(8):1040.
66. Tseng H-W, Tsai C-S, Chen Y-M, Hsiao RC, Chou F-H, Yen C-F, et al. Poor mental health in caregivers of children with attention-deficit/hyperactivity disorder and its relationships with caregivers' difficulties in managing the children's behaviors and worsened psychological symptoms during the COVID-19 pandemic. Int J Environ Res Public Health. 2021;18:9745.
67. Fernandes DV, Canavarro MC, Moreira H. Postpartum during COVID-19 pandemic: Portuguese mothers' mental health, mindful parenting, and mother–infant bonding. J Clin Psychol. 2021;77:1997–2010.
68. Lebel C, MacKinnon A, Bagshawe M, Tomfohr-Madsen L, Giesbrecht G. Elevated depression and anxiety symptoms among pregnant individuals during the COVID-19 pandemic. J Affect Disord. 2020;277:5–13. https://doi.org/10.1016/j.jad.2020.07.126.
69. Basu A, Kim IDHH, Basaldua R, Choi KW, Charron L, Kelsall N, et al. A cross-national study of factors associated with women's perinatal mental health and wellbeing during the COVID-19 pandemic. PLoS One. 2021;16(4):e0249780. https://doi.org/10.1371/journal.pone.0249780.
70. Perzow SED, Hennessey E-MP, Hoffman MC, Grote NK, Davis EP, Hankin BL. Mental health of pregnant and postpartum women in response to the COVID-19 pandemic. J Affect Disord Rep. 2021;4:100123. https://doi.org/10.1016/j.jadr.2021.100123.
71. López-Morales H, del Valle MV, Canet-Juric L, Andrés ML, Galli JI, Poó F, et al. Mental health of pregnant women during the COVID-19 pandemic: a longitudinal study. Psychiatry Res. 2021;295:113567.
72. Zhou Y, Shi H, Liu Z, Peng S, Wang R, Qi L, et al. The prevalence of psychiatric symptoms of pregnant and non-pregnant women during the COVID-19 epidemic. Transl Psychiatry. 2020;10:319.
73. Young-Wolff KC, Ray GT, Alexeeff SE, Adams SR, Does MB, Ansley D, et al. Rates of prenatal cannabis use among pregnant women before and during the COVID-19 pandemic. JAMA. 2021;326:1745–7.
74. Kahn LG, Trasande L, Liu M, Mehta-Lee SS, Brubaker SG, Jacobson MH. Factors associated with changes in pregnancy intention among women who were mothers of young children in New York City following the COVID-19 outbreak. JAMA Netw Open. 2021;4:e2124273.
75. Hawrilenko M, Kroshus E, Tandon P, Christakis D. The association between school closures and child mental health during COVID-19+ supplemental content. JAMA Netw Open. 2021;4:2124092.
76. Bray MJC, Daneshvari NO, Radhakrishnan I, Cubbage J, Eagle M, Southall P, et al. Racial differences in statewide suicide mortality trends in Maryland during the coronavirus disease 2019 (COVID-19) pandemic. JAMA Psychiat. 2021;78:444–7.
77. Mitchell TO, Li L. State-level data on suicide mortality during COVID-19 quarantine: early evidence of a disproportionate impact on racial minorities. Psychiatry Res. 2021;295:113629. https://doi.org/10.1016/j.psychres.2020.113629.
78. Friedman J, Mann NC, Hansen H, Bourgois P, Braslow J, Bui AAT, et al. Racial/ethnic, social, and geographic trends in overdose-associated cardiac arrests observed by US Emergency Medical Services during the COVID-19 pandemic. JAMA Psychiat. 2021;78:886–95.
79. Ortega AN, McKenna RM, Kemmick Pintor J, Langellier BA, Roby DH, Pourat N, et al. Health care access and physical and behavioral health among undocumented Latinos in California. Med Care. 2018;56:919–26.

80. Halford EA, Lake AM, Gould MS. Google searches for suicide and suicide risk factors in the early stages of the COVID-19 pandemic. PLoS One. 2020;15:1–8. https://doi.org/10.1371/journal.pone.0236777.
81. Substance Abuse and Mental Health Services Administration. Key substance use and mental health indicators in the United States: results from the 2018 National Survey on Drug Use and Health, Vol 170. HHS Publication No PEP19–5068, NSDUH Series H-54. Rockville, MD: Center for Behavioral Health Statistics and Quality, Substance Abuse and Mental Health Services Administration; 2019. p. 51–8. Available from: https://www.samhsa.gov/data/.
82. Dietze PM, Peacock A, Mariottini C, Ojanperä I, Kriikku P, Wang QQ, et al. Mental health, substance use, and suicidal ideation during the COVID-19. Addict Behav. 2020;29:1049–57. https://doi.org/10.1038/s41380-020-00880-7.
83. Sapara A, Shalaby R, Osiogo F, Hrabok M, Gusnowski A, Vuong W, et al. COVID-19 pandemic: demographic and clinical correlates of passive death wish and thoughts of self-harm among Canadians. J Ment Health. 2021;30:170–8.
84. Nichter B, Hill ML, Na PJ, Kline AC, Norman SB, Krystal JH, et al. Prevalence and trends in suicidal behavior among US military veterans during the COVID-19 pandemic supplemental content. JAMA Psychiat. 2021;78:1218–27.
85. Carr MJ, Steeg S, Webb RT, Kapur N, Chew-Graham CA, Abel KM, et al. Effects of the COVID-19 pandemic on primary care-recorded mental illness and self-harm episodes in the UK: a population-based cohort study. Lancet Public Health. 2021;6:e124–35.
86. Ridout KK, Alavi M, Ridout SJ, Koshy MT, Awsare S, Harris B, et al. Emergency Department encounters among youth with suicidal thoughts or behaviors during the COVID-19 pandemic. JAMA Psychiat. 2021;78(12):1319–28.
87. Knipe D, Silva T, Aroos A, Senarathna L, Hettiarachchi NM, Galappaththi SR, et al. Hospital presentations for self-poisoning during COVID-19 in Sri Lanka: an interrupted time-series analysis. Lancet Psychiatry. 2021;8:892–900. https://doi.org/10.1016/S2215-0366(21)00242-X.
88. Leske S, Kõlves K, Crompton D, Arensman E, de Leo D. Real-time suicide mortality data from police reports in Queensland, Australia, during the COVID-19 pandemic: an interrupted time-series analysis. Lancet Psychiatry. 2021;8:58–63.
89. Pirkis J, John A, Shin S, DelPozo-Banos M, Arya V, Analuisa-Aguilar P, et al. Suicide trends in the early months of the COVID-19 pandemic: an interrupted time-series analysis of preliminary data from 21 countries. Lancet Psychiatry. 2021;8:579–88. http://www.thelancet.com/article/S2215036621000912/fulltext.
90. Faust JS, Shah SB, Du C, Li SX, Lin Z, Krumholz HM. Suicide deaths during the COVID-19 stay-at-home advisory in Massachusetts, March to May 2020. JAMA Netw Open. 2021;4:2020–2.
91. Ramchand R, Gordon JA, Pearson JL. Trends in suicide rates by race and ethnicity in the United States. JAMA Netw Open. 2021;4(5):e2111563.
92. Tanaka T, Okamoto S. Increase in suicide following an initial decline during the COVID-19 pandemic in Japan. Nat Hum Behav. 2021;5(2):229–38. https://doi.org/10.1038/s41562-020-01042-z.
93. Sakamoto H, Ishikane M, Ghaznavi C, Ueda P. Assessment of suicide in Japan during the COVID-19 pandemic vs previous years. JAMA Netw Open. 2021;4:e2037378.
94. Pierce HM, Hope H, Abel KM, Pierce M, McManus S, Hope H, et al. Mental health responses to the COVID-19 pandemic: a latent class trajectory analysis using longitudinal UK data. Lancet Psychiatry. 2021;8(7):610–9.
95. Shevlin M, Butter S, McBride O, Murphy J, Gibson-Miller J, Hartman TK, et al. Refuting the myth of a ‘tsunami’ of mental ill-health in populations affected by COVID-19: evidence that response to the pandemic is heterogeneous, not homogeneous. Psychol Med. 2021;1–9. Available from: https://www.cambridge.org/core/journals/psychological-medicine/article/refuting-the-myth-of-a-tsunami-of-mental-illhealth-in-populations-affected-by-covid19-

evidence-that-response-to-the-pandemic-is-heterogeneous-not-homogeneous/7A3AD1C48EAD5BF00B84D0EF97AECA18.
96. Shevlin M, Butter S, McBride O, Murphy J, Gibson-Miller J, Hartman TK, et al. Psychological responses to the COVID-19 pandemic are heterogeneous but have stabilised over time: 1 year longitudinal follow-up of the COVID-19 Psychological Research Consortium (C19PRC) study. Psychol Med. 2021;1–3. [cited 2021 Oct 9]. Available from: https://www.cambridge.org/core/journals/psychological-medicine/article/psychological-responses-to-the-covid19-pandemic-are-heterogeneous-but-have-stabilised-over-time-1-year-longitudinal-followup-of-the-covid19-psychological-research-consortium-c19prc-study/B68D5FEC7151E294D1B9CE90B2DA0C4C.
97. Wang H, Xia Q, Xiong Z, Li Z, Xiang W, Yuan Y, et al. The psychological distress and coping styles in the early stages of the 2019 coronavirus disease (COVID-19) epidemic in the general mainland Chinese population: a web-based survey. PLoS One. 2020;15:e0233410.
98. Huang Q, Chen X, Huang S, Shao T, Liao Z, Lin S, et al. Substance and Internet use during the COVID-19 pandemic in China. Transl Psychiatry. 2021;11:1–8. https://doi.org/10.1038/s41398-021-01614-1.
99. Wang C, Pan R, Wan X, Tan Y, Xu L, Ho CS, et al. Immediate psychological responses and associated factors during the initial stage of the 2019 coronavirus disease (COVID-19) epidemic among the general population in China. Int J Environ Res Public Health. 2020;17:1729.
100. The implications of COVID-19 for mental health and substance use. KFF. [cited 2021 Jun 29]. Available from: https://www.kff.org/coronavirus-covid-19/issue-brief/the-implications-of-covid-19-for-mental-health-and-substance-use/.
101. Shuster A, O'Brien M, Luo Y, Berner LA, Perl O, Heflin M, et al. Emotional adaptation during a crisis: decline in anxiety and depression after the initial weeks of COVID-19 in the United States. Transl Psychiatry. 2021;11:1–7.
102. Kibbey MM, Fedorenko EJ, Farris SG. Anxiety, depression, and health anxiety in undergraduate students living in initial US outbreak "hotspot" during COVID-19 pandemic. Cognit Behav Ther. 2021;50:409–21.
103. Oka T, Hamamura T, Miyake Y, Kobayashi N, Honjo M, Kawato M, et al. Prevalence and risk factors of internet gaming disorder and problematic internet use before and during the COVID-19 pandemic: a large online survey of Japanese adults. J Psychiatr Res. 2021;142:218–25.
104. Geng EH, Schwab J, Foraker R, Fox B, Hoehner CM, Schootman M, et al. Outcomes associated with social distancing policies in St Louis, Missouri, during the early phase of the COVID-19 pandemic. JAMA Netw Open. 2021;4(9):e2123374.
105. Sojli E, Tham WW, Bryant R, McAleer M. COVID-19 restrictions and age-specific mental health—U.S. probability-based panel evidence. Transl Psychiatry. 2021;11:1–7. https://doi.org/10.1038/s41398-021-01537-x.
106. Özdin S, Bayrak ÖŞ. Levels and predictors of anxiety, depression and health anxiety during COVID-19 pandemic in Turkish society: the importance of gender. Int J Soc Psychiatry. 2020;66(5):504–11.
107. Vindegaard N, Benros ME. COVID-19 pandemic and mental health consequences: systematic review of the current evidence. Brain Behav Immun. 2020;89:531–42.
108. Xiong J, Lipsitz O, Nasri F, Lui LMW, Gill H, Phan L, et al. Impact of COVID-19 pandemic on mental health in the general population: a systematic review. J Affect Disord. 2020;277:55–64. https://doi.org/10.1016/j.jad.2020.08.001.
109. Zhou SJ, Zhang LG, Wang LL, Guo ZC, Wang JQ, Chen JC, et al. Prevalence and sociodemographic correlates of psychological health problems in Chinese adolescents during the outbreak of COVID-19. Eur Child Adolesc Psychiatry. 2020;29(6):749–58.
110. Zhang X, Wang F, Shen Y, Zhang X, Cen Y, Wang B, et al. Symptoms and health outcomes among survivors of COVID-19 infection 1 year after discharge from hospitals in Wuhan, China. JAMA Netw Open. 2021;4(9):e2127403.

111. Benjamin A, Kuperman Y, Eren N, Rotkopf R, Amitai M, Rossman H, et al. Stress-related emotional and behavioural impact following the first COVID-19 outbreak peak. Mol Psychiatry. 2021;26(11):6149–58. https://doi.org/10.1038/s41380-021-01219-6.
112. Mayne SL, Hannan C, Davis M, Young JF, Kelly MK, Powell M, et al. COVID-19 and adolescent depression and suicide risk screening outcomes. Pediatrics. 2021;148:e2021051507.
113. Cardel MI, Dean N, Montoya-Williams D. Preventing a secondary epidemic of lost early career scientists effects of covid-19 pandemic on women with children. Ann Am Thorac Soc. 2020;17:1366–70.
114. Gabster BP, van Daalen K, Dhatt R, Barry M. Challenges for the female academic during the COVID-19 pandemic. Lancet. 2020;395(10242):1968–70.
115. Hamadani JD, Hasan MI, Baldi AJ, Hossain SJ, Shiraji S, Bhuiyan MSA, et al. Immediate impact of stay-at-home orders to control COVID-19 transmission on socioeconomic conditions, food insecurity, mental health, and intimate partner violence in Bangladeshi women and their families: an interrupted time series. Lancet Glob Health. 2020;8:e1380–9. https://doi.org/10.1016/S2214-109X(20)30366-1.
116. Leslie E, Wilson R. Sheltering in place and domestic violence: evidence from calls for service during COVID-19. J Public Econ. 2020;189:104241. https://doi.org/10.1016/j.jpubeco.2020.104241.
117. Hao F, Tan W, Jiang L, Zhang L, Zhao X, Zou Y, et al. Do psychiatric patients experience more psychiatric symptoms during COVID-19 pandemic and lockdown? A case-control study with service and research implications for immunopsychiatry. Brain Behav Immun. 2020;87:100–6.
118. Asmundson GJG, Paluszek MM, Landry CA, Rachor GS, Mckay D, Taylor S. Do pre-existing anxiety-related and mood disorders differentially impact COVID-19 stress responses and coping? J Anxiety Disord. 2020;74:102271. https://doi.org/10.1016/j.janxdis.2020.102271.
119. Vissink CE, van Hell HH, Galenkamp N, van Rossum IW. The effects of the COVID-19 outbreak and measures in patients with a pre-existing psychiatric diagnosis: a cross-sectional study. J Affect Disord Rep. 2021;4:100102.
120. Hölzle P, Aly L, Frank W, Förstl H, Frank A. COVID-19 distresses the depressed while schizophrenic patients are unimpressed: a study on psychiatric inpatients. Psychiatry Res. 2020;291:113175. https://doi.org/10.1007/s11757-020-00599-9.
121. Boldrini T, Girardi P, Clerici M, Conca A, Creati C, di Cicilia G, et al. Consequences of the COVID-19 pandemic on admissions to general hospital psychiatric wards in Italy: reduced psychiatric hospitalizations and increased suicidality. Prog Neuro-Psychopharmacol Biol Psychiatry. 2021;110:110304.
122. Gómez-Ramiro M, Fico G, Anmella G, Vázquez M, Sagué-Vilavella M, Hidalgo-Mazzei D, et al. Changing trends in psychiatric emergency service admissions during the COVID-19 outbreak: report from a worldwide epicentre. J Affect Disord. 2021;282:26–32.
123. Li D-J, Chou L-S, Chou FH-C, Hsu S-T, Hsieh K-Y, Wu H-C, et al. COVID-related psychological distress fully mediates the association from social impact to sleep disturbance among patients with chronic schizophrenia. Sci Rep. 2021;11:1–11.
124. Montejo L, Solé B, Verdolini N, Martínez-Arán A, del Bonnín CM, Radua J, et al. Self-reported neurocognitive symptoms during COVID-19 lockdown and its associated factors in a sample of psychiatric patients. Results from the BRIS-MHC study. Eur Neuropsychopharmacol. 2021;53:7–18.
125. Serafini RA, Powell SK, Frere JJ, Saali A, Krystal HL, Kumar V, et al. Psychological distress in the face of a pandemic: an observational study characterizing the impact of COVID-19 on immigrant outpatient mental health. Psychiatry Res. 2021;295:113595. https://doi.org/10.1016/j.psychres.2020.113595.
126. di Gessa G, Maddock J, Green MJ, Thompson EJ, McElroy E, Davies HL, et al. Pre-pandemic mental health and disruptions to healthcare, economic and housing outcomes during the COVID-19 pandemic: evidence from 12 UK longitudinal studies. Br J Psychiatry. 2022;220:1–10.

127. Fond G, Nemani K, Etchecopar-Etchart D, Loundou A, Goff DC, Seung WL, et al. Association between mental health disorders and mortality among patients with COVID-19 in 7 countries: a systematic review and meta-analysis. JAMA Psychiat. 2021;78(11):1208–17.
128. Schott W, Tao S, Shea L. COVID-19 risk: adult medicaid beneficiaries with autism, intellectual disability, and mental health conditions. Autism. 2022;26(4):975–87.
129. Ceban F, Nogo D, Carvalho IP, Lee Y, Nasri F, Xiong J, et al. Association between mood disorders and risk of COVID-19 infection, hospitalization, and death: a systematic review and meta-analysis. JAMA Psychiat. 2021;78:1079–91.
130. Wang L, Wang Q, Davis PB, Nora D. Increased risk for COVID-19 breakthrough infection in fully vaccinated patients with substance use disorders in the United States between December 2020 and August 2021. World Psychiatry. 2022;21:1–9.
131. Wang QQ, Kaelber DC, Xu R, Volkow ND. COVID-19 risk and outcomes in patients with substance use disorders: analyses from electronic health records in the United States. Mol Psychiatry. 2021;26:30–9. https://doi.org/10.1038/s41380-020-00880-7.
132. Ettman CK, Cohen GH, Abdalla SM, Sampson L, Trinquart L, Castrucci BC, et al. Persistent depressive symptoms during COVID-19: a national, population-representative, longitudinal study of U.S. adults. Lancet Reg Health Am. 2021;5:100091. https://doi.org/10.1016/j.lana.2021.100091.
133. Linton SL, Leifheit KM, Mcginty EE, Barry CL, Pollack CE. Association between housing insecurity, psychological distress, and self-rated health among us adults during the COVID-19 pandemic. JAMA Netw Open. 2021;4:10–3.
134. Hansen H, Braslow J, Rohrbaugh RM. From cultural to structural competency-training psychiatry residents to act on social determinants of health and institutional racism. JAMA Psychiat. 2018;75(2):117–8.
135. Chen JA, Zhang E, Liu CH. Potential impact of COVID-19-related racial discrimination on the health of Asian Americans. Am J Public Health. 2020;110:1624–7.
136. Nguyen TT, Criss S, Dwivedi P, Huang D, Keralis J, Hsu E, et al. Exploring U.S. shifts in anti-Asian sentiment with the emergence of COVID-19. Int J Environ Res Public Health. 2020;17:1–13.
137. Cheah CSL, Wang C, Ren H, Zong X, Cho HS, Xue X. COVID-19 racism and mental health in Chinese American families. Pediatrics. 2020;146:2020021816. https://doi.org/10.1542/peds.2020-021816.
138. Woo B, Jun J. COVID-19 racial discrimination and depressive symptoms among Asians Americans: does communication about the incident matter? J Immigr Minor Health. 2022;24:1–8. https://doi.org/10.1007/s10903-021-01167-x.
139. di Giuseppe M, Zilcha-Mano S, Prout TA, Christopher Perry J, Orrù G, Conversano C, et al. Psychological impact of coronavirus disease 2019 among Italians during the first week of lockdown. Front Psych. 2020;11:576597.
140. Liang L, Gao T, Ren H, Cao R, Qin Z, Hu Y, et al. Post-traumatic stress disorder and psychological distress in Chinese youths following the COVID-19 emergency. J Health Psychol. 2020;25:1164–75. https://doi.org/10.1177/1359105320937057.
141. Gurvich C, Thomas N, Thomas EHX, Hudaib AR, Sood L, Fabiatos K, et al. Coping styles and mental health in response to societal changes during the COVID-19 pandemic. Int J Soc Psychiatry. 2021;67(5):540–9.
142. Baloran ET. Knowledge, attitudes, anxiety, and coping strategies of students during COVID-19 pandemic. J Loss Trauma. 2020;25:635–42. https://doi.org/10.1080/15325024.2020.1769300.
143. Saali A, Stanislawski ER, Kumar V, Chan C, Hurtado A, Pietrzak RH, et al. The psychiatric burden on medical students in New York city entering clinical clerkships during the COVID-19 pandemic. Psychiatry Q. 2022;93:1–16. https://doi.org/10.1007/s11126-021-09955-2.
144. Moccia L, Janiri D, Pepe M, Dattoli L, Molinaro M, de Martin V, et al. Affective temperament, attachment style, and the psychological impact of the COVID-19 outbreak: an early report on the Italian general population. Brain Behav Immun. 2020;87:75–9.

145. Eder SJ, Nicholson AA, Stefanczyk MM, Pieniak M, Martínez-Molina J, Pešout O, et al. Securing your relationship: quality of intimate relationships during the COVID-19 pandemic can be predicted by attachment style. Front Psychol. 2021;12:3016.
146. Song E, Zhang C, Israelow B, Lu-Culligan A, Vieites Prado A, Skriabine S, et al. Neuroinvasion of SARS-CoV-2 in human and mouse brain. J Exp Med. 2021;218(3):e20202135. https://doi.org/10.1084/jem.20202135.
147. Paniz-Mondolfi A, Bryce C, Grimes Z, Gordon RE, Reidy J, Lednicky J, et al. Central nervous system involvement by severe acute respiratory syndrome coronavirus-2 (SARS-CoV-2). J Med Virol. 2020;92:699–702. https://doi.org/10.1002/jmv.25915.
148. Romero-Sánchez CM, Díaz-Maroto I, Fernández-Díaz E, Sánchez-Larsen Á, Layos-Romero A, García-García J, et al. Neurologic manifestations in hospitalized patients with COVID-19: the ALBACOVID registry. Neurology. 2020;95:e1060–70.
149. Varatharaj A, Thomas N, Ellul MA, Davies NWS, Pollak TA, Tenorio EL, et al. Neurological and neuropsychiatric complications of COVID-19 in 153 patients: a UK-wide surveillance study. Lancet Psychiatry. 2020;7:875–82.
150. Helms J, Kremer S, Merdji H, Clere-Jehl R, Schenck M, Kummerlen C, et al. Neurologic features in severe SARS-CoV-2 infection. N Engl J Med. 2020;382:2268–70.
151. Lu S, Wei N, Jiang J, Wu L, Sheng J, Zhou J, et al. First report of manic-like symptoms in a COVID-19 patient with no previous history of a psychiatric disorder. J Affect Disord. 2020;277:337–40. https://doi.org/10.1016/j.jad.2020.08.031.
152. Guo Q, Zheng Y, Shi J, Wang J, Li G, Li C, et al. Immediate psychological distress in quarantined patients with COVID-19 and its association with peripheral inflammation: a mixed-method study. Brain Behav Immun. 2020;88:17–27.
153. Beach SR, Praschan NC, Hogan C, Dotson S, Merideth F, Kontos N, et al. Delirium in COVID-19: a case series and exploration of potential mechanisms for central nervous system involvement. Gen Hosp Psychiatry. 2020;65:47–53.
154. Rogers JP, Chesney E, Oliver D, Pollak TA, McGuire P, Fusar-Poli P, et al. Psychiatric and neuropsychiatric presentations associated with severe coronavirus infections: a systematic review and meta-analysis with comparison to the COVID-19 pandemic. Lancet Psychiatry. 2020;7:611–27. https://doi.org/10.1016/S2215-0366(20)30203-0.
155. Boldrini M, Canoll PD, Klein RS. How COVID-19 affects the brain. JAMA Psychiat. 2021;78:682–3.
156. Jansen van Vuren E, Steyn SF, Brink CB, Möller M, Viljoen FP, Harvey BH. The neuropsychiatric manifestations of COVID-19: interactions with psychiatric illness and pharmacological treatment. Biomed Pharmacother. 2021;135:111200.
157. Yuan N, Chen Y, Xia Y, Dai J, Liu C. Inflammation-related biomarkers in major psychiatric disorders: a cross-disorder assessment of reproducibility and specificity in 43 meta-analyses. Transl Psychiatry. 2019;9:233.
158. Delaney S, Fallon B, Alaedini A, Yolken R, Indart A, Feng T, et al. Inflammatory biomarkers in psychosis and clinical high risk populations. Schizophr Res. 2019;206:440–3. https://doi.org/10.1016/j.schres.2018.10.017.
159. Hepgul N, Cattaneo A, Agarwal K, Baraldi S, Borsini A, Bufalino C, et al. Transcriptomics in interferon-α-treated patients identifies inflammation-, neuroplasticity- and oxidative stress-related signatures as predictors and correlates of depression. Neuropsychopharmacology. 2016;41:2502–11.
160. Hou R, Garner M, Holmes C, Osmond C, Teeling J, Lau L, et al. Peripheral inflammatory cytokines and immune balance in generalised anxiety disorder: case-controlled study. Brain Behav Immun. 2017;62:212–8. https://doi.org/10.1016/j.bbi.2017.01.021.
161. Venkatesan P. NICE guideline on long COVID. Lancet Respir Med. 2021;9:129.
162. Nalbandian A, Sehgal K, Gupta A, Madhavan MV, Mc Groder C, Stevens JS, et al. Post-acute COVID-19 syndrome. Nat Med. 2021;27:601–15.
163. Logue JK, Franko NM, McCulloch DJ, McConald D, Magedson A, Wolf CR, et al. Sequelae in adults at 6 months after COVID-19 Infection. JAMA Netw Open. 2021;4:8–11.

164. El Sayed S, Shokry D, Gomaa SM. Post-COVID-19 fatigue and anhedonia: a cross-sectional study and their correlation to post-recovery period. Neuropsychopharmacol Rep. 2021;41(1):50–5.
165. Miskowiak KW, Johnsen S, Sattler SM, Nielsen S, Kunalan K, Rungby J, et al. Cognitive impairments four months after COVID-19 hospital discharge: pattern, severity and association with illness variables. Eur Neuropsychopharmacol. 2021;46:39–48.
166. Mattioli F, Stampatori C, Righetti F, Sala E, Tomasi C, de Palma G. Neurological and cognitive sequelae of Covid-19: a four month follow-up. J Neurol. 2021;1:1. https://doi.org/10.1007/s00415-021-10579-6.
167. Jacobs JJL. Persistent SARS-2 infections contribute to long COVID-19. Med Hypotheses. 2021;149:110538. https://doi.org/10.1016/j.mehy.2021.110538.
168. Voruz P, Allali G, Benzakour L, Nuber-Champier A, Thomasson M, Jacot I, et al. Long COVID neuropsychological deficits after severe, moderate or mild infection 4 5. medRxiv. 2021.
169. Ismael F, Bizario JCS, Battagin T, Zaramella B, Leal FE, Torales J, et al. Post-infection depressive, anxiety and post-traumatic stress symptoms: a retrospective cohort study with mild COVID-19 patients. medRxiv. 2020.
170. Mazza MG, de Lorenzo R, Conte C, Poletti S, Vai B, Bollettini I, et al. Anxiety and depression in COVID-19 survivors: role of inflammatory and clinical predictors. Brain Behav Immun. 2020;89:594–600.
171. Huang C, Huang L, Wang Y, Li X, Ren L, Gu X, et al. 6-month consequences of COVID-19 in patients discharged from hospital: a cohort study. Lancet. 2021;397:220–32.
172. Huang L, Yao Q, Gu X, Wang Q, Ren L, Wang Y, et al. 1-year outcomes in hospital survivors with COVID-19: a longitudinal cohort study. Lancet. 2021;398:747–58.
173. Lopez-Leon S, Wegman-Ostrosky T, Perelman C, Sepulveda R, Rebolledo PA, Cuapio A, et al. More than 50 long-term effects of COVID-19: a systematic review and meta-analysis. Sci Rep. 2021;11:1–12.
174. Taquet M, Geddes JR, Frcpsych H, Harrison PJ, et al. Articles 6-month neurological and psychiatric outcomes in 236 379 survivors of COVID-19: a retrospective cohort study using electronic health records. Lancet Psychiatry. 2021;8:416–43.
175. Taquet M, Geddes JR, Harrison PJ, Harrison PJ, et al. Bidirectional associations between COVID-19 and psychiatric disorder: retrospective cohort studies of 62 354 COVID-19 cases in the USA. Lancet Psychiatry. 2021;8:130–70.
176. Forte G, Favieri F, Tambelli R, Casagrande M. COVID-19 pandemic in the Italian population: validation of a post-traumatic stress disorder questionnaire and prevalence of PTSD symptomatology. Int J Environ Res Public Health. 2020;17:1–16.
177. Janiri D, Carfì A, Kotzalidis GD, Bernabei R, Landi F, Sani G. Posttraumatic stress disorder in patients after severe COVID-19 infection. JAMA Psychiat. 2021;78:567–9.
178. Tarsitani L, Vassalini P, Koukopoulos A, Borrazzo C, Alessi F, di Nicolantonio C, et al. Post-traumatic stress disorder among COVID-19 survivors at 3-month follow-up after hospital discharge. J Gen Intern Med. 2021;36:1702–7.
179. Conversano C, di Giuseppe M, Miccoli M, Ciacchini R, Gemignani A, Orrù G. Mindfulness, age and gender as protective factors against psychological distress during COVID-19 pandemic. Front Psychol. 2020;11:1900.
180. Wang K, Goldenberg A, Dorison CA, Miller JK, Uusberg A, Lerner JS, et al. A multi-country test of brief reappraisal interventions on emotions during the COVID-19 pandemic. Nat Hum Behav. 2021;5:1089–110.
181. Korte C, Friedberg RD, Wilgenbusch T, Paternostro JK, Brown K, Kakolu A, et al. Intolerance of uncertainty and health-related anxiety in youth amid the COVID-19 pandemic: understanding and weathering the continuing storm. J Clin Psychol Med Settings. 2021;1.
182. Ramalho R, Adiukwu F, Gashi Bytyçi D, el Hayek S, Gonzalez-Diaz JM, Larnaout A, et al. Telepsychiatry and healthcare access inequities during the COVID-19 pandemic. Asian J Psychiatr. 2020;53:102234.

183. Shore JH, Schneck CD, Mishkind MC. Telepsychiatry and the coronavirus disease 2019 pandemic-current and future outcomes of the rapid virtualization of psychiatric care. JAMA Psychiat. 2020;77(12):1211–2.
184. Wright JH, Caudill R. Remote treatment delivery in response to the COVID-19 pandemic. Psychother Psychosom. 2020;89:130–2.
185. Smith K, Edoardo O, Macdonald O, Cipriani A. COVID-19 and telepsychiatry: development of evidence-based guidance for clinicians. JMIR Ment Health. 2020;7(8):e21108.
186. Hong JS, Sheriff R, Smith K, Tomlinson A, Saad F, Smith T, et al. Digital mental health Impact of COVID-19 on telepsychiatry at the service and individual patient level across two UK NHS mental health trusts. Evid Based Ment Health. 2021;24:1–6.
187. Cuijpers P, Noma H, Karyotaki E, Cipriani A, Furukawa TA. Effectiveness and acceptability of cognitive behavior therapy delivery formats in adults with depression: a network meta-analysis. JAMA Psychiat. 2019;76:700–7.
188. Ben-Zeev D, Buck B, Meller S, Hudenko WJ, Hallgren KA. Augmenting evidence-based care with a texting mobile interventionist: a pilot randomized controlled trial. Psychiatr Serv. 2020;71:1218–24.
189. Castelnuovo G, Lamela D, Tirelli V, Bouchard S, Allard M, Robillard G, et al. Videoconferencing psychotherapy for panic disorder and agoraphobia: outcome and treatment processes from a non-randomized non-inferiority trial. Front Psychol. 2020;11:2164.
190. Tarquinio C, Brennstuhl M-J, Rydberg JA, Bassan F, Peter L, Tarquinio CL, et al. EMDR in telemental health counseling for healthcare workers caring for COVID-19 patients: a pilot study. Issues Ment Health Nurs. 2021;42:3–14.
191. Thase ME, Mccrone P, Barrett MS, Eells TD, Wisniewski SR, Balasubramani GK, et al. Improving cost-effectiveness and access to cognitive behavior therapy for depression: providing remote-ready, computer-assisted psychotherapy in times of crisis and beyond. Psychother Psychosom. 2020;89:307–13.
192. Puspitasari AJ, Heredia D, Coombes BJ, Geske JR, Gentry MT, Moore WR, et al. Feasibility and initial outcomes of a group-based teletherapy psychiatric day program for adults with serious mental illness: open, nonrandomized trial in the context of covid-19. JMIR Ment Health. 2021;8:e25542.
193. Lv Z, Li J, Zhang B, Zhang N, Wang C. The effect of computerized cognitive behavioral therapy on people's anxiety and depression during the 6 months of Wuhan's lockdown of COVID-19 epidemic: a pilot study. Front Psychol. 2021;12:687165.
194. Kwan A, Wong C, Kam F, Wong Y, Kit K, Chow S, et al. Effect of a telecare case management program for older adults who are homebound during the COVID-19 pandemic: a pilot randomized clinical trial + visual abstract + invited commentary + supplemental content. JAMA Netw Open. 2021;4:2123453.
195. Malka M, Gropp C, Jaworowski S, Oberbaum M, Katz DE. Telepsychiatry for patients with post-traumatic stress disorder during the COVID-19 outbreak. Curr Treat Options Psychiatry. 2021;8:1.
196. Li J, Yang Z, Qiu H, Wang Y, Jian L, Ji J, et al. Anxiety and depression among general population in China at the peak of the COVID-19 epidemic. World Psychiatry. 2020;19:249–50.
197. Moreira PS, Ferreira S, Couto B, Machado-Sousa M, Fernández M, Raposo-Lima C, et al. Protective elements of mental health status during the COVID-19 outbreak in the Portuguese population. Int J Environ Res Public Health. 2021;18(4):1910. https://doi.org/10.3390/ijerph18041910.
198. Zhang Y, Zhang H, Ma X, Di Q. Mental health problems during the COVID-19 pandemics and the mitigation effects of exercise: a longitudinal study of college students in China. Int J Environ Res Public Health. 2020;17(10):3722.
199. Colley RC, Bushnik T, Langlois K. Exercise and screen time during the COVID-19 pandemic. Health Rep. 2020;31(6):3–11. https://doi.org/10.25318/82-003-x202000600001-eng.

200. Puyat Id JH, Ahmad H, Avina-Galindo AM, Kazanjian A, Gupta A, Ellisid U, et al. A rapid review of home-based activities that can promote mental wellness during the COVID-19 pandemic. PLoS One. 2020;15(12):e0243125. https://doi.org/10.1371/journal.pone.0243125.
201. Liu K, Chen Y, Wu D, Lin R, Wang Z, Pan L. Effects of progressive muscle relaxation on anxiety and sleep quality in patients with COVID-19. Complement Ther Clin Pract. 2020;39:101132.
202. Wei N, Huang BC, Lu SJ, Hu JB, Zhou XY, Hu CC, et al. Efficacy of internet-based integrated intervention on depression and anxiety symptoms in patients with COVID-19. J Zhejiang Univ Sci B. 2020;21:400–4.
203. Sotoudeh HG, Alavi SS, Akbari Z, Jannatifard F, Artounian V. The effect of brief crisis intervention package on improving quality of life and mental health in patients with COVID-19. Iran J Psychiatry. 2020;15:205–12.
204. Killgore WDS, Taylor EC, Cloonan SA, Dailey NS. Psychological resilience during the COVID-19 lockdown. Psychiatry Res. 2020;291:371–9.
205. Xiao H, Zhang Y, Kong D, Li S, Yang N. The effects of social support on sleep quality of medical staff treating patients with coronavirus disease 2019(COVID-19) in January and February 2020 in China. Med Sci Monit. 2020;26:e923549–1.
206. Yu H, Li M, Li Z, Xiang W, Yuan Y, Liu Y, et al. Coping style, social support and psychological distress in the general Chinese population in the early stages of the COVID-19 epidemic. BMC Psychiatry. 2020;20:426. https://doi.org/10.1186/s12888-020-02826-3.
207. Humphreys KL, Myint T, Zeanah CH. Pre-publication release increased risk for family violence during the COVID-19 pandemic. Pediatrics. 2020;146(1):e20200982.
208. Arenas-Arroyo E, Fernandez-Kranz D, Nollenberger N. Intimate partner violence under forced cohabitation and economic stress: evidence from the COVID-19 pandemic. J Public Econ. 2021;194:104350. https://doi.org/10.1016/j.jpubeco.2020.104350.
209. Onwumere J, Creswell C, Livingston G, Shiers D, Tchanturia K, Charman T, et al. COVID-19 and UK family carers: policy implications. Lancet Psychiatry. 2021;8:929–36.
210. Susser LC, Wilkins VM, Sternberg LH. perinatal planning guide: mitigating perinatal mood and anxiety disorders during the COVID-19 pandemic. Prim Care Companion CNS Disord. 2021;23:21nr02953.
211. Golberstein E, Wen H, Miller BF. Coronavirus disease 2019 (COVID-19) and mental health for children and adolescents. JAMA Pediatr. 2020;174:819–20.
212. Duan L, Shao X, Wang Y, Huang Y, Miao J, Yang X, et al. An investigation of mental health status of children and adolescents in China during the outbreak of COVID-19. J Affect Disord. 2020;275:112–8. https://doi.org/10.1016/j.jad.2020.06.029.
213. Singh S, Roy D, Sinha K, Parveen S, Sharma G, Joshi G. Impact of COVID-19 and lockdown on mental health of children and adolescents: a narrative review with recommendations. Psychiatry Res. 2020;293:113429.
214. Zhou J, Liu L, Xue P, Yang X, Tang X. Mental health response to the COVID-19 outbreak in China. Am J Psychiatr. 2020;177:574–5.
215. Goudeau S, Sanrey C, Stanczak A, Manstead A, Darnon C. Why lockdown and distance learning during the COVID-19 pandemic are likely to increase the social class achievement gap. Nat Hum Behav. 2021;5(10):1273–81. https://doi.org/10.1038/s41562-021-01212-7.
216. Price J, Kassam-Adams N, Kazak AE. Toolkit for emotional coping for healthcare staff (TECHS): helping healthcare workers cope with the demands of COVID-19. Dela J Public Health. 2020;6:10.
217. Nourian M, Nikfarid L, Khavari AM, Barati M, Allahgholipour AR. The impact of an online mindfulness-based stress reduction program on sleep quality of nurses working in covid-19 care units: a clinical trial. Holist Nurs Pract. 2021;35:257–63.
218. Crippa JAS, Zuardi AW, Guimarães FS, Campos AC, de Osório FL, Loureiro SR, et al. Efficacy and safety of Cannabidiol Plus standard care vs standard care alone for the treatment of emotional exhaustion and burnout among frontline health care workers during the COVID-19 pandemic: a randomized clinical trial. JAMA Netw Open. 2021;4:e2120603. https://jamanetwork.com/journals/jamanetworkopen/fullarticle/2782994.

# Chapter 11
# Spatial Epidemiology of COVID-19 Pandemic: Disease Risk, Prognosis, and Complications

**Paddy Ssentongo, Claudio Fronterre, and Vernon M. Chinchilli**

## Introduction

Spatial epidemiology is the study of the spatial variation in patterns of infections and diseases and the causes and consequences of such heterogeneity [1]. From the beginning of the COVID-19 pandemic in late 2019 to the present date, the evolution of SARS-CoV-2 infection susceptibility, transmission dynamics, mortality, and the psychological and behavioral consequences such as gun violence and post-acute sequelae of SARS-CoV-2 infection (PASC), have varied geographically. The proposed chapter introduces the reader to the global and regional perspective of SARS-CoV-2 infection transmission, mortality, and PASC dynamics. The three primary objectives of this chapter are as follows.

To elucidate the global and regional evolution of the pandemic. The role of vaccination and the emergent of various strains, including the Alpha, Delta, and Omicron variant of concern (VOC), are described. Subsequently, this chapter will discuss the evolution of the COVID-19 pandemic in time and space using data-driven space-time modeling approaches with a focus on Africa. Such data-driven modeling can distinguish infections from local within- or neighbor-driven disease transmission.

P. Ssentongo (✉) · V. M. Chinchilli
Department of Public Health Sciences, Penn State College of Medicine, Hershey, PA, USA
e-mail: vchinchilli@pennstatehealth.psu.edu

C. Fronterre
Centre for Health Informatics, Computing and Statistics, Lancaster University, Lancaster, UK
e-mail: c.fronterr@lancaster.ac.uk


S. Adibi et al. (eds.), *Frontiers of COVID-19*,
https://doi.org/10.1007/978-3-031-08045-6_11

To delineate meteorological factors (temperature, humidity, UV radiation, rainfall, and air pollution) on the susceptibility of SARS-CoV-2 and mortality risk.
To assess the spatial and regional differences in psychological and societal effects of the pandemic. Specifically, we will focus on gun violence and PASC, including neuropsychiatric disorders among survivors.

This chapters' novelty lies in integrating the spatial epidemiology of COVID-19 by characterizing the transmission dynamics, risk, prognosis, and consequences of COVID-19 at the population level. This chapter is critical to the book's overarching goal to deepen our understanding of the current pandemic and provide a roadmap for preventing and treating future infectious disease pandemics.

## Global Variation in COVID-19 Case Incidence and Mortality: Impact of Vaccination and New Variants of Concern

Before vaccination was widely introduced in the population, the disease burden of COVID-19 was most significant in high-income countries (HICs). The point prevalence of COVID-19 on December 31, 2020 was 57 per 100,000 in the USA, 63 per 100,000 in the United Kingdom compared to the 1.7 and 1.7 per 100,000 in Africa and Asia, respectively [2]. The transmission dynamics changed after introducing the vaccine in late 2020 and early 2021. The mean incidence rate per population declined in HIC but increased in low- and middle-income countries (LMICs), particularly in India and South America (Fig. 11.1). However, vaccine hesitancy in the USA in mid-2021 and the emergent of the highly transmissible Delta variant that also had shorter serial intervals facilitated increased case rates in the USA and the rest of the world.

SARS-CoV-2 can generate variants with significant genomic changes [3]. These mutations alter virus attachment and entry into human cells. The emergency of new variants complicated the dynamics of infection transmission, where mutations in spike protein increased transmissibility and enhanced escape from the host immune response. Starting late 2020, several variants of concern emerged globally, including the Alpha variant (Pango lineage B.1.1.7), first detected in the UK); Beta (Pango lineage B.1.351), first detected in South Africa); Gamma (Pango lineage P.1) first detected in patients from Brazil); Delta (Pango lineage B.1.617.2), first detected in India; and Omicron (Pango lineage B.1.1.529) variant first detected in South Africa [2, 4].

The Alpha variant was first detected in southeast England in September 2020. In just a few months, it spread to become the dominant lineage in the United Kingdom (more than 98% of positive SARS-CoV-2 infections in England (Fig. 11.2) and spread to over 114 countries worldwide by April 2021 [5]. The variant had a 43–90% higher basic reproduction number than pre-existing variants. In addition to higher transmissibility, the Alpha variant had a 61% (42–82%) higher mortality risk than the original virus identified in Wuhan, China [3]. Nevertheless, the higher

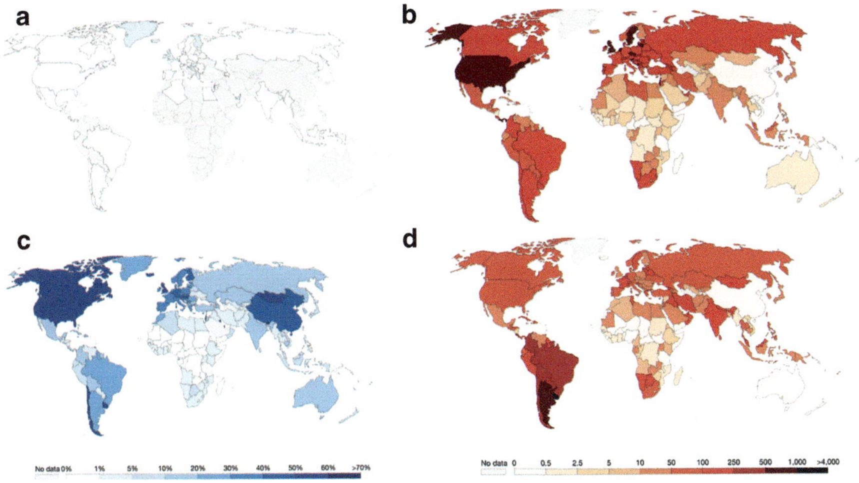


**Fig. 11.1** Disparity in vaccination rates and its effect on COVID-19 evolution and case burden. Proportion of population who received at least one dose of a COVID-19 vaccine by Dec 31, 2020 (**a**) and the corresponding daily confirmed COVID-19 cases per million people on Dec 31, 2020 (**b**). In **c** and **d**, vaccination rates by May 31, 2021, and daily confirmed COVID-19 cases per million people on May 31, 2021. Maps from Our World In Data for cases (https://ourworldindata.org/covid-cases) and vaccination (https://ourworldindata.org/covid-vaccinations)

vaccination rates in communities reduce both transmission and mortality rates. The Pfizer- BioNTech vaccine was 92% effective against this variant 2 weeks after the second dose, and two doses of the AstraZeneca vaccine were 81% effective against symptomatic disease [6]. In Europe, the dominant strain of the Alpha variant was rapidly replaced by the Delta variant. The Delta variant, also known as lineage B.1.617.2, was first identified in Maharashtra, India, in late 2020 [7]. By Mid-2021, it accounted for 99% of all infections in Europe [8]. In the USA, the Delta variant represented 30.4% of cases nationwide in June, 52% in July, and 99% by September 2021.

Compared to the Alpha variant, the risk of COVID-19 hospital admission was approximately doubled in those with the Delta variant [6, 9]. The number of pre-existing comorbidities was effect modifiers, with the risk of admission increasing in individuals with five or more comorbidities [6]. Furthermore, the Delta variant had enhanced transmissibility, was more lethal, less sensitive to serum neutralizing antibodies from recovered individuals, and less sensitive to vaccine-elicited antibodies than the wild-type SARS-CoV-2 [10]. Nevertheless, in Europe, preliminary data demonstrated the Pfizer-BioNTech and the AstraZeneca vaccine to be 79% and 60% effective against RT-PCR confirmed SARS-CoV-2 infection by the Delta strain 2 weeks after the second dose. Vaccine effectiveness against symptomatic COVID-19 at 2 weeks after the second dose was 75% and 60% for Pfizer-BioNTech and AstraZeneca, respectively. In the USA, among nursing home residents, two doses of mRNA vaccines (Pfizer-BioNTech and Moderna) were 75% effective against

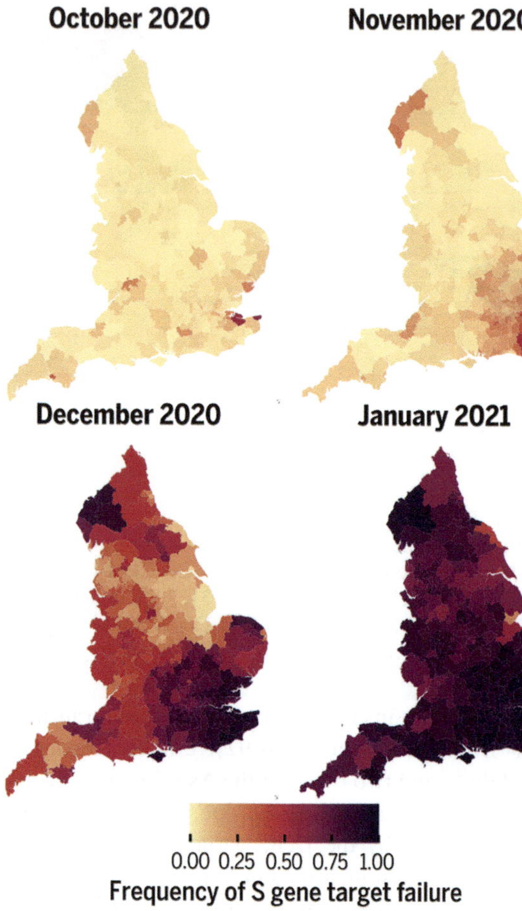


**Fig. 11.2** Spread of the Alpha variant (lineage B.1.1.7) in England. Spatial distribution of Alpha variant in England from October 2020 to January 2021 [5]. Figure from Davies et al. [5]

infection early in the vaccination program in the pre-Delta variant period (March 1 to May 9, 2021). However, waning vaccine-induced immunity was noted, evidenced by the substantial decline of vaccine effectiveness to 53% during June 21 to August 1, 2021, when the Delta variant circulation predominated the USA [11].

Vaccination roll-out was unequal globally, with HIC having over 60% of the population vaccinated by mid-June of 2021, compared to less than 5% vaccination rate in LMICs (Fig. 11.3). The vaccination rates changed the transmission dynamics of the virus and mortality globally. It is clear the burden and hotspots of COVID-19 cases increased in India, Africa, and South America by mid-2021 but decreased in North America and some countries in Europe (Fig. 11.1). Vaccine inequities might have led to the emergence of the new variant, Omicron, first identified in South Africa on November 25, 2021. Rapidly the variant spread globally. This variant was associated with an S-gene target failure and more likely to be transmissible, evade immune system compared to the Delta variant [13]. High HIV prevalence and a low vaccination rate were suggested risk factors for the emergent of Omicron [14, 15].

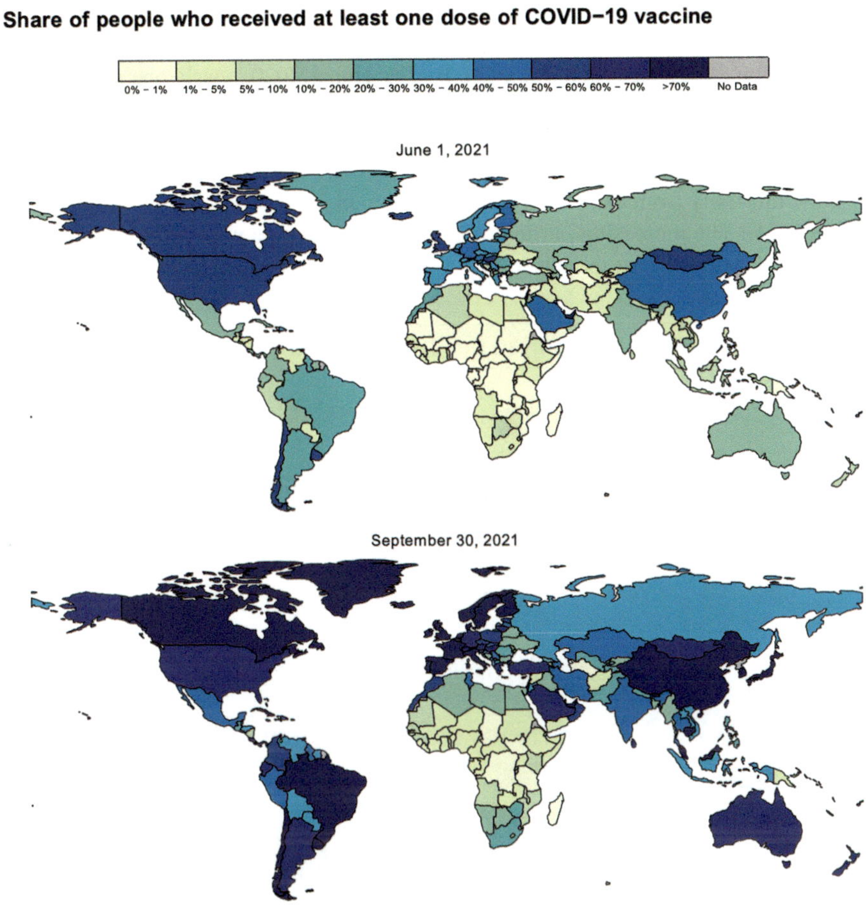


**Fig. 11.3** Disparities in SARS-CoV-2 vaccination rates. By June 1, 2021, the North America and Europe had the highest vaccination rate. Africa demonstrated the lowest vaccination rate (top panel). By the end of September of 2021, vaccination was less than 5% in majority of African countries (lower panel). Data analysis and figures from Mathieu et al. 2021 [12]

In early 2020, Africa experienced a slow trajectory in SARS-CoV-2 and death from COVID-19. The observed phenomena were explained by the overall younger population and the technical know-how of handling previous viral and bacterial outbreaks such as Ebola, Lassa fever, Polio, HIV, TB, and meningitis epidemics, endemic in the Africa meningitis belt [16]. However, in 2021, significant infection rates with associated morbidity and mortality occurred in Africa. For example, in 2021, on average attack rate in Uganda was 0.5 cases per 100,000 population. On June 19, 2021, cases had increased to 3 per 100,000 population.

Africa has a heterogeneous economy, climate, demography, and human development. These factors influenced that the dynamics of the infection and the associated mortality. Furthermore, the advent of new variants substantially impacted the dynamic of the pandemic in Africa [17]. For example, the Beta variant first recognized in South Africa was resistant to the AstraZeneca vaccine. South Africa was the most affected African country in 2020. By December 2020, nearly one million people in South Africa were infected, which accounted for approximately 50% of all known African infections according to the Africa Centres for Disease Control and Prevention (CDC) (https://africacdc.org/covid-19/). The rates of infection and the excess mortality from COVID-19 consistently remained the highest in South Africa (Fig. 11.4). The increasing burden of COVID-19 in Africa necessitated developing spatiotemporal forecast models to help mitigate disease transmission.

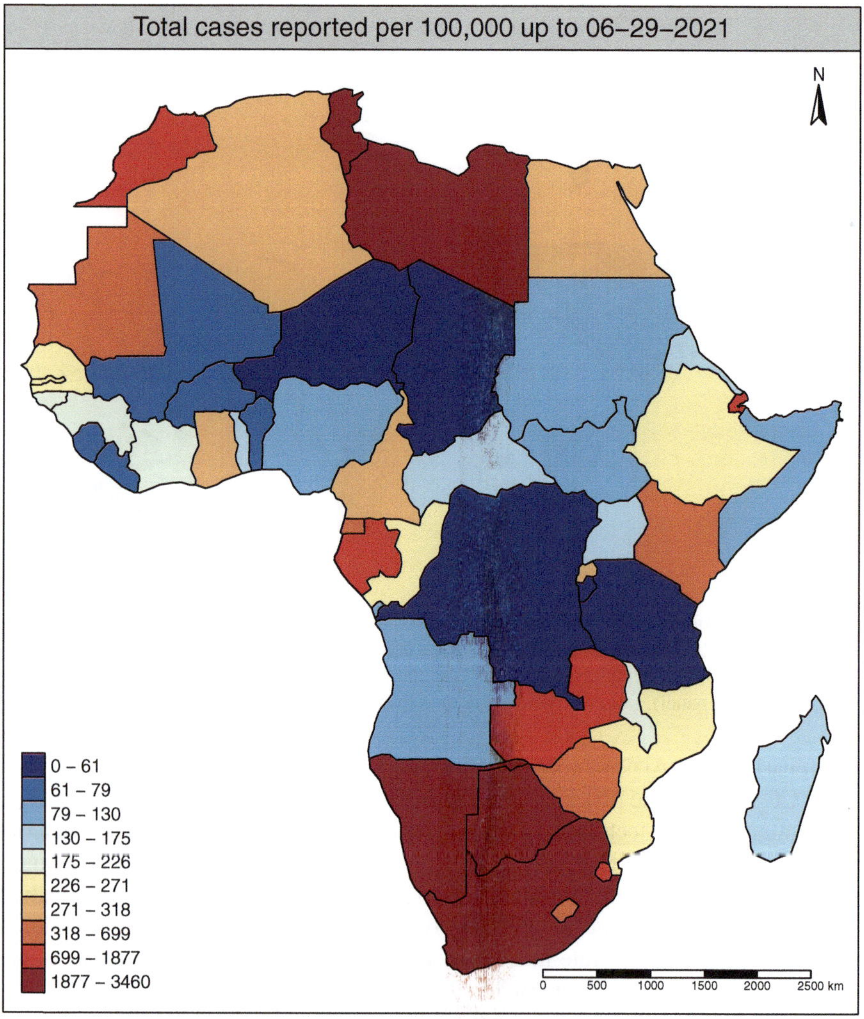


**Fig. 11.4** Geographic distribution of COVID-19 cases in up to June 29, 2021. South African region, Libya, Egypt, Djibouti showed greatest case numbers per 1,000,000. Data analysis and figures from Ssentongo et al. 2021 [18]

In their modeling framework, Ssentongo and colleagues leveraged a massive near-real-time dataset, remote-sensed temperature, precipitation, and specific humidity, and governmental response policies to create a COVID-19 tracking and prediction tool for the African continent [18]. The data-driven spatiotemporal model developed by Held and colleagues is a fusion of purely statistical and entirely mechanistic [19]. In summary, new COVID-19 cases $Y_{it}$ from country $i$ at time $t$ are assumed to be conditionally independent given past observations $Y_{i,t-d}$, $i = 1, \ldots, N$, $d = 1, \ldots, D$, and distributed according to a negative binomial distribution with mean

$\mu_{it}$ and overdispersion parameter $r > 0$ as

$$\left[Y_{it} \middle| Y_{t-1}, \ldots, Y_{t-D}\right] \sim \text{NegBin}\left(\mu_{it}, r\right)$$

The conditional variance of $Y_{it}$ is $\mu_{it}$ $(1 + \mu_{it} r)$ demonstrate the role of the overdispersion parameter to capture variability greater than the mean. The conditional mean $\mu_{it} = \epsilon_{it} + \lambda_{it} Y_{it-1} + \phi_{it} \sum_{i \neq j} w_{ij} Y_{jt-1}$ is decomposed into three additive components: (1) the endemic part ($\epsilon_{it}$), which is not driven by previous case counts but may account for factors such as seasonality, sociodemographic, animal reservoirs, and population + (2) past within-country cases ($\lambda_{it} Y_{it-1}$) + (3) past cases from all other countries $\left(\phi_{it} \sum_{i \neq j} w_{ij} Y_{jt-1}\right)$, which is the epidemic components. $w_{ij}$ is intercountry transmission susceptibility. The contributions from these various mechanisms are estimated from the data. These components depend on other factors to determine their ability to predict new cases. These factors include space-dependent: human development index (a composite index of life expectancy at birth, education, and per capita income), geographic region, access to the coastal line, and connectivity with the rest of the countries in the continent. Time-dependent factors included testing capacity, satellite-based gridded meteorological factors (daily rainfall, temperature, and specific humidity), and testing policy. The government response to the current pandemic is captured in the stringency index (lockdown measures). Stringency index combines eight policy indicators and three health measures, such as school closing, border closing, public transit, shelter in place, private gatherings, internal movement between cities/regions. This stringency index ranges from 0 (no government stringency policies) to 100 (very strict stringency). In this spatial modeling approach, 81% of landlocked countries had substantial contributions of cases from their neighboring countries (Fig. 11.5).

In countries or geographical regions with lower fiscal capacity, border closures are a challenge since they rely on open borders for needed trade revenue [20]. Nearly 30% (16 out of 54) of African countries are landlocked. These countries have 1.5 times less GDP than their non-landlocked counterparts. This modeling and forecast tool was freely available to the African countries to help them monitor and control the pandemic.

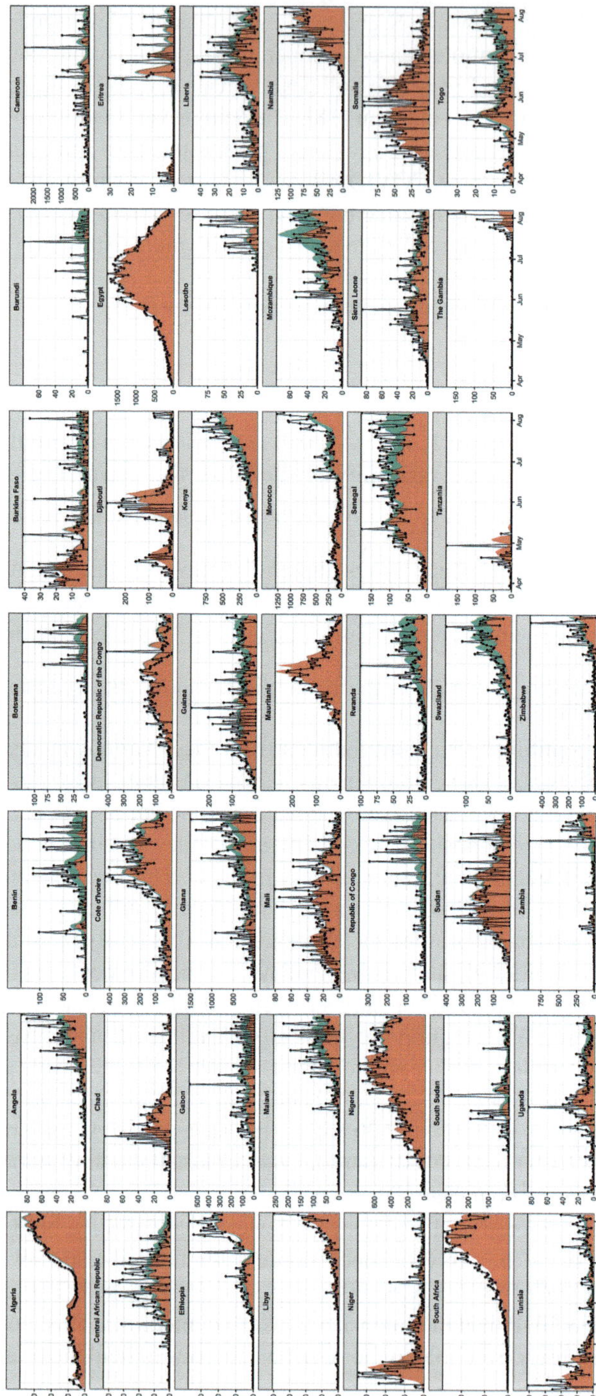


**Fig. 11.5** Model contributions by country in Africa. Observed case counts are shown with black traces. Between and within-country components are shown for the analysis period during 2020—data and figures from Ssentongo and colleagues [18]

## Spatial Variation of Risk Factors for SARS-CoV-2 Transmission and Mortality

### *Pre-existing Comorbidities and the Risk of COVID-19 Mortality*

Early in the pandemic, the transmission of SARS-CoV-2 had a predilection for the elderly. Indeed, those with pre-existing comorbidities, including cardiovascular diseases, hypertension, diabetes, congestive heart failure, cerebrovascular disease, chronic kidney disease, chronic liver disease, and cancer, had a higher risk of death from COVID-19 [21, 22]. The effect of HIV/AIDS on susceptibility, and poor prognosis of COVID-19 was not appreciated initially due to the limited data. However, as the pandemic progressed, it became increasingly clear from large systematic reviews that individuals with HIV had a higher susceptibility and risk of mortality from COVID-19 [23]. Spatially, regions with a higher burden of cardiovascular disease and HIV also demonstrated a higher mortality rate (Fig. 11.6). This geographical variation in the pre-existing conditions further increased the disparities in COVID-19 mortality. However, this relationship was moderated by the variant of the virus. For example, the Beta variant from South Africa did not respond well to the AstraZeneca vaccine in late 2020. This led to the second surge of cases in early 2021 [25].

### *Spatial Variation of Genetic Predictors of SARS-CoV-2*

Based on the global distribution of COVID-19, the cases and mortality rates in the first year of the pandemic were higher in the European and the American populations [26]. There is mounting evidence of genetic variations in various genes that code for the receptors involved in the transmission dynamics of SARS-CoV-2 and the pathogenesis of COVID-19. These include angiotensin-converting enzyme 2 (ACE2) receptors, Transmembrane Serine Protease 2 (TMPRSS2), and FURIN. The primary receptor for SARS-CoV-2 entry into the host cell is the ACE2 [27].

The entry is facilitated by FURIN cleavage [28, 29], and the spike protein of SARS-CoV-2 is primed by TMPRSS2 [30]. Interethnic and interpopulation variability in the distribution of ACE2 genetic variants associated with COVID-19 comorbidities exists globally. ACE2 variants associated with COVID-19 comorbidities are highly prevalent in the European and admixed American populations [31]. On the other hand, ACE2 variants with a protective role are more prevalent in the East and South Asian populations. A study of natural variations in the ACE2, TMPRSS2, and FURIN genes in individuals from the Middle Eastern populations (Kuwait, Qatar, and Iran) identified two activating variants (K26R and N720D) in the ACE2 gene that are more common in Europeans than in the Middle Eastern,

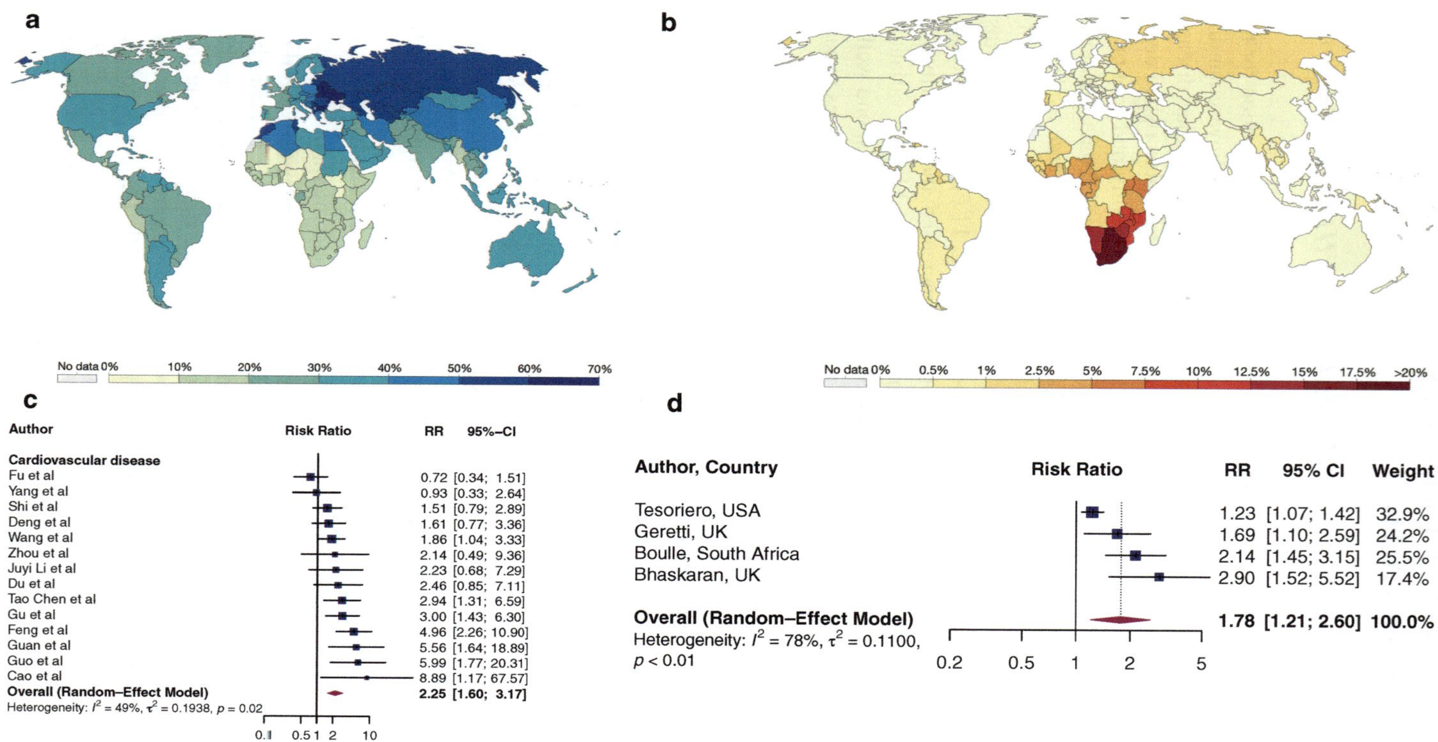


**Fig. 11.6** Geographic distribution of heart disease burden and HIV and the impact on COVID-19 mortality. The proportion of death from heart disease in 2017 (**a**). Prevalence of HIV in 2017 (**b**) [24]. The mortality risk in COVID-19 patients with heart disease compared to those without heart disease (**c**). The risk of COVID-19 mortality in individuals living with HIV compared to their HIV-negative counterparts (**d**). Maps are from Our World in Data which are open access and used under the Creative Commons license. Forest plots modified from Ssentongo et al. 2020 [21]

East Asian, and African populations [32]. It was postulated that K26R could activate ACE2 and facilitate binding to S-protein RBD, while N720D enhances TMPRSS2 cutting and, ultimately, viral entry. In addition, the study detected deleterious variants in FURIN that are frequent in the Middle Eastern but not in the European populations.

## *Meteorological and Environmental Predictors of COVID-19 Transmission and Mortality*

Seasonal variation driven by responses to a changing environment has been shown to affect the transmission intensity of several coronaviruses [33, 34]. In the USA and other countries within 30° N to 50° N latitude corridor, lower temperatures and humidity were correlated with increased SARS-CoV-2 transmission rates [35, 36]. On the other hand, studies conducted in Africa demonstrated lower temperatures to have a protective effect, but humidity had a similar relationship seen in the temperate regions [18]. Importantly, the impact of environmental predictors on transmission rate was dampened in the face of lockdowns [33]. In a dynamic metapopulation model informed by human mobility data, Ma et al. examined the effect of three meteorological factors (mean air temperature, specific humidity, and UV light) on basic reproduction number in the 2298 counties for the USA from March to December 2020 (Fig. 11.7). Lower air temperature (within the 20–40 °C range), lower specific humidity, and lower ultraviolet radiation were significantly associated with increased transmission rates of SARS-CoV-2. The attributing factor for meteorological factors was highest (21%) in December with colder and drier weather and lower UV radiation of their study period [37].

Combined effects of higher titers of viral particle shedding, greater viral stability in nasal passages, impaired nasal mucociliary clearance, viral inactivation via breakdown of their lipid layers are proposed mechanisms in which cold temperatures and high humidity impact survival and transmissibility of SARS-CoV-2 [38–41]. However, divergent behavioral patterns during higher temperatures may affect the transmission of the virus in the tropics and temperate regions. In the tropics, during higher temperatures, people spend more time indoors. But in temperate regions, people spend more time indoors during colder winter months, facilitating virus transmission [42, 43].

In addition to the meteorological factors, chronic exposure to air pollutants such as long-term (historical) PM2.5 exposure contributed to the transmission and outcomes of COVID-19. Using ecological regression analysis of United States counties, Wu and colleagues found an increase of 1 g/m$^3$ in the long-term average PM2.5 to be associated with an 11% (95% CI, 6–17%) increase in the county's COVID-19 mortality rate [44].

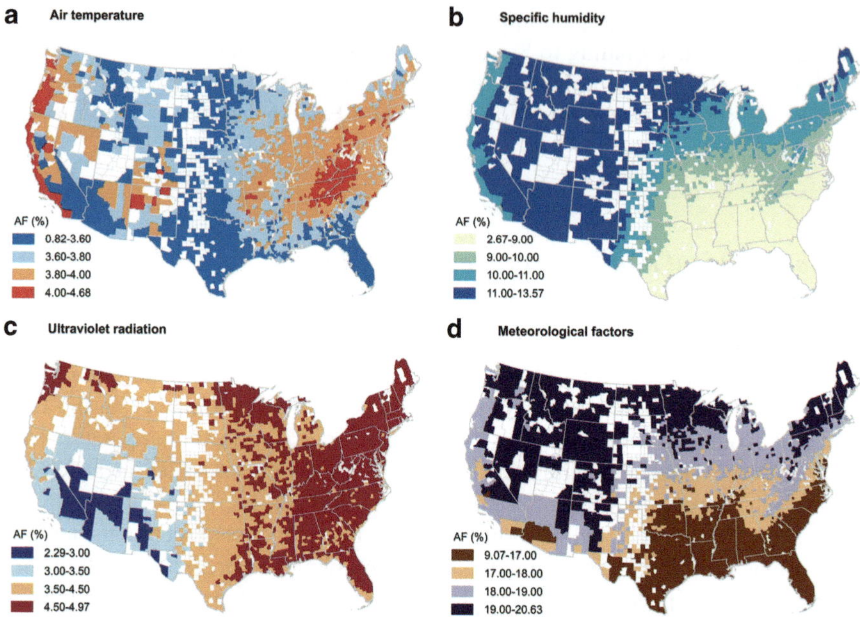


**Fig. 11.7** Fractions of basic reproduction number attributable to meteorological factors by county. The distribution of the fraction of reproduction number (Rt) attributable to temperature (**a**), specific humidity (**b**), ultraviolet radiation (**c**), or the sum of the three meteorological factors (**d**) (i.e., attributable fraction [AF]) in each county. Figure and data from Ma et al. 2021 [37]

In the first wave of the pandemic, the Italian cities of Lombardia and Emilia Romagna suffered very high mortality rates from COVID-19, perhaps one of the highest per capita in the world. Using aggregated index termed Air Quality Index (AQI), a metric for pollutants in geographical regions, it was postulated that pollution was correlated with an extremely high COVID-19 mortality rate of 12% seen in northern Italy (Lombardy and Emilia Romagna) compared to 4.5% observed in the rest of Italy which also had a lower AQI [45]. The AQI is based on concentration values for up to five key pollutants: PM10, PM2.5, $O_3$, $SO_2$, and $NO_2$. Indeed, SARS-CoV-2 RNA was found on particulate matter in samples from the Bergamo area (the epicenter of the Italian COVID-19 epidemic in Italy) [46].

Potential biological mechanisms that may explain the relationship between air pollution and COVID-19 infection outcomes include overexpression of the alveolar ACE2 receptor and the impairment of host defenses. Furthermore, air pollution-induced systemic and local inflammation leads to an innate immune system hyperactivation and endothelial injury [47, 48].

## Mental Health and Psychological Stress Consequences of COVID-19 Pandemic

While the purpose of lockdown orders was to decrease disease transmission, there were unintended consequences. The orders forced businesses to close, leaving millions unemployed. Furthermore, the physical distancing necessary to curb transmission of the virus also disrupted social support networks. Combined, these forces may have created a climate that fosters domestic violence, mental health disorders and negative psychological effects, including post-traumatic stress symptoms, confusion, and anger [49, 50].

In a study conducted early in the pandemic, the prevalence of depression symptoms was more than threefold higher during the COVID-19 pandemic than pre-pandemic [52]. In this study, lower-income, and having exposure to more stressors were contributing factors to greater risk of depression symptoms during COVID-19. In addition, unemployment, and financial strain, increased unscheduled time, and increased substance abuse may result in increased risk-taking behaviors, elevating the risk of violent crimes, homicide, and firearm-related suicides [53]. COVID-19 pandemic had alarming implications for emotional and social functioning, leading to increased aggression and possibly gun violence. Ssentongo and colleagues estimated the rate of gun violence in the USA during the pandemic and compared it to the similar months pre-pandemic. They found an overall 30% increase in the rate of GV [51]. Spatially, there were clusters of increased risk. They indicated that psychological stress and the panic induced by the pandemic might have led to increased gun purchase, translating to increased events (Fig. 11.8).

Among survivors of COVID-19, the rate of post-acute sequelae of SARS-CoV-2 infection (long-COVID) is 50% [54]. Mental health disorders are one of the manifestations of long-COVID. The mechanisms that lead to neuropsychiatric symptoms in survivors of COVID-19 are not well understood. However, widespread acute injury to cortical/sub-cortical and white matter fiber bundles may impact brain function and impede distal brain connectivity, respectively [55, 56], leading to neuropsychiatric sequelae in the survivors. The burden of these PASC is predicted to be higher in LMIC than HICs [54].

## Conclusion

In summary, the transmission, mortality, and consequences of the global COVID-19 pandemic displayed regional and national heterogeneity. Population genetic variation, environmental factors, health access disparities, and the burden of preexisting conditions were drivers and modifiers of the spatial epidemiology of the pandemic. Emphasis should be placed on global public health to identify risk factors of heightened disease risk to create strategies to prevent, control, and treat the acute and post-acute cases of COVID-19 and other future pandemics.

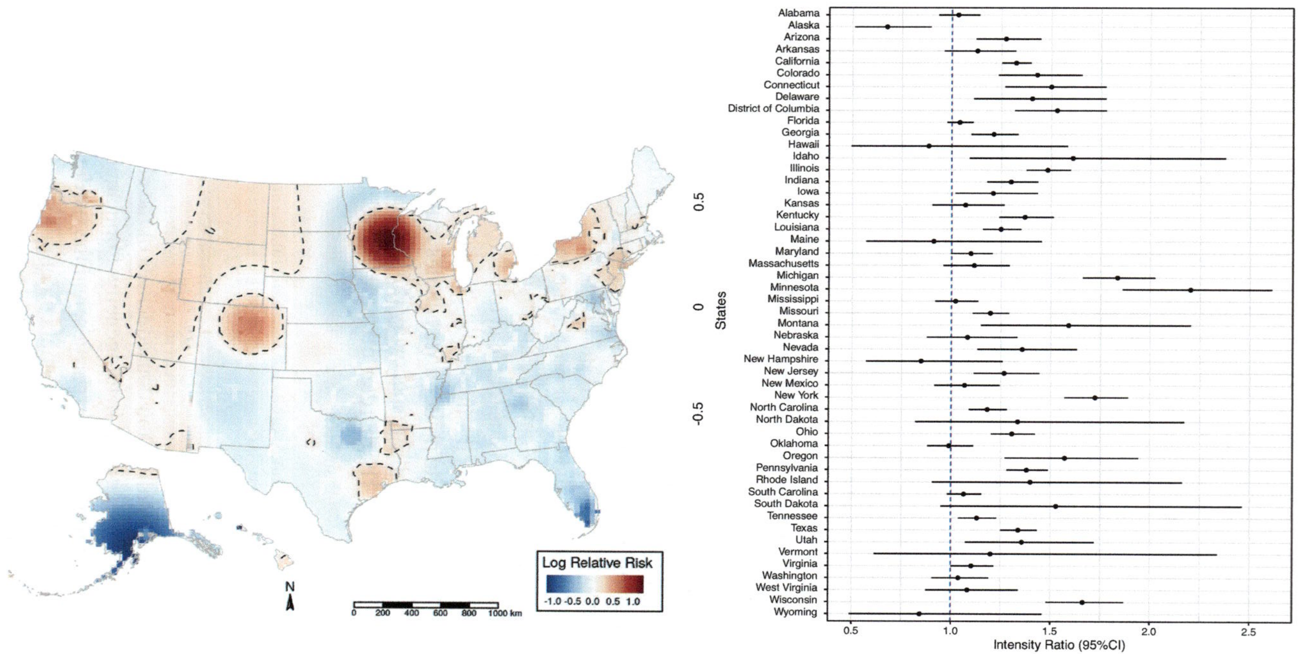


**Fig. 11.8** Spatial relative risk of gun violence during the pandemic vs. pre-pandemic. Left figure shows the intensity (or risk) difference which was estimated by comparing the smoothed intensity of GV events during the pandemic (March 01, 2020, through March 31, 2021) vs. before the pandemic (February 01, 2019, through February 29, 2020) across 50 States and (50) Washington D.C. If the difference is 0, the risk of GV is unrelated to spatial location. Evidence of spatial variation in risk occurs where the intensities differ. Difference values >0 indicate increased risk and values <0 indicate lower risk. Dotted lines highlight the areas of significantly increased risk of GV during the pandemic. (Right) The state-specific intensity of GV during and before the pandemic. State-specific intensity ratio (IR) and their 95% confidence intervals of GV. The dashed blue vertical line in the forest plots represents the null estimate. IR greater than one indicates the higher intensity of GV during the COVID-19 pandemic compared to the pre-pandemic. Figures modified from Ssentongo et al. 2021 [51]

## References


1. Brooker S. Spatial epidemiology of human schistosomiasis in Africa: risk models, transmission dynamics and control. Trans R Soc Trop Med Hyg. 2007;101(1):1–8.
2. Hannah Ritchie EM, Rodés-Guirao L, Appel C, Giattino C, Ortiz-Ospina E, Hasell J, MacDonald B, Beltekian D, Dattani S, Roser M. Coronavirus pandemic (COVID-19). Our World in Data; 2020. https://ourworldindata.org/coronavirus. Accessed 9 Dec 2021.
3. Lauring AS, Hodcroft EB. Genetic variants of SARS-CoV-2—what do they mean? JAMA. 2021;325(6):529–31.
4. The World Health Organization. Tracking SARS-CoV-2 variants. Geneva: WHO; 2020. https://www.who.int/en/activities/tracking-SARS-CoV-2-variants/. Accessed 9 Dec 2021.
5. Davies NG, Abbott S, Barnard RC, et al. Estimated transmissibility and impact of SARS-CoV-2 lineage B.1.1.7 in England. Science. 2021;372(6538):eabg3055.
6. Sheikh A, McMenamin J, Taylor B, Robertson C. SARS-CoV-2 delta VOC in Scotland: demographics, risk of hospital admission, and vaccine effectiveness. Lancet. 2021;397(10293):2461–2.
7. Ferreira IA, Kemp SA, Datir R, et al. SARS-CoV-2 B.1.617 mutations L452R and E484Q are not synergistic for antibody evasion. J Infect Dis. 2021;224(6):989–94.
8. Alizon S, Haim-Boukobza S, Foulongne V, et al. Rapid spread of the SARS-CoV-2 Delta variant in some French regions, June 2021. Eur Secur. 2021;26(28):2100573.
9. Twohig KA, Nyberg T, Zaidi A, et al. Hospital admission and emergency care attendance risk for SARS-CoV-2 delta (B.1.617. 2) compared with alpha (B.1.1.7) variants of concern: a cohort study. Lancet Infect Dis. 2022;22(1):35–42.
10. Mlcochova P, Kemp SA, Dhar MS, et al. SARS-CoV-2 B.1.617.2 Delta variant replication and immune evasion. Nature. 2021;599:1–6.
11. Nanduri S, Pilishvili T, Derado G, et al. Effectiveness of Pfizer-BioNTech and Moderna vaccines in preventing SARS-CoV-2 infection among nursing home residents before and during widespread circulation of the SARS-CoV-2 B. 1.617. 2 (Delta) variant—National Healthcare Safety Network, March 1–August 1, 2021. Morbid Mortal Weekly Rep. 2021;70(34):1163.
12. Mathieu E, Ritchie H, Ortiz-Ospina E, et al. A global database of COVID-19 vaccinations. Nat Hum Behav. 2021;5:1–7.
13. Karim SSA, Karim QA. Omicron SARS-CoV-2 variant: a new chapter in the COVID-19 pandemic. Lancet. 2021;398(10317):2126–8.
14. Dyer O. Covid-19: South Africa's surge in cases deepens alarm over omicron variant. BMJ. 2021;375:n3013.
15. Msomi N, Lessells R, Mlisana K, de Oliveira T. Africa: tackle HIV and COVID-19 together. Nature. 2021;600(7887):33–6.
16. Loembé MM, Tshangela A, Salyer SJ, Varma JK, Ouma AEO, Nkengasong JN. COVID-19 in Africa: the spread and response. Nat Med. 2020;26:1–4.
17. Tegally H, Wilkinson E, Giovanetti M, et al. Detection of a SARS-CoV-2 variant of concern in South Africa. Nature. 2021;592(7854):438–43.
18. Ssentongo P, Fronterre C, Geronimo A, et al. Pan-African evolution of within-and between-country COVID-19 dynamics. Proc Natl Acad Sci. 2021;118(28):e2026664118.
19. Held L, Höhle M, Hofmann M. A statistical framework for the analysis of multivariate infectious disease surveillance counts. Stat Model. 2005;5(3):187–99.
20. Bonaccorsi G, Pierri F, Cinelli M, et al. Economic and social consequences of human mobility restrictions under COVID-19. Proc Natl Acad Sci. 2020;117(27):15530–5.
21. Ssentongo P, Ssentongo AE, Heilbrunn ES, Ba DM, Chinchilli VM. Association of cardiovascular disease and 10 other pre-existing comorbidities with COVID-19 mortality: a systematic review and meta-analysis. PLoS One. 2020;15(8):e0238215.
22. Ssentongo A, Ssentongo P, Heilbrunn ES, et al. Renin-angiotensin-aldosterone system inhibitors and mortality in patients with hypertension hospitalized for COVID-19: a systematic review and meta-analysis. medRxiv. 2020.

23. Ssentongo P, Heilbrunn ES, Ssentongo AE, et al. Epidemiology and outcomes of COVID-19 in HIV-infected individuals: a systematic review and meta-analysis. Sci Rep. 2021;11(1):1–12.
24. Roser M, Ritchie H. HIV/AIDS. Our World in Data; 2019. https://ourworldindata.org/hiv-aids. Accessed 11 Dec 2021.
25. Salyer SJ, Maeda J, Sembuche S, et al. The first and second waves of the COVID-19 pandemic in Africa: a cross-sectional study. Lancet. 2021;397(10281):1265–75.
26. Dong E, Du H, Gardner L. An interactive web-based dashboard to track COVID-19 in real time. Lancet Infect Dis. 2020;20(5):533–4.
27. Yan R, Zhang Y, Li Y, Xia L, Guo Y, Zhou Q. Structural basis for the recognition of SARS-CoV-2 by full-length human ACE2. Science. 2020;367(6485):1444–8.
28. Coutard B, Valle C, de Lamballerie X, Canard B, Seidah NG, Decroly E. The spike glycoprotein of the new coronavirus 2019-nCoV contains a furin-like cleavage site absent in CoV of the same clade. Antivir Res. 2020;176:104742.
29. Papa G, Mallery DL, Albecka A, et al. Furin cleavage of SARS-CoV-2 spike promotes but is not essential for infection and cell-cell fusion. PLoS Pathog. 2021;17(1):e1009246.
30. Hoffmann M, Kleine-Weber H, Schroeder S, et al. SARS-CoV-2 cell entry depends on ACE2 and TMPRSS2 and is blocked by a clinically proven protease inhibitor. Cell. 2020;181(2):271–280.e8.
31. Shoily SS, Ahsan T, Fatema K, Sajib AA. Disparities in COVID-19 severities and casualties across ethnic groups around the globe and patterns of ACE2 and PIR variants. Infect Genet Evol. 2021;92:104888.
32. Al-Mulla F, Mohammad A, Al Madhoun A, et al. ACE2 and FURIN variants are potential predictors of SARS-CoV-2 outcome: a time to implement precision medicine against COVID-19. Heliyon. 2021;7(2):e06133.
33. Smith TP, Flaxman S, Gallinat AS, et al. Temperature and population density influence SARS-CoV-2 transmission in the absence of nonpharmaceutical interventions. Proc Natl Acad Sci. 2021;118(25):e2019284118.
34. Merow C, Urban MC. Seasonality and uncertainty in global COVID-19 growth rates. Proc Natl Acad Sci. 2020;117(44):27456–64.
35. Sajadi MM, Habibzadeh P, Vintzileos A, Shokouhi S, Miralles-Wilhelm F, Amoroso A. Temperature, humidity, and latitude analysis to estimate potential spread and seasonality of coronavirus disease 2019 (COVID-19). JAMA Netw Open. 2020;3(6):e2011834.
36. Wang J, Tang K, Feng K, et al. Impact of temperature and relative humidity on the transmission of COVID-19: a modelling study in China and the United States. BMJ Open. 2021;11(2):e043863.
37. Ma Y, Pei S, Shaman J, Dubrow R, Chen K. Role of meteorological factors in the transmission of SARS-CoV-2 in the United States. Nat Commun. 2021;12(1):1–9.
38. Chan K-H, Peiris JM, Lam S, Poon L, Yuen K, Seto WH. The effects of temperature and relative humidity on the viability of the SARS coronavirus. Adv Virol. 2011;2011:734690.
39. Matson MJ, Yinda CK, Seifert SN, et al. Effect of environmental conditions on SARS-CoV-2 stability in human nasal mucus and sputum. Emerg Infect Dis. 2020;26(9):2276.
40. Morris DH, Yinda KC, Gamble A, et al. Mechanistic theory predicts the effects of temperature and humidity on inactivation of SARS-CoV-2 and other enveloped viruses. elife. 2021;10:e65902.
41. Moriyama M, Hugentobler WJ, Iwasaki A. Seasonality of respiratory viral infections. Ann Rev Virol. 2020;7(1):83–101.
42. Qian H, Miao T, Liu L, Zheng X, Luo D, Li Y. Indoor transmission of SARS-CoV-2. Indoor Air. 2021;31(3):639–45.
43. Shaman J, Galanti M. Will SARS-CoV-2 become endemic? Science. 2020;370(6516):527–9.
44. Wu X, Nethery RC, Sabath M, Braun D, Dominici F. Air pollution and COVID-19 mortality in the United States: strengths and limitations of an ecological regression analysis. Sci Adv. 2020;6(45):eabd4049.

45. Conticini E, Frediani B, Caro D. Can atmospheric pollution be considered a co-factor in extremely high level of SARS-CoV-2 lethality in northern Italy? Environ Pollut. 2020;261:114465.
46. Setti L, Passarini F, De Gennaro G, et al. SARS-Cov-2RNA found on particulate matter of Bergamo in northern Italy: first evidence. Environ Res. 2020;188:109754.
47. Yang J, Chen Y, Yu Z, Ding H, Ma Z. The influence of PM2.5 on lung injury and cytokines in mice. Exp Ther Med. 2019;18(4):2503–11.
48. Pope CA III, Bhatnagar A, McCracken JP, Abplanalp W, Conklin DJ, O'Toole T. Exposure to fine particulate air pollution is associated with endothelial injury and systemic inflammation. Circ Res. 2016;119(11):1204–14.
49. Brooks SK, Webster RK, Smith LE, et al. The psychological impact of quarantine and how to reduce it: rapid review of the evidence. Lancet. 2020;395(10227):912–20.
50. Leslie E, Wilson R. Sheltering in place and domestic violence: evidence from calls for service during COVID-19. J Public Econ. 2020;189:104241.
51. Ssentongo P, Fronterre C, Ssentongo AE, et al. Gun violence incidence during the COVID-19 pandemic is higher than before the pandemic in the United States. Sci Rep. 2021;11(1):1–8.
52. Ettman CK, Abdalla SM, Cohen GH, Sampson L, Vivier PM, Galea S. Prevalence of depression symptoms in US adults before and during the COVID-19 pandemic. JAMA Netw Open. 2020;3(9):e2019686.
53. Sutherland M, McKenney M, Elkbuli A. Gun violence during COVID-19 pandemic: paradoxical trends in New York city, Chicago, Los Angeles and Baltimore. Am J Emerg Med. 2021;39:225–6.
54. Groff D, Sun A, Ssentongo AE, et al. Short-term and long-term rates of postacute sequelae of SARS-CoV-2 infection: a systematic review. JAMA Netw Open. 2021;4(10):e2128568.
55. Baig AM, Khaleeq A, Ali U, Syeda H. Evidence of the COVID-19 virus targeting the CNS: tissue distribution, host–virus interaction, and proposed neurotropic mechanisms. ACS Chem Neurosci. 2020;11(7):995–8.
56. Parsons N, Outsikas A, Parish A, et al. Modelling the anatomic distribution of neurologic events in patients with COVID-19: a systematic review of MRI findings. Am J Neuroradiol. 2021;42(7):1190–5.

# Chapter 12
# Eye Disorders and Neuro-ophthalmic Manifestations of COVID-19

**Elias Premi, Roberto Acampora, Greta Karen Wood, Ingrid Andreea Ilie, Benedict Daniel Michael, and Francesco Lanfranchi**

## Introduction

Since the start of the coronavirus (COVID-19) pandemic, numerous works have described ocular involvement [1–3]. The quality of evidence has often been limited by difficulty performing ophthalmic clinical evaluation and instrumental

E. Premi
Ophthalmology Unit, ASST Sette Laghi, Circolo Hospital and Macchi Foundation, Varese, Italy

Department of Biotechnologies and Life Sciences, University of Insubria, Varese, Italy

R. Acampora
Milan Center for Neuroscience (NeuroMI), Milan, Italy

Neurology and Stroke-Unit, Hospital Ospedale del Mare, Naples, Italy

G. K. Wood · B. D. Michael
Department of Neurology, The Walton Centre NHS Foundation Trust, Liverpool, UK

Clinical Infection Microbiology and Neuroimmunology, Institute of Infection, Veterinary and Ecological Science, Liverpool, UK

The NIHR Health Protection Research Unit for Emerging and Zoonotic Infection, Liverpool, UK
e-mail: greta.wood@liverpool.ac.uk; benedict.michael@liverpool.ac.uk

I. A. Ilie
Department of Life Sciences and Biotechnology, School of Biology, University of Ferrara, Ferrara, Italy

F. Lanfranchi (✉)
Department of Health Sciences (DISSAL), University of Genoa, Genoa, Italy
e-mail: flanfranchi@hotmail.com


S. Adibi et al. (eds.), *Frontiers of COVID-19*,
https://doi.org/10.1007/978-3-031-08045-6_12

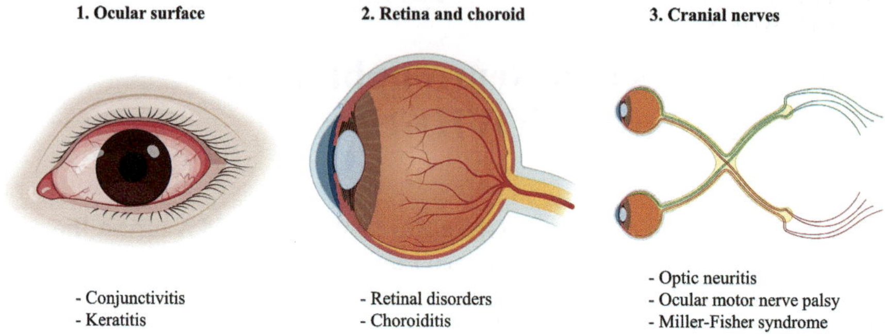


**Fig. 12.1** Graphical summary of eye disorders and neuro-ophthalmic manifestations associated with SARS-CoV-2 infection. Created with BioRender.com

examination in the pandemic period. Initial investigations focused upon the potential mechanisms that could lead to infection of ocular tissues by severe acute respiratory distress coronavirus 2 (SARS-COV-2). The aim of this chapter (graphically summarized in Fig. 12.1) was to display current evidence about ocular involvement in patients presenting SARS-CoV-2 infection, describing possible underlying mechanisms and illustrating the most common manifestations occurring in both superficial and profound eye structures as well as neuro-ophthalmic presentations. Topic of interest included clinically detectable signs and symptoms, reliable methods for early diagnosis, and proper treatments of these complications.

## Pathophysiological Mechanisms

Polymerase chain reaction (PCR) testing of ocular samples has shown an extremely variable detection rate between different studies, ranging from 0% to 57.1% [4, 5], potentially because of varying sample collection methods. As suggested by experiments conducted on Rhesus macaques [6], eye exposure and subsequently systemic infection could follow three main different pathways. Despite these hypotheses are recurrent in different clinical and preclinical studies, available data suggest multiple mechanisms but do not establish a confirmed pathway [6].

The direct infection of the eye surface from droplets or from the contact with contaminated hand or objects is supported by the expression on conjunctival cells of many virus-bindable receptors [6, 7], such as angiotensin converting enzyme 2 (ACE-2), furin, transmembrane serine protease 2 (TMPRSS-2), A disintegrin and metalloproteinase 17 (ADAM-17), the cluster of differentiation 147 (CD-147), cathepsin L and dipeptidyl peptidase 4 (DPP-4) (Fig. 12.2). In fact, ACE-2 and TMPRSS-2 are the main expressed co-factors in epithelial superficial cells of the cornea (namely, basal corneal epithelium, limbal niche, corneal wing cells, transit amplifying cells, limbal superficial cells, corneal epithelial superficial cells, and

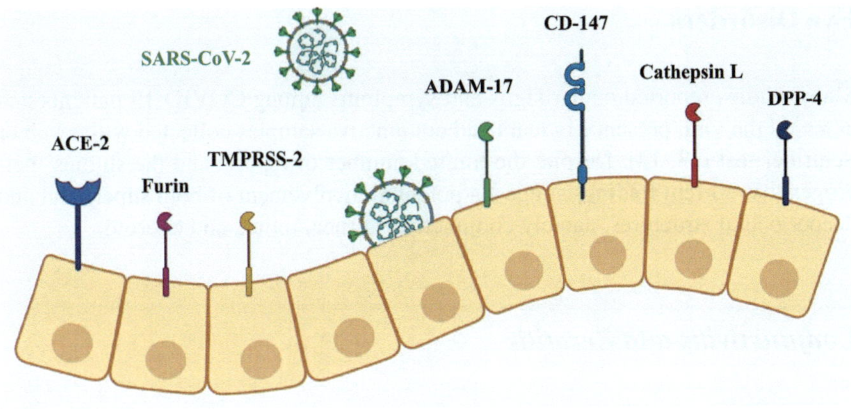


**Fig. 12.2** Overview of SARS-CoV-2 entry molecules expressed by conjunctival cells. Figure and caption modified from Kitazawa et al. [7] and licensed under Creative Common License CC BY 4.0 (https://creativecommons.org/licenses/by/4.0/)

limbal stem cells), potentially allowing SARS-CoV-2 to entry. This hypothesis is further corroborated by a study conducted on cornea-explanted patients, showing more than 80% of patients being positive for SARS-CoV-2 ribonucleic acid (RNA) [8]. However, in the same study viral isolation was unsuccessful. Regarding the eye-driven transmissibility, the most notable evidence is provided by an observational clinical study [9], reporting that among hospitalized patient there was a lower prevalence (5.8%; 95% CI: 3.0–8.6%) of subject wearing glasses for more than 8 h per day compared to age-matched general population (31.5%). Despite limitations in the study design, the results are consistent with the involvement of the eye in transmitting the disease, probably by direct contagion from air and self-touching with hands [4, 6].

Moreover, a post-viremia secretion of the virus from the lacrimal glands has been proposed as a possible mechanism [4], supported by analogous findings in other viral infections [10]. SARS-CoV-2 could penetrate aqueous humor fluid through cornea or trough ciliary body secretion. The apparently contrasting detection of viral mRNA in aqueous humor in patients with negative nasopharyngeal swab [8] could suggest the SARS-COV-2 persistence in immunoprivileged spaces in absence of systemic involvement [11].

Considering the high vascularization of structures such as retina and choroid, a third hypothesis is hematogenous dissemination in the eye. A case-control study linked alteration in vascular density of the choroid and a cystoid degeneration of the retina with the microanatomical changes in the retina and choroid in post-mortem COVID-19 patients [12]. Evidence of the presence of SARS-CoV-2 in lens, vitreous humor, retinal and choroidal tissues is limited by the difficulty taking in vivo samples, however, a dedicated study [8] detected SARS-CoV-2 RNA in vitreous humor in 3 of 11 patients.

## Eye Disorders

Many studies reported ocular signs and symptoms among COVID-19 patients and assessed the viral presence in tears and conjunctiva samples collected with swab or Schirmer test [13, 14]. Despite the limited number of reports and the studies' heterogeneity, current findings suggest a potential involvement of both superficial and deeper ocular structures, namely conjunctiva, cornea, retina, and choroid.

### *Conjunctivitis and Keratitis*

Most studies have been performed on heterogeneous patient groups with a small proportion of PCR-positive cases and infrequent ocular manifestations [3, 13–22]. Despite a low prevalence of ocular signs and symptoms, one study [4] has shown a high prevalence of SARS-COV-2 positive conjunctival samples among 91 COVID-19 patients (57.1%; 95% CI: 46.3–67.5%). Thus, from available data, no correlation between the viral presence on ocular surface and ophthalmic signs and symptoms seems to be demonstrated.

The metanalysis conducted by Nasiri and co-colleagues [2], including 38 studies with a cumulative number of 8219 COVID-19 patients, the pooled prevalence of ocular manifestations was to be 11.03% (95% CI: 5.71–17.72%). The most common ocular symptoms were dry eye or foreign body sensation (16%), redness (13.3%), tearing (12.8%), itching (12.6%), eye pain (9.6%), and discharge (8.8%). Among patients with ocular symptoms, conjunctivitis was the most prevalent (88.8%). A previous metanalysis by Loffredo and co-authors [23], based on three studies including 1167 patients, showed an increased incidence of conjunctivitis in hospitalized patients (odds ratio: 3.4; 95% CI: 1.1–10.2) and an association between COVID-19 severity and the frequency of conjunctiva inflammation (3% and 0.7% in severe and non-severe COVID-19 patients, respectively).

Keratitis seems to be a very rare presentation of COVID-19 involving the eye, reported in only one study describing a young patient presenting to the emergency department with COVID-19 respiratory symptoms and keratitis diagnosed at slit lamp examination [24].

### *Retinal Disorders and Choroiditis*

Retinal vascular disorders reported in COVID-19 patients included central (Fig. 12.3) or branch retinal artery occlusion [25–27] presenting with typical manifestations, such as a reduction in best corrected visual acuity (BCVA) and a low recovery. However, all the described patients had a medical history predisposing to both ocular and vascular complications, such as hypertension, smoking, and arterial

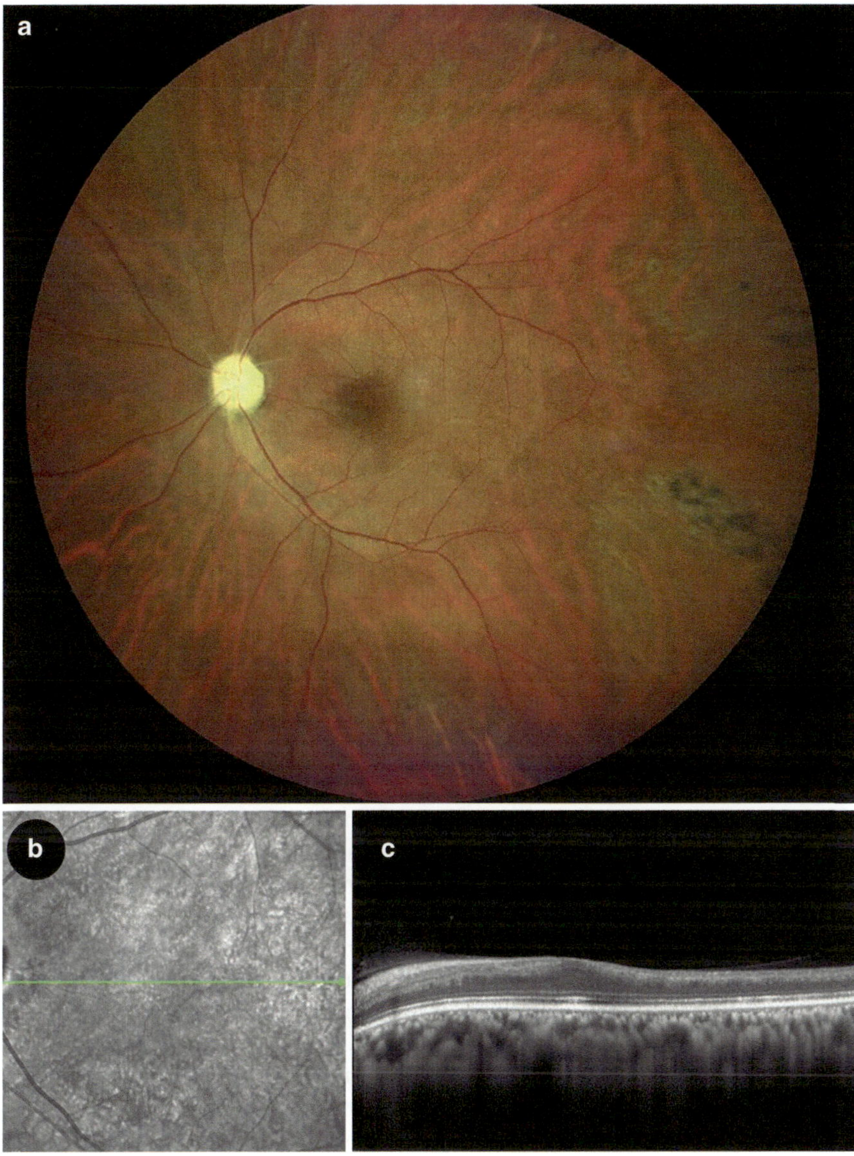


**Fig. 12.3** (**a**) Fundus photography of the left eye showing the presence of a pale optic disc, diffuse arterial narrowing, a mild "cherry-red spot" macula and peripheral areas of retinal pigmented epithelium hyperpigmentation. (**b**, **c**) Infrared reflectance and spectral domain optical coherence tomography acquisition over the macular region of the same eye denoting atrophy of the inner retina layers with loss of foveal depression and temporal macular thinning. Figure and caption modified from Montesel et al. [25] and licensed under Creative Common License CC BY 4.0 (https://creativecommons.org/licenses/by/4.0/)

hypertension. A single study [28] reported a young patient with the classic pattern of a branch retinal vein occlusion in the absence of known thrombotic risk factors. Ophthalmologic examination revealed no visual loss except a paracentral scotoma and fundus examination of the affected eye showed rare, scattered hemorrhages in the inferior part of the retina and dilated and tortuous vessels, while the other eye appeared normal. Fluorescein angiography (FA) demonstrated marked delay in filling of the inferior venous arcade and a late vessel staining. Optical coherence tomography (OCT) evaluation showed no sign of central macular edema. Higher quality evidence is required to correlate SARS-CoV-2 infection with retinal vascular illnesses.

A rare clinical entity potentially associated with retinal microvascular capillary micro-thrombotic phenomena is paracentral acute middle maculopathy (PAMM) [29, 30], an acute onset disease characterized by paracentral scotoma, potential reduction of BCVA, and typical OCT alterations. PAMM has previously been associated with viral infections [30] and has been described in a small number of COVID-19 patients presenting with paracentral scotoma [31, 32]. At ophthalmic evaluation, small white lesions can be seen at fundus examination and the definitive diagnosis is based on OCT findings (Fig. 12.4), including focal hyper-reflective changes in the inner and outer plexiform layers with inner nuclear layer volume loss in the parafoveal region. Recovery is typically spontaneous, but a minority of cases have persistent paracentral scotoma and various degrees of visual impairment [30]. Thromboembolic events are a well-recognized complication of COVID-19 [34], and vascularized tissue in the retina and choroid could be susceptible to this phenomenon. The current literature is limited to retinal vessel alterations observed in a small number of case reports. Thus, it is not possible to establish a causal relationship with SARS-CoV-2 given the very limited number of patients described and the high risk of a misinterpretation due to confounding.

There is currently a single report of potential choroid involvement which describes atypical manifestations of choroiditis in a young patient with monocular vision loss in the right eye after 5 days of systemic symptoms in confirmed SARS-CoV-2 infection [35]. Fundus examination revealed multiple yellow-whitish placoid lesions at the posterior pole. At FA, lesions showed early and mild late staining, and no neovascularization signs were detected. OCT scans demonstrated irregular retinal pigment epithelial elevation, diffuse interruption of the outer retinal layers, and the retinal pigment epithelium and choroid thickness. After 11 days of corticosteroid treatment, there was clinical improvement and lesion resolution. Given the very limited evidence, it is impossible to demonstrate an association between choroid alterations and SARS-CoV-2 infection.

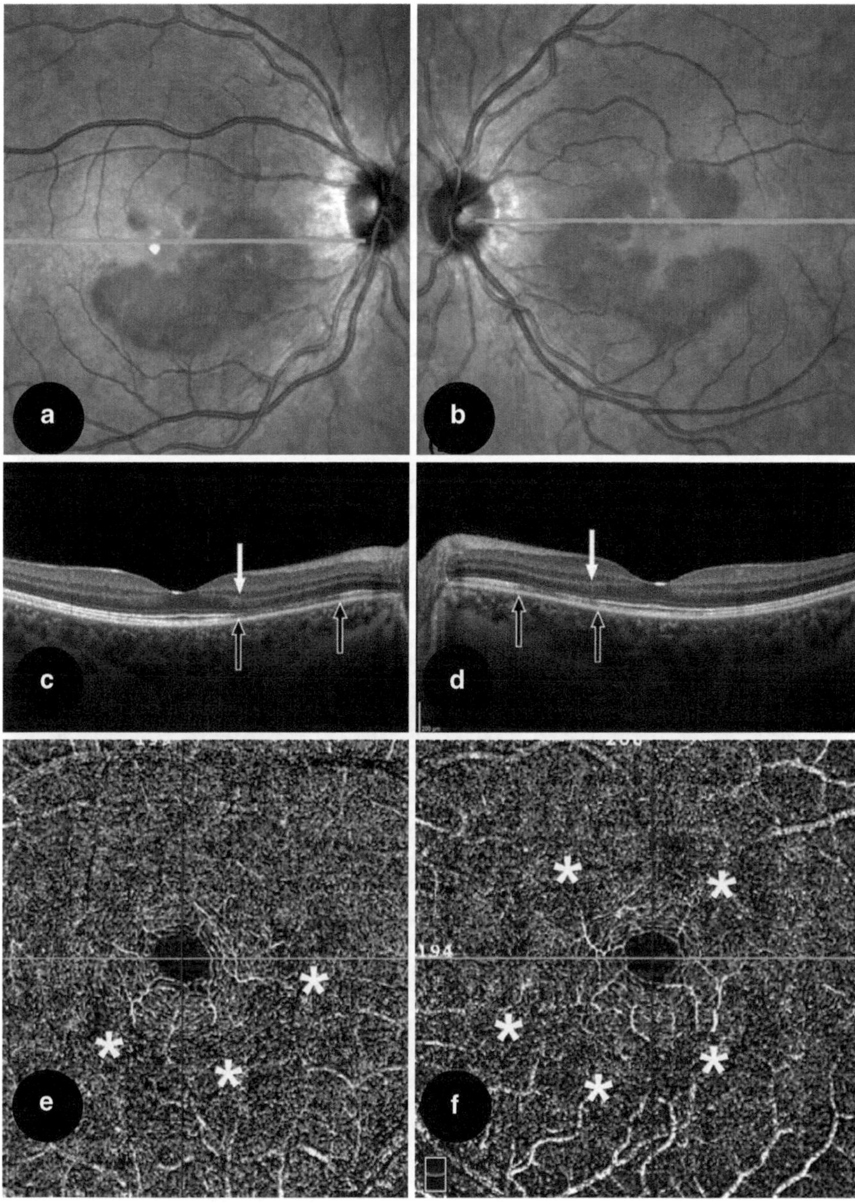


**Fig. 12.4** (**a**, **b**) Near-infrared imaging of right eye (**a**) and left eye (**b**) show multiple hyporeflective lesions in the paracentral macula in both eyes. The small lesions have a petaloid shape, but the majority of lesions are large and confluent, almost forming a ring around the fovea. (**c**, **d**) Spectral-domain OCT of right eye (**c**) and left eye (**d**) at the level of the green line in Fig. **a**, **b**, shows interruption of the ellipsoid zone and the interdigitation zone (black arrows). There are also hyperreflective changes (white arrow) within the outer nuclear layers. (**e**, **f**) OCT angiography of the right eye (**e**) and left eye (**f**) shows multiple areas of decreased vascular flow signal (asterisks) at the level of the deep capillary plexus corresponding to the lesions visible in the near-infrared reflectance imaging. Figure and caption modified from Giacuzzo, Eandi, and Kawasakiet [33] and licensed under Creative Common License CC BY 4.0 (https://creativecommons.org/licenses/by/4.0/)

## Neuro-ophthalmic Manifestations

### *Optic Neuritis*

There are several studies reporting optic neuritis (ON) in patients with a positive PCR for SARS-CoV-2 and a single case diagnosed by positive IgM [36]. Ophthalmic symptoms are most frequently described after respiratory illness, however, Benito-Pascual and co-authors [37] presented a case of ON as a possible first manifestation of SARS-CoV-2 infection, occurring 10 days prior to respiratory symptom onset. Ophthalmic pathology is unilateral in most reports, with a small number of cases demonstrating involvement of both optic nerves and a full recovery after treatment with corticosteroids [22, 38]. In some cases, patients with concomitant neurological symptoms [39–41], as well as reports of myelin oligodendrocyte glycoprotein antibody detection [22, 36].

A small number of studies have reported neuroimaging abnormalities in ON, including hyperintensity and gadolinium enhancement of the optic nerve in brain magnetic resonance imaging (MRI) [38, 39, 42] and orbit MRI [38, 43, 44] (Fig. 12.5). In all other reports, MRI was negative or non-specific. Burgos-Blasco

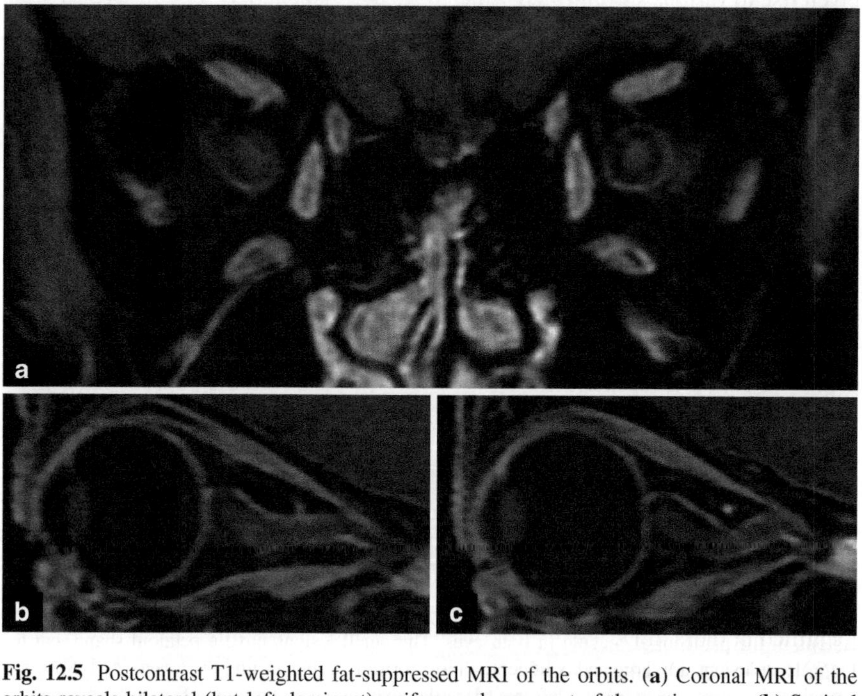


**Fig. 12.5** Postcontrast T1-weighted fat-suppressed MRI of the orbits. (**a**) Coronal MRI of the orbits reveals bilateral (but left dominant) uniform enhancement of the optic nerve. (**b**) Sagittal MRI of the right orbit reveals a slightly ill-defined appearance of the optic nerve and slight enhancement of optic nerve sheaths. (**c**) Sagittal MRI of the left orbit reveals uniform enhancement along with optic nerve sheaths. Figure and caption modified from Kogure et al. [43] and licensed under Creative Common License CC BY 4.0 (https://creativecommons.org/licenses/by/4.0/)

and co-authors additionally demonstrated [45] an increase in retinal nerve fiber layer thickness at OCT in patients with a positive PCR test, including in the absence of clinical ocular manifestations. There is, however, no evidence of alterations in optic nerve vascular density in patients recovered from SARS-CoV-2 infection [46].

## *Ocular Motor Nerves Palsy*

Involvement of cranial nerves innervating the ocular muscles has also been reported in COVID-19 patients, including abnormalities detected on imaging [42, 47]. There are a series of reports of oculomotor nerve palsy with typical symptoms and SARS-CoV-2 confirmed by PCR or serology in most cases [48–52]. A unique case of isolated monocular fourth nerve palsy has been described by Pascual-Prieto and colleagues [53], presenting with diplopia after respiratory symptoms onset. The patient had a positive PCR test, and favorably recovered. Unilateral abducens nerve palsy with typical symptoms has been reported in multiple PCR-confirmed SARS-CoV-2 infections [53–56]. A rare case of internuclear ophthalmoplegia in a COVID-19 PCR-positive patient with a typical and unilateral clinical presentation has been described [57]. After off-label treatment with vitamin B12, vitamin C, and ivermectin, the patient fully recovered. In contrast to findings from an MRI case series of cranial nerve palsy in COVID-19 patients conducted by Corrêa and co-authors [42], few studies have detected neuroimaging abnormalities in patients with clinical ocular motor cranial nerve pathology [54, 56].

Despite a growing number of reported cases, the association between ocular cranial nerve manifestations and SARS-CoV-2 infection remains weak. Further neuroimaging studies including routine brain or orbital MRI would be particularly valuable, alongside studies into the potential underlying pathophysiological mechanisms including direct neuroinvasion and immune-mediated phenomena [58].

## *Miller Fisher Syndrome*

Classified as a rare variant of the Guillain–Barré syndrome (GBS) spectrum [59, 60], Miller Fisher syndrome (MFS) has been observed with typical symptoms including ataxia and areflexia [61]. The most common neuro-ophthalmic symptoms detected in these patients were palsy of the oculomotor [62, 63] and abducens [62, 64] cranial nerves, ophthalmoparesis or ophthalmoplegia [63, 65–67], and impairment in pupillary reflex [68]. A minority of studies have reported positive anti-ganglioside (GD)-1b immunoglobulin G (IgG) antibodies [62], or abnormal neuroimaging findings including gadolinium enhancement and T2-weighted hyperintensity of the clinically involved ocular motor nerve on MRI [63]. In most studies evaluating these parameters, anti-GD1b-IgG results have been borderline [63] or negative [62, 64, 65, 67], and no abnormality has been detected on neuroimaging [64–66, 68].

Most commonly, SARS-CoV-2 infection diagnosis was performed by PCR [62, 63, 66, 67]; in one recently exposed patient presenting a negative molecular test, the diagnosis was based on serological assay [64]. In all cases, patients recovered either after intravenous immunoglobulin (IVIG) administration [62–65, 67, 68] or, less frequently, even without a specific treatment [62, 66]. Lowery and colleagues [69] described an atypical variant of GBS with positive anti-ganglioside antibodies in an immunosuppressed COVID-19 patient with concurrent severe respiratory illness requiring intensive care and intubation. Despite treatment with IVIG, the patient reported long-term sequelae.

Available findings suggest GBS occurs in association with SARS-CoV-2 infection and has a typical clinical picture [70–72]. Epidemiological data on MFS in association with SARS-CoV-2 are limited by the small number of reported cases and heterogeneous nature of diagnostic assessments [73]. Well-designed case-control studies and investigations into disease mechanisms would enhance the evidence base.

## Looking to the Future

It is necessary to find effective remote procedures for assessing and monitoring suspected or confirmed COVID-19 patients. De Arrigunaga and colleagues [74] reported teleophthalmology as providing excellent results in visual acuity examination, although the self-administrable test accuracy has not been clearly validated. Additionally, a mobile application for pupil assessment showed great concordance with traditional examination [75]. As expected, remote examination of the anterior segment resulted easier and more reliable than tools for assessing the posterior chamber [74]. Newman-Casey and co-authors [76] reported that appropriately remote-conducted triages appeared to be a safe way to reduce in-person assessments. High patient satisfaction rates in teleophthalmology were described by several studies [77–80], especially for video consultation. Less than 20 percent of patients under 65 years old requested a face-to-face visit [78]. Moreover, physicians reported high rate of satisfaction in using remote tools [77]. Available evidence for teleophthalmology is therefore encouraging, and further implementation research should be conducted to verify the role of the practice [74].

Evidence suggestive of ocular involvement in COVID-19 patients are growing [1–3]; however, the lack of standardized prospective studies, the heterogeneity of inclusion criteria and diagnostic assessment, and small number of patients included in any single study represent a major limitation [2]. Further studies should investigate the underlying mechanisms and sequelae of potential acute and post-acute ocular complications of SARS-CoV-2. This could include functional imaging such as positron emission tomography [81–83], which has not yet been conducted in COVID-19 patients with neuro-ophthalmic manifestations as well as routine post-mortem analyses of the ocular tissues. Correlation of clinical phenotypes with neuroimaging, pathology results as well as metabolic and immune markers of disease, will be central to improve current understanding about disease mechanisms.

**Acknowledgments** All the authors are thankful to their teammates and collaborators. They also thank all health workers around the world who are dealing with this pandemic; all the authors express their deepest condolences and offer a heartfelt thanks to all colleagues fallen fighting against this invisible enemy, as well as to their families.

**Funding** This research received no external funding.

**Disclosure Statement** E.P., R.A., G.K.W., I.A.I., and F.L. declare no conflict of interest, and do not receive any financial aid. B.D.M. is supported to conduct COVID-19 neuroscience research by the UKRI/MRC (MR/V03605X/1); for additional neurological inflammation research due to viral infection B.D.M. is also supported by grants from the MRC/UKRI (MR/V007181//1), MRC (MR/T028750/1), and Wellcome (ISSF201902/3).

**Author Contributions** Conceptualization: E.P., R.A., B.D.M. and F.L.; literature research, screening, and selection: E.P., R.A., G.K.W. and I.A.I.; original draft preparation: E.P. and F.L.; review: G.K.W. and I.A.I.; writing and editing: all authors.

All authors have read and approved the definitive version of the manuscript.

## References

1. Badawi AE, Elsheikh SS, Addeen SZ, Soliman MA, Abd-Rabu R, Abdella WS, Gad EA. An ophthalmic insight into novel coronavirus 2019 disease: a comprehensive review of the ocular manifestations and clinical hazards. J Curr Ophthalmol. 2020;32(4):315–28. https://doi.org/10.4103/JOCO.JOCO_255_20.
2. Nasiri N, Sharifi H, Bazrafshan A, Noori A, Karamouzian M, Sharifi A. Ocular manifestations of COVID-19: a systematic review and meta-analysis. J Ophthalmic Vis Res. 2021;16(1):103–12. https://doi.org/10.18502/JOVR.V16I1.8256.
3. Wu P, Duan F, Luo C, Liu Q, Xingguang Q, Liang L, Kaili W. Characteristics of ocular findings of patients with coronavirus disease 2019 (COVID-19) in Hubei Province, China. JAMA Ophthalmol. 2020;138(5):575. https://doi.org/10.1001/jamaophthalmol.2020.1291.
4. Azzolini C, Donati S, Premi E, Baj A, Siracusa C, Genoni A, Grossi PA, et al. SARS-CoV-2 on ocular surfaces in a cohort of patients with COVID-19 from the Lombardy region, Italy. JAMA Ophthalmol. 2021;139(9):1–9. https://doi.org/10.1001/jamaophthalmol.2020.5464.
5. Deng C, Yang Y, Chen H, Chen W, Chen Z, Ma K, Wang J. Ocular detection of SARS-CoV-2 in 114 cases of COVID-19 pneumonia in Wuhan, China: an observational study. SSRN Electron J. 2020; https://doi.org/10.2139/ssrn.3543587.
6. Qu JY, Xie HT, Zhang MC. Evidence of SARS-CoV-2 transmission through the ocular route. Clin Ophthalmol. 2021;15:687–96. https://doi.org/10.2147/OPTH.S295283.
7. Kitazawa K, Deinhardt-Emmer S, Inomata T, Deshpande S, Sotozono C. The transmission of SARS-CoV-2 infection on the ocular surface and prevention strategies. Cell. 2021;10(4):796. https://doi.org/10.3390/cells10040796.
8. Casagrande M, Fitzek A, Spitzer MS, Püschel K, Glatzel M, Krasemann S, Nörz D, Lütgehetmann M, Pfefferle S, Schultheiss M. Presence of SARS-CoV-2 RNA in the cornea

of Viremic patients with COVID-19. JAMA Ophthalmol. 2021;139(4):383–8. https://doi.org/10.1001/jamaophthalmol.2020.6339.
9. Zeng W, Wang X, Li J, Yang Y, Qiu X, Song P, Jianjun X, Wei Y. Association of dailywear of eyeglasses with susceptibility to coronavirus disease 2019 infection. JAMA Ophthalmol. 2020;138(11):1196–9. https://doi.org/10.1001/jamaophthalmol.2020.3906.
10. Han Y, Ning W, Zhu W, Li Y, Zuo L, Ye J, Qiu Z, Xie J, Li T. Detection of HIV-1 viruses in tears of patients even under long-term HAART. AIDS. 2011;25(15):1925–7. https://doi.org/10.1097/QAD.0b013e32834b3578.
11. Reinhold A, Tzankov A, Matter M, Mihic-Probst D, Scholl HPN, Meyer P. Ocular pathology and occasionally detectable intraocular SARS-CoV-2 RNA in five fatal COVID-19 cases. Ophthalmic Res. 2021;64:785–92. https://doi.org/10.1159/000514573.
12. Jidigam VK, Singh R, Batoki JC, Milliner C, Sawant OB, Bonilha VL, Rao S. Histopathological assessments reveal retinal vascular changes, inflammation and gliosis in patients with lethal COVID-19. MedRxiv. 2021. https://doi.org/10.1101/2021.02.25.21251531.
13. Arora R, Goel R, Kumar S, Chhabra M, Saxena S, Manchanda V, Pumma P. Evaluation of SARS-CoV-2 in tears of patients with moderate to severe COVID-19. Ophthalmology. 2021;128(4):494–503. https://doi.org/10.1016/j.ophtha.2020.08.029.
14. Yan Y, Zeng B, Zhang Z, Cheng H, Yan M, Li B, Zhang X, Chen X. Detection of SARS-CoV-2 in simultaneously collected tear and throat swab samples from the patients with 2019- new SARS-CoV-2 infection disease: a single center cross-sectional study. Ophthalmic Epidemiol. 2021;28(5):369–75. https://doi.org/10.1080/09286586.2021.1875011.
15. Chen L, Deng C, Chen X, Zhang X, Chen B, Huimin Y, Qin Y, Xiao K, Zhang H, Sun X. Ocular manifestations and clinical characteristics of 535 cases of COVID-19 in Wuhan, China: a cross-sectional study. Acta Ophthalmol. 2020;98(8):e951–9. https://doi.org/10.1111/aos.14472.
16. Güemes-Villahoz N, Burgos-Blasco B, Arribi-Vilela A, Arriola-Villalobos P, Rico-Luna CM, Cuiña-Sardiña R, Delgado-Iribarren A, García-Feijoó J. Detecting SARS-CoV-2 RNA in conjunctival secretions: is it a valuable diagnostic method of COVID-19? J Med Virol. 2021;93(1):383–8. https://doi.org/10.1002/jmv.26219.
17. Kocamış Ö, Örnek K, Aşıkgarip N, Hızmalı L, Sezgin FM, Şahin Y. Evaluation of nasopharyngeal and conjunctival swab samples of hospitalised patients with confirmed COVID-19. Ocul Immunol Inflamm. 2021;29:1–4. https://doi.org/10.1080/09273948.2020.1838558.
18. Li M, Yang Y, He T, Wei R, Shen Y, Qi T, Han T, et al. Detection of SARS-CoV-2 in the ocular surface in different phases of COVID-19 patients in Shanghai, China. Ann Transl Med. 2021;9(2):100. https://doi.org/10.21037/atm-20-6026.
19. Savastano MC, Gambini G, Savastano A, Falsini B, De Vico U, Sanguinetti M, Cattani P, et al. Evidence-based of conjunctival COVID-19 positivity: an Italian experience: Gemelli against COVID group. Eur J Ophthalmol. 2021;31(6):2886–93. https://doi.org/10.1177/1120672120976548.
20. Seah I, Agrawal R. Can the coronavirus disease 2019 (COVID-19) affect the eyes? A review of coronaviruses and ocular implications in humans and animals. Ocul Immunol Inflamm. 2020;28(3):391–5. https://doi.org/10.1080/09273948.2020.1738501.
21. Zhang X, Chen X, Chen L, Deng C, Zou X, Liu W, Huimin Y, Chen B, Sun X. The evidence of SARS-CoV-2 infection on ocular surface. Ocul Surf. 2020;18(3):360–2. https://doi.org/10.1016/j.jtos.2020.03.010.
22. Zhou Y, Duan C, Zeng Y, Tong Y, Nie Y, Yang Y, Chen Z, Chen C. Ocular findings and proportion with conjunctival SARS-COV-2 in COVID-19 patients. Ophthalmology. 2020;127(7):982–3. https://doi.org/10.1016/j.ophtha.2020.04.028.
23. Loffredo L, Pacella F, Pacella E, Tiscione G, Oliva A, Violi F. Conjunctivitis and COVID-19: a meta-analysis. J Med Virol. 2020;92(9):1413–4. https://doi.org/10.1002/jmv.25938.
24. Cheema M, Aghazadeh H, Nazarali S, Ting A, Hodges J, McFarlane A, Kanji JN, Zelyas N, Damji KF, Solarte C. Keratoconjunctivitis as the initial medical presentation of the novel

coronavirus disease 2019 (COVID-19). Can J Ophthalmol. 2020;55(4):e125–9. https://doi.org/10.1016/j.jcjo.2020.03.003.
25. Montesel A, Bucolo C, Mouvet V, Moret E, Eandi CM. Case report: central retinal artery occlusion in a COVID-19 patient. Front Pharmacol. 2020;11(December):2149. https://doi.org/10.3389/fphar.2020.588384.
26. Bapaye MM, Nair AG, Bapaye CM, Bapaye MM, Shukla JJ. Simultaneous bilateral central retinal artery occlusion following COVID-19 infection. Ocul Immunol Inflamm. 2021;29(4):671–4. https://doi.org/10.1080/09273948.2021.1891262.
27. Murchison AP, Sweid A, Dharia R, Theofanis TN, Tjoumakaris SI, Jabbour PM, Bilyk JR. Monocular visual loss as the presenting symptom of COVID-19 infection. Clin Neurol Neurosurg. 2021;201:106440. https://doi.org/10.1016/j.clineuro.2020.106440.
28. Finn AP, Khurana RN, Chang LK. Hemi-retinal vein occlusion in a young patient with COVID-19. Am J Ophthalmol Case Rep. 2021;22(June):101046. https://doi.org/10.1016/j.ajoc.2021.101046.
29. Bakhoum MF, Bailey Freund K, Dolz-Marco R, Leong BCS, Baumal CR, Duker JS, Sarraf D. Paracentral acute middle maculopathy and the ischemic Cascade associated with retinal vascular occlusion. Am J Ophthalmol. 2018;195(November):143–53. https://doi.org/10.1016/j.ajo.2018.07.031.
30. Moura-Coelho N, Gaspar T, Ferreira JT, Dutra-Medeiros M, Cunha JP. Paracentral acute middle maculopathy—review of the literature. Graefes Arch Clin Exp Ophthalmol. 2020;258(12):2583–96. https://doi.org/10.1007/s00417-020-04826-1.
31. Padhy SK, Dcruz RP, Kelgaonkar A. Paracentral acute middle maculopathy following SARS-CoV-2 infection: the D-dimer hypothesis. BMJ Case Rep. 2021;14(3):e242043. https://doi.org/10.1136/bcr-2021-242043.
32. Turedi N, Onal Gunay B. Paracentral acute middle maculopathy in the setting of central retinal artery occlusion following COVID-19 diagnosis. Eur J Ophthalmol. 2021;32(3):NP62–6. https://doi.org/10.1177/1120672121995347.
33. Giacuzzo C, Eandi CM, Kawasaki A. Bilateral acute macular neuroretinopathy following COVID-19 infection. Acta Ophthalmol. 2022;100(2):e611–2. https://doi.org/10.1111/aos.14913.
34. Tan BK, Mainbourg S, Friggeri A, Bertoletti L, Douplat M, Dargaud Y, Grange C, Lobbes H, Provencher S, Lega JC. Arterial and venous thromboembolism in COVID-19: a study-level meta-analysis. Thorax. 2021:76, 1–10. https://doi.org/10.1136/thoraxjnl-2020-215383.
35. Souza EC, De VE, Campos D, Duker JS. Atypical unilateral multifocal choroiditis in a COVID-19 positive patient. Am J Ophthalmol Case Rep. 2021;22:101034. https://doi.org/10.1016/j.ajoc.2021.101034.
36. Žorić L, Rajović-Mrkić I, Čolak E, Mirić D, Kisić B. Optic neuritis in a patient with seropositive myelin oligodendrocyte glycoprotein antibody during the post-COVID-19 period. Int Med Case Rep J. 2021;14:349–55. https://doi.org/10.2147/IMCRJ.S315103.
37. Benito-Pascual B, Gegúndez JA, Díaz-Valle D, Arriola-Villalobos P, Carreño E, Culebras E, Rodríguez-Avial I, Benitez-Del-Castillo JM. Panuveitis and optic neuritis as a possible initial presentation of the novel coronavirus disease 2019 (COVID-19). Ocul Immunol Inflamm. 2020;28(6):922–5. https://doi.org/10.1080/09273948.2020.1792512.
38. Sawalha K, Adeodokun S, Kamoga GR. COVID-19-induced acute bilateral optic neuritis. J Investig Med High Impact Case Rep. 2020;8:2324709620976018. https://doi.org/10.1177/2324709620976018.
39. Rodrigo-Armenteros P, Uterga-Valiente JM, Zabala-Del-Arco J, Taramundi-Argüeso S, Antón-Méndez L, Gómez-Muga JJ, Garcia-Monco JC. Optic neuropathy in a patient with COVID-19 infection. Acta Neurol Belg. 2022;122(3):789–91. https://doi.org/10.1007/s13760-021-01600-w.
40. Shaw VC, Chander G, Puttanna A. Neuromyelitis optica spectrum disorder secondary to COVID-19. Br J Hosp Med. 2020;81(9):1–3. https://doi.org/10.12968/hmed.2020.0401.

41. Zhou S, Jones-Lopez EC, Soneji DJ, Azevedo CJ, Patel VR. Myelin oligodendrocyte glycoprotein antibody-associated optic neuritis and myelitis in COVID-19. J Neuroophthalmol. 2020;40(3):398–402. https://doi.org/10.1097/WNO.0000000000001049.
42. Corrêa DG, Hygino LC, da Cruz F, Lopes CR, de Carvalho C, Rangel AL, de Tessarollo AH, Coelho KCG, Brandão RZ, et al. Magnetic resonance imaging features of COVID-19-related cranial nerve lesions. J Neurovirol. 2021;27(1):171–7. https://doi.org/10.1007/s13365-020-00934-0.
43. Kogure C, Kikushima W, Fukuda Y, Hasebe Y, Takahashi T, Shibuya T, Sakurada Y, Kashiwagi K. Myelin oligodendrocyte glycoprotein antibody-associated optic neuritis in a COVID-19 patient: a case report. Medicine. 2021;100(19):e25865. https://doi.org/10.1097/MD.0000000000025865.
44. Rodríguez-Rodríguez MS, Romero-Castro RM, Alvarado-de C, la Barrera M, González-Cannata G, García-Morales AK, Ávila-Ríos S. Optic neuritis following SARS-CoV-2 infection. J Neurovirol. 2021;27(2):359–63. https://doi.org/10.1007/s13365-021-00959-z.
45. Burgos-Blasco B, Güemes-Villahoz N, Donate-Lopez J, Vidal-Villegas B, García-Feijóo J. Optic nerve analysis in COVID-19 patients. J Med Virol. 2021;93(1):190–1. https://doi.org/10.1002/jmv.26290.
46. Burgos-Blasco B, Güemes-Villahoz N, Vidal-Villegas B, Garcia-Feijoo J, Donate-Lopez J, Martin-Sanchez FJ, Gonzalez-Armengol JJ, Mendez-Hernandez CD. Optic nerve head vessel density assessment in recovered COVID-19 patients: a prospective study using optical coherence tomography angiography. J Glaucoma. 2021;30(8):711–7. https://doi.org/10.1097/IJG.0000000000001858.
47. Roussel A, Germanaud D, Bouchoucha Y, Ouldali N, Vedrenne-Cloquet M, Castelle M, Baruchel A. Cranial polyneuropathy as the first manifestation of a severe COVID-19 in a child. Pediatr Blood Cancer. 2021;68(3):e28707. https://doi.org/10.1002/pbc.28707.
48. Belghmaidi S, Nassih H, Boutgayout S, El Fakiri K, El Qadiri R, Hajji I, Bourahouate A, Moutaouakil A. Third cranial nerve palsy presenting with unilateral diplopia and strabismus in a 24-year-old woman with COVID-19. Am J Case Rep. 2020;21:1–5. https://doi.org/10.12659/AJCR.925897.
49. Douedi S, Naser H, Mazahir U, Hamad AI, Sedarous M. Third cranial nerve palsy due to COVID-19 infection. Cureus. 2021;13(4):e14280. https://doi.org/10.7759/cureus.14280.
50. Fitzpatrick JC, Comstock JM, Longmuir RA, Donahue SP, Fitzpatrick JM, Bond JB. Cranial nerve III palsy in the setting of COVID 19 infection. J Neuroophthalmol. 2021;41(3):e286–7. https://doi.org/10.1097/WNO.0000000000001160.
51. Lonardi V, Meneghesso D, Debertolis G, Pin JN, Nosadini M, Sartori S. Isolated third cranial nerve palsy and COVID-19 infection in a child. Pediatr Neurol. 2021. https://doi.org/10.1016/j.pediatrneurol.2021.03.011.
52. Oliveira MR, De AR, Lucena VP, Higino TMM, Ventura CV. Oculomotor nerve palsy in an asymptomatic child with COVID-19. J AAPOS. 2021;25(3):169–70. https://doi.org/10.1016/j.jaapos.2021.02.001.
53. Pascual-Prieto J, Narváez-Palazón C, Porta-Etessam J, Gómez-de-Liaño R. COVID-19 epidemic: should ophthalmologists be aware of oculomotor paresis? Arch Soc Esp Oftalmol. 2020;95(7):361–2. https://doi.org/10.1016/j.oftal.2020.05.002.
54. Falcone MM, Rong AJ, Humberto Salazar D, Redick W, Falcone S, Cavuoto KM. Acute Abducens nerve palsy in a patient with the novel coronavirus disease (COVID-19). J AAPOS. 2020;24(4):216–7. https://doi.org/10.1016/j.jaapos.2020.06.001.
55. Greer CE, Bhatt JM, Oliveira CA, Dinkin MJ. Isolated cranial nerve 6 palsy in 6 patients with COVID-19 infection. J Neuroophthalmol. 2020;40(4):520–2. https://doi.org/10.1097/WNO.0000000000001146.
56. Pascual-Goñi E, Fortea J, Martínez-Domeño A, Rabella N, Tecame M, Gómez-Oliva C, Querol L, Gómez-Ansón B. COVID-19-associated Ophthalmoparesis and hypothalamic involvement. Neurol Neuroimmunol Neuroinflamm. 2020;7(5):e823. https://doi.org/10.1212/NXI.0000000000000823.

57. Vasanthpuram VH, Badakere A. Internuclear Ophthalmoplegia as a presenting feature in a COVID-19-positive patient. BMJ Case Rep. 2021;14(4):e241873. https://doi.org/10.1136/bcr-2021-241873.
58. Costello F, Dalakas MC. Cranial neuropathies and COVID-19: neurotropism and autoimmunity. Neurology. 2020;95(5):195–6. https://doi.org/10.1212/WNL.0000000000009921.
59. Al Othman B, Raabe J, Kini A, Lee AG. Update: the miller fisher variants of Guillain-Barré syndrome. Curr Opin Ophthalmol. 2019;30(6):462–6. https://doi.org/10.1097/ICU.0000000000000611.
60. Teener JW. Miller Fisher's syndrome. Semin Neurol. 2012;32(5):512–6. https://doi.org/10.1055/s-0033-1334470.
61. Mori M, Kuwabara S, Fukutake T, Yuki N, Hattori T. Clinical features and prognosis of miller fisher syndrome. Neurology. 2001;56(8):1104–6. https://doi.org/10.1212/WNL.56.8.1104.
62. Gutiérrez-Ortiz C, Méndez-Guerrero A, Rodrigo-Rey S, Pedro-Murillo ES, Bermejo-Guerrero L, Gordo-Mañas R, de Aragón-Gómez F, Benito-León J. Miller fisher syndrome and polyneuritis Cranialis in COVID-19. Neurology. 2020;95(5):e601–5. https://doi.org/10.1212/WNL.0000000000009619.
63. Lantos JE, Strauss SB, Lin E. COVID-19-associated miller fisher syndrome: MRI findings. Am J Neuroradiol. 2020;41(7):1184–6. https://doi.org/10.3174/AJNR.A6609.
64. Reyes-Bueno JA, García-Trujillo L, Urbaneja P, Ciano-Petersen NL, Postigo-Pozo MJ, Martínez-Tomás C, Serrano-Castro PJ. Miller-fisher syndrome after SARS-CoV-2 infection. Eur J Neurol. 2020;27(9):1759–61. https://doi.org/10.1111/ene.14383.
65. Manganotti P, Bellavita G, D'Acunto L, Tommasini V, Fabris M, Sartori A, Bonzi L, Stella AB, Pesavento V. Clinical neurophysiology and cerebrospinal liquor analysis to detect Guillain-Barré syndrome and polyneuritis Cranialis in COVID-19 patients: a case series. J Med Virol. 2021;93(2):766–74. https://doi.org/10.1002/jmv.26289.
66. Ray A. Miller fisher syndrome and COVID-19: is there a link? BMJ Case Rep. 2020;13(8):e236419. https://doi.org/10.1136/bcr-2020-236419.
67. Senel M, Abu-Rumeileh S, Michel D, Garibashvili T, Althaus K, Kassubek J, Otto M. Miller-fisher syndrome after COVID-19: neurochemical markers as an early sign of nervous system involvement. Eur J Neurol. 2020;27(11):2378–80. https://doi.org/10.1111/ene.14473.
68. Fernández-Domínguez J, Ameijide-Sanluis E, García-Cabo C, García-Rodríguez R, Mateos V. Miller–fisher-like syndrome related to SARS-CoV-2 infection (COVID 19). J Neurol. 2020;267(9):2495–6. https://doi.org/10.1007/s00415-020-09912-2.
69. Lowery MM, Malik MT, Seemiller J, Tsai CS. Atypical variant of Guillain Barre syndrome in a patient with COVID-19. J Crit Care Med. 2020;6(4):231–6. https://doi.org/10.2478/jccm-2020-0038.
70. Abu-Rumeileh S, Abdelhak A, Foschi M, Tumani H, Otto M. Guillain–Barré syndrome spectrum associated with COVID-19: an up-to-date systematic review of 73 cases. J Neurol. 2021;268(4):1133–70. https://doi.org/10.1007/s00415-020-10124-x.
71. Sansone P, Giaccari LG, Aurilio C, Coppolino F, Esposito V, Fiore M, Paladini A, Passavanti MB, Pota V, Pace MC. Post-infectious Guillain–Barré syndrome related to Sars-Cov-2 infection: a systematic review. Life. 2021;11(2):167. https://doi.org/10.3390/life11020167.
72. Sheikh AB, Chourasia PK, Javed N, Chourasia MK, Suriya SS, Upadhyay S, Ijaz F, Pal S, Moghimi N, Shekhar R. Association of Guillain-Barre Syndrome with COVID-19 infection: an updated systematic review. J Neuroimmunol. 2021;355:577577. https://doi.org/10.1016/j.jneuroim.2021.577577.
73. Li Z, Li X, Shen J, Chan MTV, Wu WKK. Miller fisher syndrome associated with COVID-19: an up-to-date systematic review. Environ Sci Pollut Res. 2021;28(17):20939–44. https://doi.org/10.1007/s11356-021-13233-w.
74. De Arrigunaga S, Aziz K, Lorch AC, Friedman DS, Armstrong GW. A review of ophthalmic telemedicine for emergency department settings. Semin Ophthalmol. 2022;37:1–8. https://doi.org/10.1080/08820538.2021.1922712.

75. McAnany JJ, Smith BM, Garland A, Kagen SL. IPhone-based pupillometry: a novel approach for assessing the pupillary light reflex. Optom Vis Sci. 2018;95(10):953–8. https://doi.org/10.1097/OPX.0000000000001289.
76. Newman-Casey PA, De Lott L, Cho J, Ballouz D, Azzouz L, Saleh S, Woodward MA. Telehealth-based eye care during the COVID-19 pandemic: utilization, safety and the patient experience. Am J Ophthalmol. 2021;230:234–42. https://doi.org/10.1016/j.ajo.2021.04.014.
77. Arntz A, Khaliliyeh D, Cruzat A, Rao X, Rocha G, Grau A, Altschwager P, Azócar V. Open-care telemedicine in ophthalmology during the COVID-19 pandemic: a pilot study. Arch Soc Esp Oftalmol. 2020;95(12):586–90. https://doi.org/10.1016/j.oftal.2020.09.005.
78. Golash V, Athwal S, Khandwala M. Teleophthalmology and COVID-19: the patient perspective. Future Healthc J. 2021;8(1):e54–9. https://doi.org/10.7861/fhj.2020-0139.
79. Kalavar M, Hua HU, Sridhar J. Teleophthalmology: an essential tool in the era of the novel coronavirus 2019. Curr Opin Ophthalmol. 2020;31(5):366–73. https://doi.org/10.1097/ICU.0000000000000689.
80. Kilduff CLS, Thomas AAP, Dugdill J, Casswell EJ, Dabrowski M, Lovegrove C, Sim DA, Hay GR, Thomas PBM. Creating the Moorfields' virtual eye casualty: video consultations to provide emergency teleophthalmology care during and beyond the COVID-19 pandemic. BMJ Health Care Informat. 2020;27(3):e100179. https://doi.org/10.1136/bmjhci-2020-100179.
81. Donegani MI, Miceli A, Pardini M, Bauckneht M, Chiola S, Pennone M, Marini C, et al. Brain metabolic correlates of persistent olfactory dysfunction after SARS-Cov2 infection. Biomedicine. 2021;9(3):287. https://doi.org/10.3390/biomedicines9030287.
82. Guedj E, Campion JY, Dudouet P, Kaphan E, Bregeon F, Tissot-Dupont H, Guis S, et al. 18F-FDG brain PET Hypometabolism in patients with long COVID. Eur J Nucl Med Mol Imaging. 2021;48:1–11. https://doi.org/10.1007/s00259-021-05215-4.
83. Sollini M, Morbelli S, Ciccarelli M, Cecconi M, Aghemo A, Morelli P, Chiola S, Gelardi F, Chiti A. Long COVID hallmarks on [18F]FDG-PET/CT: a case-control study. Eur J Nucl Med Mol Imaging. 2021;48(10):3187–97. https://doi.org/10.1007/s00259-021-05294-3.

# Chapter 13
# Evaluation and Management of Dysphagia During the COVID-19 Pandemic

**Peter K. M. Ku, Alexander C. Vlantis, Raymond Fong, Zenon W. C. Yeung, Erin P. L. So, Thomas Law, Ryan H. W. Cho, Jason Y. K. Chan, Becky Y. T. Chan, Eddy W. Y. Wong, Kathy Y. S. Lee, Andrew van Hasselt, and Michael C. F. Tong**

## Introduction

The global healthcare system has faced an unprecedented challenge since the declaration of the global novel coronavirus disease 2019 (COVID-19) pandemic by the World Health Organization (WHO) on March 12, 2020. On June 13, 2021 the number of confirmed COVID-19 cases had exceeded the number of cases that were reported as of April 1, 2020 by over 218-fold, which were 800,000 [1]. Although

P. K. M. Ku (✉) · Z. W. C. Yeung · R. H. W. Cho
Department of Otorhinolaryngology, Head and Neck Surgery, United Christian Hospital and Tseung Kwan O Hospital, Hong Kong, China

Department of Otorhinolaryngology, Head and Neck Surgery, The Chinese University of Hong Kong, Shatin, New Territories, Hong Kong

A. C. Vlantis · R. Fong · T. Law · J. Y. K. Chan · K. Y. S. Lee · A. van Hasselt · M. C. F. Tong
Department of Otorhinolaryngology, Head and Neck Surgery,
The Chinese University of Hong Kong, Shatin, New Territories, Hong Kong
e-mail: lexvlantis@ent.cuhk.edu.hk; raymondfong@ent.cuhk.edu.hk; thomaslaw@ent.cuhk.edu.hk; leeys@ent.cuhk.edu.hk; andrewvan@ent.cuhk.edu.hk; mtong@ent.cuhk.edu.hk

E. P. L. So · B. Y. T. Chan
Department of Speech Therapy, Prince of Wales Hospital,
Shatin, New Territories, Hong Kong
e-mail: cyt628@ha.org.hk

E. W. Y. Wong
Department of Otorhinolaryngology, Head and Neck Surgery,
The Chinese University of Hong Kong, Shatin, New Territories, Hong Kong

Department of Ear, Nose and Throat, Prince of Wales Hospital,
Shatin, New Territories, Hong Kong


S. Adibi et al. (eds.), *Frontiers of COVID-19*,
https://doi.org/10.1007/978-3-031-08045-6_13

this pandemic has commanded tremendous resources from healthcare systems, it must be remembered that patients with other illnesses still require medical attention.

Dysphagia is a global healthcare burden that requires multidisciplinary care. In 2019, Hong Kong public hospitals reported 101,840 inpatient and 8,736 outpatient attendances for dysphagia management. Patients with strokes, degenerative neurological diseases, cancers, trauma, head and neck infections, and musculoskeletal diseases may experience dysphagia and aspiration which require evaluation. Besides bedside assessment, a fiberoptic endoscopic evaluation of swallowing (FEES) and a videofluoroscopic swallow study (VFSS) are commonly used to assess the swallowing function of patients. As FEES and VFSS both have advantages and limitations in the assessment of swallowing, they can supplement each other.

During the COVID-19 pandemic, most elective services performed in hospitals have been suspended to accommodate patients with confirmed COVID-19. On January 28, 2020 the dysphagia clinic at the Prince of Wales Hospital was suspended due to the onset of the local outbreak of COVID-19 in Hong Kong and the subsequent global shortage of personal protective equipment (PPE). As the duration of the COVID-19 pandemic has exceeded that of the 2003 severe acute respiratory syndrome (SARS) pandemic, a practical workflow has become necessary to manage dysphagia and to avoid a backlog of patients while protecting the safety of patients and healthcare workers.

## Mode of Transmission of SARS-CoV-2 Infection

Reports of severe acute respiratory syndrome coronavirus 2 (SARS-CoV-2) transmission by droplets and aerosol production may be confusing and seem to imply differing risks of viral transmission, which would then require different specifications for PPE. In fact, aerosols are smaller-sized droplets (usually <5 μm in diameter) that may penetrate surgical masks and can remain suspended in air for longer and travel further than larger droplets can. For these reasons, high-level PPE such as an N95 respirator is required during any aerosol-generating procedure (AGP). However, few studies have attempted to verify specific AGPs other than by generalization and rationalization at the beginning of the outbreak, and according to observation and expert opinion [2]. Therefore, we have conducted our clinical work according to current evidence.

The SARS-CoV-2 virus spreads primarily through droplets of saliva when an infected person coughs or through droplets of nasal mucus when an infected person sneezes, and so it is important to take precautions seriously and to practice respiratory etiquette. Current evidence indicates that coughing can generate droplets ranging from 0.1 to 100 μm in size, which includes the range of aerosol generation [3]. Consequently, we can simply categorize a FEES as a procedure that induces coughing as an aerosol generating procedure, and accordingly we should adopt a high level of PPE including a face shield or goggles and an N95. This is especially important when testing laryngeal sensation using an air-pulse stimulator, which fires air pulses with pressures of 2–10 mmHg at 50 ms intervals to elicit reflexive vocal cord twitching prior to an endoscopic swallowing examination [4]. Air pulses may either create a pharyngeal air current or induce coughing if the air pressure is high, both of which can generate droplets and aerosols.

The risk of transmission of SARS-Co-2, the pathogen responsible for COVID-19, during nasal endoscopic surgery has elicited concerns from neurosurgeons, otolaryngologists and respiratory physicians regarding the level of PPE required during any trans-nasal procedure. These concerns increased further after reports of healthcare workers being infected during trans-nasal endoscopic intracranial surgery [5], which suggests a potentially higher level of viral shredding in the nasal cavity. Recent reports of hyposmia, anosmia, and dysgeusia in many confirmed that COVID-19 cases further support this observation [6]. Recent reports suggest R0 values of 5.71–7.23 for SARS-CoV-2 [7], which are higher than the values reported for SARS-CoV in 2003 [8]. Therefore, SARS-CoV-2 is far more infectious than SARS was, which may explain the seemingly uncontrolled pandemic situation in many countries.

## The Characteristics of Dysphagia in Patients After Recovery from COVID-19

Several studies [9–13] have been published recently which provide an understanding of the characteristics of dysphagia post COVD-19 as the attention in the pandemic shifts from acute critical care to care along a continuum including rehabilitation. Early studies on this issue have used observational cohort studies [9, 10, 14] and case reports [11, 13, 15]. The methodology varied but most described the prevalence and characteristics of dysphagia based on clinical evaluation and functional outcomes of swallowing [9, 10, 14]. This is understandable as it has been stated in guidelines that instrumental assessment of swallowing should only be considered when necessary during the pandemic [16].

In one of the largest cohorts studied, 208 COVID-19 patients who were referred for swallowing assessment were profiled in terms of dysphagia presentation and management [10]. Of the 208 patients, 49.0% (102/208) were admitted to an intensive care unit and 39.4% (82/208) underwent a tracheostomy [10]. Of the patients assessed, 21% (39/193) were recommended altered (thickened) fluids while 76% (145/193) were recommended modified diets [10]. The longitudinal data for this cohort is not available as many of them were transferred to community rehabilitation beds. The study concluded that patients with a tracheostomy require more speech language therapy sessions than those without or who were not admitted to an intensive care unit [10]. In a study from Ireland, 100 patients who had been intubated were studied. In the cohort 90% (90/100) had some alteration of their oral intake, 59% (59/100) were on tube feeding and 36% (36/100) could not tolerate any oral feeding [14]. Risk factors were analyzed and age, pre-existing respiratory conditions prior to COVID-19 and the use of the prone position during treatment of the respiratory system were predictors of severe dysphagia [14]. In this group, 37% (37/100) of patients received dysphagia rehabilitation and 27% (27/100) voice rehabilitation. On discharge from hospital, 27% (27/100) had residual dysphagia and 37% (37/100) residual dysphonia [14]. Although the prevalence varied across studies and the studied populations were not homogeneous, there is a general consensus that patients with COVID-19 are at risk of subsequently developing dysphagia.

Several case studies of COVID-19 patients with dysphagia have been published. In one report, a patient needed a tracheostomy for a right vocal fold paralysis and a left vocal fold paresis due to an undetermined cause post COVD-19 [11]. The patient received medical therapy and swallowing rehabilitation and eventually the patient resumed oral feeding and was decannulated after the function of the left hemilarynx returned [11]. Another case study reported impaired sensation of the pharynx and larynx which was postulated to contribute to swallowing dysfunction [13].

In summarizing the findings of published literature, the mechanisms of dysphagia in COVID-19 patients include pharyngo-laryngeal trauma and prolonged intubation associated with mechanical ventilation, neuromuscular, and neurosensory pathology associated with disuse and critical illness, the use of the prone position, and respiration-swallow discoordination in patients with respiratory compromise. In one of the cohort studies, there was a significant positive correlation ($p < 0.01$) between number of days intubated and the latency to resuming oral intake (from the intubation date) in patients with or without tracheostomy [10]. In another study of 164 patients, of which 78.7% (129/164) had been intubated and 52.4% (86/164) had been tracheostomized, it was concluded that both intubation and premorbid impairment were important factors as to whether dysphagia would persist or not, although it could not be established statistically that patients with dysphagia had been intubated for longer [9].

Neuromuscular weakness and sensory problems were also present in some patients with dysphagia post COVID-19. One study found that 13.4% (19/164) of patients developed new neurological deficits compared with their baselines [9]. In a treatment study using pharyngeal stimulation, it was reported that the stimulation level was abnormally high at the first session, which could be due to impaired pharyngeal sensation [15]. This was also supported by a case report of a patient with neurosensory dysphagia who had no sensation as indicated by the absence of a cough reflex when an endoscope was introduced into the laryngeal inlet [13]. The authors of that study postulated that a common pathogenic background could exist that accounted for the sensory problem in the pharynx and larynx, together with anosmia and ageusia, which are common symptoms of COVID-19 patients [13]. Disuse atrophy, a long sedation period and the use of neuromuscular blockers were also hypothesized to lead to muscle weakness, which could lead to impaired bolus propulsion in the oral cavity and the pharynx, impaired laryngeal closure and ultimately aspiration [11]. This was supported by the hypothesis that stroke, encephalopathy, critical illness neuropathy, and skeletal muscle injury were all possible as a direct or indirect consequence of COVID-19 [17]. With such causes, the swallowing pathway from the cortical level to the central pattern generator in the brainstem, cranial nerves, and muscles responsible for swallowing could all be affected [17].

Some authors have proposed that the use of the prone position, which is a strategy to improve oxygen saturation levels in COVID-19 patients [12], could have negative effects on the swallowing mechanism and increase the risk of aspiration pneumonia. The rationale is that the position predisposes patients to aspiration of saliva and secretions and makes it difficult for healthcare workers to perform regular oral hygiene [12]. However, this was not confirmed in a study of 164 patients and proning did not affect the prevalence of dysphonia or dysphagia [9]. The authors suggested that further investigation of the duration of proning and its effects on swallowing and voice should be studied [9]. In conclusion, the causes of dysphagia in patients with COVID-19 are likely to be multi-factorial. The clinical course of patients could affect the outcome of swallowing, while the neurological involvement by the disease and the treatment provided for the respiratory system could also affect swallowing to differing degrees.

## Videofluoroscopic Swallowing Study Findings After Severe COVID-19

A VFSS has often been used to assess swallow function as it is able to visualize the swallowing process across phases. Reports of swallowing function using videofluoroscopy in patients with COVID-19 are limited, presumably due to the novel disease and the risks of infection in conducting the examination [16]. In a cohort of 164 patients who were referred for speech and swallowing management, only 4.3% (7/164) had undergone a VFSS [9]. In a study of 21 patients with COVID-19, VFSS was performed just before or at most 14 days after discharge from the intensive care unit [18]. It was found that 90.5% (19/21) of the patients had dysphagia. Findings confirmed that patients were likely to have sensory problems in their pharynx and larynx, as was found in 71.4% (15/21) of patients with penetration/aspiration during swallowing who did so silently, and in 23.8% (5/21) who had penetration/aspiration after swallowing of pharyngeal residue and who also did so silently [18]. In terms of swallowing physiology, results showed problems in the oral phase with lip seal impairment (14.3%; 3/21), impaired tongue control leading to posterior spillage (42.9%; 9/21), and a prolonged oral phase (23.8%; 5/21) [18]. In the pharyngeal phase, delayed initiation of swallow (71.4%; 15/21) and reduced tongue base retraction (57.1%; 12/21) were prominent, while impaired pharyngeal contraction (33.3%; 7/21) and laryngeal vestibule closure (42.9%; 9/21) were also present in some patients [18].

The preliminary findings of this study were that swallowing was affected in both oral and pharyngeal phases. The most significant finding that concurred with the hypothesis and case reports was the high prevalence of penetration/aspiration without response in the cohort, which could suggest sensory deficits may be one of the main factors for dysphagia [18]. As instrumental assessment is needed to confirm the presence of such "silent" penetration or aspiration, the use of FEES and VFSS should be considered once the risk of infection to the healthcare workers has been taken into account. It has been recommended that FEES could be considered for patients 7–10 days after extubation as this would strike a balance between the patient's condition and their clinical needs [13].

## Clinic Setup and Precautions Necessary When Assessing Patients with Dysphagia During the COVID-19 Pandemic

In our experience with FEES procedures at the Prince of Wales Hospital, relatively few patients experience intense intraprocedural sneezing and coughing that led to the termination of the investigation. In a review of 982 patients seen at our dysphagia clinic, we found that 78% had an impaired laryngeal protective reflex while a similar proportion had lost their gag reflex. The incidence of coughing and sneezing should be low in these patients when the pharynx is not over sensitive to instrumentation and when using fiberoptic endoscopes of a smaller diameter. However, researchers have noted that even oral speaking can transmit SARS-CoV-2 via droplets, especially important when patients are generally not able to wear face masks during swallowing evaluations [19]. Therefore, healthcare workers must be mindful of this when considering endoscopic examinations during this critical period. If possible, FEES and VFSS procedures for high-risk patients with COVID-19 (according to their history and symptomatology) should be postponed until the patient is no longer considered to be infectious and reconsidered for a swallowing study when safe and at a later date. For urgent cases, a polymerase chain reaction (PCR) test for SARS-CoV-2 should be done prior to any swallowing evaluation. Here, VFSS is superior to FEES because it does not involve intraprocedural instrumentation and the operators can maintain a distance from the patient. However, VFSS must be performed in a radiology suite. In contrast, FEES is more ambulatory, has lower setup costs and can be conducted at the bedside. We prefer to perform FEES and VFSS with IQAir® HealthPro® (Incen AG, Switzerland) facilities with a high efficiency particulate air or HEPA class H13 filtration system which can filter out 99.97% of all particles >0.3 μm (Fig. 13.1). The number of healthcare workers in the consultation room at any one time should be minimized. All healthcare workers should wear personal protective equipment with an N95 respirator and a face shield if an AGP is anticipated in the swallowing clinic. Direct vision through the flexible endoscope by clinicians should be avoided, instead a monitor should be used to observe the findings during endoscopic assessment of the pharyngo-larynx and swallowing functions. This helps to keep a distance between the endoscopist and the patient to minimize the risk of cross-infection. Figure 13.2 summarizes our workflow for swallowing evaluations in patients with dysphagia during the COVID-19 pandemic.

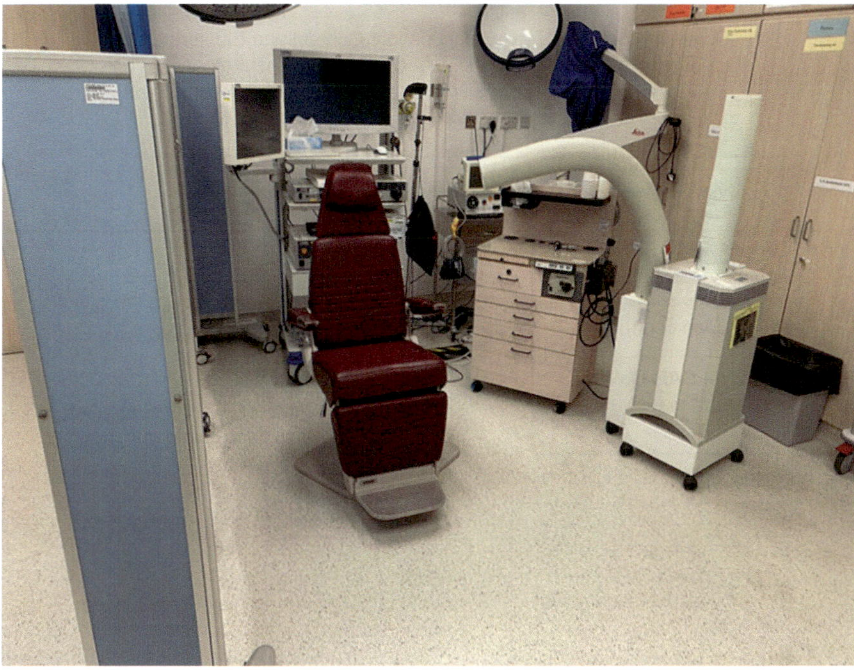

**Fig. 13.1** Audiovisual facilities for fiberoptic endoscopic evaluation of swallowing with an IQAir® air filter in the room

## The Selection of Patients with Dysphagia and the Selection of Their Assessment During the COVID-19 Pandemic

In certain facilities, screening tests are carried out as routine procedures. Patients who fail are referred to speech-language pathologists (SLPs) for clinical swallowing evaluation. Patients who pass or are in facilities without routine screening tests may also be referred if there are any concerns indicating the need for a more detailed assessment. For instance, if family members express concerns related to swallowing and feeding or if physicians need to elucidate the relationship between dysphagia and a medical condition including but not limited to dehydration, malnutrition, weight loss, and recurrent pneumonia [20].

A bedside swallowing examination is the first step in the swallowing assessment done by SLPs for almost all patients. There are several circumstances that prompt SLPs to proceed with an instrumental examination after a clinical swallowing evaluation. First, when a patient's signs of oropharyngeal dysphagia are inconsistent with their swallowing physiologies of the bedside examination. Second, when silent aspiration is strongly suspected. Third, when there is an unexplained repeated chest infection. Fourth, when documentation of progress is required before/ during/ after

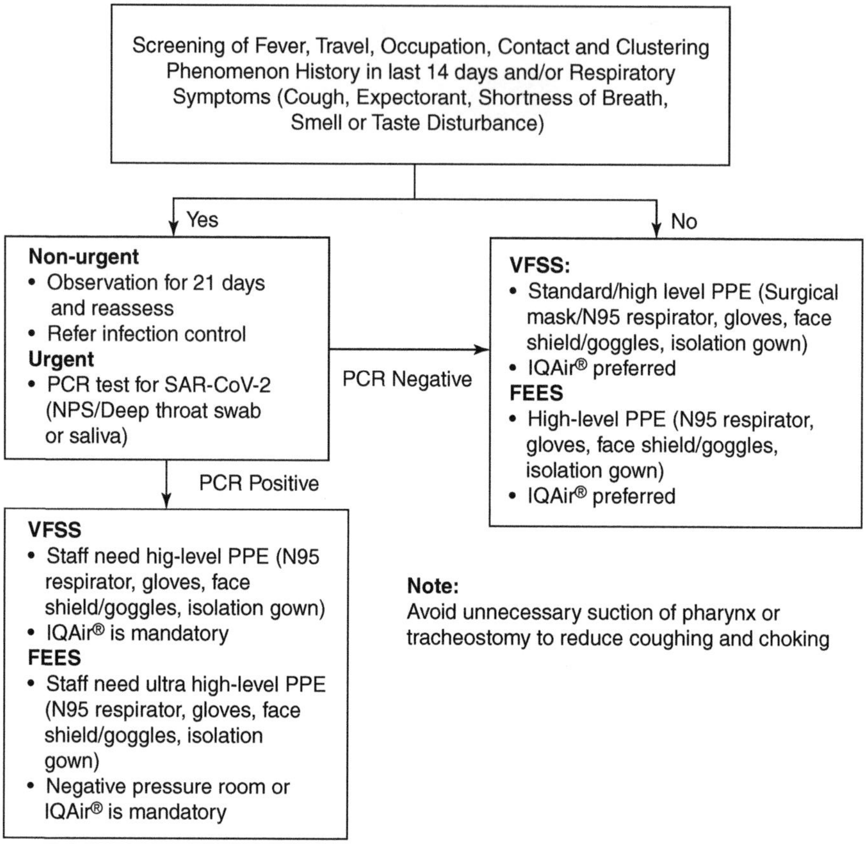


**Fig. 13.2** Workflow for swallowing studies in patients during the COVID-19 pandemic. *NPS* nasopharyngeal swab, *PPE* personal protective equipment, *PCR* polymerase chain reaction, *PAPR* positive airway pressure respirator, *SAR-CoV-2* novel coronavirus

rehabilitation. Lastly, when appropriate intervention strategies need to be determined [21]. Objective information and measurements are required for all these conditions, and are applicable for both FEES and VFSS.

There are occasions when SLPs prefer FEES to VFSS or vice versa. The selection of FEES is considered more appropriate if a direct or apparent visualization of nasopharyngeal and laryngeal structures is required, e.g., patients with suspected vocal cord pathology, asymmetrical pharyngeal contraction or a history of head and neck surgery, or if clinicians aim to clearly assess pharyngeal stasis post-swallow [24]. Nevertheless, contraindications include bilateral choanal atresia, a history of epistaxis and laryngospasm on insertion of the endoscope, severe confusion or poor cooperation for the procedure [22].

VFSS can be adopted if a patient is intolerant of FEES. Other indications favoring VFSS over FEES include the SLP's interest in the entire swallowing anatomy from the oral cavity to the upper esophagus, the function of the upper esophageal sphincter, and the exclusion of an anatomical anomaly such as an esophageal diverticulum [23]. Likewise, there are contraindications to VFSS, in particular, patients who are pregnant, who find it difficult to maintain the required physical position during the study, or who have a known history of an allergic reaction to contrast media [24].

If signs and symptoms of dysphagia persist after oropharyngeal dysphagia is ruled out as above, patients should be further assessed for possible esophageal dysphagia if symptoms are suggestive. Endoscopy is recommended as the first instrumental examination to exclude the presence of structural problems or inflammation. If found unremarkable, manometry is then suggested to evaluate for any esophageal dysmotility [25].

## Management of Dysphagia in Head and Neck Cancer Patients During the COVID-19 Pandemic: A Practical Strategy

While our routine clinical service has been reduced during the COVID-19 pandemic due to the global shortage of personal protective equipment and to minimize cross transmission of the SARS-CoV-2, our head and neck cancer service has been maintained as it has in numerous countries [26–30]. One of the common presentations of advanced head and neck cancer is dysphagia, occurring in up to 53–59% [31, 32] of patients with an associated mortality rate of 9% due to aspiration [32]. These dysphagic patients are often elderly, malnourished, immunocompromised and have multiple medical comorbidities such as diabetes, cardiovascular or cerebrovascular diseases, and who are more likely to suffer severe COVID-19 if they develop a SARS-CoV-2 infection [33]. Therefore, otolaryngologists and speech-language pathologists must stringently adhere to infection control measures to prevent cross transmission of infection while assessing and managing patients with dysphagia.

To minimize the chance of nosocomial infection, all patients who are admitted for head and neck cancer surgeries or swallowing assessments at our institution must be tested and confirmed to be negative for SARS-CoV-2 1–2 days prior to admission. The assessment of swallowing involves a wide range of tools including a bedside swallowing assessment, a fiberoptic endoscopic evaluation of swallowing, a videofluoroscopic swallowing study and cough reflex testing. These dysphagia screening tools may have the potential to lead to the generation of aerosols [16, 34]. Moreover, dysphagia rehabilitation and nursing care, for instance, feeding tube insertion or oral care, may also lead to aerosol generation, and potentially also cause cross transmission of infection to healthcare workers and other patients [33, 35, 36]. When direct patient contact is necessary, a distance of between 1 and 2 m (3–6 ft) should be maintained [16, 37, 38]. The highest level of personal protective equipment with a face shield or goggles, an N95 respirator, a waterproof gown and gloves should be worn. Assessment should be conducted by a skilled speech language pathologist with extensive experience in endoscopic procedures and be completed within a time frame of 10–15 min [16, 38]. Careful donning and doffing of isolation gowns is critical to minimize potential contamination. Hand hygiene should be carefully performed before and after attending to each patient using liquid soap and water when hands are visibly dirty or soiled with body fluid. When hands are not visibly soiled, hand hygiene with a 70–80% alcohol-based hand rub is an effective alternative [39].

Fiberoptic endoscopic evaluation of swallowing (FEES) and videofluoroscopic swallowing studies (VFSS) remain the two standard swallowing assessment tools for head and neck cancer patients. FEES involves the use of a fiberoptic endoscope to dynamically assess the anatomy of the pharynx, larynx and the presence of laryngeal penetration and aspiration of food materials into the airway [40]. FESS is considered to carry a higher risk of aerosolization when compared to VFSS, which involves the use of real-time X-ray to assess swallowing and aspiration into the airway. Therefore, VFSS is a preferable option to FEES in the context of the COVID-19 outbreak. During any swallowing assessment procedure, patients may sneeze and/or cough due to aspiration of food material, which may cause aerosolization, requiring proper personal protective equipment including N95 respirators to be worn by clinical staff.

A tracheostomy is prevalent in head and neck cancer patients. It is recommended that a closed suction system and a heat moisture exchanger should be used to protect clinical staff who are involved in nursing care. Nursing staff should be reminded that a tracheostomy wound dressing and a tracheostomy tube change are high risk procedures, necessitating personal protective equipment to be worn at these times. During suctioning, splashes must be anticipated due to coughing. Nursing staff should stand at the side of patients and not in front of patients to avoid tracheal secretions being coughed onto them by patients [33]. When in doubt, a tracheostomy tube or dressing change can be postponed until the COVID-19 status is confirmed to be negative unless there are obvious signs of soiling or infection [33]. When a tracheostomy tube is in place, the use of a close proximity IQAir HealthPro (Incen AG, Thal, Switzerland) air-filter is recommended. Such a filter is capable of removing 99.97% of all particles >0.3 μm from the environment and thus reduce environmental contamination by respiratory droplets [40].

## Implementation of Rehabilitation of Swallowing During the COVID-19 Pandemic: From the Acute Hospital to the Old Age Home

For the protection of patients and healthcare workers, guidelines for swallowing assessment and dysphagia management during the COVID-19 pandemic have been published by professional bodies and societies across the globe [35, 41, 42]. Early guidelines published by professional bodies such as the European Society for Swallowing Disorder recommended that no cough inducing techniques should be used for swallowing rehabilitation [41]. As a cough is an aerosol generating event, the avoidance of a cough in techniques such as the supraglottic swallow is advocated [41]. The guidelines also recommend that clinicians adopt primarily compensatory techniques such as postural modification, and fluid and diet modification instead of active rehabilitation exercises [41]. It also recommends that the treatment session duration should be as short as possible to minimize risk to healthcare workers. Guidelines from various societies have been reviewed [16] and conclude that, for dysphagia rehabilitation, techniques such as thermal tactile stimulation, and expiratory and inspiratory muscle strength training should also be avoided in patients diagnosed with COVID-19.

Apart from measures to reduce transmission risk, the review also advocated the change from an oxygen mask to a nasal cannula during oral feeding and rehabilitation if the patient's condition allows [16]. The importance of oral hygiene was stressed, as this could possibly reduce the risk of aspiration pneumonia [16]. Guidelines have also suggested that patients perform oral hygiene independently, if possible, to minimize the risk of transmission to healthcare workers during the process [41, 43]. On discharge from hospital, it is recommended that patients are followed up to normalize swallowing function as much as possible [16], as swallowing dysfunction in the long run could affect nutrition, hydration and quality of life. The use of telehealth technologies to facilitate follow-up of discharged patients is also recommended [40].

## Telemedicine and the Evaluation and Management of Patients with Dysphagia

Clinical swallowing evaluation should include instrumental and quantitative swallowing measures to allow objective documentation of swallowing functions. Many validated patient-reported outcome (PRO) measures and clinician-rated scales are available to assess the swallowing condition of patients suffering from dysphagia after treatment of a head and neck cancer. This assessment can also be implemented through telecare and is offered to patients who have no access to inpatient or outpatient care during the outbreak of COVID-19. The MD Anderson Dysphagia Inventory is a 20-item PRO that helps to assess the patient's perception of their dysphagia and is widely used in head and neck cancer patients [44, 45]. Other available swallowing specific PROs that can be used include the Royal Brisbane Hospital Outcome Measure for Swallowing (RBHOMS) [46], the Sydney Swallow Questionnaire [47] and EAT-10 [48]. There are several clinician related tools that can be applied to assess dysphagia and its outcomes in subjects presenting with swallowing difficulties. The Performance Status Scale Head and Neck (PSSHN) [49] is commonly used in head and neck cancer patients to evaluate the impact of dysphagia on their lives. Moreover, the Food Intake Level Scale (FILS) [50] and the

Functional Oral Intake Scale (FOIS) [51] can be used to document the level of their dysphagia diet based on the subject's swallowing status. All these measures provide invaluable information to clinicians when combined with the clinical history and findings on examination which guide the treatment plan and recommendations to allow for safe swallowing.

Swallowing therapy is also an important rehabilitation that should be implemented during the COVID-19 pandemic. This can be safely offered to subjects through telecare to minimize the risk of transmission of COVID-19, especially when mobile communication devices are so ubiquitous nowadays. There is further evidence which demonstrates the benefits of the application of telecare in swallowing training that has good compliance compared to traditional on-site therapy [52]. Clinicians should optimize the application of telecare to the patient's needs while it is not possible for them to access onsite clinical care and provide them with the same quality and standard. In Hong Kong, patients with a history of nasopharyngeal cancer and radiotherapy may find such mobile apps and telecare beneficial as they are relatively younger, knowledgeable in technology and open minded to innovative ideas [53]. While telecare does not allow routine oro-motor examination and other endoscopic procedures, they can still be offered in subsequent follow-ups during swallowing rehabilitation to review the progress and receive feedback from patients. Thus, clinicians may also adopt a more conservative approach to dysphagia management with close attention to potential markers of complications such as increased cough, fever and weight loss. Table 13.1 summarizes the guidelines for telemedicine for speech therapy and swallowing management.

**Table 13.1** Guidelines for telemedicine in speech therapy for voice and swallowing management

| | |
|---|---|
| *Type of patients* | 1. *Inpatient*<br>Active cases<br>2. *Outpatient/Day Hospital patients/CST patients*<br>Active cases<br>New cases with history known to the clinicians |
| *Selection criteria* | 1. Patients/carers receptive to tele-care<br>2. Problems that can be tackled by education, advice, monitoring and indirect training. For example:<br>*Dysphagia/feeding problem*<br>Monitoring of diet tolerance, meal observation, swallowing exercises, oromotor exercises, education on feeding techniques, and diet modification<br>*Voice disorder*<br>Voice therapy, vocal hygiene, alaryngeal speech training<br>*Acquired speech and language disorder*<br>Dysarthria and aphasia therapy, oromotor exercises<br>*Developmental speech and language disorder*<br>Articulation training, parent education on language facilitation skills |
| *Intervention* | Patient and career education and advice, home exercise and program prescription, home program delivery and monitoring, communication for discharge planning |

## Management of Dysphagia in the COVID-19 Era: A Multidisciplinary Approach

Dysphagia is more common than dysphonia in COVID-19 patients and may be associated with other symptoms such as choking, sore throat, shortness of breath, and copious sputum. Any patient who suffers from aspiration pneumonia after previous endotracheal intubation should be worked up properly by endoscopy and swallowing studies to rule out silent aspiration. The management of dysphagia requires a multidisciplinary approach to yield the optimal outcome of diagnostic and therapeutic measures. Otolaryngologists and speech language pathologists are two specialties who receive referrals for patients with oropharyngeal dysphagia and who can coordinate or manage the evaluation process [54]. Other members of the healthcare team such as neurologists, respiratory physicians, surgeons, radiologists, physiotherapists, and occupational therapists can be consulted for subsequent evaluation depending on the initial assessment on history, physical examination, bed-side swallowing examination, and specific swallowing studies such as FEES and VFSS. In the era of the COVID-19 pandemic, when a joint consultation is not feasible due to the potential risk of transmission of infection, a telecare consultation that involves multiple specialties is still possible based on existing technology and electronic communication devices [55]. This allows each member of the healthcare team to work together to accomplish the goal in the patient's care but still function independently [56]. This transdisciplinary model of service also allows a team member from different hospitals to participate in a patient's care and to solve difficult and complex swallowing problems [57].

## Conclusions

During the current COVID-19 pandemic with healthcare systems under unprecedented pressure, priority must be given to the safety of healthcare workers and patients. Dysphagia can result in complications such as aspiration pneumonia and should be addressed in patients following decannulation after endotracheal intubation or tracheostomy. Asymptomatic carriers can be screened with a suitable PCR test prior to swallowing assessment. An instrumental swallowing study of a high-risk COVID-19 patient with acute respiratory symptoms can be safely performed with suitable precautions. Alternatively, in high-risk patients, the assessment of their swallowing function can be possible through tele-medicine using various non-instrumental methods. Telecare can also be used to implement swallowing training, monitoring and progress review during rehabilitation.

## References


1. World Health Organization. Coronavirus disease 2019 (COVID): situation report 72. World Health Organization; 2020. https://www.who.int/docs/default-source/coronaviruse/situation-reports/20200401-sitrep-72-covid-19.pdf?sfvrsn=3dd8971b_2. Accessed 17 June 2021.
2. Thamboo A, Lea J, Sommer DD, et al. Clinical evidence based review and recommendations of aerosol generating medical procedures in otolaryngology—head and neck surgery during the COVID-19 pandemic. J Otolaryngol Head Neck Surg. 2020;49(1):28.
3. Lindsley WG, Pearce TA, Hudnall JB, et al. Quantity and size distribution of cough-generated aerosol particles produced by influenza patients during and after illnesses. J Occup Environ Hyg. 2012;9(7):443–9.
4. Ku PK, Vlantis AC, Leung SF, et al. Laryngopharyngeal sensory deficits and impaired pharyngeal motor function predict aspiration in patients irradiated for nasopharyngeal carcinoma. Laryngoscope. 2010;120(2):223–8.
5. China Newsweek. Recovering the infective route of "super-spreaders". Published January 25, 2020. http://view.inews.qq.com/a/20200125A07TT200?uid=&devid=BDFE70CD-5BF1-4702-91B7-329F20A6E839&qimei=bdfe70cd-5bf1-4702-91b7-329f20a6e839. Accessed 17 June 2021.
6. Patel ZM, Fernandez-Miranda J, Hwang PH, et al. Precautions for endoscopic transnasal skull base surgery during the COVID-19 pandemic. American Academy of Otolaryngology-Head and Neck Surgery, Coronavirus Disease 2019: resources. Published March 23, 2020. https://www.entnet.org/sites/default/files/uploads/covid-19_endosb_lettertoeditor_neurosurgery_update3.23.20.pdf. Accessed 17 June 2021.
7. Tang B, Wang X, Li Q, et al. Estimation of the transmission risk of the 2019-nCoV and its implication for public health interventions. J Clin Med. 2020;9(2):462.
8. World Health Organization. Consensus document on the epidemiology of SARS. Wkly Epidemol Rec. 2003;78:373–5. https://www.who.int/csr/sars/en/WHOconsensus.pdf. Accessed 17 June 2021.
9. Archer SK, Iezzi CM, Gilpin L. Swallowing and voice outcomes in patients hospitalized with COVID-19: an observational cohort study. Arch Phys Med Rehabil. 2021;102(6):1084–90.
10. Dawson C, Capewell R, Ellis S, Matthews S, Adamson S, Wood M, et al. Dysphagia presentation and management following COVID-19: an acute care tertiary centre experience. J Laryngol Otol. 2020;1–6. https://doi.org/10.1017/S0022215120002443.
11. De Vincentis G, Ferrari C, Rocco DG. Severe oropharyngeal dysphagia following COVID-19: a case report. Clin Case Rep. 2021;9(3):1539–43.
12. Mohan R, Mohapatra B. Shedding light on dysphagia associated with COVID-19: the what and why. OTO Open. 2020;4(2):2473974X20934770. https://doi.org/10.1177/2473974X20934770.
13. Zanon A, Cacciaguerra L, Martelli G, Filippi M. Neurosensory dysphagia in a COVID-19 patient. J Neurol. 2021;19:1–3. https://doi.org/10.1007/s00415-021-10541-6.
14. Regan J, Walshe M, Lavan S, Horan E, Gillivan-Murphy P, Healy A, et al. Post-extubation dysphagia and dysphonia amongst adults with COVID-19 in the Republic of Ireland: a prospective multi-site observational cohort study. Clin Otolaryngol. 2021;46(6):1290–9.
15. Traugott M, Hoepler W, Kitzberger R, Pavlata S, Seitz T, Baumgartner S, et al. Successful treatment of intubation-induced severe neurogenic post-extubation dysphagia using pharyngeal electrical stimulation in a COVID-19 survivor: a case report. J Med Case Rep. 2021;15(1):148.
16. Vergara J, Skoretz SA, Brodsky MB, Miles A, Langmore SE, Wallace S, et al. Assessment, diagnosis, and treatment of dysphagia in patients infected with SARS-CoV-2: a review of the literature and international guidelines. Am J Speech Lang Pathol. 2020;29(4):2242–53.
17. Dziewas R, Warnecke T, Zurcher P, Schefold JC. Dysphagia in COVID-19 -multilevel damage to the swallowing network? Eur J Neurol. 2020;27(9):e46–7.
18. Lagier A, Melotte E, Poncelet M, Remacle S, Meunier P. Swallowing function after severe COVID-19: early videofluoroscopic findings. Eur Arch Otorhinolaryngol. 2021;3:1–5. https://doi.org/10.1007/s00405-020-06522-6.

19. Eiche T, Kuster M. Aerosol release by healthy people during speaking: possible contribution to the transmission of SARS-CoV-2. Int J Environ Res Public Health. 2020;17(23):9088.
20. Goodwich SJ, Walker AI. Clinical swallow evaluation. In: Leonard R, Kendall K, editors. Dysphagia assessment and treatment planning: a team approach. Plural Publishing; 2017. p. 37–52.
21. Hong Kong Institute of Speech Therapists Limited. Guideline of Videofluoroscopic Swallowing Study (VFSS) in speech therapy. Published September 17, 2019. https://hkist.org.hk/static/guideline-of-videofluoroscopic-swallowing-study-vfss-in-speech-therapy.pdf. Accessed 28 Apr 2021.
22. Birchall O, Bennett M, Lawson N, Cotton S, Vogel AP. Fiberoptic endoscopic evaluation of swallowing and videofluoroscopy swallowing assessment in adults in residential care facilities; a scoping review protocol. JBI Evid Synth. 2020;18(3):599–609.
23. Erman A, Chhetri DK. Modified barium swallow study. In: Dysphagia evaluation and management in otolaryngology. Elsevier; 2019. p. 63–72.
24. Royal College of Speech and Language Therapists. Videofluoroscopic evaluation of oropharyngeal swallowing function (VFS): the role of speech and language therapists RCSLT position paper 2013. 2013. Published June 1, 2021. https://rcslt.org/wp-content/uploads/media/Project/RCSLT/videofluoroscopic-position-paper.pdf. Accessed 17 June 2021.
25. Liu LW, Andrews CN, Armstrong D, et al. Clinical practice guidelines for the assessment of uninvestigated esophageal dysphagia. J Can Assoc Gastroenterol. 2018;1(1):5–19.
26. Lee AK, Cho RH, Lau EH, Cheng HK, Wong EW, Ku PK, et al. Mitigation of head and neck cancer service disruption during COVID-19 in Hong Kong through telehealth and multi-institutional collaboration. Head Neck. 2020;42(7):1454–9.
27. COVIDSurg Collaborative. Head and neck cancer surgery during the COVID-19 pandemic: an international, multicenter, observational cohort study. Cancer. 2020;127(14):2476–88. https://doi.org/10.1002/cncr.33320.
28. Fakhry N, Schultz P, Moriniere S, Breuskin I, Bozec A, Vergez S, et al. French consensus on management of head and neck cancer surgery during COVID-19 pandemic. Eur Ann Otorhinolaryngol Head Neck Dis. 2020;137(3):159–60.
29. Jain S, Gupta S, Singh TP, Chhabra K, Jain R, Sohi AS, et al. Short term outcomes of head and neck oncology surgery during COVID-19 pandemic: experience from a tertiary cancer care centre in North India. Indian J Otolaryngol Head Neck Surg. 2021;8:1–5.
30. Riva G, Pizzo C, Fassone E, Pecorari G. Head and neck cancer surgery in COVID-19 pandemic in northern Italy. Oral Oncol. 2020;107:104835. https://doi.org/10.1016/j.oraloncology.2020.104835.
31. Langerman A, Maccracken E, Kasza K, Haraf DJ, Vokes EE, Stenson KM. Aspiration in chemoradiated patients with head and neck cancer. Arch Otolaryngol Head Neck Surg. 2007;133(12):1289–95.
32. Nguyen NP, Frank C, Moltz CC, Vos P, Smith HJ, Bhamidipati PV, et al. Aspiration rate following chemoradiation for head and neck cancer: an underreported occurrence. Radiother Oncol. 2006;80(3):302–6.
33. Kimura Y, Ueha R, Furukawa T, Oshima F, Fujitani J, Nakajima J, et al. Society of swallowing and dysphagia of Japan: position statement on dysphagia management during the COVID-19 outbreak. Auris Nasus Larynx. 2020;47(5):715–26.
34. Bolton L, Mills C, Wallace S, Brady MC, Royal College of S, Language Therapists C-AG. Aerosol generating procedures, dysphagia assessment and COVID-19: a rapid review. Int J Lang Commun Disord. 2020;55(4):629–36.
35. American Speech-Language-Hearing Association. ASHA guidance to SLPs regarding aerosol generating procedures. Published April 12, 2021. https://www.asha.org/SLP/healthcare/ASHA-Guidance-to-SLPs-Regarding-Aerosol-Generating-Procedures/. Accessed 17 June 2021.
36. Dysphagia Research Society. COVID-19 information and resources: risk management of AGPs for dysphagia care. Published October 1, 2020. https://www.dysphagiaresearch.org/page/COVID19AGPs. Accessed 17 June 2021.

37. Mattei A, Amy de la Breteque B, Crestani S, Crevier-Buchman L, Galant C, Hans S, et al. Guidelines of clinical practice for the management of swallowing disorders and recent dysphonia in the context of the COVID-19 pandemic. Eur Ann Otorhinolaryngol Head Neck Dis. 2020;137(3):173–5.
38. Royal College of Speech and Language Therapists. Speech and language therapist-led endoscopic procedures: considerations for all patents during the COVID-19 pandemic. Published April 2021. Accessed 17 June 2021.
39. Centre for Health Protection. Perform hand hygiene properly. Hong Kong Special Administration Region. Published January 2020. Accessed 17 June 2021.
40. Ku PK, Holsinger FC, Chan JY, et al. Management of dysphagia in the patient with head and neck cancer during COVID-19 pandemic: practical strategy. Head Neck. 2020;42(7):1491–6.
41. Schindler A, Baijens LW, Clave P, et al. ESSD commentary on dysphagia management during COVID pandemia. Dysphagia. 2021;36:1–4. https://doi.org/10.1007/soo455-020-10194-z.
42. Speech Pathology Australia. Speech Pathology Australia guidance for service delivery, clinical procedures and infection control during COVID-19 pandemic. Published August 24, 2020. Accessed 17 June 2021.
43. Miles A, Connor NP, Desai RV, et al. Dysphagia care across the continuum: a multidisciplinary dysphagia research society taskforce report of service-delivery during the COVID-19 global pandemic. Dysphagia. 2021;36(2):170–82.
44. Chen AY, Frankowski R, Bishop-Leone J, et al. The development and validation of a dysphagia-specific quality-of-life questionnaire for patients with head and neck cancer: the M.D. Anderson dysphagia inventory. Arch Otolaryngol Head Neck Surg. 2001;127(7):870–6.
45. Zhang LJ, Jiang N, Li Z, et al. Psychometric properties of the Chinese version of the M.D. Anderson dysphagia inventory for head and neck cancer patients. Cancer Nurs. 2017;40(3):E9–E16.
46. Ward EC, Conroy AL. Validity, reliability and responsivity of the Royal Bisbrane hospital outcome measure for swallowing. Asian Pacific J Speech Lang Hear. 1999;4(2):109–29.
47. Dwivedi RC, St Rose S, Roe JW, et al. Validation of the Sydney swallow questionnaire (SSQ) in a cohort of head and neck cancer patients. Oral Oncol. 2010;46(4):e10–4.
48. Belafsky PC, Mouadeb DA, Rees CJ, et al. Validity and reliability of the eating assessment tool (EAT-10). Ann Otol Rhinol Laryngol. 2008;117(12):919–24.
49. List MA, D'Antonio LL, Cella DF, et al. The performance status scale for head and neck cancer patients and the functional assessment of cancer therapy-head and neck scale. A study of utility and validity. Cancer. 1996;77(11):2294–301.
50. Kunieda K, Ohno T, Fujishima I, Hojo K, Morita T. Reliability and validity of a tool to measure the severity of dysphagia: the food intake LEVEL scale. J Pain Symptom Manag. 2013;46(2):201–6.
51. Crary MA, Mann GD, Groher ME. Initial psychometric assessment of a functional oral intake scale for dysphagia in stroke patients. Arch Phys Med Rehabil. 2005;86(8):1516–20.
52. Wall LR, Ward EC, Cartmill B. Adherence to a prophylactic swallowing therapy program during (chemo) radiotherapy: impact of service delivery model and patient factors. Dysphagia. 2017;32(2):279–92.
53. Starmer HM, Abrams R, Webster K, et al. Feasibility of a mobile application to enhance swallowing therapy for patients undergoing radiation-based treatment for head and neck cancer. Dysphagia. 2018;33(2):227–33.
54. Coutts KA. Dysphagia services in the era of COVID-19: are speech-language therapists essential? S Afr J Commun Disord. 2020;67(1):e1–6.
55. Ward EC, Burns CL, Theodoros DG, Russell TG. Impact of dysphagia severity on clinical decision making via telerehabilitation. Telemed J E Health. 2014;20(4):296–303.
56. Magnus VS, Turkington L. Communication interaction in ICU—patient and staff experiences and perceptions. Intensive Crit Care Nurs. 2006;22(3):167–80.
57. Van Bewer V. Transdisciplinarity in health care: a concept analysis. Nurs Forum. 2017;52(4):339–47.

# Chapter 14
# Gastrointestinal Manifestations of COVID-19 and Inflammatory Bowel Disease in the COVID-19 Era: Clinical Overview and Updated Guidelines

**Sarah El-Nakeep**

## Abbreviations

| | |
|---|---|
| ACE-2 | Angiotensin-converting enzyme 2 |
| AGA | American Gastroenterology Association |
| APAGE | Asian Pacific Association of Gastroenterology |
| B0AT1 | Neutral amino acid transporter |
| CD | Crohn's disease |
| COVID | Coronavirus disease |
| ECCO | European Crohn's and Colitis Organization |
| GI | Gastrointestinal |
| GIP | Gastric inhibitory peptide |
| GIT | Gastrointestinal tract |
| GLP-1 | Glucagon like peptide-1 |
| IBD | Inflammatory bowel disease |
| IOIBD | International Organization for the Study of Inflammatory Bowel Disease |
| OR | Odds ratio |
| PCR | Polymerase chain reaction |
| SARS-CoV2 | Severe acute respiratory syndrome coronavirus 2 |
| SECURE-IBD | Surveillance Epidemiology of Coronavirus Under Research Exclusion |
| TMPRSS2 | Transmembrane protease, serine 2 enzyme |
| TNF-α | Tumor necrosis factor alpha |
| UC | Ulcerative colitis |

S. El-Nakeep (✉)
Gastroenterology and Hepatology Unit, Internal Medicine Department, Faculty of Medicine, Ain Shams University, Cairo, Egypt
e-mail: sarahnakeep@med.asu.edu.eg


S. Adibi et al. (eds.), *Frontiers of COVID-19*,
https://doi.org/10.1007/978-3-031-08045-6_14

## Gastrointestinal Manifestations

### *Clinical Background and Pathogenesis of Gastrointestinal Manifestations in COVID-19*

The clinical concentration when dealing with the current coronavirus pandemic is always shifted to the respiratory manifestations, including pneumonia, and respiratory failure associated with the systemic inflammatory response of the virus. However, GI manifestations are a common presentation of the disease, either initially before the respiratory symptoms or concurrent with them, and they could help in establishing the severity of the illness and its prognosis. Several studies researched the viral shedding and GI infectivity of the COVID-19 disease and their effect on the disease course [1, 2]. This chapter aims to discuss the current situation regarding the GI manifestation presented in COVID-19 infection.

Recurrent GI manifestations association with coronaviruses' infection was previously explained in the literature by "Tropism" to the gastrointestinal tract observed in coronavirus infection [3]. The colon, terminal ileum, and esophageal mucosa possess the highest prevalence of angiotensin-converting enzyme 2 (ACE-2) receptors expression reaching 30%, thus these areas are at high risk for SARS-CoV-2 infection. In contrast, the liver and the stomach show a lower receptor expression prevalence of <1%, with lower risk of infection [4, 5].

Viral shedding causes spreading of infection, which takes place through fecal-oral or fecal-aerosol respiratory routes [6], *please see* Fig. 14.1. This viral shedding is apparent through the presence of the virus in the stool and anal samples of 43%

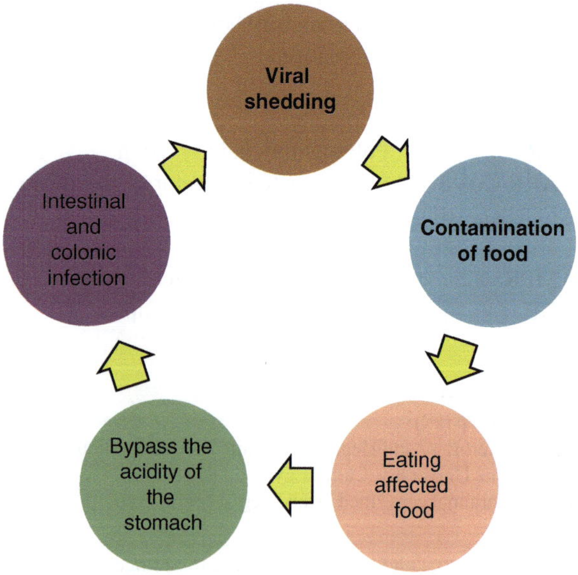


**Fig. 14.1** Showing vicious circle of feco-oral infection

of infected patients, as detected by viral polymerase chain reaction (PCR) [7]. Moreover, acidity of the stomach does not appear to cause destruction of the corona viral particles, as live virus is present in the stool of the patients, which renders the feco-oral route for COVID-19 infection a plausible one. However, gut infection does not result in systemic viremia as in the case of respiratory infection [8, 9].

Furthermore, ACE-2 receptors have an important role in amino acid metabolism, as the entry of tryptophan through the *B0AT1* (*neutral amino acid transporter*) receptors causes the induction of an antimicrobial response, along with the induction of incretins' release (glucagon like peptide-1 (GLP-1) and gastric inhibitory peptide (GIP) responsible for glucose metabolism). As a result, deficiency of tryptophan metabolism and cellular entry causes dysbiosis and hyperglycemia in COVID-19 patients. This dysbiosis enhances the growth of opportunistic bacteria, increases lipopolysaccharides, and induces GI inflammatory response [9–11].

A well-established theory in COVID-19 is "*The Gut-Lung Axis*"; known as the interaction between the gut and lung where an inflammatory response in one organ affects the other. Clinically, COVID-19 patients with GI manifestations presented with more severe respiratory symptoms, than those without GI manifestations [12]. *Please see* Fig. 14.2.

A recent meta-analysis on global metabolomics datasets showed that other metabolites such as propanoate and selenocompound could be affected by the gut microbiota and could change in the severity of COVID-19 infection as well [13].

Regarding hepatic manifestation, normally the liver possesses a low amount of ACE-2 receptors, but in case of chronic inflammatory conditions, the ACE-2 receptors level rises due to the associated hepatocellular hypoxemia. SARS-CoV-2 causes a decrease in ACE receptors level and consequently causes elevation of liver enzymes and induction of hepatocyte inflammation [10].

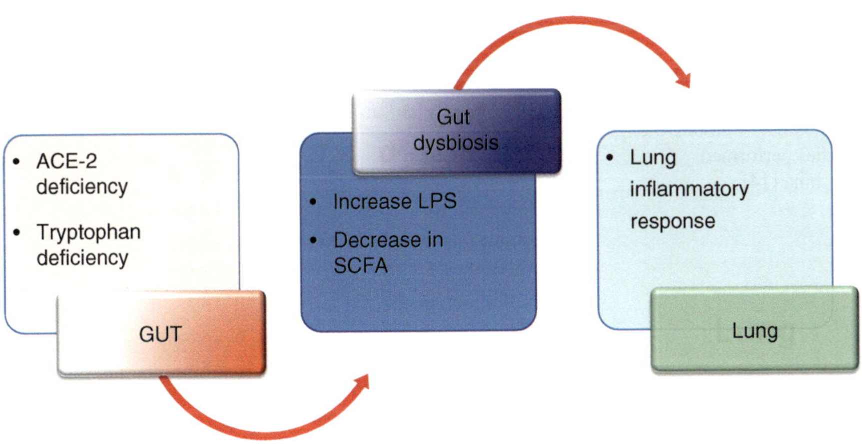


**Fig. 14.2** The GUT-LUNG axis and the effect of dysbiosis

## *Gastrointestinal and Hepatic Presentations of COVID-19*

Gastrointestinal and hepatic manifestations that present in COVID-19 patients are shown in Table 14.1 [14]. The commonest GIT manifestations with COVID-19 are abdominal pain, diarrhea, and vomiting [3]. A study by Wang et al. showed that only abdominal pain is associated with increased risk of ICU admission [15]. Moreover, Wong et al. showed that diarrhea was the most prevalent symptom in SARS-CoV-2 infection studies (ranging from 13.8 to 73.3%) [16], with pooled diarrhea prevalence of 13.8% [17] and 10.4% in two different meta-analyses [18]. Patients with diarrhea symptom tend to have longer disease course of COVID-19, but with more enhanced immunity. Besides, viral shedding in their stool tends to lag for a longer duration after resolving their symptoms [19]. In addition, COVID-19 severity of infection and mortality incidence differ according to the presence of GIT symptoms. The severity of COVID-19 disease's risk increases with presence of GIT manifestations, odds ratio (OR) of 2.07. The risk of mortality increases with presence of hepatic manifestations, OR of 1.26, but not with presence of GIT manifestations, OR 0.92 [3]

In a recent meta-analysis the pooled prevalence of GIT manifestations included diarrhea 16.5%, nausea 9.7%, elevated liver enzymes 5.6%, abdominal pain 4.5%, while vomiting, loss of taste, and anorexia were < 2%. Furthermore, GI related mortality was 3.5% and GI related ICU admission had odds ratio of 1.01. But the GI related mortality was different from one country to another (<1% in China and > 10% in the USA) [20].

The hepatic interaction with COVID-19 includes hepatotoxicity from drug regimens, viral entry through the ACE-2 receptors, hepatocellular hypoxia due to respiratory failure, increased inflammatory markers in systemic inflammatory response, and exacerbation of preexisting chronic liver disease [21]. This is shown in Fig. 14.3.

**Table 14.1** GIT and hepatic manifestations of COVID-19 among the studies performed in China [14]

| Symptom or lab variation | Prevalence in studies (minimum to maximum) |
|---|---|
| Diarrhea | 2–75% |
| Nausea | 1–29.4% |
| Vomiting | 1–18.6% |
| Jaundice (increased bilirubin) | 2–18% |
| Anorexia | 1–78.6% |
| Abdominal pain | 2–13% |
| ALT elevation | 6–28% |
| AST elevation | 2–18% |

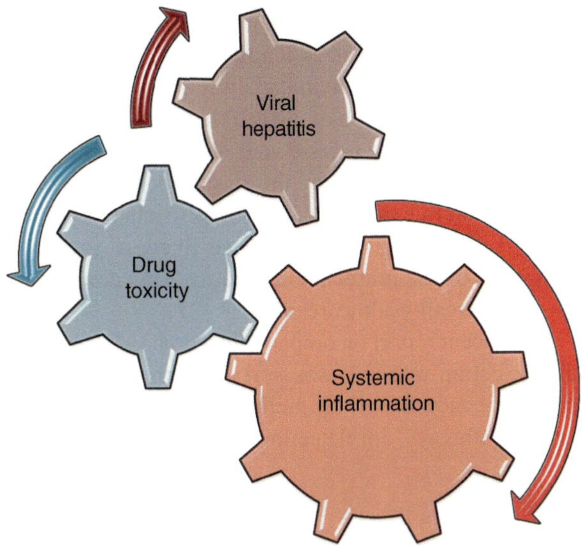


**Fig. 14.3** Different interactions between COVID-19 and the liver [14]

## *Diagnosis and Treatment of GIT and Hepatic Manifestations of COVID-19*

Laboratory diagnosis for hepatitis includes assessment by liver enzymes and abdominal ultrasound.

Viral PCR of the diarrhea stool samples shows viral shedding was validated by many studies. Although, recent Chinese guidelines are using this method as their gold standard for diagnosis, it is still not widely accepted. A recent meta-analysis of the reported Chinese cases by Cheung et al. found an overall viral prevalence of 48.1% in stool samples [22], with the presence of live virus in fecal PCR samples [23]. The great variability in viral detection among studies was attributed to direct freezing of stool samples, which causes disintegration of the viral particles and lower yield [8, 24]. This problem could be resolved simply by adding a special buffer to the stool samples before freezing, in order to preserve the viral particles [25].

## *Protection of the Health Care Workers*

Viral shedding through the GIT in latent SARS-CoV2 virus causes spread of infection among healthcare workers during certain procedures that involve contact with gastrointestinal fluids as with: dentists during dental procedures, gastroenterologists during endoscopies (upper GIT endoscopy or colonoscopy), and otolaryngologists.

At the beginning of the pandemic, all elective procedures were halted, even calprotectin testing for inflammatory activity was prohibited due to the risk of infection from stool samples, and a significant reduction in therapeutic drug monitoring was noticed in patients receiving adalimumab (75%) and infliximab (36%) [26].

The risk of infection of the health care workers depends on the degree of application of the protective measures. It was found that physicians, although directly interacting with the patients, are the least infected with infection rate of 13.3%. Whereas the infection rate in the cleaning staff reached 33.3% and in the administrative staff reached 42.9%, thus they are more likely to get infected, owing to the less strict follow-up of the protective measures. This confirms the importance of awareness spreading to all healthcare workers [27].

In a recent report on outpatients who had GI endoscopy procedures, it was found that infection rate risk was very low, providing that the patients follow stringent protective measures [28], including "minimization" of airborne infection [29] and "green pathways" for detection of infection before preparation to endoscopy.

## Inflammatory Bowel Disease (IBD) in the COVID-19 Era

### *Clinical Background of the Condition*

IBD is an autoimmune disease involving the gastrointestinal tract with two subtypes: Crohn's disease and ulcerative colitis. Crohn's disease (CD) affects mainly the intestine but could also affect the whole GI tract. The main presentations of the disease include diarrhea, abdominal pain, fistula or intestinal obstruction. CD pathology is transmural, with three subtypes: intestinal inflammation, stricturing, or fistulizing disease. Ulcerative colitis (UC) mainly affects the colorectal part of the GIT and could present with bleeding per rectum, diarrhea, and abdominal pain. UC pathology is transmembranous with crypt abscess. UC could be complicated with toxic megacolon or associated with high risk of colon cancer [30].

Both CD and UC have extra-gastrointestinal manifestations such as hypercoagulable state, uveitis, hepatitis, arthritis, secondary biliary cholangitis, etc. [31].

Surveillance Epidemiology of Coronavirus Under Research Exclusion (SECURE)-IBD is a worldwide registry (https://covidibd.org/) which depends on the voluntary collaboration of physicians, reporting on IBD patients worldwide [32]. It helps in documenting the cases and providing clinical updates across its platform, thus offering valuable information for decision-making worldwide.

### *Effect of COVID-19 on IBD*

During the pandemic, COVID-19 could alter the management of IBD patients. So, we have to weigh the benefits versus the risks of acquiring COVID-19 infection with respect to the following measures, administering subcutaneous instead of intravenous biologics; using telemedicine instead of actual clinical examination; delaying initiation of therapy; delaying follow-up of elective GI endoscopies, delaying elective surgeries related to the condition; among others [33]. Furthermore, we have to consider certain measures in the medical treatment of IBD. For example, we found that Infliximab (a drug used for induction and maintenance of remission in IBD), when received in active IBD patients was associated with ameliorating of the cytokine storm and pulmonary manifestations of COVID-19 [34].

Patients, who continue their maintenance biologic regimens of vedolizumab or Infliximab, still have no increase in the risk of COVID-19 infection [35]. It was proposed that the use of mesalamine/sulfasalazine does not affect the severity of COVID-19 infection and can be used safely in IBD patients [36]. However, clinical data presented by a metaanalysis included 525 cases on the SECURE-IBD database from 33 countries. The study showed that any of the following factors could trigger the occurrence of severe manifestations including increase in age, presence of ≥2 comorbidities, and treatment with sulfasalazine, 5-aminosalicylate, or systemic corticosteroids, while tumor necrosis factor alpha (TNF-α) antagonists did not [37]. In addition, using azathioprine either in mono or combination therapy is associated with severe COVID-19 [38].

The IBD patients' perspectives are crucial when dealing with COVID-19. First, they are more aware of the risk of acquiring infections from their immunosuppressive medications, so they are more cautious. Second, they seek advice through different media and consultations, so their level of awareness is higher than the general population. Third, their maintenance of biological therapy could be delayed out of fear of "going to the hospital," thus they need specific formulated measures to guide them and follow their adherence to medications [39]. These measures include cancellation or rescheduling of elective visits and procedures as follow-up colonoscopy while enhancing the telemedicine communication with the patients such as email, telephone, WhatsApp, video calls, etc. [40].

Telemedicine showed tremendous benefit during the pandemic when compared to the standard of care, providing a safe and efficient medium of interaction between the IBD patients and the specialists, resulting in reduction of hospital admissions.

Conversely, limitations include the low availability of IBD specialists using telemedicine and the unclear health insurance policies covering this online method. Moreover, concerns about the ideal methods of drug delivery to the patients need further assessment when using telemedicine in IBD patients [41].

## *Effect of IBD on COVID-19*

COVID infection risk is ameliorated in IBD due to patients' awareness of the protective measures, and their avoidance of hospital visits unless they have severe disease presentations, physicians postponing elective endoscopies and surgeries, and tapering of the steroid dose or even complete withholding for fear of lowering the immunity of the patients [34].

A recent systematic review examined the vulnerability of IBD patients to COVID-19 infection and concluded that there is no increased risk associated. However, they stated that COVID-19 could exacerbate IBD symptoms [5]. With most reports showing that there is no increase in the incidence of acquiring COVID-19 in IBD patients, it remains important to differentiate IBD exacerbation from COVID-19 GI manifestation [32].

The risk of COVID-19 infection in IBD was 0.3%, similar to the infection rate in the general population [34, 42]. The presence of bowel inflammation and the administration of immunosuppressives will not increase the expression of ACE-2 receptors in the gut, hence no increase in the risk of COVID-19 infection [43]. Furthermore, no increase in the severity of COVID-19 infection is detected in IBD patients as compared to the general population [37].

The differentiation between gastrointestinal symptoms caused by IBD flare versus COVID-19 infection is important. Mostly, we follow the "*Wait And See*" policy, where after 5–7 days the COVID-19 GI manifestations resolve, while GI manifestations of the IBD flare increase. Calprotectin could help differentiate between the two illnesses [34]. This is shown in Fig. 14.4.

Gastrointestinal manifestations in IBD patients are triggered by many factors including: IBD exacerbation, incompliance to medications, low or ineffective dose of IBD medication, antibiotic associated dysbiosis, side effects of the IBD medications, or concomitant COVID-19 infection [5, 44]. This is shown in Fig. 14.5.

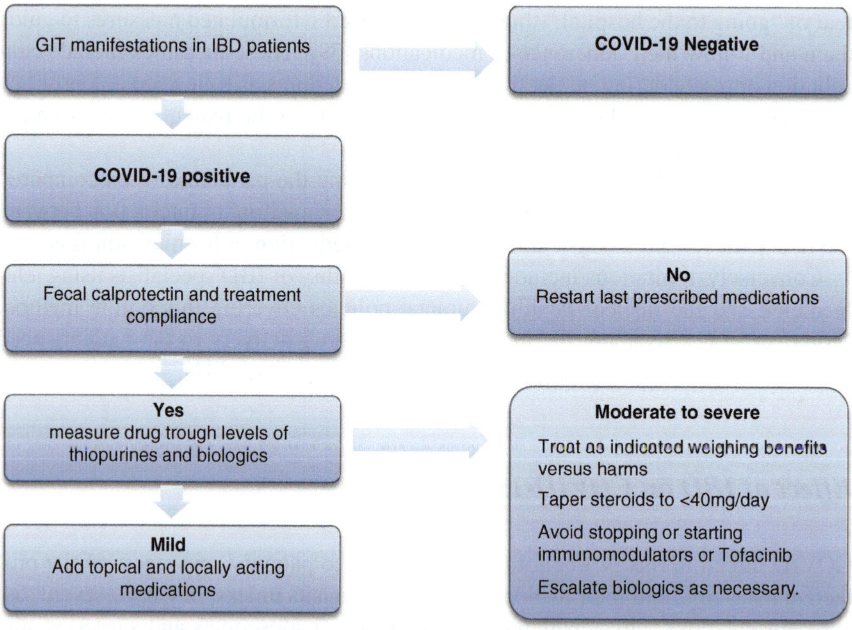


**Fig. 14.4** Flow diagram of the treatment algorithm of IBD patients presenting with GI manifestations during the COVID-19 pandemic

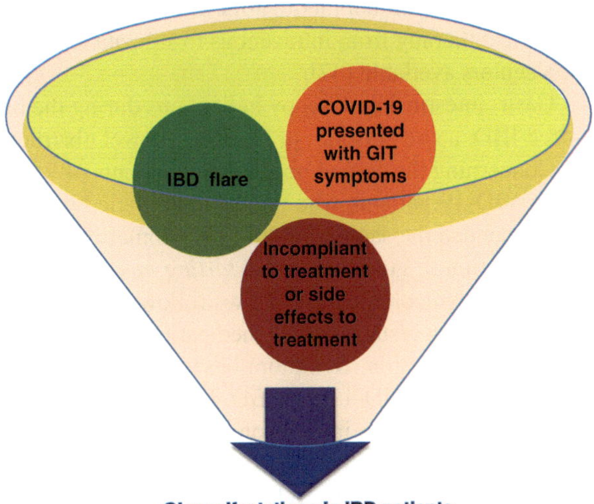


**Fig. 14.5** The causes of GI manifestations in IBD patients during the pandemic

## *Guidelines for IBD Treatment and Follow-Up, Dilemmas, and Differences*

When designing the guidelines for IBD patients during the pandemic, our data and clinical experience with this new virus are still limited. Thus, we have to weigh the benefits of decreasing the IBD medication doses to enhance the patient's immunity versus the risk of exacerbating the disease but could increase the risk of relapse and hospitalization.

*European Crohn's and Colitis Organization (ECCO)* guidelines stated that all immunomodulators are to be stopped on confirmation of infection (contact with a patient) including thioprine, methotrexate, tofacitinib, TNF, vedolizumab, ustekinumab. However, nonimmune modulators such as antibiotics, local budesonide, aminosalicylate, or rectal therapy could be continued. As for *American Gastroenterology Association* (AGA), and *International Organization for the Study of Inflammatory Bowel Disease* (IOIBD), they recommended applying the same measures for both confirmed or suspected cases (exposed to COVID-19 patients) [34].

*American Gastroenterological Association (AGA)* recommendations state that as patients with IBD are not in an increased risk of acquiring COVID-19 infection, there is no need for withholding the maintenance therapy for fear of being infected by SARS-CoV-2 as this will burden the health care system, with consequent relapse of the IBD disease [45].

We need strict following of the protective measures the infusion centers [46], along with mandatory screening of patients. Moreover, infusion centers should consider shifting to subcutaneous drug alternatives and shorten the duration of infusion in their centers [46].

*Asian Pacific Association of Gastroenterology (APAGE)* guidelines are similar to the ECCO and IOIBD in tapering the steroids dosage and withholding the JAK inhibitors and immunomodulators. But, they do not recommend switching of the biological therapy from intravenous to subcutaneous, unless there are no open infusion centers available [47].

Gastrointestinal endoscopy indications during the pandemic include newly diagnosed IBD, acute episodes of bleeding, bowel obstruction, or UC flare [48].

Concerning the care of hospitalized patients [49], ECCO added another category of COVID-19 patients who are asymptomatic but have positive PCR testing; they recommended the same as mildly symptomatic disease. Please see Table 14.2.

In relation to guidance *for restarting medications after a period of withholding them*, ECCO recommended that we follow the "Symptom-based" and "Test-based" strategies when restarting IBD medications after a period of withholding, caused by COVID-19 infection. Symptom-based strategy depends on the severity of symptoms of both COVID-19 and IBD. It was shown that the more clinically severe the COVID-19, the more inclination to delay restarting of IBD medications, whereas the more severe or hard to control the IBD, the more inclination to fasten the restarting of IBD medications. While test-based strategy depends on two consecutive (24-h apart) negative PCR tests for SARS-CoV-2 and then restart [50].

Regarding *thromoprophylaxis*, it is given to patients with high-risk factors or presenting with severe COVID-19 infection requiring hospitalization, this is independent of their IBD stage (mild, moderate, or severe) [34]. These patients have a double risk for hypercoagulability, from both IBD and severe COVID-19 [51]. Please see Table 14.2. Furthermore, adding thromboprophylaxis in pregnant IBD patients is empirical, whether the patient is infected with COVID-19 or not, with avoiding steroids administration if possible [52].

**Table 14.2** Areas of agreement across the current IBD treatment guidelines in mild and moderate-severe COVID-19 infection

| Drug | Effect on immune system | Mild COVID-19 Infection decision | Moderate to severe COVID-19 infection decision |
|---|---|---|---|
| *Budesonide* | Do not increase the risk of infection | Continue | Continue |
| *5-aminosalicylic acid* | Do not increase the risk of infection | Continue | Continue |
| *Corticosteroids* | Increase the risk of infection | Withdraw or taper to <20 mg/day<br>Shift to local steroids | Withdraw or taper to <20 mg/day |
| *Thiopurines/ methotrexate* | Cause leukopenia | Withhold | Withhold |
| *Tofacitinib/JAK inhibitors* | Decrease interferon alpha | Withhold | Withhold |
| *Biologics* | Anti-TNF<br>Anti-integrins | Delay for 2 weeks and monitor clinical symptoms | Delay for 2 weeks and monitor clinical symptoms |
| *Anticoagulation* | Protection from thromboembolism risk | None | 4 weeks of heparin or direct oral anticoagulants |

## *Guidelines for Vaccination*

Vaccination is recommended in the IBD management guidelines including influenza and pneumococcal vaccines and is imperative during the pandemic [47]. The IBD management guidelines recommends influenza vaccination to IBD patients during the COVID-19 pandemic. This vaccination will protect IBD patients from acquiring infleunza infection by elevating the protecting antibody levels against the hemagglutinin portion of the virus. Also, the influenza vaccine plays an important protective role in COVID-19 infection itself [5]. Gastroenterologists should be aware of the vaccination history of IBD patients, especially when commencing a new immunosuppressive regimen, and vaccinations should be administered only during the disease remission [53].

A recent survey found that half of IBD patients are willing to receive COVID-19 vaccination. This could be due to patients' concerns about safety and long term side effects [54]. Moreover, there is a debate, whether vaccination in IBD patients could achieve desirable effects on immunity, as the immunosuppressive and immunomodulatory drugs may prohibit the antibody and cellular protective response of the vaccine. However, it was noticed that new biological therapies such as ustekinumab or vedolizumab do not affect the immunological response to flu vaccination, and increasing the dose of flu vaccine in patients receiving anti-TNF-a elucidates an effective response. Thus, the IOIBD panel recommends vaccination of all IBD patients regardless of the type of treatment received, without stopping their medications; but the administration of live (viral vector) or attenuated virus vaccines is forbidden [34, 55].

Furthermore, both the British Society of Gastroenterology IBD section and IBD clinical research group recommend vaccination for IBD patients independent of their TNF-a medications. They stated that vaccination is safe in this population and benefits outweigh the risks [56].

However, IBD could induce a hypercoagulable state, increasing the risk of thromboembolism and affecting both the arterial and venous systems [57]. As safety concerns have risen recently from the AstraZeneca vaccine, with hypercoagulable state noticed in some patients receiving the vaccine, we have to be more cautious when dealing with high-risk populations such as IBD patients [58].

## *Future Research Points*

More data becomes available each day on IBD patients; this will help modify the existing guidelines during the pandemic and after. In addition, clinical trials will expand our therapeutic armamentarium in both IBD and COVID-19. It goes without question that patient's safety is a priority when conducting clinical trials [59]. Special populations such as pregnant women or children with IBD will have more cohorts and clinical trials to know more about their management with SARS-CoV2 especially the vaccination issue, hence most of the recommendations for this category is based on expert or theoretical opinions from previous outbreaks.

As awareness of the disease overcomes the initial "disease scare," and the disease pathophysiology becomes more understandable, these will help build more structural and easy protective measures, which could be easily followed and also cost-effective.

Data are updated on a daily basis for IBD patients. This will help modify the existing guidelines during the pandemic and after. In addition, clinical trials will expand our therapeutic armamentarium in both IBD and COVID-19. However, since the patient's safety is the main priority when conducting clinical trials [59], special populations such as pregnant women or children with IBD will need more cohorts and clinical trials to establish their management plans regarding SARS-CoV2, especially the vaccination issue. Hence, most of the recommendations for this category are based on expert or theoretical opinions from previous outbreaks.

As awareness of the disease overcomes the initial "disease scare," and the disease pathophysiology becomes more understandable, more structural, cost-effective, and easier protective measures will be available.

Scarce data could be found on the difference between the two IBD subtypes (UC and CD) and their association with COVID-19. In a large cohort by Singh et al. UC had more severe presentation of COVID-19 than CD. However, further studies are needed for confirmation. This difference in presentation between the subtypes could be explained by many factors, UC patients tend to be older than CD patients; CD patients tend to receive biological therapy earlier in their disease, while UC patients could try a lot of regimens or be controlled on ASA-5, which is an associated with more severe COVID-19 disease. In addition, the different distributions of ACE-2 and transmembrane protease, serine 2 enzyme (TMPRSS2) receptors in the two subtypes may play an important role in COVID-19 presentation [60, 61]. We need further research in this area.

The implementation of virtual clinical practice technologies (i.e. telemedicine) gained a tremendous usage expansion in the COVID-19 pandemic [61]. As for the impact of COVID-19 on telemedicine efficiency in antenatal care of IBD patients, a cohort of 244 pregnant IBD patients showed that nevertheless most of the antenatal care was conducted through telephone, there was no deterioration in the level of medical care, no increment in maternal or fetal complications, while there was a higher rate of biological therapy maintenance. But more research is required in this special category of IBD patients [62].

Regarding the relation between IBD and COVID-19 risk of infection, a cohort of 500 IBD patients showed no COVID-19 cases [63]. However, the tendency towards hasty conclusions, after small cohorts or weak conducted studies, is not recommended. We must examine the level of evidence at each step and request more research with high quality evidence. In addition, we should consider the epidemiological factors, including the proper sample size calculation *before* conducting the study, and the balance between different confounders as a source for possible bias [64].

Special categories such as pregnant women and children are always excluded from the clinical initial trials of vaccines and drugs because we have to establish all the safety issues first. Fortunately, children with IBD have low risk of COVID-19 infection. In addition, recent data from the Pfizer vaccine trials on children with IBD aging 12–15 years are promising in their safety profile, and an emergency authorization for this special age group was approved in the USA. Moreover, there is an ongoing trial on the vaccination of 6 months to 11 years old children with IBD. Moreover, recent data on COVID-19 vaccination in pregnant women showed a high safety profile [65].

Furthermore, as of August 11, 2021, the Centers for Disease Control and Prevention (CDC) has updated its recommendations for vaccination of all children of 12 years or older and pregnant women, especially high-risk patients [66].

## Conclusions

Gastrointestinal manifestations of COVID-19 infection are common, and COVID-19 diagnosis should be suspected upon presentation of GI symptoms. Inflammatory bowel disease flare or activity could be confused with COVID-19 GI presentation. Patients with IBD should follow strict protective measures during the pandemic, along with the recommended vaccinations. Medications should be adjusted according to both the severity of IBD and COVID-19.

## References

1. El Ouali S, Achkar JP, Lashner B, Regueiro M. Gastrointestinal manifestations of COVID-19. Cleve Clin J Med. 2021. https://doi.org/10.3949/ccjm.87a.ccc049. Online ahead of print.
2. Leal T, Costa E, Arroja B, Gonçalves R, Alves J. Gastrointestinal manifestations of COVID-19: results from a European Centre. Eur J Gastroenterol Hepatol. 2021;33(5):691–4.
3. Menon T, Sharma R, Earthineni G, Iftikhar H, Sondhi M, Shams S, et al. Association of gastrointestinal system with severity and mortality of COVID-19: a systematic review and meta-analysis. Cureus. 2021;13(2):e13317.
4. Zou X, Chen K, Zou J, Han P, Hao J, Han Z. Single-cell RNA-seq data analysis on the receptor ACE2 expression reveals the potential risk of different human organs vulnerable to 2019-nCoV infection. Front Med. 2020;14(2):185–92.
5. Barbalho SM, Matias JN, Flato UAP, Pilon JPG, Bitelli P, Pagani Junior MA, et al. What do influenza and COVID-19 represent for patients with inflammatory bowel disease? Gastroenterology Res. 2021;14(1):1–12.
6. Song M, Li ZL, Zhou YJ, Tian G, Ye T, Zeng ZR, et al. Gastrointestinal involvement of COVID-19 and potential faecal transmission of SARS-CoV-2. J Zhejiang Univ Sci B. 2020;21(9):749–51.

7. van Doorn AS, Meijer B, Frampton CMA, Barclay ML, de Boer NKH. Systematic review with meta-analysis: SARS-CoV-2 stool testing and the potential for faecal-oral transmission. Aliment Pharmacol Ther. 2020;52(8):1276–88.
8. Bwire GM, Majigo MV, Njiro BJ, Mawazo A. Detection profile of SARS-CoV-2 using RT-PCR in different types of clinical specimens: a systematic review and meta-analysis. J Med Virol. 2021;93(2):719–25.
9. Penninger JM, Grant MB, Sung JJY. The role of angiotensin converting enzyme 2 in modulating gut microbiota, intestinal inflammation, and coronavirus infection. Gastroenterology. 2021;160(1):39–46.
10. Banu N, Panikar SS, Leal LR, Leal AR. Protective role of ACE2 and its downregulation in SARS-CoV-2 infection leading to macrophage activation syndrome: therapeutic implications. Life Sci. 2020;256:117905.
11. Santacroce L, Inchingolo F, Topi S, Del Prete R, Di Cosola M, Charitos IA, et al. Potential beneficial role of probiotics on the outcome of COVID-19 patients: an evolving perspective. Diabetes Metab Syndr. 2021;15(1):295–301.
12. Chhibber-Goel J, Gopinathan S, Sharma A. Interplay between severities of COVID-19 and the gut microbiome: implications of bacterial co-infections? Gut Pathogens. 2021;13(1):14.
13. Pang Z, Zhou G, Chong J, Xia J. Comprehensive meta-analysis of COVID-19 global metabolomics datasets. Metabolites. 2021;11(1):44.
14. Patel KP, Patel PA, Vunnam RR, Hewlett AT, Jain R, Jing R, et al. Gastrointestinal, hepatobiliary, and pancreatic manifestations of COVID-19. J Clin Virol. 2020;128:104386.
15. Wang D, Hu B, Hu C, Zhu F, Liu X, Zhang J, et al. Clinical characteristics of 138 hospitalized patients with 2019 novel coronavirus-infected pneumonia in Wuhan, China. JAMA. 2020;323(11):1061–9.
16. Wong SH, Lui RN, Sung JJ. Covid-19 and the digestive system. J Gastroenterol Hepatol. 2020;35(5):744–8.
17. Villamizar-PeÑA R, Gutiérrez-Ocampo E, Rodríguez-Morales AJ. Pooled prevalence of diarrhea among COVID-19 patients. Clin Gastroenterol Hepatol. 2020;18(10):2385–7.
18. D'Amico F, Baumgart DC, Danese S, Peyrin-Biroulet L. Diarrhea during COVID-19 infection: pathogenesis, epidemiology, prevention, and management. Clin Gastroenterol Hepatol. 2020;18(8):1663–72.
19. Han C, Duan C, Zhang S, Spiegel B, Shi H, Wang W, et al. Digestive symptoms in COVID-19 patients with mild disease severity: clinical presentation, stool viral RNA testing, and outcomes. Am J Gastroenterol. 2020;115(6):916–23.
20. Shehab M, Alrashed F, Shuaibi S, Alajmi D, Barkun A. Gastroenterological and hepatic manifestations of patients with COVID-19, prevalence, mortality by country, and intensive care admission rate: systematic review and meta-analysis. BMJ Open Gastroenterol. 2021;8(1):e000571.
21. Cichoż-Lach H, Michalak A. Liver injury in the era of COVID-19. World J Gastroenterol. 2021;27(5):377–90.
22. Cheung KS, Hung IFN, Chan PPY, Lung KC, Tso E, Liu R, et al. Gastrointestinal manifestations of SARS-CoV-2 infection and virus load in fecal samples from a Hong Kong cohort: systematic review and meta-analysis. Gastroenterology. 2020;159(1):81–95.
23. Cuicchi D, Lazzarotto T, Poggioli G. Fecal-oral transmission of SARS-CoV-2: review of laboratory-confirmed virus in gastrointestinal system. Int J Color Dis. 2021;36(3):437–44.
24. Xing X-C, Qi B, Deng K. SARS-CoV-2 RNA detection in gastrointestinal sample displays poor performance. Gastroenterology. 2021;160(3):972–3.e1.
25. Natarajan A, Han A, Zlitni S, Brooks EF, Vance SE, Wolfe M, et al. Standardized and optimized preservation, extraction and quantification techniques for detection of fecal SARS-CoV-2 RNA. medRxiv. 2021.
26. Shields S, Dunlop A, Seenan JP, Macdonald J. Disease monitoring of biologic treatment in IBD: early impact and future implications of COVID-19 pandemic. Frontline Gastroenterol. 2021;12(4):345.

27. Kassem AM, Talaat H, Shawky S, Fouad R, Amer K, Elnagdy T, et al. SARS-CoV-2 infection among healthcare workers of a gastroenterological service in a tertiary care facility. Arab J Gastroenterol. 2020;21(3):151–5.
28. Hayee B, Hussain BP, Rees CJ, Penman I. COVID-19 transmission following outpatient endoscopy during pandemic acceleration phase involving SARS-CoV-2 VOC 202012/01 variant in UK. Gut. 2021;70(12):2227–9.
29. Morawska L, Tang JW, Bahnfleth W, Bluyssen PM, Boerstra A, Buonanno G, et al. How can airborne transmission of COVID-19 indoors be minimised? Environ Int. 2020;142:105832.
30. Seyedian SS, Nokhostin F, Malamir MD. A review of the diagnosis, prevention, and treatment methods of inflammatory bowel disease. J Med Life. 2019;12(2):113–22.
31. Rusoniene S, Urbonas V, Avcin T. Extraintestinal manifestations of inflammatory bowel disease. In: Cimaz R, editor. Periodic and non-periodic fevers. Cham: Springer International Publishing; 2020. p. 177–213.
32. Mak JWY, Weng MT, Wei SC, Ng SC. Zero COVID-19 infection in inflammatory bowel disease patients: findings from population-based inflammatory bowel disease registries in Hong Kong and Taiwan. J Gastroenterol Hepatol. 2021;36(1):171–3.
33. Kotze PG, Peyrin-Biroulet L, Danese S. Balancing risks and benefits in inflammatory bowel disease patients during the COVID-19 pandemic. Gastroenterology. 2021;160(1):472–3.
34. Chebli JMFQN, Damião AOMC, Chebli LA, Costa MHM, Parra RS. How to manage inflammatory bowel disease during the COVID-19 pandemic: a guide for the practicing clinician. World J Gastroenterol. 2021;27(11):1022–42.
35. McGregor CG, Adams A, Sadler R, Arancibia-Cárcamo CV, Palmer R, Ambrose T, et al. Maintenance therapy with infliximab or vedolizumab in IBD is not associated with increased SARS-CoV-2 seroprevalence: UK experience in the 2020 pandemic. Gut. 2021.
36. Attauabi M, Seidelin J, Burisch J. Association between 5-aminosalicylates in patients with IBD and risk of severe COVID-19: an artefactual result of research methodology? Gut. 2021;70(10):2020–2.
37. Brenner EJ, Ungaro RC, Gearry RB, Kaplan GG, Kissous-Hunt M, Lewis JD, et al. Corticosteroids, but not TNF antagonists, are associated with adverse COVID-19 outcomes in patients with inflammatory bowel diseases: results from an international registry. Gastroenterology. 2020;159(2):481–91.e3.
38. Ungaro RC, Brenner EJ, Gearry RB, Kaplan GG, Kissous-Hunt M, Lewis JD, et al. Effect of IBD medications on COVID-19 outcomes: results from an international registry. Gut. 2021;70(4):725–32.
39. Grunert PC, Reuken PA, Stallhofer J, Teich N, Stallmach A. Inflammatory bowel disease in the COVID-19 pandemic: the patients' perspective. J Crohn's Colitis. 2020;14(12):1702–8.
40. Martin Arranz E, Suarez Ferrer C, García Ramírez L, Rueda García JL, Sánchez-Azofra M, Poza Cordón J, et al. Management of COVID-19 pandemic in Spanish inflammatory bowel disease units: results from a National Survey. Inflamm Bowel Dis. 2020;26(8):1149–54.
41. Zhang YF, Qiu Y, He JS, Tan JY, Li XZ, Zhu LR, et al. Impact of COVID-19 outbreak on the care of patients with inflammatory bowel disease: a comparison before and after the outbreak in South China. J Gastroenterol Hepatol. 2021;36(3):700–9.
42. Aziz M, Fatima R, Haghbin H, Lee-Smith W, Nawras A. The incidence and outcomes of COVID-19 in IBD patients: a rapid review and meta-analysis. Inflamm Bowel Dis. 2020;26(10):e132–e3.
43. Burgueño JF, Abreu MT. Reply to the letter to the editor: the incidence and outcomes of COVID-19 in patients with IBD: a rapid review and meta-analysis. Inflamm Bowel Dis. 2020;26(10):e127.
44. Nitzan O, Elias M, Peretz A, Saliba W. Role of antibiotics for treatment of inflammatory bowel disease. World J Gastroenterol. 2016;22(3):1078–87.
45. Rubin DT, Feuerstein JD, Wang AY, Cohen RD. AGA clinical practice update on Management of Inflammatory Bowel Disease during the COVID-19 pandemic: expert commentary. Gastroenterology. 2020;159(1):350–7.

46. Dotan I, Panaccione R, Kaplan GG, O'Morain C, Lindsay JO, Abreu MT, et al. Best practice guidance for adult infusion Centres during the COVID-19 pandemic: report from the COVID-19 International Organization for the Study of IBD [IOIBD] task force. J Crohn's Colitis. 2020;14(Supplement_3):S785–S90.
47. Ling KL, Hilmi I, Raja Ali RA, Leong RWL, Leung WK, Ng SC, et al. Asian Pacific Association of Gastroenterology (APAGE) inflammatory bowel disease (IBD) working party guidelines on IBD management during the COVID-19 pandemic. JGH Open. 2020;4(3):320–3. https://doi.org/10.1002/jgh3.12362.
48. Ng SC, Mak JWY, Hitz L, Chowers Y, Bernstein CN, Silverberg MS, et al. COVID-19 pandemic: which IBD patients need to be scoped—who gets scoped now, who can wait, and how to resume to Normal. J Crohn's Colitis. 2020;14(Supplement_3):S791–S7.
49. Allez M, Fleshner P, Gearry R, Lakatos PL, Rubin DT, On behalf of the International Organization for the Study of inflammatory bowel D. Care of the Patient with IBD requiring hospitalisation during the COVID-19 pandemic. J Crohn's Colitis. 2020;14(Supplement_3):S774–S9.
50. Siegel CA, Christensen B, Kornbluth A, Rosh JR, Kappelman MD, Ungaro RC, et al. Guidance for restarting inflammatory bowel disease therapy in patients who withheld immunosuppressant medications during COVID-19. J Crohn's Colitis. 2020;14(Supplement_3):S769–S73.
51. Tan CW, Tan JY, Wong WH, Cheong MA, Ng IM, Conceicao EP, et al. Clinical and laboratory features of hypercoagulability in COVID-19 and other respiratory viral infections amongst predominantly younger adults with few comorbidities. Sci Rep. 2021;11(1):1793.
52. De Lima-Karagiannis A, Juillerat P, Sebastian S, Pedersen N, Bar-Gil Shitrit A, van der Woude CJ. Management of Pregnant Inflammatory Bowel Disease Patients during the COVID-19 pandemic. J Crohn's Colitis. 2020;14(Supplement_3):S807–S14.
53. Manser CN, Maillard MH, Rogler G, Schreiner P, Rieder F, Bühler S. Vaccination in patients with inflammatory bowel diseases. Digestion. 2020;101 Suppl 1(suppl 1):58–68.
54. Caron B, Neuville E, Peyrin-Biroulet L. Inflammatory bowel disease and COVID-19 vaccination: a patients' survey. Dig Dis Sci. 2022;67(6):2067–73.
55. Siegel CA, Melmed GY, McGovern DPB, Rai V, Krammer F, Rubin DT, et al. SARS-CoV-2 vaccination for patients with inflammatory bowel diseases: recommendations from an international consensus meeting. Gut. 2021;70(4):635.
56. Alexander JL, Moran GW, Gaya DR, Raine T, Hart A, Kennedy NA, et al. SARS-CoV-2 vaccination for patients with inflammatory bowel disease: a British Society of Gastroenterology Inflammatory Bowel Disease section and IBD clinical research group position statement. Lancet Gastroenterol Hepatol. 2021;6(3):218–24.
57. Owczarek D, Cibor D, Głowacki MK, Rodacki T, Mach T. Inflammatory bowel disease: epidemiology, pathology and risk factors for hypercoagulability. World J Gastroenterol. 2014;20(1):53–63.
58. Oldenburg J, Klamroth R, Langer F, Albisetti M, von Auer C, Ay C, et al. Diagnosis and management of vaccine-related thrombosis following AstraZeneca COVID-19 vaccination: guidance statement from the GTH. Hamostaseologie. 2021;41(3):184–9.
59. Reinisch W, Danese S, Peyrin-Biroulet L, Loftus EV Jr, On behalf of the International Organization for the Study of inflammatory bowel D. Clinical trials for inflammatory bowel disease: global guidance during the COVID-19 pandemic. J Crohn's Colitis. 2020;14(Supplement_3):S815–S9.
60. Singh S, Khan A, Chowdhry M, Bilal M, Kochhar GS, Clarke K. Risk of severe coronavirus disease 2019 in patients with inflammatory bowel disease in the United States: a multicenter research network study. Gastroenterology. 2020;159(4):1575–8.e4.
61. Kumric M, Ticinovic Kurir T, Martinovic D, Zivkovic PM, Bozic J. Impact of the COVID-19 pandemic on inflammatory bowel disease patients: a review of the current evidence. World J Gastroenterol. 2021;27(25):3748–61.
62. Selinger CP, Fraser A, Collins P, Gunn M, Chew TS, Kerry G, et al. Impact of the coronavirus infectious disease (COVID-19) pandemic on the provision of inflammatory bowel

disease (IBD) antenatal care and outcomes of pregnancies in women with IBD. BMJ Open Gastroenterol. 2021;8(1):e000603.
63. Norsa L, Indriolo A, Sansotta N, Cosimo P, Greco S, D'Antiga L. Uneventful course in patients with inflammatory bowel disease during the severe acute respiratory syndrome coronavirus 2 outbreak in northern Italy. Gastroenterology. 2020;159(1):371–2.
64. Gower-Rousseau C, Fumery M, Pariente B. Inflammatory bowel disease and the SARS-CoV-2 pandemic: more speed, less haste. Gastroenterology. 2021;160(1):473–4.
65. Shimabukuro TT, Kim SY, Myers TR, Moro PL, Oduyebo T, Panagiotakopoulos L, et al. Preliminary findings of mRNA Covid-19 vaccine safety in pregnant persons. N Engl J Med. 2021;384(24):2273–82.
66. CDC. COVID-19 vaccines while pregnant or breastfeeding. Centers for Disease Control and Prevention (CDC). 2021; 11 August.

# Chapter 15
# Post COVID-19 Conditions: The New Challenge to Mankind

**Iana Simova, Denis Nikolov, Denislava Hristova, Hristina Tzanovska, Anyuta Ivanova, Maria-Magdalena Pintova, Diliana Iakova, Vladimir Kornovski, Todor Kundurzhiev, and Toni Vekov**

## The Post COVID-19 Syndrome

Post COVID-19 conditions include all signs and symptoms of COVID-19 that persist after the end of the acute phase (3–4 weeks), without a limit of duration (as for the knowledge we have so far). Another term for these conditions, introduced by

I. Simova (✉)
Heart and Brain Centre of Excellence, Pleven, Bulgaria

Bulgarian Cardiac Institute, Sofia, Bulgaria

Medical University, Pleven, Bulgaria

D. Nikolov · D. Hristova · H. Tzanovska · A. Ivanova · M.-M. Pintova
Heart and Brain Centre of Excellence, Pleven, Bulgaria

D. Iakova
Heart and Brain Centre of Excellence, Pleven, Bulgaria

Medical University, Pleven, Bulgaria

V. Kornovski
Heart and Brain Centre of Excellence, Burgas, Bulgaria

T. Kundurzhiev
Medical University, Sofia, Bulgaria

T. Vekov
Bulgarian Cardiac Institute, Sofia, Bulgaria

Medical University, Pleven, Bulgaria


S. Adibi et al. (eds.), *Frontiers of COVID-19*,
https://doi.org/10.1007/978-3-031-08045-6_15

Antoni Fauci, is "Post-Acute Consequences of SARS-CoV-2 Infection" (PASC) [1]. The available data demonstrates that the consequences after the infection can be just as serious and continue for an unusually long period of time after the onset of the disease. It is the long persistence of complaints and manifestations after the acute phase of the infection that are known as post COVID-19 conditions. So far there is no precise scientific definition for the reason, duration, and prognosis of PASC [2]. The severity of the acute phase of the disease does not determine the onset of post COVID-19 syndrome. There are reported cases of patients with PASC who were with mild or even asymptomatic infection. There is no age limit for the manifestation of post COVID-19 conditions, but the reported frequency is higher in the elderly population [3, 4]. According to the latest data from the World Health Organization, the consequences of an infectious disease can last for 2–3 years [5].

One of the many pathogenetic hypotheses for PASC is direct cell damage by binding of SARC-CoV-2 to ACE2 receptors, initiating an immune response, leading to increased cytokine production, and triggering procoagulation states. It was later discovered that the reason for prolonged viral replication is the fact that SARS-CoV-2 can be transmitted through a different pathway—the gastrointestinal tract, which could be considered a second hypothesis. The gastrointestinal tract has its own specific microbiome and a disturbance in it leads to dysbacteriosis. Furthermore, intestinal inflammation increases the expression of ACE2, and the virus stays in the gut for much longer, which in turn modulates immune responses and causes prolonged symptoms. This has been proven by an intestinal biopsy, which detects the presence of the virus. In some cases, SARS-CoV-2 can cause autoimmune reactions, leading to a more severe course of the disease and the development of post COVID-19 conditions [6, 7].

The suboptimal immune response leads to a higher viral load and is associated with disturbances in interferon production. In severe cases of the disease the body lacks IFN-beta, and the level of IFN-alpha and IFN-lambda is reduced. Lymphopenia and unregulated inflammation have been observed in patients with severe COVID-19 and prolonged persistence of the infection as a result of decreased production of granular lymphocytes (NK cells), CD16 + monocytes, plasmacytoid dendritic cells, which are responsible for innate immunity [7, 8].

The range of the symptoms can vary from mild to inability of performing normal daily activities. All systems can be involved, with a typical changing of symptoms over the course of time. Prolonged exposure to viral load can cause multisystem inflammatory syndrome (MIS) or trigger autoimmune conditions. The involvement in PASC is multi-organ, with the most common being complaints from the nervous system [9]. Post COVID-19 conditions are more common among people with chronic diseases such as hypertension, kidney diseases, diabetes mellitus, obesity. Genetic predisposition to the disease has not yet been described. The most frequent systems to be affected are the nervous, cardiovascular, pulmonary, and excretory systems, musculoskeletal system, and integumentary. Many healthcare centers are opening specialized wards to provide clinical care for people with persistent symptoms after COVID-19. It is important to note that most patients who have COVID-19 recover successfully. The scientific community should focus on that part of the people in whom the effects of the disease leave persisting traces and worsen their quality of life. The duration of PASC is still not known. In approximately 30% of COVID-19 survivors, symptoms may persist indefinitely. 76% of patients reported persistence of at least one symptom of PASC for at least 6 months after the acute phase [10]. Many COVID-19 survivors cannot return to their normal lifestyle. At this stage, there is no accurate scientific data on whether these long symptoms can lead to a chronification of the disease.

In conclusion, understanding the pathogenesis of PASC may provide answers and guide the medical community to the right management of the condition. The loss of human lives, the disability of the population, the increase in the costs of health care and services burden the health care systems. Persistence of post COVID-19 conditions affects various levels of medical and social life, and the negative effects on healthcare and the economy may be fully appreciated in the future. The psychological and social consequences of ongoing COVID-19 should be considered as part of clinical care models [10].

## Cardiovascular Involvement in COVID-19

The primary target for SARS-CoV-2 is the respiratory system, but the cardiovascular system can be involved as well. Apart from the mild flu-like symptoms, COVID-19 often causes serious damage to the cardiovascular system—endotheliitis, microangiopathy, thrombosis, heart failure, myocarditis, pericarditis, cardiac arrhythmias, and acute coronary syndromes. Once in the nasopharynx, the SARS-CoV-2 enters the body by binding through its S-binding protein to angiotensin I-converting enzyme 2 receptors (ACE2-r), found predominantly in the lungs, cardiomyocytes, and endothelial cells. ACE2 is known to have protective effects by catalyzing the hydrolysis of angiotensin II and therefore lowers the activation of the renin–angiotensin–aldosterone system (RAAS), which occurs in conditions of cardiovascular disease (CVD) such as hypertension, congestive heart failure, and atherosclerosis. Entering the cells via endocytosis, the virus begins to replicate, causing widespread infection. Since ACE2 converts angiotensin I and II to cardioprotective peptides, angiotensin 1–9 and angiotensin 1–7, its loss on cell surface may potentiate cardiac damage, resulting in endothelial dysfunction, inflammation, and thrombosis. ACE2 activity is known to be reduced in vessels with established atherosclerotic plaques and diabetes, while it is increased in women and young people due to the action of estrogens [11–14]. Reduction in ACE2 activity may potentiate the so-called cytokine storm. It involves elevated levels of circulating cytokines and immune cell hyperactivation caused by dysregulating RAAS and activating ACE2/bradykinin axis. The overproduction of cytokines and hyperinflammation leads to exacerbation of underlying cardiovascular diseases or triggering new ones. According to the latest epidemiological data, about 80% of patients with COVID-19 have mild symptoms, about 45% require hospitalization, while 5% of patients need mechanical ventilation. The difference in the course of the disease is related to the degree of viral load, host immune response, age of the patient, and the presence of other diseases such as hypertension, diabetes, and coagulation abnormalities. Aging is associated with increased oxidative stress and reduced role of endogenous defense mechanisms. With aging there is a reduced efficiency of thrombolysis, lower protection against myocardial ischemia, and more frequent manifestation of heart failure and other CVD. It has not yet been established whether the patient's older age or greater immune response to the virus or both are responsible for myocardial damage with consecutive complications [15–18].

## Cardiovascular Complications in COVID-19

Direct viral infection, cytokine dysregulation, and direct cardiomyocyte involvement can lead to acute myocardial injury in patients with COVID-19. Thus except for the high levels of CRP (C-reactive protein), elevated troponin levels suggest acute myocardial injury. It can be a result of myocarditis, ischemic injury, Takotsubo's cardiomyopathy, septic cardiomyopathy, pulmonary embolism [7, 19, 20].

Acute coronary syndromes can be a manifestation of imbalance between myocardial supply and demand as a result of systemic changes—hypoxemia, tachycardia, hypotension, vasoconstriction, or acute thrombosis in the coronary arteries. Often, when the right coronary artery is affected a complete atrioventricular heart block can be provoked. Other location of the coronary lesion may lead to severe ischemic cardiomyopathy, left ventricular aneurysm formation with apical thrombosis [21–23]. The most frequent arrhythmia seen in COVID-19 patients is atrial fibrillation, which is a result of acute respiratory failure. Electrolyte imbalance such as low levels of potassium or magnesium can also lead to arrhythmic states [24]. Some of the medications used in the treatment of COVID-19 have proarrhythmogenic effects and should be used with caution, as they can provoke long QT interval, ventricular tachycardia, and sudden cardiac death [25, 26].

A hypercoagulable state and thrombotic events, that are related to markedly elevated D-dimer and fibrin degradation products, are thought to be secondary to systemic inflammatory response [27, 28].

Takotsubo cardiomyopathy is mainly a result of increased stimulation of the sympathetic nervous system, which is usually observed in patients with COVID-19. It can be due to physical and psychological stress. This state can mimic acute coronary syndrome, which can develop within severe sepsis, hypoxemia, or metabolic acidosis [29–31].

Acute myocarditis due to myocardial inflammation can lead to ventricular dysfunction because of focal or global myocarditis or necrosis [25]. Life-threatening arrhythmias can be a consequence of myocarditis. When linked with pericardial effusion, further deteriorating of the hemodynamics might lead to acute heart failure (HF) and cardiogenic shock [26, 32].

## Life After COVID-19: Results of the First National Campaign in Bulgaria

Bulgarian Cardiac Institute (BCI) is an organization for cardiac treatment, which leads the largest and fastest growing medical group in Bulgaria. Covering 2/3 of the patient flow and 3/4 from the territory of the country, BCI is a leading center in medical activity, applying the most modern methods and equipment for diagnosis and treatment in the field of cardiology, cardiac surgery, neurology, neurosurgery, vascular surgery, oncology, surgery, orthopedics, genetics, immunology, radiotherapy, and radiosurgery. In correlation with this, maintaining the trend of laying the foundations for innovation, we launched the first national, free, and long-term campaign "Life after COVID-19."

The campaign focused on all citizens who had suffered from COVID-19, regardless of the form of the disease. Through a survey available on an Internet platform or conducted through a telephone conversation, participants reported their health status. The questions they answered were closed-ended, with two possible answers—yes (i.e. there is a problem) or no (i.e. no problem). The data was processed and every citizen with at least one persistent symptom was offered a free-of-charge medical examination. It was conducted by leading cardiologists in the country and included a detailed history, status, blood pressure measurement, electrocardiogram. In case of pathological deviations, additional examinations, treatment, and consultations were performed. The participants were followed up for a long time and in case of persistent symptoms, despite the performed medical-diagnostic procedures, they were hospitalized in high-tech hospitals for continuous treatment.

The overwhelming interest in the campaign led to the participation of over 2300 citizens who survived COVID-19. We found that 75% of the respondents received treatment at home, while 25% had a more severe course of the disease, which required treatment in a hospital (1% in the intensive care unit). Of all respondents, 68% reported persistent complaints months and even a year later. The main questions that received a positive answer (yes, i.e. there is a problem) were those related to signs and symptoms of fatigue (62%), palpitations (39%), shortness of breath (32%), chest pain (28%), joint pain (25%), headache (20%), impaired concentration (16%), dizziness (16%), persistent cough (14%) (Fig. 15.1).

A medical examination was performed on 1547 patients (57% women and 43% men). The most common pathological finding was destabilization of blood pressure control (52%), among which hypertension was predominant (95%), followed by hypotension (3%), and instability in blood pressure values (2%). Cardiac arrhythmias were found in more than 1/3 of those examined—manifesting as tachycardia (96%) or bradycardia (4%). Manifestations of decompensated heart failure were observed in 16% of cases.

These pathological abnormalities necessitated additional examinations in 61% of those examined. The main instrumental method supporting the diagnostic process was echocardiography, performed in 43%. It was followed by Holter ECG (4%) and radiography (3%). Laboratory tests were performed in 10% of cases.

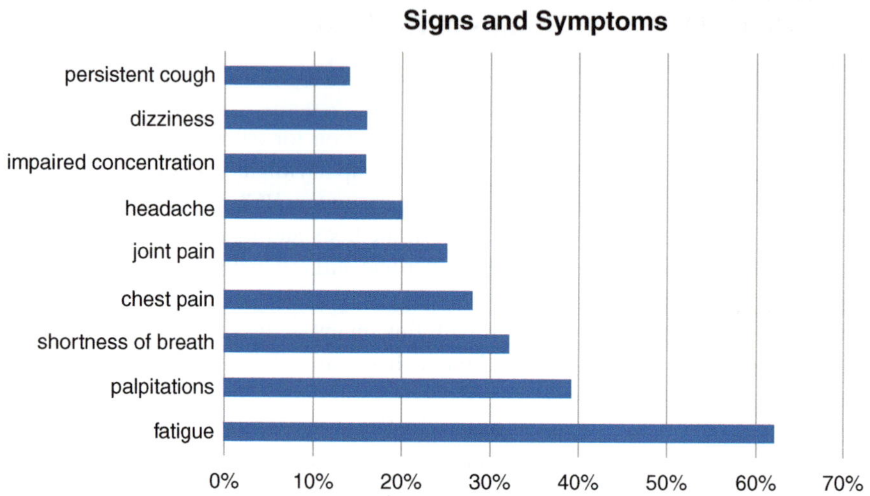


**Fig. 15.1** Persistent signs and symptoms after COVID-19

These included complete blood count, NT-proBNP, D-dimer, blood sugar profile. The various signs and symptoms determined the need for multidisciplinary medical care (9%). Consultations were conducted with a neurologist (30%), pulmonologist (24%), endocrinologist (12%), vascular surgeon (6%), rheumatologist (5%), and others. Summarizing the results of the medical examination, a change in therapy was required for 56% of those followed.

At the secondary examination, new studies were performed in 6% and a change in therapy in 3%. Despite the performed medical-diagnostic procedures, in 10% of the cases the symptoms persisted, which necessitated hospital treatment.

Our experience showed that the care of patients with COVID-19 did not stop with the control of the acute phase of the disease. Most of the citizens who took part in the campaign suffered from a mild form of the disease and were treated in an outpatient setting. However, the signs and symptoms persisted in 68% of cases, and their duration could reach a year after the illness. The most common complaints were fatigue, palpitations, shortness of breath, chest pain, joint pain, headache, impaired concentration, dizziness, and persistent cough. High values of blood pressure, tachycardia, and manifestations of heart failure were the leading objective changes. In half of the cases additional examinations were needed, and treatment was changed. The various symptoms required the collaboration of doctors with different specialties. Despite the dedicated medical care, every tenth citizen with persistent symptoms required re-hospitalization and hospital treatment.

COVID-19 does not stop spreading. If at the beginning of the pandemic the virus mainly affected the countries in the northern hemisphere, today it is a fact that even the warmest countries have been diagnosed with cases. The increase in the number of affected children is another alarming statistic, alerting that along with newly diagnosed cases, post-COVID conditions will increase in waves and will be among the leading problems in healthcare systems. That is why it is extremely important to identify health problems, methods for diagnosis and treatment of post-COVID conditions. Only in this way we will deal with the disease after the disease.

## Imaging Methods of Choice in COVID-Related Cardiovascular Complications

As COVID-19 is a highly contagious disease, clinical personnel should use methods of imaging that minimize the risk of spreading the infection. Most suitable are transthoracic echocardiography and point of care ultrasound (POCUS). They are the first-line cardiac imaging techniques in this clinical setting, due to their portability, bedside feasibility in emergency settings, and low cost [33]. Ultrasound is a diagnostic method for imaging the heart structures, valves, and regional wall motion. According to the European Association of Cardiovascular Imaging (EACVI) it is recommended to perform echocardiography in patients with abnormally high levels of cardiac biomarkers and/or ECG signs of myocardial damage, while acknowledging that other imaging diagnostic tests are not routinely used in the emergency context of the COVID-19 pandemic [34, 35]. CT scan and MRI can also be used for distinguishing cardiovascular complications, but they have higher cost and lower availability [36, 37].

Every hospital should develop appropriate protocols for rapid diagnosis, triage, isolation, and management of patients with COVID-19 and concomitant cardiovascular complications. These protocols should be well-rehearsed for proper use of health services and to minimize the exposure of the medical staff [38].

Transthoracic echocardiography (TTE) is the most frequently used imaging method, which gives us information about the heart function. Global longitudinal strain (GLS) is an important additive method for evaluation of LV function at global and regional levels. It is a more sensitive method for detecting myocardial dysfunction, compared with left ventricular ejection fraction (LVEF) [39]. MRI is also an informative method; however, it is not used that often, due to higher expenses and due to the fact that it is more time-consuming. Almost all patients with severe COVID-19 and most of the patients with moderate disease have a certain degree of myocardial damage. Echocardiography usually does not show significant changes in the LVEF and LV sizes in patients with mild or moderate COVID-19. However, in one trial in China, 78.3% of the patients with mild infection and 98% of the patients who were in critical condition had echocardiographic deviations. For example, the motion of the LV walls was abnormal, and the wall thickness was slightly thickened, particularly for the septum. But in patients who were in critical state, lower LVEF was found. The changes are in correlation with elevated serum levels of cardiac troponin I (cTnI) and N-terminal pro-B-type natriuretic peptide (NT-proBNP), pulse oxygen saturation ($SpO_2$), and inflammatory markers, such as C-reactive protein and cytokines [40, 41]. Even though echocardiographic deviations are found mostly in patients with severe COVID-19, GLS can identify subclinical myocardial dysfunction. Moreover, measuring GLS gives us the opportunity for earlier diagnosis of myocardial injury, even before a reduction in the LVEF occurs. Studies showed that reduced LV-GLS is more frequent, occurring in 80% of the patients, while LV function parameters such as reduced EF and wall motion abnormalities were less frequent findings. 2D-speckle tracking echocardiography is a method, which evaluates myocardial function at global and regional levels. It shows the percentage of deformation between two points in the myocardium. Studies in COVID-19 patients show that the abnormal GLS predominantly involves the basal-septal and basal-lateral segments of the left ventricle. This pattern reminded of a "reverse Takotsubo" morphology and is not typical for other viral myocarditis. Another interesting finding is that the reduction of the LV-GLS is usually reversible, with normalization of the findings for 1–3 months [42, 43].

Cardiac magnetic resonance (CMR) is currently the gold standard for evaluation of cardiac morphology and function. It has higher sensitivity for detecting occult cardiac dysfunction than hs-cTnI. With its mapping techniques, such as T1, T2, extracellular volume (ECV), and late gadolinium enhancement (GLE), this method can assess quantitatively diffuse or local myocardial fibrosis and edema [44]. One study in Frankfurt with patients recently recovered from COVID-19 showed that 78% of them had abnormal CMR findings, more specifically—lower LVEF, higher left ventricle volumes, raised signals in native T1 and T2 mapping, which illustrates edema and changes in LGE, showing myocardial fibrosis. Endomyocardial biopsy was performed in patients with severe findings which revealed active lymphocytic inflammation [30].

Our experience in "Life after COVID" campaign shows that about two-thirds of PASC patients referred for echocardiography have the typical post COVID-19 GLS impairment, involving predominantly the basal segments. We observe such findings in severe as well as non-severe COVID-19 cases. Our management strategy in these cases includes prolongation of antiaggregant therapy, initiation of cardioprotective therapy (could include some or all of the following: beta-blocker, trimetazidine, molsidomine), antiviral therapy (hydroxychloroquine), and advice to reduce vigorous physical activity, although maintaining moderate physical activity. Our initial experience with 3-month follow-up of these patients shows a resolution of the abnormality in about 80% of the cases in this period.

## Acute Coronary Syndrome as Part of the Post COVID-19 Conditions

Apart from the direct damage to the lungs, COVID-19 is associated with damage to other systems and organs, including the heart, and causes conditions such as congestive heart failure, myocarditis, conduction abnormalities, arrhythmias, and acute coronary syndromes [45, 46]. The SARS-CoV-2 infection can also induce coagulation abnormalities that are associated with cardiopulmonary damage and therefore worsening the prognosis.

The range of clinical complications to COVID-19 is extremely broad. Endothelial injury is an underlying mechanism that precedes the inflammation and consequent thrombosis [47, 48]. It is currently hypothesized that the ACE-2 receptor is the entry way for the virus to invade and infect tissues [49]. The vascular endothelium appears to be targeted directly by the virus as ACE-2 is expressed extensively in the blood vessels and the heart. The result is exocytosis of multiple endothelial granules containing vWF (von Willebrand's factor), P-selectin, and other proinflammatory cytokines, which mediate platelets adhesion, aggregation, and leukocyte adherence to the vessel wall, leading to intravascular thrombosis [50].

Many patients with severe COVID-19 face thromboembolic events, due to this coagulopathy [51, 52]. One of the most life-threatening types of this coagulation abnormality is the one involving the coronary blood flow and provoking a heart attack. In this situation many additional problems arise—for example: access to a Cath lab, exposure of additional medical personnel during the additional procedures needed, more complications, and increased mortality for the patients. Coronary angiography for COVID-19 patients is a logistic challenge and, in some cases, there is not a need for intervention since the main problem is the thrombosis and the dysfunction in the microcirculation.

Hence, we evaluated in detail a case series of 26 patients referred for primary percutaneous coronary intervention (pPCI) for MI in our catheterization laboratory during COVID-19 infection. The main goal we set ourselves was to evaluate if there are parameters that could predict the presence of an interventional target, infarct related artery (IRA), prior to catheterization, and to determine their sensitivity and specificity.

During the period between November 2020 and April 2021 twenty-six patients were referred to the Cath lab with MI defined by the fourth universal definition [53]. Most of the patients in our study were sent to our hospital due to acute coronary syndrome, while others developed ACS during their stay in the COVID-19 department.

After coronary angiography, we found that 17 patients (65.38%) had an IRA, and they underwent pPCI. The other 9 (34.62%) did not have an IRA, they did not require pPCI, and the diagnosis of myocardial infarction with no obstructive coronary arteries (MINOCA) was made, most probably due to myocarditis or microvascular dysfunction.

Comparing the patients with IRA to those without we found that the subjects who required pPCI had significantly higher hsTRI values, and more often typical chest pain. The other observed variables did not differ significantly between the two groups (Table 15.1).

We performed a ROC analysis for hsTrI values and we found that hsTrI cut-off >2.63 showed sensitivity of 70.6%, specificity of 77.8%, positive predictive value (PPV) of 85.7%, and negative predictive value (NPV) of 58.3% for detecting the presence of IRA and need for pPCI in ACS COVID-19 patients (area under the curve—AUC 0.771; 95% confidence interval 0.59–0.96; $p = 0.025$), Fig. 15.2.

**Table 15.1** Comparison between the groups with and without an IRA and need for a PCI

| Variable | Patients with IRA and pPCI *n* = 17 | Patients w/o IRA and pPCI *n* = 9 | *p* value |
|---|---|---|---|
| Age (years) (mean ± SD) | 68.35 ± 10.92 | 64.33 ± 9.62 | 0.363 |
| Male (*n*, %) | 9 (52.9) | 6 (66.7) | 0.683 |
| AH (*n*, %) | 17 (100.0) | 8 (88.9) | 0.346 |
| DLP (*n*, %) | 14 (82.4) | 8 (88.9) | 1.000 |
| DM (*n*, %) | 5 (29.4) | 2 (22.2) | 1.000 |
| *Typical chest pain (n, %)* | *17 (100.0)* | *2 (22.2)* | *<0.001* |
| ST elevation (*n*, %) | 11 (73.3) | 5 (55.6) | 0.635 |
| Symptoms of HF (*n*, %) | 9 (52.9) | 3 (33.3) | 0.429 |
| Symptom onset (days) (mean ± SD) | 12.00 ± 7.51 | 14.8 ± 8.7 | 0.725 |
| Home treatment (*n*, %) | 4 (23.5) | 1 (11.1) | 0.628 |
| $SatO_2$ at admission (%) (mean ± SD) | 79.50 ± 8.39 | 83.80 ± 12.46 | 0.843 |
| Hospital stay (days) (median, IQR) | 4.50 (5.00) | 5.00 (4.00) | 0.863 |
| ICU stay (days) (median, IQR) | 3.50 (12.00) | 3.00 (5.00) | 1.000 |
| Mechanical ventilation (*n*, %) | 8 (47.1) | 1 (11.1) | 0.098 |
| *hsTrI (ng/ml) (median, IQR)* | *7.13 (61.00)* | *1.28 (2.94)* | *0.025* |
| CK (U/l) (median, IQR) | 348.00 (1028.50) | 227.00 (281.50) | 0.319 |
| CK-MB (U/l) (median, IQR) | 51.00 (154.50) | 25.40 (29.15) | 0.131 |
| D-dimer (ng/ml) (median, IQR) | 960.00 (1460.50) | 221.00 (1319.00) | 0.195 |
| hsCRP (mg/l) (median, IQR) | 36.90 (131.65) | 55.50 (159.93) | 0.771 |
| Leu (× $10^9$ g/l) (mean ± SD) | 13.34 ± 5.56 | 10.94 ± 5.98 | 0.324 |
| Lym (× $10^9$ g/l) (median, IQR) | 1.03 (1.13) | 0.55 (0.64) | 0.295 |
| LDH (U/l) (mean ± SD) | 846.00 ± 610.58 | 775.33 ± 391.49 | 0.800 |
| ASAT (U/l) (median, IQR) | 136.00 (221.50) | 39.00 (73.50) | 0.063 |
| ALAT (U/l) (median, IQR) | 55.00 (70.25) | 25.00 (124.00) | 0.403 |

We performed a binary logistic regression and we found that hsTrI values >2.63 was the only independent predictive factor for the presence of IRA and need for pPCI (odds ratio 8.4; 95% CI 1.27–55.39, $p = 0.027$).

According to our published data search, we were not able to find another study analyzing the predictors for the presence of IRA and the need for pPCI in COVID-19 MI patients.

So in conclusion, most of the patients in our study group (34.62%) with MI during the acute or post-acute COVID-19 infection did not have an IRA and hence did not need a coronary intervention. Patients with MI and IRA had significantly higher hsTrI values and exclusively typical chest pain compared to patients with MI but without an IRA, whose hsTrI values were lower and chest pain was atypical or non-stenocardic. ECG changes had no statistical significance for distinguishing between MI patients with or without IRA. Our results suggested that in patients with

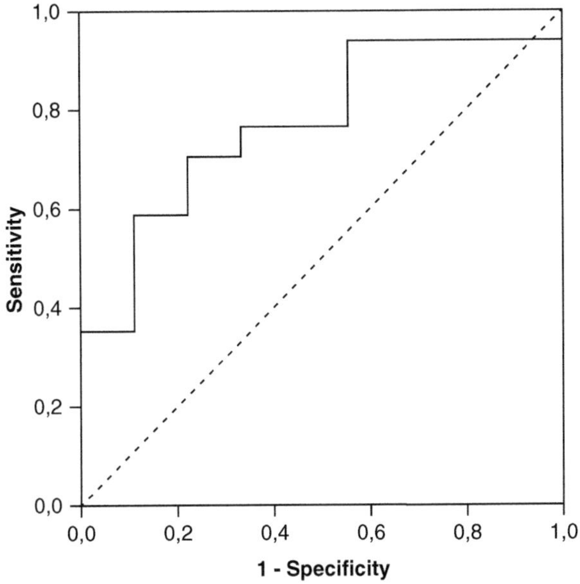


**Fig. 15.2** ROC analysis for hsTrI values as a predictor for the presence of IRA

COVID-19 and acute coronary syndrome, the diagnostic accuracy for identifying type 1 MI with an indication for pPCI could be significantly increased using a higher cut-off value for hsTrI.

## Pulmonary Embolism in COVID-19 Patients

Due to procoagulant effects SARS-CoV-2 infection can in some cases be the cause of a pulmonary thromboembolism (PE) [54, 55]. Due to the lack of large prospective studies, little is known about the pathogenesis underlying PE, caused by COVID-19 (80). Additional conditions complicating the diagnosis are the presence of risk factors for PE in almost all patients with COVID-19, as well as the overlap of the clinical presentation between PE and COVID-19.

We designed a single-center study, conducted at the Heart and Brain Center of Clinical Excellence Hospital, Pleven in the period Dec 2020 to Feb 2021, to try and find the indicators that predict the presence of PE in patients with COVID-19. It included 27 consecutively hospitalized patients with recent pneumonia caused by COVID-19 and clinical presentation suggesting PE. The patients were divided into two groups—with and without definite PE, confirmed by CT pulmoangiography.

Our results showed that 8 patients from the group had PE, and 19 did not have PE. The mean age of the group was 65 years. Eighteen of the patients were women. The two groups did not differ significantly in age and distribution between the sexes. In the two groups statistically significant differences were observed in the electrocardiographic findings. In patients without PE, 18 (94.7%) had no S-waves greater than 1.5 mm in I, aVL. In the group with PE in 3 (37.5%) this ECG criteria was not present, and in 5 (62.5%) it was present ($p = 0.004$). Similar ratios were found in terms of the presence of Q-wave in III, aVF. In patients without PE, 18 (94.7%) did not have this ECG sign, while it was present in half of the patients with PE ($p = 0.017$). In patients without PE, the median value of oxygen saturation was 92.0% (69–97), and in those with PE 88.5% (83–95) ($p < 0.001$). Statistically significant differences between the two groups were observed in the indicator—the ratio RV/LV diameters ≥1.0 ($p = 0.001$). In patients without PE there was none with an increase in the ratio ≥ 1 in favor of the right ventricle, while in the group of patients with massive form 5 (62.5%) had the ratio RV/LV diameters ≥1.0, and 3 (37, 5%) did not have it. Right ventricular dysfunction was more prevalent in the PE group, and none of the patients in the non-PE group had right ventricular dysfunction ($p = 0.001$). The RV/LV diameter ratios ≥1.0 as well as right ventricular dysfunction showed both a sensitivity of 62.5%, specificity 100%, positive predictive value 100% and negative such 86.4% to verify the PE diagnosis.

D-dimer values differed significantly in the two groups. In patients without PE, the mean D-dimer value was 1546 ng/ml (109–8840), while in those with PE 6489.75 ng/ml (570–17,051) ($p = 0.021$). For our laboratory, the upper limit of the normal range is 500 ng/ml. As a result of the ROC analysis, we found that the D-dimer cut-off value of 1032 ng/ml (2064 times higher above the upper limit of the normal range) had an optimal sensitivity (Se) of 87.5%, specificity (Sp) of 57.9%, positive predictive value (PPV) of 46.7%, and negative predictive value (NPV) of 91.7% for the diagnosis of PE ($p = 0.021$) (Fig. 15.3). Having D-dimer as a binary variable (cut-off 1032 ng/ml), we found that in the group without PE, in 11 (57.9%) of patients the D-dimer was ≤1032 ng/ml, while in 8 (42.1%) it was >1032 ng/ml.

**Fig. 15.3** ROC analysis for D-dimer values and the probability of PE

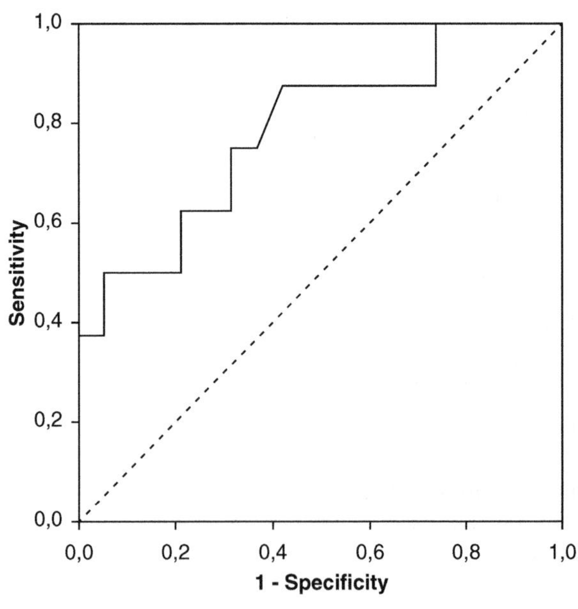

Of the patients with massive PE, only 1 (12.5%) had a D-dimer ≤1032 ng/ml, and the remaining 7 (87.5%) were >1032 ng/ml (Fisher's exact tests, $p = 0.043$).

When performing binary logistic regression, part of the ECG criteria, S-wave over 1.5 mm in I lead and aVL ($p = 0.007$), Q-wave in III and aVF ($p = 0.020$), as well as the D-dimer as quantitative variable ($p = 0.025$) proved to be independent predictors of PE.

Our results show that against the background of acute and post-acute COVID-19 conditions ECG and echocardiographic criteria remain predictive of PE. As for the D-dimer values, we found that a cut-off concentration with optimal Se, Sp, PPV, and NPV for diagnosis of PE is two times higher than the upper limit of normal, with high Se and NPV. Our study suggests that a higher D-dimer cut-off value should be applied in COVID-19 and post-COVID-19 patients to raise a significant suspicion for the presence of PE.

## Conclusion

The conclusion we can make from everything we have observed and experienced during the past 2 years is that the COVID-19 pandemic is not something mankind cannot handle. We have learned a lot from our mistakes and now we have a new understanding about the disease and its treatment. With the massive vaccination programs combined with adequate medical treatment, the number of casualties and the spreading of the disease will soon decline to a point, where it will become a memory of a dire part of our history. Unfortunately, here comes the next challenge—we are yet to face the long-term complications. This is a topic not to be underestimated and is of crucial importance for the near future of the mankind. We still have a lot of research and clinical work to answer many unanswered questions, regarding the exact prevalence, range, and duration of long-term COVID-19 consequences, our possibilities to predict, prevent, and treat them, questions about the immunological response, coagulation status, and genetic susceptibility. But as we all know—a journey of a thousand miles begins with a single step.

## References

1. COVID-19 rapid guideline: managing the long-term effects of COVID-19. NICE guideline [NG188]. 18 Dec 2020. https://www.nice.org.uk/guidance/ng188
2. Nalbandian A, Sehgal K, Gupta A, et al. Post-acute COVID-19 syndrome. Nat Med. 2021;27:601–15. https://doi.org/10.1038/s41591-021-01283-z.
3. Logue JK, Franko NM, McCulloch DJ, et al. Sequelae in adults at 6 months after COVID-19 infection. JAMA Netw Open. 2021;4(2):e210830. https://doi.org/10.1001/jamanetworkopen.2021.0830.
4. McNamara D. Infectious COVID-19 can persist in gut for weeks, September 11, 2020, MedScape.

5. World Health Organization (WHO). COVID-19 clinical management living guidance. WHO; 2021. 25 January 2021.
6. Mason RJ. Pathogenesis of COVID-19 from a cell biology perspective. Eur Respir J. 2020;55:2000607. https://doi.org/10.1183/13993003.00607-2020.
7. Yeoh YK, Zuo T, Lui GC, et al. Gut microbiota composition reflects disease severity and dysfunctional immune responses in patients with COVID-19. Gut. 2021;70:698–706.
8. Murthy S, Lee TC. IL-6 blockade for COVID-19: a global scientific call to arms. Lancet Respir Med. 2021;9(5):438–40. https://doi.org/10.1016/S2213-2600(21)00127-2.
9. Huang C, Huang L, Wang Y. 6-month consequences of COVID-19 in patients discharged from hospital: a cohort study. Lancet. 2021;397(10270):220–32. https://doi.org/10.1016/S0140-6736(20)326568.
10. CDC. Post-COVID conditions, centers for disease control and prevention, vol. 2021. CDC; 2021. https://www.cdc.gov/.
11. Bansal M. Cardiovascular disease and COVID-19. Diabetes Metab Syndr. 2020;14(3):247–50.
12. Napoli C, Tritto I, Benincasa G, Mansueto G, Ambrosioc G. Cardiovascular involvement during COVID-19 and clinical implications in elderly patients. A review. Ann Med Surg. 2020;57:236–43. https://doi.org/10.1016/j.amsu.2020.07.054.
13. Hoffmann M, Kleine-Weber H, Schroeder S, Krüger N, Herrler T, Erichsen S. SARS-CoV-2 cell entry depends on ACE2 and TMPRSS2 and is blocked by a clinically proven protease inhibitor. Cell. 2020;181(271–80):e8.
14. Sattar Y, Ullah W, Rauf H, Virk H-u-H, Yadav S, Chowdhury M, Connerney M, Mamtani S, Pahuja M, Patel RD, Mir T, Almas T, Pacha HM, Alraiesg MC. COVID-19 cardiovascular epidemiology, cellular pathogenesis, clinical manifestations and management. Int J Cardiol Heart Vasc. 2020;29:100589. https://doi.org/10.1016/j.ijcha.2020.100589.
15. Ksiazek TG, Erdman D, Goldsmith CS, et al. A novel coronavirus associated with severe acute respiratory syndrome. N Engl J Med. 2003;348:1953–66.
16. Wang D, Hu B, Hu C, Zhu F, Liu X, Zhang J, Wang B, Xiang H, Cheng Z, Xiong Y, Zhao Y, Li Y, Wang X, Peng Z. Clinical characteristics of 138 hospitalized patients with 2019 novel coronavirus-infected pneumonia in Wuhan, China. J Am Med Assoc. 2020;323:1061–9. https://doi.org/10.1001/jama.2020.1585.
17. Huang C, Wang Y, Li X. Clinical features of patients infected with 2019 novel coronavirus in Wuhan, China. Lancet. 2020;395:497–506. https://doi.org/10.1016/S0140-6736(20)30183-5.
18. Chen N, Zhou M, Dong X, Qu J, Gong F, Han Y, Qiu Y, Wang J, Liu Y, Wei Y, Xia J, Yu T, Zhang X, Zhang L. Epidemiological and clinical characteristics of 99 cases of 2019 novel coronavirus pneumonia in Wuhan, China: a descriptive study. Lancet. 2020;395:507–13. https://doi.org/10.1016/S0140-6736(20)30211-7.
19. Li B, Yang J, Zhao F. Prevalence and impact of cardiovascular metabolic diseases on COVID-19 in China. Clin Res Cardiol. 2020;109(5):531–8.
20. Zhou F, Yu T, Du R. Clinical course and risk factors for mortality of adult inpatients with COVID-19 in Wuhan, China: a retrospective cohort study. Lancet. 2020;
21. Mihatov N, Januzzi JL, Gaggin HK. Type 2 myocardial infarction due to supply-demand mismatch. Trends Cardiovasc Med. 2017;27(6):408–17.
22. Asrress KN, Williams R, Lockie T, Khawaja MZ, De Silva K, Lumley M, Patterson T, Arri S, Ihsan S, Ellis H, Guilcher A, Clapp B, Chowienczyk PJ, Plein S, Perera D, Marber MS, Redwood SR. Physiology of angina and its alleviation with nitroglycerin: insights from invasive catheter laboratory measurements during exercise. Circulation. 2017;136(1):24–34.
23. Xiong TY, Redwood S, Prendergast B, Chen M. Coronaviruses and the cardiovascular system: acute and long-term implications. Eur Heart J. 2020;41(19):1798–800.
24. Chen D, Li X, Song Q, Hu C, Su F, Dai J. Hypokalemia and clinical implications in patients with coronavirus disease 2019 (COVID-19). medRxiv. 2020. https://doi.org/10.1101/2020.02.27.20028530.

25. Puntmann VO, Carerj ML, Wieters I, Fahim M, Arendt C, Hoffmann J. Outcomes of cardiovascular magnetic resonance imaging in patients recently recovered from coronavirus disease 2019 (COVID-19). JAMA Cardiol. 2020;5(11):1265–73.
26. Hua A, O'Gallagher K, Sado D, Byrne J. Life-threatening cardiac tamponade complicating myo-pericarditis in COVID-19. Eur Heart J. 2020;41(22):2130.
27. Gómez-Mesa JE, Galindo-Coral S, Montes MC, Muñoz Martin AJ. Thrombosis and coagulopathy in COVID-19. Curr Probl Cardiol. 2021;46(3):100742. https://doi.org/10.1016/j.cpcardiol.2020.100742.
28. Tang N, Li D, Wang X, Sun Z. Abnormal coagulation parameters are associated with poor prognosis in patients with novel coronavirus pneumonia. J Thromb Haemostasis. 2020;18(4):844–7.
29. Knight DS, Kotecha T, Razvi Y, Chacko L, Brown JT, Jeetley PS. COVID-19: myocardial injury in survivors. Circulation. 2020;142(11):1120–2.
30. Guo T, Fan Y, Chen M, Wu X, Zhang L, He T. Cardiovascular implications of fatal outcomes of patients with coronavirus disease 2019 (COVID-19). JAMA Cardiol. 2020;5(7):811–8.
31. Sala S, Peretto G, Gramegna M, Palmisano A, Villatore A, Vignale D. Acute myocarditis presenting as a reverse Tako-Tsubo syndrome in a patient with SARS-CoV-2 respiratory infection. Eur Heart J. 2020;41(19):1861–2.
32. Manka R, Karolyi M, Polacin M, Holy EW, Nemeth J, Steiger P. Myocardial edema in COVID-19 on cardiac MRI. J Heart Lung Transplant. 2020;39(7):730–2.
33. Zhang L, Wang B, Zhou J, Kirkpatrick J, Xie M, Johri AM. Bedside focused cardiac ultrasound in COVID-19 from the Wuhan epicenter: the role of cardiac point-of-care ultrasound, limited transthoracic echocardiography, and critical care echocardiography. J Am Soc Echocardiogr. 2020;33(6):676–82.
34. Skulstad H, Cosyns B, Popescu BA, Galderisi M, Salvo GD, Donal E. COVID-19 pandemic and cardiac imaging: EACVI recommendations on precautions, indications, prioritization, and protection for patients and healthcare personnel. Eur Heart J Cardiovasc Imaging. 2020;21(6):592–8.
35. Cosyns B, Lochy S, Luchian ML, Gimelli A, Pontone G, Allard SD. The role of cardiovascular imaging for myocardial injury in hospitalized COVID-19 patients. Eur Heart J Cardiovasc Imaging. 2020;21(7):709–14.
36. Motwani M, Kidambi A, Greenwood JP, Plein S. Advances in cardiovascular magnetic resonance in ischaemic heart disease and non-ischaemic cardiomyopathies. Heart. 2014;100(21):1722–33.
37. Citro R, Pontone G, Bellino M, Silverio A, Iuliano G, Baggiano A, Manka R, Iesu S, Vecchione C, Asch FM, Ghadri JR, Templinf C. Role of multimodality imaging in evaluation of cardiovascular involvement in COVID-19. Trends Cardiovasc Med. 2021;31(1):8–16. https://doi.org/10.1016/j.tcm.2020.10.001.
38. Tam CF, Cheung KS, Lam S. Impact of coronavirus disease 2019 (COVID-19) outbreak on ST-segment-elevation myocardial infarction care in Hong Kong, China. Circ Cardiovasc Qual Outcomes. 2020;13:CIRCOUTCOMES120006631.
39. Karlsen S, Dahlslett T, Grenne B, Sjøli B, Smiseth O, Edvardsen T, Karlsen HB, et al. Global longitudinal strain is a more reproducible measure of left ventricular function than ejection fraction regardless of echocardiographic training. Cardiovasc Ultrasound. 2019;17:18.
40. Li R, Wang H, Ma F, et al. Widespread myocardial dysfunction in COVID-19 patients detected by myocardial strain imaging using 2-D speckle-tracking echocardiography. Acta Pharmacol Sin. 2021;42:1–8.
41. Li SS, Cheng CW, Fu CL, et al. Left ventricular performance in patients with severe acute respiratory syndrome: a 30-day echocardiographic follow-up study. Circulation. 2003;108(15):1798–803.
42. Shmueli H, Shah M, Ebinger J, et al. Left ventricular global longitudinal strain in identifying subclinical myocardial dysfunction among patients hospitalized with COVID-19. Int J Cardiol Heart Vasc. 2021;32:100719.

43. St S, Richter S, Seige M. Echocardiographic characteristics of patients with SARS-CoV-2 infection. Clin Res Cardiol. 2020;109:1549–66.
44. Huang L, Zhao P, Tang D, et al. Cardiac involvement in recovered COVID-19 patients identified by magnetic resonance imaging. JACC Cardiovasc Imaging. 2020;13(11):2330–9. https://doi.org/10.1016/j.jcmg.2020.05.004.
45. Rattka M, Dreyhaupt J, Winsauer C, et al. Effect of the COVID-19 pandemic on mortality of patients with STEMI: a systematic review and meta-analysis. Heart. 2021;107:482–7.
46. Samidurai A, Das A. Cardiovascular complications associated with COVID-19 and potential therapeutic strategies. Int J Mol Sci. 2020;21(18):6790. https://doi.org/10.3390/ijms21186790.
47. ZsuzsannaVarga AJ, Flammer PS, Haberecker M, Andermatt R, Zinkernagel AS, et al. Endothelial cell infection and endotheliitis in COVID-19. Lancet. 2020;395(10234):1417–8. https://doi.org/10.1016/S0140-6736(20)30937-5. Epub 2020 Apr 21.
48. Lowenstein CJ, Solomon SD. Severe COVID-19 is a microvascular disease. Circulation. 2020;142:1609–11.
49. Kasal DA, De Lorenzo A, Tibiriçá E. COVID-19 and microvascular disease: pathophysiology of SARS-CoV-2 infection with focus on the renin- angiotensin system. Heart Lung Circ. 2020;29(11):1596–602. https://doi.org/10.1016/j.hlc.2020.08.010.
50. McFadyen JD, Stevens H, Peter K. The emerging threat of (micro)thrombosis in COVID-19 and its therapeutic implications. Circ Res. 2020;127:571–87. https://doi.org/10.1161/CIRCRESAHA.120.317447.
51. Asakura H, Ogawa H. COVID-19-associated coagulopathy and disseminated intravascular coagulation. Int J Hematol. 2021;113:45–57. https://doi.org/10.1007/s12185-020-03029-y.
52. Schiavone M, Gobbi C, Biondi-Zoccai G, et al. Acute coronary syndromes and Covid-19: exploring the uncertainties. J Clin Med. 2020;9(6):1683. https://doi.org/10.3390/jcm9061683.
53. Thygesen K, Alpert JS, Jaffe AS, Chaitman BR, Bax JJ, Morrow DA, White HD, ESC Scientific Document Group. Fourth universal definition of myocardial infarction (2018). Eur Heart J. 2019;40(3):237–69. https://doi.org/10.1093/eurheartj/ehy462.
54. Sakr Y, Giovini M, Leone M, et al. Pulmonary embolism in patients with coronavirus disease-2019 (COVID-19) pneumonia: a narrative review. Ann Intensive Care. 2020;10:124.
55. Rouhezamin MR, Haseli S. Diagnosing pulmonary thromboembolism in COVID-19: a stepwise clinical and imaging approach. Acad Radiol. 2020;27(6):896–7.

# Chapter 16
# Association of Alpha 1 Antitrypsin Deficiency with COVID-19 Mortality: Basis for Clinical Trials

**Atanu Kumar Dutta and Kalyan Goswami**

## Introduction

COVID-19 has emerged as a major cause of suffering and destruction of life and livelihood for mankind with 177,439,911 cases and 3,842,439 deaths as of 18th June 2021 [1]. Though the pandemic has hardly spared any nations there have been significant differences in the case fatality ratio globally with Asian and African countries reporting lower mortality statistics compared to other continents [1] (Fig. 16.1).

This difference has been confounded by several factors like the availability of testing resources and medical care, stage of the epidemic wave, the prevalence of co-morbidities like diabetes mellitus, heart disease, cancer, chronic respiratory diseases, a higher percentage of the population over the age 70 years, kidney diseases, outdoor air pollution, and smoking [2]. However, the contribution of viral and host genotypes also has a definitive impact on the observed difference. It has been shown that based on hierarchical clustering for various established mutational signatures of SARS-CoV-2, countries can be classified into different clusters which correlate with the case fatality rate [3]. A systematic review identified C14408T and A23403G variants to be the most prominent causes of life-threatening infections [4].

A. K. Dutta (✉) · K. Goswami
Department of Biochemistry, All India Institute of Medical Sciences,
Kalyani, West Bengal, India
e-mail: atanu.biochem@aiimskalyani.edu.in; kalyan.biochem@aiimskalyani.edu.in


S. Adibi et al. (eds.), *Frontiers of COVID-19*,
https://doi.org/10.1007/978-3-031-08045-6_16

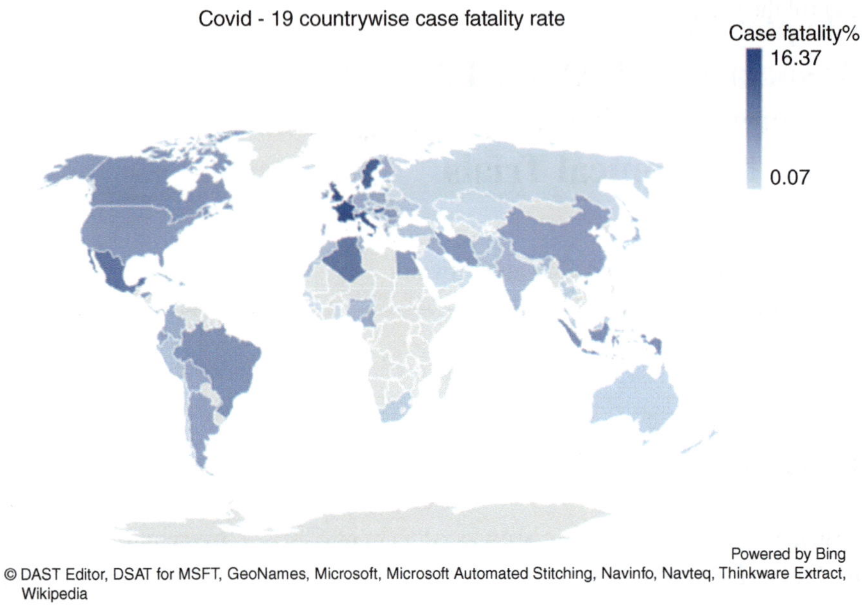


**Fig. 16.1** World map showing country specific case fatality rates as on 7th May 2020 highlighting low case fatality rate in East Asia

## Host Genetics of COVID-19

Since the start of the pandemic, major international efforts have been focused on pooling human genotype data from multiple research groups across the world to find out both common and rare variants to establish any possible correlation with the severity and clinical outcome of SARS-CoV-2 infections [5]. The recent-most genome-wide association meta-analysis data release 6 released by this group included 61 studies from 25 countries leading to a combined sample size of 126,621 COVID-19 infected cases, 25,027 hospitalized cases, and 2,575,347 controls [6]. The most recent data release 6 identified 20 loci associated with severity of disease in hospitalized COVID-19 patients, which include genes involved in antimicrobial defense (*OAS1*, *TAC4*, *DPP9*, *IFNAR2*, *SFTPD*), transport of ions (*SLC6A20*, *SLC22A31*), transcription (*FOXP4*, *KANSL1*, *RAVER1*, *FBRSL1*, *NR1H2*), cellular differentiation (*ELF5*), adhesion (*RPL24*, *THBS3*), cilium assembly (*LZTFL1*), regulation of cardiac conduction (*TMEM65*), glycosylation (*ABO*, *MUC5B*), and lipid biosynthesis (*PLEKHA4*). This data release also identified *HLA-DPB1* and *ACE2* locus to be associated with susceptibility to SARS-CoV-2 infection. For the *ACE2* rs190509934 polymorphism, the minor allele decreases the expression of ACE2, thereby decreasing the risk of severe disease [7]. Incidentally, this variant is most common in South Asians with the allele frequency of 0.02 in gnomAD which could partially explain the lower case fatality rate in South Asians. Similarly, the

*ELF5* rs766826 is also a protective polymorphism where the minor allele decreases the expression of *ELF5*. *ELF5* is co-regulated with *TMPRSS2* in the publicly available RNAseq data [8]. Both the genes are co-expressed in the lung, as reported in the GTEx portal data [9] (Fig. 16.2).

## Targeting TMPRSS2 to Treat COVID-19

Thus, *TMPRSS2* is associated with the risk of severe COVID-19. TMPRSS2 or transmembrane protease serine 2 is an androgen-induced membrane-bound serine protease that is expressed in the prostate, stomach, colon, pancreas, lung, and small intestine in the gradual lower order of magnitude [9]. TMPRSS2 is essential for processing both the ACE2 receptor and SARS-CoV-2 spike protein, thereby facilitating the interaction between them and consequent viral entry into the host cell [10]. Mice lacking TMPRSS2 did not have reduced fertility or life span [11]. Targeting TMPRSS2, therefore, is considered as an approach to decrease the viral entry as both ACE2 and TMPRSS2 are expressed in the lung [12]. Camostat mesylate which is a synthetic TMPRSS2 inhibitor [13] has already been approved in Japan for the treatment of pancreatitis and reflux esophagitis. The predominant circulating serine protease inhibitor alpha 1 antitrypsin (A1AT) is protecting against viral entry both in the broncho-alveolar lavage fluid [14] and in cell-based assays [15]. Therefore, A1AT as an innate immune defense against SARS-CoV-2 can be readily repurposed for treating patients with COVID-19. Conversely, patients with AlAT deficiency were found to be both at higher risk of infection as well as adverse outcomes [16] highlighting the urgent need to screen for A1AT deficiency for population risk stratification and prioritization of vaccine delivery [17].

## Correlation of COVID-19 Case Fatality Rate with A1AT Deficiency

Many studies were able to correlate the geographical differences of COVID-19 severity with the prevalence of A1AT deficiency. For example, early in the pandemic, the northern Lombardy region of Italy with the highest burden of the mutant PI*ZZ allele was having the highest case fatality rate [18]. Using the estimated countrywide carrier frequency of PI*Z and PI*S mutations [19] it was shown that the prevalence of mutation carrier status correlated with the severity of COVID-19 and case fatality rate with a correlation coefficient of 0.87 for the PI*Z mutation [20]. The correlation also persisted when adjusted for confounders like testing strategy, urbanization, and population age distribution [21]. As the PI*Z mutation was rare in South Asia, we used a different approach and estimated the ethnicity-specific combined frequency of all pathogenic *SERPINA1* mutation in the gnomAD v2.1.1

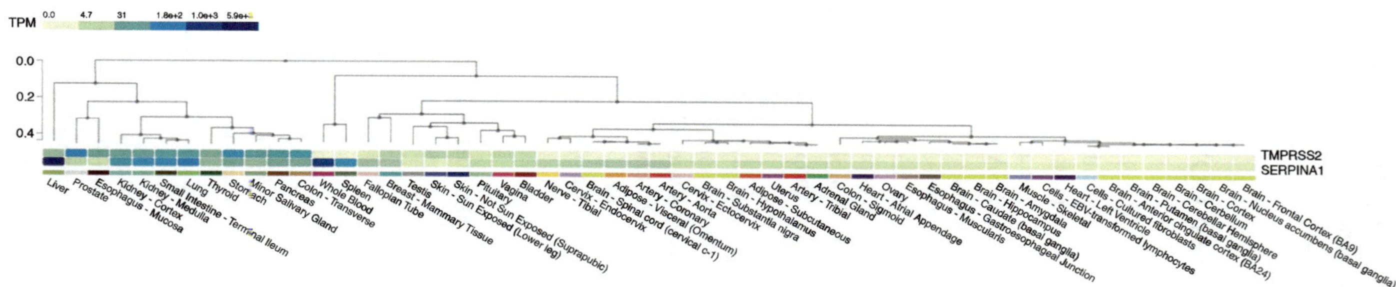


**Fig. 16.2** Coexpression of SERPINA1 and TMPRSS2 lung tissue in GTEx database

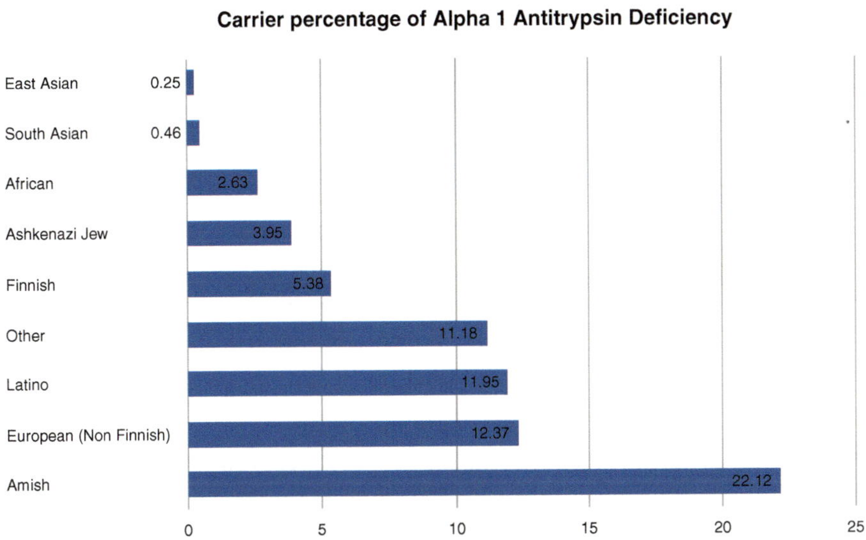


**Fig. 16.3** Carrier percentage of alpha 1 antitrypsin deficiency among ethnic groups represented in gnomAD data retrieved on 9th May 2020

database [22] as per ACMG criteria [23]. We found the combined allele frequency of 32 pathogenic variants was highest in Amish (0.12) and lowest in East Asians (0.001) [24] (Fig. 16.3).

Our findings also corroborated with the finding that countries with the highest case fatality rate also had the highest A1AT pathogenic mutation rate as Europeans have a mutation frequency of 0.066 and Latins have 0.064 [24]. Consistent with these findings it was also shown that the SARS-CoV-2 mutant subtype 614G spread much slower in East Asian countries with lower A1AT deficiency [25]. The 614G substitution created a neutrophil elastase cleavage site in the viral spike protein which enabled faster viral spread in the population with higher neutrophil elastase activity due to a higher burden of A1AT deficiency [25].

## Mechanism of the Protective Effect of A1AT

The mechanism of protective action of A1AT is not just limited to inhibition of TMPRSS2 but also its general anti-inflammatory role (Fig. 16.4).

The biological mechanisms of A1AT protective effects range from antiviral to immunomodulatory effects. These are as follows:

1. A1AT is known to inhibit RNA viruses like HIV 1 [26], influenza A and B [27]. The various antiviral mechanisms include blockage of viral entry and induction of autophagy.

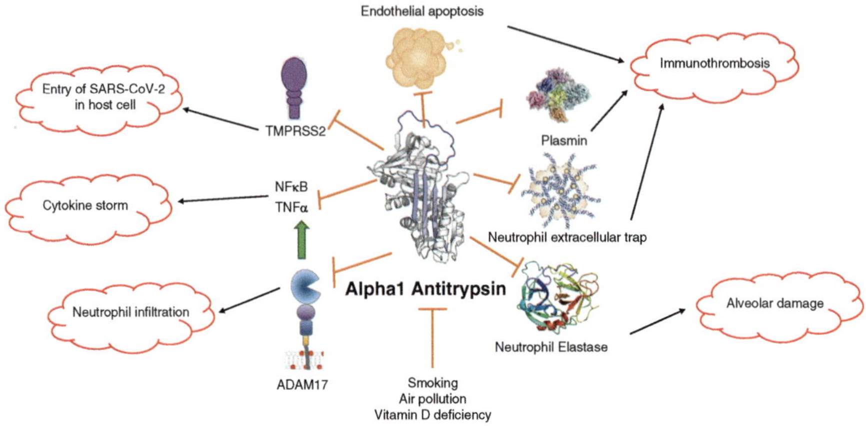


**Fig. 16.4** Alpha 1 antitrypsin inhibits TMPRSS2, NFκB/TNFα, ADAM17, neutrophil elastase, neutrophil extracellular traps, plasmin, and endothelial apoptosis, thereby preventing viral entry, cytokine storm, neutrophil infiltration, alveolar damage, and immunothrombosis. Smoking, air pollution, and vitamin D deficiency in turn inhibit alpha 1 antitrypsin

2. A1AT decreases the level of proinflammatory cytokines like IL-6 [28] by inhibiting the NfκB signaling [29]; caspase 3,6,7 [30]; binding of TNF-α to TNFR1 and TNFR2 [31]. A1AT inhibits the caspase 3 induced lung damage [32]. Interestingly IL-6 is implicated in the cytokine storm seen in COVID-19 patients [33].
3. A1AT also binds IL-8, thereby preventing it from binding CXCR1 receptors which in turn blocks the activation of the Akt signaling pathway [34]. This effect also blocks cytokine storm [33].
4. A1AT also inhibits the TGFβ signaling, thereby mitigating inflammation and fibrosis in COVID-19 patients [35].
5. Another protease, ADAM17, is involved in SARS-CoV-2 infection [36]. Through its membrane shedding function, ADAM17 cleaves ACE2 and thereby increasing its serum level which is a poor prognostic factor for COVID-19 [37]. ADAM17 increases pulmonary inflammation by activation of TNF-α and cleavage of IL6 receptors [38], leading to a cytokine storm. A1AT is known to inhibit ADAM17, independent of its effect on neutrophil elastase [39].
6. Neutrophil elastase, which is also a serine protease, has a significant role in viral pathogenesis by damaging the alveolar elastin and collagen [40]. A1AT has the physiological role of inhibiting the neutrophil elastase activity in the alveoli.
7. A1AT mediated inhibition of ADAM17 and consequent decrease in the shedding of ACE2 preserves the inhibition of bradykinin production and thereby prevents neutrophil infiltration [41].
8. Due to such effect ACE mediated conversion of angiotensin II to angiotensin (1–7) and (1–9) is retained, both of which have anti-inflammatory properties [42, 43].
9. Both pulmonary and venous thromboembolisms are the leading causes of mortality due to COVID-19 [44]. This is also the major cause of hypoxia seen in

this disease [45]. As most of the coagulation factors belong to the serine protease class, hence A1AT has the potential to circumvent this immunothrombosis [46]. Neutrophil extracellular traps (NETs) consisting of neutrophil products like elastase, cathepsin, etc. play a central role in immunothrombosis [47]. A1AT has been shown to decrease the adherence of NETs preventing the thrombotic effects [48].

10. In addition A1AT also inhibits neutrophil chemotaxis and thereby its recruitment in COVID-19 [34].
11. A1AT also inhibits endothelial apoptosis [32] and therefore can decrease the endothelial cell injury leading to lung damage, increased vascular permeability, and also severe pre-eclampsia [49] in pregnant women with COVID-19.
12. A1AT modulates macrophage cell polarization to the M2 phenotype which is critical for tissue repair in SARS-CoV2 infection [50]. The M1 phenotype in turn secretes proinflammatory cytokines [51].
13. A1AT also helps in the differentiation of T cells to Treg subtype [52] which helps in modulating the immune response away from the cytokine storm [53].
14. Some of the environmental co-morbidities associated with the severity of COVID-19 can also interfere with the biological effects of A1AT like damage due to smoking [30] and/or air pollution [54] and vitamin D deficiency [55].

## Clinical Trials of A1AT in COVID-19

To date, there are eight clinical trials registered in the https://clinicaltrials.gov using A1AT/Prolastin as an intervention in COVID-19 or using A1AT as a biomarker for disease severity (NCT04799873, NCT04547140, NCT04495101, NCT04675086, NCT04385836, NCT04473170, NCT04348396, and NCT04366089). One small study that has published results showed beneficial effects of intravenous or inhaled A1AT [56]. Following positive results in 2D and 3D respiratory epithelial organoid cultures, A1AT was administered in nine patients with mild to moderate COVID-19. The CRP level fell within a day in all the patients and all patients recovered without any adverse event. The investigators underlined the utility of A1AT either in the early disease as an antiviral agent or in severe disease as an immunomodulator [56]. Results of double-blind placebo-controlled trials are awaited [57]. Apart from a therapeutic role A1AT also has substantial utility as a prognostic marker with low levels correlating with higher mortality in severe COVID-19 patients [55].

## Conclusion

With this perspective, it appears that A1AT, due to its crucial role in the prevention of the pathogenesis of the COVID-19 infection and associated complications, has the significant potential not only in predicting the susceptibility and prognosis but also demands its justified place in the anti-COVID therapeutic repertoire.

## References

1. Dong E, Du H, Gardner L. An interactive web-based dashboard to track COVID-19 in real-time. Lancet Infect Dis. 2020;20:533–4. https://doi.org/10.1016/S1473-3099(20)30120-1.
2. Sorci G, Faivre B, Morand S. Explaining among-country variation in COVID-19 case fatality rate. Sci Rep. 2020;10:18909. https://doi.org/10.1038/s41598-020-75848-2.
3. Toyoshima Y, Nemoto K, Matsumoto S, Nakamura Y, Kiyotani K. SARS-CoV-2 genomic variations associated with mortality rate of COVID-19. J Hum Genet. 2020;65:1075–82. https://doi.org/10.1038/s10038-020-0808-9.
4. SeyedAlinaghi S, Afsahi AM, MohsseniPour M, Behnezhad F, Salehi MA, Barzegary A, Mirzapour P, Mehraeen E, Dadras O. Late complications of COVID-19; a systematic review of current evidence. Arch Acad Emerg Med. 2021;20;9(1):e14. https://doi.org/10.22037/aaem.v9i1.1058.
5. The COVID-19 Host Genetics Initiative. The COVID-19 host genetics initiative, a global initiative to elucidate the role of host genetic factors in susceptibility and severity of the SARS-CoV-2 virus pandemic. Eur J Hum Genet. 2020;28:715–8. https://doi.org/10.1038/s41431-020-0636-6.
6. COVID-19 Host Genetics Initiative. Mapping the human genetic architecture of COVID-19. Nature. 2021;600(7889):472–7. https://doi.org/10.1038/s41586-021-03767-x.
7. Horowitz JE, Kosmicki JA, Damask A, Sharma D, Roberts GHL, Justice AE, Banerjee N, Coignet MV, Yadav A, Leader JB, Marcketta A, Park DS, Lanche R, Maxwell E, Knight SC, Bai X, Guturu H, Sun D, Baltzell A, Kury FSP, Backman JD, Girshick AR, O'Dushlaine C, McCurdy SR, Partha R, Mansfield AJ, Turissini DA, Li AH, Zhang M, Mbatchou J, Watanabe K, Gurski L, McCarthy SE, Kang HM, Dobbyn L, Stahl E, Verma A, Sirugo G; Regeneron Genetics Center, Ritchie MD, Jones M, Balasubramanian S, Siminovitch K, Salerno WJ, Shuldiner AR, Rader DJ, Mirshahi T, Locke AE, Marchini J, Overton JD, Carey DJ, Habegger L, Cantor MN, Rand KA, Hong EL, Reid JG, Ball CA, Baras A, Abecasis GR, Ferreira MAR. Genome-wide analysis provides genetic evidence that ACE2 influences COVID-19 risk and yields risk scores associated with severe disease. Nat Genet. 2022;54(4):382–92. https://doi.org/10.1038/s41588-021-01006-7.
8. Deelen P, van Dam S, Herkert JC, Karjalainen JM, Brugge H, Abbott KM, van Diemen CC, van der Zwaag PA, Gerkes EH, Zonneveld-Huijssoon E, Boer-Bergsma JJ, Folkertsma P, Gillett T, van der Velde KJ, Kanninga R, van den Akker PC, Jan SZ, Hoorntje ET, te Rijdt WP, Vos YJ, Jongbloed JDH, van Ravenswaaij-Arts CMA, Sinke R, Sikkema-Raddatz B, Kerstjens-Frederikse WS, Swertz MA, Franke L. Improving the diagnostic yield of exome-sequencing by predicting gene–phenotype associations using large-scale gene expression analysis. Nat Commun. 2019;10:2837. https://doi.org/10.1038/s41467-019-10649-4.
9. The GTEx Consortium. The GTEx consortium atlas of genetic regulatory effects across human tissues. Science. 2020;369:1318–30. https://doi.org/10.1126/science.aaz1776.
10. Hoffmann M, Kleine-Weber H, Schroeder S, Krüger N, Herrler T, Erichsen S, Schiergens TS, Herrler G, Wu N-H, Nitsche A, Müller MA, Drosten C, Pöhlmann S. SARS-CoV-2 cell entry depends on ACE2 and TMPRSS2 and is blocked by a clinically proven protease inhibitor. Cell. 2020;181:271–280.e8. https://doi.org/10.1016/j.cell.2020.02.052.
11. Kim TS, Heinlein C, Hackman RC, Nelson PS. Phenotypic analysis of mice lacking the *Tmprss2*-encoded protease. Mol Cell Biol. 2006;26:965–75. https://doi.org/10.1128/MCB.26.3.965-975.2006.
12. Baughn LB, Sharma N, Elhaik E, Sekulic A, Bryce AH, Fonseca R. Targeting TMPRSS2 in SARS-CoV-2 infection. Mayo Clin Proc. 2020;95:1989–99. https://doi.org/10.1016/j.mayocp.2020.06.018.
13. Zhou Y, Vedantham P, Lu K, Agudelo J, Carrion R, Nunneley JW, Barnard D, Pöhlmann S, McKerrow JH, Renslo AR, Simmons G. Protease inhibitors targeting coronavirus and filovirus entry. Antivir Res. 2015;116:76–84. https://doi.org/10.1016/j.antiviral.2015.01.011.

14. Wettstein L, Weil T, Conzelmann C, Muller JA, Gross R, Hirschenberger M, Seidel A, Klute S, Zech F, Prelli Bozzo C, Preising N, Fois G, Lochbaum R, Knaff PM, Mailander V, Standker L, Thal DR, Schumann C, Stenger S, Kleger A, Lochnit G, Mayer B, Ruiz-Blanco YB, Hoffmann M, Sparrer KMJ, Pohlmann S, Sanchez-Garcia E, Kirchhoff F, Frick M, Munch J. Alpha-1 antitrypsin inhibits TMPRSS2 protease activity and SARS-CoV-2 infection. Nat Commun. 2021;12(1):1726. https://doi.org/10.1038/s41467-021-21972-0.
15. Azouz NP, Klingler AM, Callahan V, Akhrymuk IV, Elez K, Raich L, Henry BM, Benoit JL, Benoit SW, Noe F, Kehn-Hall K, Rothenberg ME. Alpha 1 antitrypsin is an inhibitor of the SARS-CoV-2-priming protease TMPRSS2. Pathog Immun. 2021;6(1):55–74. https://doi.org/10.20411/pai.v6i1.408.
16. Ferrarotti I, Ottaviani S, Balderacchi AM, Barzon V, De Silvestri A, Piloni D, Mariani F, Corsico AG. COVID-19 infection in severe alpha 1-antitrypsin deficiency: looking for a rationale. Respir Med. 2021;183:106440. https://doi.org/10.1016/j.rmed.2021.106440.
17. Yang C, Chapman KR, Wong A, Liu M. Alpha1-antitrypsin deficiency and the risk of COVID-19: an urgent call to action. Lancet Respir Med. 2021;9(4):337–9. https://doi.org/10.1016/S2213-2600(21)00018-7.
18. Vianello A, Braccioni F. Geographical overlap between alpha-1 antitrypsin deficiency and COVID-19 infection in Italy: casual or causal? Arch Bronconeumol. 2020;56(9):609–10. https://doi.org/10.1016/j.arbr.2020.05.011.
19. de Serres FJ, Blanco I. Prevalence of α1-antitrypsin deficiency alleles PI*S and PI*Z worldwide and effective screening for each of the five phenotypic classes PI*MS, PI*MZ, PI*SS, PI*SZ, and PI*ZZ: a comprehensive review. Ther Adv Respir Dis. 2012;6:277–95. https://doi.org/10.1177/1753465812457113.
20. Yoshikura H. Epidemiological correlation between COVID-19 epidemic and prevalence of α-1 antitrypsin deficiency in the world. Glob Health Med. 2021;3(2):73–81. https://doi.org/10.35772/ghm.2020.01068.
21. Shapira G, Shomron N, Gurwitz D. Ethnic differences in alpha-1 antitrypsin deficiency allele frequencies may partially explain national differences in COVID-19 fatality rates. FASEB J. 2020;34(11):14160–5. https://doi.org/10.1096/fj.202002097.
22. Genome Aggregation Database Consortium, Karczewski KJ, Francioli LC, Tiao G, Cummings BB, Alföldi J, Wang Q, Collins RL, Laricchia KM, Ganna A, Birnbaum DP, Gauthier LD, Brand H, Solomonson M, Watts NA, Rhodes D, Singer-Berk M, England EM, Seaby EG, Kosmicki JA, Walters RK, Tashman K, Farjoun Y, Banks E, Poterba T, Wang A, Seed C, Whiffin N, Chong JX, Samocha KE, Pierce-Hoffman E, Zappala Z, O'Donnell-Luria AH, Minikel EV, Weisburd B, Lek M, Ware JS, Vittal C, Armean IM, Bergelson L, Cibulskis K, Connolly KM, Covarrubias M, Donnelly S, Ferriera S, Gabriel S, Gentry J, Gupta N, Jeandet T, Kaplan D, Llanwarne C, Munshi R, Novod S, Petrillo N, Roazen D, Ruano-Rubio V, Saltzman A, Schleicher M, Soto J, Tibbetts K, Tolonen C, Wade G, Talkowski ME, Neale BM, Daly MJ, MacArthur DG. The mutational constraint spectrum quantified from variation in 141,456 humans. Nature. 2020;581:434–43. https://doi.org/10.1038/s41586-020-2308-7.
23. On behalf of the ACMG Laboratory Quality Assurance Committee, Richards S, Aziz N, Bale S, Bick D, Das S, Gastier-Foster J, Grody WW, Hegde M, Lyon E, Spector E, Voelkerding K, Rehm HL. Standards and guidelines for the interpretation of sequence variants: a joint consensus recommendation of the American College of Medical Genetics and Genomics and the Association for Molecular Pathology. Genet Med. 2015;17:405–23. https://doi.org/10.1038/gim.2015.30.
24. Dutta AK, Goswami K. Host genomics of COVID-19: evidence point towards alpha 1 antitrypsin deficiency as a putative risk factor for higher mortality rate. Med Hypotheses. 2021;147:110485.
25. Bhattacharyya C, Das C, Ghosh A, Singh AK, Mukherjee S, Majumder PP, Basu A, Biswas NK. SARS-CoV-2 mutation 614G creates an elastase cleavage site enhancing its spread in high AAT-deficient regions. Infect Genet Evol. 2021;90:104760. https://doi.org/10.1016/j.meegid.2021.104760.

26. Shapiro RS. COVID-19 vaccines and nanomedicine. Int J Dermatol. 2021;60(9):1047–52. https://doi.org/10.1111/ijd.15673.
27. Harbig A, Mernberger M, Bittel L, Pleschka S, Schughart K, Steinmetzer T, Stiewe T, Nist A, Böttcher-Friebertshäuser E. Transcriptome profiling and protease inhibition experiments identify proteases that activate H3N2 influenza A and influenza B viruses in murine airways. J Biol Chem. 2020;295:11388–407. https://doi.org/10.1074/jbc.RA120.012635.
28. Kaner Z, Ochayon DE, Shahaf G, et al. Acute phase protein 1-antitrypsin reduces the bacterial burden in mice by selective modulation of innate cell responses. J Infect Dis. 2015;211(9):1489–98.
29. Shapiro L, Pott BG, Ralston AH. Alpha-1-antitrypsin inhibits human immunodeficiency virus type 1. FASEB J. 2001;15:115–22. https://doi.org/10.1096/fj.00-0311com.
30. Lockett AD, Van Demark M, Gu Y, Schweitzer KS, Sigua N, Kamocki K, Fijalkowska I, Garrison J, Fisher AJ, Serban K, Wise RA, Flotte TR, Mueller C, Presson RG, Petrache HI, Tuder RM, Petrache I. Effect of cigarette smoke exposure and structural modifications on the α-1 antitrypsin interaction with caspases. Mol Med. 2012;18:445–54. https://doi.org/10.2119/molmed.2011.00207.
31. Van Molle W, Libert C, Fiers W, Brouckaert P. Alpha 1-acid glycoprotein and alpha 1-antitrypsin inhibit TNF-induced but not anti-Fas-induced apoptosis of hepatocytes in mice. J Immunol. 1997;1950(159):3555–64.
32. Petrache I, Fijalkowska I, Zhen L, Medler TR, Brown E, Cruz P, Choe K-H, Taraseviciene-Stewart L, Scerbavicius R, Shapiro L, Zhang B, Song S, Hicklin D, Voelkel NF, Flotte T, Tuder RM. A novel Antiapoptotic role for $\alpha_1$-antitrypsin in the prevention of pulmonary emphysema. Am J Respir Crit Care Med. 2006;173:1222–8. https://doi.org/10.1164/rccm.200512-1842OC.
33. Chen LY, Hoiland RL, Stukas S, Wellington CL, Sekhon MS. Confronting the controversy: interleukin-6 and the COVID-19 cytokine storm syndrome. Eur Respiratory Soc. 2020;56(4):2003006.
34. Bergin DA, Reeves EP, Meleady P, et al. α-1 antitrypsin regulates human neutrophil chemotaxis induced by soluble immune complexes and IL-8. J Clin Invest. 2010;120(12):4236–50.
35. Cho J-H, Ryu H-M, Oh E-J, et al. Alpha1-antitrypsin attenuates renal fibrosis by inhibiting TGF-1-induced epithelial mesenchymal transition. PLoS One. 2016;11(9):e0162186.
36. Haga S, Yamamoto N, Nakai-Murakami C, Osawa Y, Tokunaga K, Sata T, Yamamoto N, Sasazuki T, Ishizaka Y. Modulation of TNF-α-converting enzyme by the spike protein of SARS-CoV and ACE2 induces TNF-α production and facilitates viral entry. Proc Natl Acad Sci. 2008;105:7809–14. https://doi.org/10.1073/pnas.0711241105.
37. Heurich A, Hofmann-Winkler H, Gierer S, Liepold T, Jahn O, Pohlmann S. TMPRSS2 and ADAM17 cleave ACE2 differentially and only proteolysis by TMPRSS2 augments entry driven by the severe acute respiratory syndrome coronavirus spike protein. J Virol. 2014;88:1293–307. https://doi.org/10.1128/JVI.02202-13.
38. Gooz M. ADAM-17: the enzyme that does it all. Crit Rev Biochem Mol Biol. 2010;45:146–69. https://doi.org/10.3109/10409231003628015.
39. Lee S, Lee Y, Hong K, Hong J, Bae S, Choi J, Jhun H, Kwak A, Kim E, Jo S, Dinarello CA, Kim S. Effect of recombinant α1-antitrypsin fc-fused (AAT-fc) protein on the inhibition of inflammatory cytokine production and Streptozotocin-induced diabetes. Mol Med. 2013;19:65–71. https://doi.org/10.2119/molmed.2012.00308.
40. Watanabe R, Matsuyama S, Shirato K, Maejima M, Fukushi S, Morikawa S, Taguchi F. Entry from the cell surface of severe acute respiratory syndrome coronavirus with cleaved S protein as revealed by pseudotype virus bearing cleaved S protein. J Virol. 2008;82:11985–91. https://doi.org/10.1128/JVI.01412-08.
41. Sodhi CP, Wohlford-Lenane C, Yamaguchi Y, Prindle T, Fulton WB, .Wang S, McCray PB, Chappell M, Hackam DJ, Jia H. Attenuation of pulmonary ACE2 activity impairs inactivation of des-Arg$^9$ bradykinin/BKB1R axis and facilitates LPS-induced neutrophil infiltration. Am J Physiol Lung Cell Mol Physiol. 2018;314:L17–31. https://doi.org/10.1152/ajplung.00498.2016.

42. Zhong J, Guo D, Chen CB, Wang W, Schuster M, Loibner H, Penninger JM, Scholey JW, Kassiri Z, Oudit GY. Prevention of angiotensin II-mediated renal oxidative stress, inflammation, and fibrosis by angiotensin-converting enzyme 2. Hypertension. 2011;57(2):314–22. https://doi.org/10.1161/HYPERTENSIONAHA.110.164244.
43. Gonzalez-Torres, Diego C, Centurion R, Macias M, Lara G, Carrasco R, Almendral J. Angiotensin-neprilysin inhibition further reverses cardiac remodeling as compared to angiotensin inhibition in reduced heart failure patients. Clin Cardiol J. 2018;2(1):6–9.
44. Wichmann D, Sperhake J-P, Lütgehetmann M, Steurer S, Edler C, Heinemann A, Heinrich F, Mushumba H, Kniep I, Schröder AS, Burdelski C, de Heer G, Nierhaus A, Frings D, Pfefferle S, Becker H, Bredereke-Wiedling H, de Weerth A, Paschen H-R, Sheikhzadeh-Eggers S, Stang A, Schmiedel S, Bokemeyer C, Addo MM, Aepfelbacher M, Püschel K, Kluge S. Autopsy findings and venous thromboembolism in patients with COVID-19: a prospective cohort study. Ann Intern Med. 2020;173:268–77. https://doi.org/10.7326/M20-2003.
45. Ackermann M, Verleden SE, Kuehnel M, Haverich A, Welte T, Laenger F, Vanstapel A, Werlein C, Stark H, Tzankov A, Li WW, Li VW, Mentzer SJ, Jonigk D. Pulmonary vascular endothelialitis, thrombosis, and angiogenesis in Covid-19. N Engl J Med. 2020;383:120–8. https://doi.org/10.1056/NEJMoa2015432.
46. Gans H, Tan BH. α1-antitrypsin, an inhibitor for thrombin and plasmin. Clin Chim Acta. 1967;17:111–7. https://doi.org/10.1016/0009-8981(67)90104-0.
47. Middleton EA, He X-Y, Denorme F, Campbell RA, Ng D, Salvatore SP, Mostyka M, Baxter-Stoltzfus A, Borczuk AC, Loda M, Cody MJ, Manne BK, Portier I, Harris ES, Petrey AC, Beswick EJ, Caulin AF, Iovino A, Abegglen LM, Weyrich AS, Rondina MT, Egeblad M, Schiffman JD, Yost CC. Neutrophil extracellular traps contribute to immunothrombosis in COVID-19 acute respiratory distress syndrome. Blood. 2020;136:1169–79. https://doi.org/10.1182/blood.2020007008.
48. Frenzel E, Korenbaum E, Hegermann J, Ochs M, Koepke J, Koczulla AR, Welte T, Köhnlein T, Janciauskiene S. Does augmentation with alpha1-antitrypsin affect neutrophil extracellular traps formation? Int J Biol Sci. 2012;8:1023–5. https://doi.org/10.7150/ijbs.4701.
49. Cruz Melguizo S, de la Cruz Conty M, Carmona Payán P, Abascal-Saiz A, Pintando Recarte P, González Rodríguez L, Cuenca Marín C, Martínez Varea A, Oreja Cuesta A, Rodríguez P, Fernández Buhigas I, Rodríguez Gallego M, Fernández Alonso A, López Pérez R, Broullón Molanes J, Encinas Pardilla M, Ramírez Gómez M, Gimeno M, Sánchez Muñoz A, Martínez-Pérez O, on behalf of the Spanish Obstetric Emergency Group (S.O.E.G.). Pregnancy outcomes and SARS-CoV-2 infection: the Spanish obstetric emergency group study. Viruses. 2021;13:853. https://doi.org/10.3390/v13050853.
50. Guttman O, Freixo- Lima GS, Lewis EC. Alpha1-antitrypsin, an endogenous immunoregulatory molecule: distinction between local and systemic effects on tumor immunology. Integr Cancer Sci Therap. 2015;2(6):272–80.
51. Gracia-Hernandez M, Sotomayor EM, Villagra A. Targeting mac-rophages as a therapeutic option in COVID-19. Front Pharmacol. 2020;11:1659.
52. Baranovski BM, Freixo- Lima GS, Lewis EC, Rider P. T helper subsets, peripheral plasticity, and the acute phase protein, 1-antitrypsin. Biomed Res Int. 2015;2015:184574.
53. Stephen-Victor E, Das M, Karnam A, Pitard B, Gautier J-F, Bayry J. Potential of regulatory T-cell-based therapies in the management of severe COVID-19. Eur Respir J. 2020;56(3):2002182.
54. Murgia N, Corsico AG, D'Amato G, Maesano CN, Tozzi A, Annesi-Maesano I. Do gene-environment interactions play a role in COVID-19 distribution? The case of Alpha-1 antitrypsin, air pollution and COVID-19. Multidiscip Respir Med. 2021;16(1):741. https://doi.org/10.4081/mrm.2021.741.
55. Shimi G, Zand H. Association of alpha-1-antitrypsin deficiency with vitamin D status: who is most at risk of getting severe COVID-19? Inflamm Res. 2021;70(4):375–7. https://doi.org/10.1007/s00011-021-01456-z.

56. Ritzmann F, Chitirala P, Kruger N, Hoffmann M, Zuo W, Lammert F, Smola S, Tov N, Alagem N, Lepper PM, Pohlmann S, Beisswenger C, Herr C, Bals R. Therapeutic application of alpha-1-antitrypsin in COVID-19. Am J Respir Crit Care Med. 2021;204(2):224–7. https://doi.org/10.1164/rccm.202104-0833LE.
57. McEvoy NL, Clarke JL, Mc Elvaney OJ, Mc Elvaney OF, Boland F, Hyland D, Geoghegan P, Donnelly K, Friel O, Cullen A, Collins AM, Fraughen D, Martin-Loeches I, Hennessy M, Laffey JG, Mc Elvaney NG, Curley GF. A randomised, double-blind, placebo-controlled, pilot trial of intravenous plasma purified alpha-1 antitrypsin for SARS-CoV-2-induced acute respiratory distress syndrome: a structured summary of a study protocol for a randomised, controlled trial. Trials. 2021;22:288. https://doi.org/10.1186/s13063-021-05254-0.

# Chapter 17
# Social Cognition Approaches to Understanding and Changing COVID-19 Preventive Behaviors

**Stephanie R. Smith, Martin S. Hagger, Jacob J. Keech, Susette A. Moyers, and Kyra Hamilton**

S. R. Smith
School of Applied Psychology, Griffith University, Brisbane, QLD, Australia

Menzies Health Institute Queensland, Griffith University, Brisbane, QLD, Australia
e-mail: stephanie.smith@griffith.edu.au

M. S. Hagger
School of Applied Psychology, Griffith University, Brisbane, QLD, Australia

Health Sciences Research Institute, University of California, Merced, CA, USA

Department of Psychological Sciences, University of California, Merced, CA, USA

Faculty of Sport and Health Sciences, University of Jyväskylä, Jyväskylä, Finland
e-mail: mhagger@ucmerced.edu

J. J. Keech
School of Applied Psychology, Griffith University, Brisbane, QLD, Australia

School of Health and Behavioral Sciences, University of the Sunshine Coast, Sunshine Coast, QLD, Australia
e-mail: jkeech@usc.edu.au

S. A. Moyers
Department of Psychological Sciences, University of California, Merced, CA, USA

Center for Health Sciences, Oklahoma State University, Tulsa, OK, USA
e-mail: susette.moyers@okstate.edu

K. Hamilton (✉)
School of Applied Psychology, Griffith University, Brisbane, QLD, Australia

Menzies Health Institute Queensland, Griffith University, Brisbane, QLD, Australia

Health Sciences Research Institute, University of California, Merced, CA, USA
e-mail: kyra.hamilton@griffith.edu.au


S. Adibi et al. (eds.), *Frontiers of COVID-19*,
https://doi.org/10.1007/978-3-031-08045-6_17

## Introduction

While global COVID-19 cases and deaths continue to decrease as a result of COVID-19 vaccines and other measures, daily infection and mortality rates remain a public health threat in many nations, particularly those with low vaccination rates. Most countries have seen a decrease in infection and mortality rates since April 2021, but cases in countries with high population densities and limited access to vaccinations continue to increase, such as India, Brazil, Argentina, and Columbia. According to the World Health Organization, in June 2021, over 2.6 million new cases and 72,000 deaths attributed to COVID-19 were reported globally [1]. Until sufficient widespread immunity from mass inoculation is achieved, promotion of engagement in behaviors that prevent the spread of infections (e.g., physical distancing, hand hygiene practices, reducing mass gatherings) remains important for virus containment [2, 3]. While recent meta-analytic evidence supports the efficacy of behavioral measures in stemming COVID-19 infections [4], the success of behavioral strategies depends on behavioral compliance. There is therefore a necessity for public health organizations to develop behavioral interventions that are efficacious in promoting uptake and continued maintenance of COVID-19 preventive behaviors.

Behavioral scientists have advocated the application of behavioral theories, particularly social cognition theories, to inform the development of behavior change interventions [5], including in the context of a pandemic [6, 7]. The application of these theories is predicated on the recognition that producing efficacious interventions requires a fundamental understanding of human behavior. The theories enable the identification of determinants that are reliably related to the behavior of interest which then become targets for intervention by matching evidence-based behavior change strategies proposed to affect change in the targeted determinants [8–10]. The identification of modifiable determinants of COVID-19 preventive behaviors is, therefore, central to informing public health efforts aimed at stemming COVID-19 infections [6].

Social cognition approaches, such as the theory of planned behavior [11] and health action process approach [12, 13], have been applied extensively to predict health behavior and to inform the development of behavior change interventions [8]. These theories have had demonstrable efficacy in accounting for variance in health behavior [14–16]. Although research applying these models to identify the determinants of COVID-19 preventive behaviors and associated mechanism is, by comparison, limited, there is emerging evidence that they can be effective in accounting for variance in COVID-19 preventive behaviors [17–25]. For example, prospective correlational evidence indicates the utility of many social cognition constructs that reflect motivational, volitional, and automatic processes in explaining physical distancing behavior in samples of Australian and USA community members [21, 22], with longitudinal evidence supporting the sustained effects of these constructs on behavior over time [26]. Research has also tested the efficacy of interventions utilizing persuasive communication, imagery, and implementation intention techniques to target social cognition determinants of hand hygiene practices during the COVID-19 pandemic [25]. This growing body of research provides useful preliminary data that can inform public health communications promoting performance of COVID-19 preventive behaviors.

The purpose of this chapter is to provide an overview of research applying key theoretical frameworks to explain and predict COVID-19 preventive behaviors and the mechanisms involved. The chapter also outlines how this research may inform potential interventions to promote engagement in these preventive behaviors. Building on this evidence, the chapter provides example materials used in behavior change interventions based on social cognition theories, which may have application across a broad range of COVID-19 preventive behaviors. This is followed by a discussion of future directions and challenges in moving behavior change research forward, and bridging divides between theory, practice, and research.

## Social Cognition Theories Used to Explain and Change Behavior

Research examining the determinants of health behavior has commonly applied social cognition theories, which consider enactment of future health behavior is the consequence of a reasoned process determined by beliefs about the behavior and its outcomes, and the associated social conditions and constraints [8]. The theory of planned behavior typifies social cognition theories and has been widely applied to predicting health behavior and used to inform interventions [16, 27]. The theory of planned behavior [11] posits that behavioral intention is the most proximal determinant of a given target behavior. *Behavioral intention* is a motivational construct reflecting how hard a person is willing to try to perform the behavior. Behavioral intention is a function of three sets of belief-based constructs: attitudes toward the behavior, subjective norm, and perceived behavioral control. *Attitudes* are individuals' positive and negative evaluations of the behavior. *Subjective norms* are perceptions of social approval or pressure to engage or not engage in the behavior. *Perceived behavioral control* are individuals' beliefs in their ability and confidence, and the resources they have to perform the behavior. To the extent that perceived behavioral control reflects actual behavioral control, perceived behavioral control is also proposed to directly predict behavior, although original theorizing suggested a moderation effect [11, 28]. The theory has successfully been applied to explaining a diverse range of health behaviors; a meta-analysis of prospective studies found theory of planned behavior constructs predicted 44.3% of the variance in intention and 19.3% of the variance in behavior [16].

Another prominent social cognition approach that has widely been applied to understanding health behavior is the health action process approach [12]. The health action process approach is a *dual-phase* model that includes constructs that represent two key processes or *phases* relating to intentional action: a *motivational phase*, in which an individual engages in deliberative or reasoned consideration of the future performance of a target behavior leading to the formation of goals and intentions. In this phase, intentions are considered to be the key determinant of behavior and are a function of three belief-based constructs: outcome expectancies, action self-efficacy, and risk perceptions. *Outcome expectancies* are beliefs that performing the behavior will lead to the desired health outcomes. *Action self-efficacy* refers to beliefs about personal capacity to perform the behavior. *Risk perceptions* refer to perceived vulnerability to, and severity of, any health condition that may arise due to performing, or avoiding, the behavior. When an individual has formed an intention to perform the behavior, the theory predicts that individuals then enter a *volitional phase*. In the volitional phase, key determinants of behavior include self-regulatory strategies and volitional stage-specific forms of self-efficacy. Regulatory strategies encompass *action planning*, which is plans formed detailing when, where, and how to enact the behavior; *coping planning*, which is plans formed that detail strategies to overcome obstacles to engaging in the behavior; and action control, which reflects maintenance of behavior—which is achieved through the use of self-regulatory skills to regulate the behavior, with self-monitoring being the key component of action control. Volitional stage-specific forms of self-efficacy include coping self-efficacy, which is beliefs about one's capacity to overcome obstacles to maintaining the behavior; and *recovery self-efficacy*, which is beliefs about one's ability to get back on track after performing the behavior has been derailed. The health action process approach has successfully been applied to understanding and increasing engagement in a range of health behaviors [13]. A recent meta-analysis [15] found that the health action process approach constructs explained 26.1% of the variance in intentions and 17.5% of the variance in behavior. However, risk perceptions are suggested to only be relevant in certain contexts and only tend to exhibit small effects on intention with limited association with behavior.

## Social Cognition Determinants of COVID-19 Preventive Behaviors

Researchers have begun to apply social cognition theories to identify the determinants of COVID-19 preventive behaviors such as physical distancing, mask wearing, and hand hygiene practices [17–25]. For example, a recent prospective correlational study applied the health action process approach to predict physical distancing behavior in Australia and USA samples during the pandemic [22]. Health action process approach constructs with respect to physical distancing and behavior were measured at an initial point in time and again 1 week later. Results indicated that the motivational and volitional constructs from the model including self-efficacy, intention, and action control predicted physical distancing behavior in both samples. Such findings are consistent with other research on physical distancing behavior [17], hand hygiene behavior [29], mask wearing [30, 31], or an aggregate of multiple COVID-19 preventive behaviors [18, 24, 32, 33]. However, although risk perception and volitional processes, such as action and coping planning, were not identified as important predictors of physical distancing, it does not preclude them as important predictors of other COVID-19 preventive behaviors. For example, action planning and coping planning may be better predictors of mask wearing than physical distancing—and risk perception and planning have been shown to significantly predict aggregate COVID-19 preventive behaviors [23]. Taken together, these findings provide preliminary support for the proposed effects of the constructs reflecting both processes in the health action process approach on behaviors to protect against COVID-19.

Another recent study applied an integrated social cognition model to identify the determinants of physical distancing behavior and the processes involved [18, 22]. The integrated model was based on the theory of planned behavior and augmented to include additional predictors including moral norm and habit. The study adopted a three-wave longitudinal survey design with measures taken over a 4-month period. Results indicated that subjective norm, moral norm, and perceived behavioral control, but not attitude, were consistent predictors of physical distancing intention on each occasion, and intention and habit were consistent predictors of subsequent physical distancing behavior. Other studies have identified perceived behavioral control, normative beliefs, and attitude as significant correlates or predictors of COVID-19 preventive intentions and/or behaviors, including physical distancing [34], mask wearing [30, 31], vaccination against COVID-19 [35–37], or aggregate measures of COVID-19 behaviors [18–20, 24, 38, 39].

Overall, evidence from studies applying social cognition theories indicates their efficacy in accounting for variance in intentions or behaviors in a number of COVID-19 preventive behaviors including physical distancing, mask wearing, vaccination, and hand hygiene practices. The most prominent predictors include normative beliefs (e.g., subjective and moral norms), control perceptions (e.g., self-efficacy and perceived behavioral control), and volitional processes (e.g., action control and planning). This research provides useful guidance for the development of future behavioral interventions aimed at promoting COVID-19 preventive behaviors by providing indication of the constructs that should be targeted for change.

## An Application of Theory- and Evidence-Based Strategies to Promote a COVID-19 Preventive Behavior

The identification of potentially modifiable psychological constructs of COVID-19 preventive behavior may provide some indication of the constructs that might need to change in order to bring about behavior change. It might also signal potential intervention techniques that might have utility in changing behavior. This is predicated on the assumption that techniques that have been verified through consensus and evidence synthesis as potentially being able to bring about change in these constructs may work in the context of changing COVID-19 behaviors [40, 41]. Identification of determinants that are reliably related to the behavior of interest through theory and formative research is a first step in intervention development.

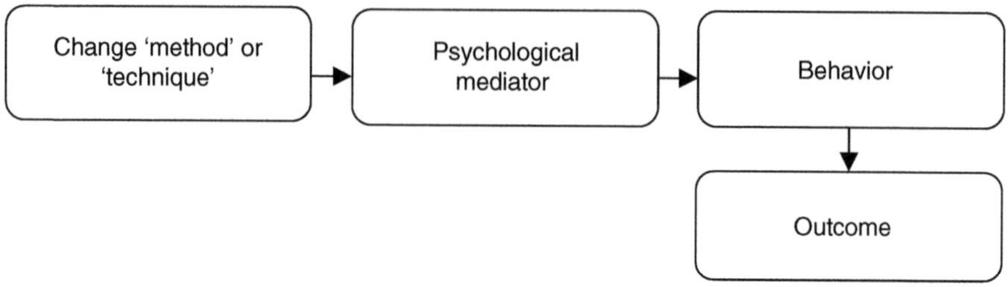


**Fig. 17.1** Basic process model of health behavior change

Matching evidence-based behavior change strategies or techniques proposed to affect change with the targeted determinants forms the second step [8–10]. Together, these steps imply a *mechanism of action*, which is illustrated in the basic process model in Fig. 17.1. In the figure, behavior change technique is applied in an intervention setting to initiate change in the theoretical construct (i.e., the psychological mediator); with change in the determinant of the behavior expected to result in change of the behavior itself. Over time, change in the behavior is expected to lead to specific adaptive health outcomes.

A recent study provides an illustration of an intervention developed through this process, and its evaluation, in the context of COVID-19 preventive behaviors. The intervention targeted increased engagement in hand hygiene practices to prevent COVID-19 infection through the "mapping" of behavior change strategies on theoretical predictors of behavior [25]. Specifically, the target behavior was *avoidance of touching the face with unwashed hands*, based on international guidelines advocating for regular handwashing with soap and water and avoiding touching the face, particularly the eyes, nose, and mouth, to avoid infection through transfer of the virus from contaminated surfaces [42]. The key constructs targeted were attitudes, subjective norms, and perceived behavioral control from the theory of planned behavior; and risk perceptions and action planning from the health action process approach. Given the relative novelty of engaging in avoidance of touching one's face with unwashed hands to prevent COVID-19 transmission, and the dearth of research identifying its determinants from social cognition theories, the theoretical targets of the intervention were informed by research identifying the theoretical predictors of other COVID-19 preventive behaviors (e.g., physical distancing) [21–23] and prior research in other health behaviors [15, 16]. Behavior change techniques derived from previous theory and evidence that were expected to target change in the identified determinants were selected. Table 17.1 provides a summary of the behavior change methods and the corresponding theoretical constructs adopted in the intervention. Specifically, the intervention adopted persuasive communication, mental imagery, and implementation intention techniques to target change in the theory of planned behavior and health action process approach constructs.

One aspect of the intervention comprised persuasive communication techniques, which are designed to guide individuals toward the adoption of an attitude or action

**Table 17.1** Behavior change methods, targeted theoretical constructs, and intervention content from [43]

| Intervention component | Behavior change technique(s) | Content of component | Target theory construct |
|---|---|---|---|
| Education | Information provision | Provide information about the risks of contracting COVID-19 by touching face with unwashed hands | Attitude, risk perception |
| Formation of a goal intention | Personalize risk; scenario-based risk; information provision; provide opportunities for social comparison; goal setting | Providing information about the personal risk and risk to others; performance of the behavior described as rewarding for oneself, desirable to others, and achievable; formation of goal to perform behavior | Intention, attitude, subjective norm, perceived behavioral control, risk perception |
| Implementation intentions | If-then contingency plans; goal setting | Provide examples of scenarios in which behavior should be performed; record if-then plan | Intention, action planning |
| Process mental imagery | Planning behavioral responses; guided practice; using imagery | Imagine steps involved in performing the behavior when in the relevant scenario(s); process mental simulation exercise; record summary of process imagery | Intention, perceived behavioral control, action planning |
| Outcome mental imagery | Personalize risk; information about others' approval; provide contingent rewards; using imagery | Encouragement to think about benefits and risks of performing and not performing the behavior, respectively; imagine what important others will think. Outcome mental simulation exercise; record summary of outcome imagery | Intention, attitude, subjective norm, perceived behavioral control, risk perception |

by presenting arguments which highlight the advantages and disadvantages of engaging in, or failing to engage in, a behavior. Evidence supports the use of persuasive communication to promote attitude, intention, and behavior change [44], with meta-analyses showing that such interventions promote simultaneous change in attitudes and behavior in health contexts [44–46]. The way in which the strategy was applied was that participants were guided through a slideshow that included images and messages designed to highlight the potential risks of touching the face with unwashed hands (e.g., contracting the virus themselves; transmitting the virus to others) and to facilitate the visualization of virus transference through hand-to-face contact (e.g., image of a hand touching an escalator handrail contaminated with the virus; an image of a contaminated hand with exaggerated magnification so the virus is visible on the skin). This was developed to target intention, attitudes, and risk perception toward avoiding touching the face with unwashed hands. The slides also included messages describing avoidance of touching the face with unwashed hands as rewarding (targeting attitude), achievable (targeting perceived behavioral control), and desirable in the eyes of others (targeting subjective norm).

Another aspect of the intervention consisted of implementation intentions, a technique in which individuals are prompted to form plans about when, where, and how to enact an intended behavior to achieve a specific goal [47]. This strategy was designed to target change in constructs intention and action planning. Research supports the effectiveness of implementation intentions in promoting effective enactment of intended behaviors beyond mere formation of a goal intention [48]. Participants were guided through a planning exercise in which they were instructed to consider when, where, and how they will avoid touching their face with unwashed hands in the next week. Then, to increase the likelihood of following through on their intention, participants recorded their plan using an "If-then" format consistent with suggested guidelines [49, 50]. An example of an "If-then" plan to avoid touching the face with unwashed hands is "If… *I visit the supermarket during the next week,* then I will… *ensure that I avoid touching my face until I have washed my hands afterwards.*"

A final component of the intervention comprised mental imagery techniques, in which participants were instructed to mentally represent and rehearse future actions and consequences [51–53]. Imagery is proposed to target change in attitudes and perceived behavioral control or self-efficacy toward the behavior. Meta-analytic evidence and previous intervention studies support the effectiveness of mental imagery techniques on behaviors and social cognition constructs [51, 54–58]. The study instructed participants to imagine the *process* of performing the behavior of avoiding touching their face with unwashed hands in relevant scenarios in a very vivid manner, using their senses and imagination to make the imagery as realistic as possible. The process imagery exercise was designed to target intention and perceived behavioral control with respect to avoiding touching the face with unwashed hands. Participants were then guided through a second imagery exercise, this time imagining the *outcomes* of avoiding touching their face with unwashed hands. Participants were instructed to imagine the benefits of performing the behavior, and the consequences of failing to perform the behavior, which targeted attitudes and risk perception; to picture themselves successfully avoiding touching their face with unwashed hands and imagining the satisfaction that comes with it, which targeted perceived behavioral control; and to imagine how their significant others will feel about their successful performance of the behavior, which targeted subjective norms.

Taken together, the process described above provides an illustration of how interventionists might develop a theory-based intervention targeting change in COVID-19 preventive behavior.

## Key Challenges and Future Directions

Effective large-scale behavior change strategies aimed at mitigating the effects of the COVID-19 pandemic should be informed by behavioral science [59]. While the body of literature applying theories of social cognition to predict and change

COVID-19 preventive behaviors is growing, there are challenges that still need to be addressed. First, there is a need for more longitudinal research to model changes in COVID-19 preventive behaviors and the social cognition constructs over time and to specify temporal order in model predictions. Second, while prospective correlational research is useful for identifying the theoretical predictors of COVID-19 preventive behaviors, the design precludes causal inference about the relationships between the constructs. This is a problem for intervention design because targeting change in constructs correlated with behavior may not lead to behavior changes if changes in the constructs have not also been shown to be associated with changes in behavior. Researchers are encouraged to use the findings of preliminary prospective correlational research as a basis for developing studies that test change through experimental or intervention designs. Intervention or experimental studies that show how techniques that target change in theory constructs in the context of COVID-19 preventive behaviors are therefore paramount to providing this evidence. This would permit evaluation of the extent to which such techniques lead to change in the constructs themselves and, particularly, change in the respective COVID-19 preventive behaviors.

A further problem is that studies applying social cognition theories to COVID-19 preventive behaviors often adopt aggregate behavior measures. This is problematic given that the determinants of the types of COVID-19 preventive behaviors may differ. For example, descriptive norms, which refer to the extent to which people perceive others are engaging in a behavior, are likely to be a stronger determinant of high-visibility behaviors such as mask wearing, compared to behaviors that are not as easily observable in a public setting, such as handwashing. When different preventive behaviors are grouped together, it makes identification of the salient predictors, and subsequent selection of behavior change strategies that target change in the salient predictors, of specific COVID-19 preventive behaviors, difficult. As such, to optimize the utility of research applying theories of behavior change to predict COVID-19 preventive behaviors, it is recommended researchers ensure individual measurement, and modeling, of different COVID-19 behaviors and their related social cognition constructs.

Finally, there is likely to be variability in individuals' responses to interventions, which may be explained by any number of sociodemographic characteristics (e.g., age, sex, education, income, relationship status, ethnicity, location, etc.), individual trait differences, or individuals' current and previous experience with COVID-19 preventive behaviors. For example, there are subgroups within a population who are likely to need greater encouragement to adhere to recommended behavioral guidelines than others, such as those that are vaccine hesitant [60]. In order to improve the efficacy of interventions moving forward, it is suggested that identification of the individual differences likely to influence individuals' responses to messaging and interventions is needed. This information can be used to tailor messaging to target subgroups with the lowest behavioral compliance.

## Conclusion

The goal of this chapter has been to provide an overview of some of the research applying social cognition theories to predict COVID-19 preventive behaviors, and how interventions based on these theories to promote and maintain COVID-19 preventive behaviors may be developed. The chapter provides example materials that have been used in behavior change interventions based on social cognition theories and may be efficacious in changing COVID-19 preventive behaviors in interventions going forward. This information is important as public health organizations seek to develop messaging and strategies that promote population-level compliance with preventive behavioral strategies for current and future pandemics.

## References

1. World Health Organization. Weekly epidemiological update on COVID-19 - 15 June 2021. Geneva: WHO; 2021. https://www.who.int/publications/m/item/weekly-epidemiological-update-on-covid-19%2D%2D-15-june-2021.
2. Hodgson SH, Mansatta K, Mallett G, Harris V, Emary KRW, Pollard AJ. What defines an efficacious COVID-19 vaccine? A review of the challenges assessing the clinical efficacy of vaccines against SARS-CoV-2. Lancet Infect Dis. 2021;21(2):e26–35. https://doi.org/10.1016/S1473-3099(20)30773-8.
3. Moghadas SM, Vilches TN, Zhang K, Wells CR, Shoukat A, Singer BH, Meyers LA, Neuzil KM, Langley JM, Fitzpatrick MC, Galvani AP. The impact of vaccination on COVID-19 outbreaks in the United States. medRxiv. 2021;2020.11.27.20240051. https://doi.org/10.1101/2020.11.27.20240051.
4. Chu DK, Akl EA, Duda S, Solo K, Yaacoub S, Schünemann HJ, Chu DK, Akl EA, El-harakeh A, Bognanni A, Lotfi T, Loeb M, Hajizadeh A, Bak A, Izcovich A, Cuello-Garcia CA, Chen C, Harris DJ, Borowiack E, Chamseddine F, Schünemann F, Morgano GP, Muti Schünemann GEU, Chen G, Zhao H, Neumann I, Chan J, Khabsa J, Hneiny L, Harrison L, Smith M, Rizk N, Giorgi Rossi P, AbiHanna P, El-khoury R, Stalteri R, Baldeh T, Piggott T, Zhang Y, Saad Z, Khamis A, Reinap M, Duda S, Solo K, Yaacoub S, Schünemann HJ. Physical distancing, face masks, and eye protection to prevent person-to-person transmission of SARS-CoV-2 and COVID-19: a systematic review and meta-analysis. Lancet. 2020;395:1973–87. https://doi.org/10.1016/S0140-6736(20)31142-9.
5. Michie S, Prestwich A. Are interventions theory-based? Development of a theory coding scheme. Health Psychol. 2010;29:1–8. https://doi.org/10.1037/a0016939.
6. West R, Michie S, Rubin GJ, Amlôt R. Applying principles of behaviour change to reduce SARS-CoV-2 transmission. Nat Hum Behav. 2020;4(5):1–9. https://doi.org/10.1038/s41562-020-0887-9.
7. Weston D, Ip A, Amlôt R. Examining the application of behaviour change theories in the context of infectious disease outbreaks and emergency response: a review of reviews. BMC Public Health. 2020;20:1483. https://doi.org/10.1186/s12889-020-09519-2.
8. Hagger MS, Cameron LD, Hamilton K, Hankonen N, Lintunen T. The handbook of behavior change. Cambridge: Cambridge University Press; 2020. https://doi.org/10.1017/9781108677318.046.
9. Rothman AJ, Klein WMP, Sheeran P. Moving from theoretical principles to intervention strategies: applying the experimental medicine approach. In: Hagger MS, Cameron L, Hamilton K,

Hankonen N, Lintunen T, editors. The handbook of behavior change. Cambridge: Cambridge University Press; 2020. p. 285–99. https://doi.org/10.1017/9781108677318.020.
10. Sheeran P, Klein WMP, Rothman AJ. Health behavior change: moving from observation to intervention. Annu Rev Psychol. 2017;68:573–600. https://doi.org/10.1146/annurev-psych-010416-044007.
11. Ajzen I. The theory of planned behavior. Organ Behav Hum Decis Process. 1991;50:179–211. https://doi.org/10.1016/0749-5978(91)90020-T.
12. Schwarzer R. Modeling health behavior change: how to predict and modify the adoption and maintenance of health behaviors. Appl Psychol. 2008;57:1–29. https://doi.org/10.1111/j.1464-0597.2007.00325.x.
13. Schwarzer R, Hamilton K. Changing behaviour using the health action process approach. Cambridge: Cambridge University Press; 2020. https://doi.org/10.1017/9781108677318.007.
14. Hagger MS, Chatzisarantis NLD. Integrating the theory of planned behaviour and self-determination theory in health behaviour: a meta-analysis. Br J Health Psychol. 2009;14:275–302. https://doi.org/10.1348/135910708X373959.
15. Zhang CQ, Zhang R, Schwarzer R, Hagger MS. A meta-analysis of the health action process approach. Health Psychol. 2019;38:623–37. https://doi.org/10.1037/hea0000728.
16. McEachan RRC, Conner M, Taylor NJ, Lawton RJ. Prospective prediction of health-related behaviours with the theory of planned behaviour: a meta-analysis. Health Psychol Rev. 2011;5:97–144. https://doi.org/10.1080/17437199.2010.521684.
17. Beeckman M, De Paepe A, Van Alboom M, Maes S, Wauters A, Baert F, Kissi A, Veirman E, Van Ryckeghem DML, Poppe L. Adherence to the physical distancing measures during the COVID-19 pandemic: a HAPA-based perspective. Appl Psychol Heal Well Being. 2020;12:1224–43. https://doi.org/10.1111/aphw.12242.
18. Bogg T, Milad E. Demographic, personality, and social cognition correlates of coronavirus guideline adherence in a U.S. sample. Health Psychol. 2020;39:1026–36. https://doi.org/10.1037/hea0000891.
19. Clark C, Davila A, Regis M, Kraus S. Predictors of COVID-19 voluntary compliance behaviors: an international investigation. Glob Transitions. 2020;2:76–82. https://doi.org/10.1016/j.glt.2020.06.003.
20. Gibson Miller J, Hartman TK, Levita L, Martinez AP, Mason L, McBride O, McKay R, Murphy J, Shevlin M, Stocks TVA, Bennett KM, Bentall RP. Capability, opportunity, and motivation to enact hygienic practices in the early stages of the COVID-19 outbreak in the United Kingdom. Br J Health Psychol. 2020;25(4):856–64. https://doi.org/10.1111/bjhp.12426.
21. Hagger MS, Smith SR, Keech JJ, Moyers SA, Hamilton K. Predicting social distancing behavior during the COVID-19 pandemic: an integrated social cognition model. Ann Behav Med. 2020;54:713–27. https://doi.org/10.1093/abm/kaaa073.
22. Hamilton K, Smith S, Keech JJ, Moyers S, Hagger MS. Application of the health action process approach to social distancing behavior during COVID-19. Appl Psychol Heal Well Being. 2020;12(4):1244–69. https://doi.org/10.1111/aphw.12231.
23. Lin C, Imani V, Majd NR, Ghasemi Z, Griffiths MD, Hamilton K, Hagger MS, Pakpour AH. Using an integrated social cognition model to predict COVID-19 preventive behaviours. Br J Health Psychol. 2020;25(4):981–1005. https://doi.org/10.1111/bjhp.12465.
24. Moussaoui LS, Ofosu ND, Desrichard O. Social psychological correlates of protective Behaviours in the COVID-19 outbreak: evidence and recommendations from a nationally representative sample. Appl Psychol Heal Well Being. 2020;12:1183–204. https://doi.org/10.1111/aphw.12235.
25. Smith SR, Hagger MS, Keech JJ, Moyers SA, Hamilton K. Improving hand hygiene behavior using a novel theory-based intervention during the COVID-19 pandemic. https://doi.org/10.31219/osf.io/uzhvx.
26. Hagger MS, Smith SR, Keech JJ, Moyers SA, Hamilton K. Predicting physical distancing over time during COVID-19: testing an integrated model. Psychol Health. 2021;1–21. https://doi.org/10.1080/08870446.2021.1968397.

27. Hamilton K, van Dongen A, Hagger MS. An extended theory of planned behavior for parent-for-child health behaviors: a meta-analysis. Health Psychol. 2020;39(10):863–78. https://doi.org/10.1037/hea0000940.
28. Ajzen I, Schmidt P. Changing behavior using the theory of planned behavior. In: Hagger MS, Cameron L, Hamilton K, Hankonen N, Lintunen T, editors. The handbook of behavior change. Cambridge: Cambridge University Press; 2020. p. 17–31. https://doi.org/10.1017/9781108677318.002.
29. Derksen C, Keller FM, Lippke S. Obstetric healthcare workers' adherence to hand hygiene recommendations during the COVID-19 pandemic: observations and social-cognitive determinants. Appl Psychol Heal Well Being. 2020;12:1286–305. https://doi.org/10.1111/aphw.12240.
30. Sun Y, Qin B, Hu Z, Li H, Li X, He Y, Huang H. Predicting mask-wearing behavior intention among international students during COVID-19 based on the theory of planned behavior. Ann Palliat Med. 2021;10(4):3633–47.
31. Barile JP, Guerin RJ, Fisher KA, Tian LH, Okun AH, Vanden Esschert KL, Jeffers A, Gurbaxani BM, Thompson WW, Prue CE. Theory-based behavioral predictors of self-reported use of face coverings in public settings during the COVID-19 pandemic in the United States. Ann Behav Med. 2021;55:82–8. https://doi.org/10.1093/abm/kaaa109.
32. Yıldırım M, Güler A. COVID-19 severity, self-efficacy, knowledge, preventive behaviors, and mental health in Turkey. Death Stud. 2022;46:1–8. https://doi.org/10.1080/07481187.2020.1793434.
33. Shahnazi H, Ahmadi-Livani M, Pahlavanzadeh B, Rajabi A, Hamrah MS, Charkazi A. Assessing preventive health behaviors from COVID-19: a cross sectional study with health belief model in Golestan Province, Northern of Iran. Infect Dis Poverty. 2020;9:157. https://doi.org/10.1186/s40249-020-00776-2.
34. Das AK, JMM AK, Uddin MS, Uddin MA, Ghosh AK. Fighting ahead: adoption of social distancing in COVID-19 outbreak through the lens of theory of planned behavior. J Hum Behav Soc Environ. 2021;31:373–93. https://doi.org/10.1080/10911359.2020.1833804.
35. Graupensperger S, Abdallah DA, Lee CM. Social norms and vaccine uptake: college students' COVID vaccination intentions, attitudes, and estimated peer norms and comparisons with influenza vaccine. Vaccine. 2021;39:2060–7. https://doi.org/10.1016/j.vaccine.2021.03.018.
36. Zampetakis LA, Melas C. The health belief model predicts vaccination intentions against COVID-19: a survey experiment approach. Appl Psychol Heal Well Being. 2021;13:469–84. https://doi.org/10.1111/aphw.12262.
37. Shmueli L. Predicting intention to receive COVID-19 vaccine among the general population using the health belief model and the theory of planned behavior model. BMC Public Health. 2021;21:804. https://doi.org/10.1186/s12889-021-10816-7.
38. Anaki D, Sergay J. Predicting health behavior in response to the coronavirus disease (COVID-19): worldwide survey results from early March 2020. PLoS One. 2021;16:e0244534.
39. Prasetyo YT, Castillo AM, Salonga LJ, Sia JA, Seneta JA. Factors affecting perceived effectiveness of COVID-19 prevention measures among Filipinos during enhanced community quarantine in Luzon, Philippines: integrating protection motivation theory and extended theory of planned behavior. Int J Infect Dis. 2020;99:312–23. https://doi.org/10.1016/j.ijid.2020.07.074.
40. Hagger MS, Moyers S, McAnally K, McKinley LE. Known knowns and known unknowns on behavior change interventions and mechanisms of action. Health Psychol Rev. 2020;14:199–212. https://doi.org/10.1080/17437199.2020.1719184.
41. Connell LE, Carey RN, de Bruin M, Rothman AJ, Johnston M, Kelly MP, Michie S. Links between behavior change techniques and mechanisms of action: an expert consensus study. Ann Behav Med. 2019;53:708–20. https://doi.org/10.1093/abm/kay082.
42. World Health Organization. Coronavirus disease (COVID-19) advice for the public. Geneva: WHO. https://www.who.int/emergencies/diseases/novel-coronavirus-2019/advice-for-public.
43. Smith SR, Hagger MS, Keech JJ, Moyers SA, Hamilton K. Improving hand hygiene behavior using a novel theory-based intervention during the covid-19 pandemic. Annals of Behavioral Medicine. 2022. https://doi.org/10.1093/abm/kaac041.

44. Hamilton K, Johnson BT. Attitudes and persuasive communication interventions. In: Hagger MS, Cameron L, Hamilton K, Hankonen N, Lintunen T, editors. The handbook of behavior change. Cambridge: Cambridge University Press; 2020. p. 445–60. https://doi.org/10.1017/9781108677318.031.
45. Sheeran P, Maki A, Montanaro E, Avishai-Yitshak A, Bryan A, Klein WMP, Miles E, Rothman AJ. The impact of changing attitudes, norms, and self-efficacy on health-related intentions and behavior: a meta-analysis. Health Psychol. 2016;35:1178–88. https://doi.org/10.1037/hea0000387.
46. Steinmetz H, Knappstein M, Ajzen I, Schmidt P, Kabst R. How effective are behavior change interventions based on the theory of planned behavior? A three-level meta analysis. Z Psychol. 2016;224:216–33. https://doi.org/10.1027/2151-2604/a000255.
47. Gollwitzer PM. Implementation intentions: strong effects of simple plans. Am Psychol. 1999;54:493–503. https://doi.org/10.1037/0003-066X.54.7.493.
48. Gollwitzer PM, Sheeran P. Implementation intentions and goal achievement: a meta-analysis of effects and processes. Adv Exp Soc Psychol. 2006;38:69–119. https://doi.org/10.1016/S0065-2601(06)38002-1.
49. Armitage CJ. Effectiveness of experimenter-provided and self-generated implementation intentions to reduce alcohol consumption in a sample of the general population: a randomized exploratory trial. Health Psychol. 2009;28:545–53. https://doi.org/10.1037/a0015984.
50. Gollwitzer PM. Weakness of the will: is a quick fix possible? Motiv Emot. 2014;38:305–22. https://doi.org/10.1007/s11031-014-9416-3.
51. Conroy D, Hagger MS. Imagery interventions in health behavior: a meta-analysis. Health Psychol. 2018;37:668–79. https://doi.org/10.1037/hea0000625.
52. Kavanagh DJ, Andrade J, May J. Imaginary relish and exquisite torture: the elaborated intrusion theory of desire. Psychol Rev. 2005;112:446–67. https://doi.org/10.1037/0033-295X.112.2.446.
53. Pham LB, Taylor SE. From thought to action: effects of process-versus outcome-based mental simulations on performance. Personal Soc Psychol Bull. 1999;25:250–60. https://doi.org/10.1177/0146167299025002010.
54. Hagger MS, Lonsdale A, Chatzisarantis NLD. A theory-based intervention to reduce alcohol drinking in excess of guideline limits among undergraduate students. Br J Health Psychol. 2012;17:18–43. https://doi.org/10.1111/j.2044-8287.2010.02011.x.
55. Koka A, Hagger MS. A brief intervention to increase physical activity behavior among adolescents using mental simulations and action planning. Psychol Health Med. 2017;22:701–10. https://doi.org/10.1080/13548506.2016.1211298.
56. Knäuper B, Roseman M, Johnson PJ, Krantz LH. Using mental imagery to enhance the effectiveness of implementation intentions. Curr Psychol. 2009;28:181–6. https://doi.org/10.1007/s12144-009-9055-0.
57. Knäuper B, McCollam A, Rosen-Brown A, Lacaille J, Kelso E, Roseman M. Fruitful plans: adding targeted mental imagery to implementation intentions increases fruit consumption. Psychol Health. 2011;26:601–17. https://doi.org/10.1080/08870441003703218.
58. Hamilton K, Keech JJ, Peden AE, Hagger MS. Protocol for developing a mental imagery intervention: a randomised controlled trial testing a novel implementation imagery e-health intervention to change driver behaviour during floods. BMJ Open. 2019;9:e025565. https://doi.org/10.1136/bmjopen-2018-025565.
59. Michie S, West R, Rogers MB, Bonell C, Rubin GJ, Amlôt R. Reducing SARS-CoV-2 transmission in the UK: a behavioural science approach to identifying options for increasing adherence to social distancing and shielding vulnerable people, vol. 25; 2020. p. 945–56. https://doi.org/10.1111/bjhp.12428.
60. Murphy J, Vallières F, Bentall RP, Shevlin M, McBride O, Hartman TK, McKay R, Bennett K, Mason L, Gibson-Miller J, Levita L, Martinez AP, Stocks TVA, Karatzias T, Hyland P. Psychological characteristics associated with COVID-19 vaccine hesitancy and resistance in Ireland and the United Kingdom. Nat Commun. 2021;12:29. https://doi.org/10.1038/s41467-020-20226-9.

# Chapter 18
# Neurological Complications of COVID-19

**Dean Walton, Roberto Acampora, Greta Karen Wood, Elias Premi, Ingrid Andreea Ilie, Francesco Lanfranchi, and Benedict Daniel Michael**

D. Walton
Department of Neurology, The Walton Centre NHS Foundation Trust, Liverpool, UK

R. Acampora
Milan Center for Neuroscience (NeuroMI), Milan, Italy

Neurology and Stroke-Unit, Hospital Ospedale del Mare, Naples, Italy

G. K. Wood · B. D. Michael (✉)
Department of Neurology, The Walton Centre NHS Foundation Trust, Liverpool, UK

Clinical Infection Microbiology and Neuroimmunology, Institute of Infection, Veterinary and Ecological Science, Liverpool, UK

The NIHR Health Protection Research Unit for Emerging and Zoonotic Infection, Liverpool, UK
e-mail: greta.wood@liverpool.ac.uk; benedict.michael@liverpool.ac.uk

E. Premi
Ophthalmology Unit, ASST Sette Laghi, Circolo Hospital and Macchi Foundation, Varese, Italy

Department of Biotechnologies and Life Sciences, University of Insubria, Varese, Italy

I. A. Ilie
Department of Life Sciences and Biotechnology, School of Biology, University of Ferrara, Ferrara, Italy

F. Lanfranchi
Department of Health Sciences (DISSAL), University of Genoa, Genoa, Italy
e-mail: flanfranchi@hotmail.com


S. Adibi et al. (eds.), *Frontiers of COVID-19*,
https://doi.org/10.1007/978-3-031-08045-6_18

## Introduction

Ever since novel coronavirus disease (COVID-19), neurological complications have been observed in patients at all stages of the disease [1–3], even if it is a predominantly respiratory virus. At the beginning of the pandemic, evidence was limited to case reports and case series [4, 5], but their rising prevalence has been detected quicker, and they appeared to be strongly linked with severe acute respiratory syndrome coronavirus-2 (SARS-CoV-2) infection, to exert a detrimental effect on COVID-19 morbidity, and to increase patients' mortality.

The prevalence of neurological symptoms in general has been documented extensively, highlighted by large retrospective and prospective cohort studies [1, 6, 7]. This has been taken further with a large meta-analysis highlighting the ubiquity of neurological and neuropsychiatric symptoms [5]. However, considering the heterogeneity of the diagnostic criteria adopted, it is quite tough to predict their real prevalence. A projection based on neurological complications seen with previous coronaviruses was performed, but they did not incorporate neurovascular syndromes, strongly witnessed in COVID-19, in their calculations [8, 9].

More recently, cohort studies are highlighting the prevalence of specific neurological complications. Overall, the prevalence of neurological complications seems to range from less than 0.1% to 13.5% [10–15]. Stroke and encephalopathy consistently feature as the most common complications, even across different countries and continents [11, 12, 14, 16–19]. This was closely followed by neuromuscular disorders and peripheral nervous system (PNS), such as Guillain-Barré syndrome (GBS), and central nervous system (CNS) inflammatory syndromes.

The demographics and clinical characteristics at higher risk are difficult to ascertain. The cohort studies available enrolled selected populations, often represented by patients hospitalized or admitted to intensive therapy units (ITU), producing a selection bias. However, it is clear that severe COVID-19 patients have a greater risk of developing neurological complications [20, 21].

Consistent findings across studies have shown that neurological complications, in particular stroke, increase the risk of mortality and prolong the hospitalization time [10, 11, 20]. As with COVID-19 in general, age and frailty also correlate with negative outcomes. Furthermore, the mortality rate from neurological complications alone was found to be 4.1% in one Spanish cohort study [7].

The aim of the present chapter was to discuss neurological manifestations associated with previously known respiratory viruses and to classify and describe the large spectrum of neurological complications of COVID-19 (Neuro-COVID), in order to increase awareness about current and potential emerging complications, to facilitate their early recognition and effective management, and to evaluate adequate surveillance protocols and preventive strategies for the future.

## Neurological Manifestations and Neuropathophysiology of Respiratory Viruses

The first association between influenza virus and encephalitis was documented during the H2N2 Asian influenza pandemic of 1958 by Anderson and Jaros [22]. More recently, neurological disorders such as encephalitis, meningitis, meningoencephalitis, GBS, and polyneuropathy have been associated with H1N1 influenza A pandemic of 2009, in both adults and children [23–25]. Moreover, current evidence has linked even the common seasonal influenza to influenza associated encephalopathy, especially in pediatric age; however, non-specific confounding symptoms are common and there is a lack of direct signs of central nervous system involvement [26, 27].

In addition, several coronaviruses have been associated with neurological complications [28]. Epidemic SARS coronavirus (renamed SARS-CoV-1 after the identification of the novel coronavirus 2019) was isolated in brain culture and cerebrospinal fluid (CSF) by polymerase chain reaction (PCR) [29–31], and Middle Eastern respiratory syndrome (MERS) is associated with neurological complications ranging from encephalitis, acute disseminated encephalomyelitis (ADEM), and GBS [32, 33]. Beyond epidemic coronaviruses, even HCoV-OC43, a common seasonal coronavirus, has been identified in some children affected by neurological conditions; in particular, the virus has been detected in the CSF of a child with ADEM [34], in the nasopharyngeal swab of a three-year-old boy with GBS [35], and in the brain biopsy samples of two little children with encephalitis [36, 37].

Looking at previous evidence and reports, it is not surprising that SARS-CoV-2 infection could lead to a wide array of neurological manifestations. However, the major question is whether these complications are caused by the viral infection, or they are merely coincidental [8, 9]. Nowadays, to clearly establish if the Hill key domains (strength of the association, specificity, consistency, temporality, and plausibility) are satisfied [38], further robust and detailed research are necessary. Conversely, probably the first way for clarifying this topic is to assess the exact mechanisms underlying Neuro-COVID multifaceted symptoms; as suggested by the variability in temporal relationship, severity, and site of neurological complications with COVID-19, this goal seems to be as intriguing as complex.

The first step of this process is to discriminate the direct effect of SARS-CoV-2 on CNS and the ones related to the host immune response. If complications arising acutely with incipient infection are more likely a para-infectious phenomenon, delayed neurological manifestations and sequelae likely represent a post-infectious process mediated by immune pathways.

There is significant evidence that SARS-CoV-2 disrupts the integrity of the blood–brain barrier (BBB), allowing systemic pro-inflammatory cytokines and cellular populations to migrate across it, and so causing neuroinflammation [39–41].

The importance of this mechanism is highlighted by the direct correlation between prevalence of neurological complications and illness severity. The process seems to be independent from direct viral neuroinvasion; in fact, it is demonstrated even in patients without viral detection in the CSF [42, 43]. Moreover, even post-mortem data support this hypothesis, showing a variety of inflammatory neuropathological findings like microglial activation, especially in the medulla oblongata [44, 45]. However, this may represent a sign of critical illness encephalopathy rather than a specific COVID-19 finding [46].

Direct viral invasion is substantiated by SARS-CoV-2 detection by using a variety of methods in CNS tissue [44]. However, this is not ubiquitous across all studies, it is not often correlated with the severity of neuroinflammation, and the sensitivity of applied detection methods is questionable [44, 45]. Moreover, there are a lot of mechanisms proposed as potentially responsible for this phenomenon [8, 9, 47], but it is still not clear their relevance and the potential impact on clinical manifestations.

One of the first hypothesis was that the virus could enter via the olfactory bulb, the only part of the CNS not protected by the dural meningeal membrane; this theory is supported by the high prevalence of anosmia in COVID-19 patients, an early symptom even in mild stages of the disease, and by murine evidence with prior coronaviruses [48–50]. Conversely, the virus is frequently not detected in the olfactory bulb [44]. Another hypothesis is that the virus could pass the BBB through infected cells. Endothelial cells are evidenced as a potential source of viral penetration through hematogenous spreading, and this theory is enhanced by the documentation of the virus in this kind of cell [51–53]. Even infected immune cells could be responsible for SARS-CoV-2 neuroinvasion, and their cross through the BBB may be facilitated by the aforementioned disruption of the barrier itself [48]. While this mechanism has been documented with other coronaviruses [54], studies focused on SARS-CoV-2 are missing or still ongoing [44].

Beyond specific mechanism of neuroinvasion, cytokines storm and critical illness could determine neurological complications independently by their etiology, and because of the frequency of this phenomena in COVID-19, this infection should be considered a relevant potential cause of CNS disorders.

## Classification of COVID-19 Neurological Complications

The operative importance of characterizing and defining CNS complications was strongly highlighted by Varatharaj and colleagues [3]. By performing this, they provide clear and consistent case definitions for various neurological disorders, allowing the harmonization of data collection and analysis [55, 56]. This tentative attempt of standardization is particularly relevant, because a lot of early published data consists of case reports and studies often lacking uniform investigations, imaging findings, and CSF analysis, leading to unreliable diagnoses [4, 8, 9].

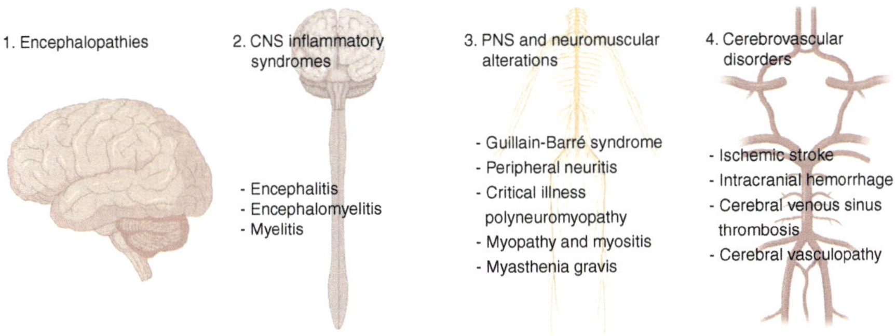


**Fig. 18.1** Graphical summary of the current classification of neuro-COVID manifestations. Created with BioRender.com

The need for a standardized classification was a concept stressed by Ellul and co-authors [8, 9] that suggests the definitions for confirmed, probable, and possible neurological complications related to SARS-CoV-2 infection, according to the World Health Organization (WHO) definition of COVID-19 case. While debate may occur over the minutia of these classifications, early implementation and adherence will aid future research and data sets [8, 9, 57].

According to these definitions, Neuro-COVID manifestations (graphically summarized in Fig. 18.1) could be classified as follows: (1) encephalopathies, (2) CNS inflammatory syndromes, (3) PNS and neuromuscular alterations, and (4) cerebrovascular disorders. In general, our discussion of neurological complications will follow these topics, including also early sensitive symptoms.

## Anosmia and Ageusia

Ever since the beginning of COVID-19 pandemic, the loss of smell (anosmia) and taste (ageusia) has been repeatedly reported in a growing number of COVID-19 patients worldwide. To date, scientific evidence shows that anosmia along with ageusia are common findings in a relevant percentage of both symptomatic and paucisymptomatic COVID-19 patients. In these subjects they could be the first and often the only clinical presentation [58–60]. Systematic review data [61] including 27 studies and 20,451 cumulative COVID-19 patients reported a pooled prevalence of 48.5% for anosmia and of 41.5% for ageusia, and the combined prevalence of the two symptoms was 35%.

Regarding the clinical onset of anosmia and ageusia, an Italian cohort study [58–60] conducted during the first wave of the pandemic and recruiting patients affected by COVID-19 at every stage of severity has demonstrated that such chemo-sensitive disorders occur in the first three days in the cohort of symptomatic patients in about two-third of all cases and represent the first symptom of COVID-19 in about one-third of the population investigated. In addition, the same study suggested a higher severity of hypo/anosmia and in the first four days from the clinical onset of the disease.

Considering the prognosis of these disorders, several COVID-19 case series [62, 63] showed a remarkable recovery of olfactory function within 1 or 2 weeks after the onset of the dysfunction, while a multicenter questionnaire study [64] conducted on 417 mild to moderate COVID-19 patients affected by anosmia and ageusia revealed that 25% of the patients completely recovered both their sense of smell and taste during 2 weeks following resolution of COVID-19 general symptoms. Nevertheless, in the sample of patients investigated who recovered, at least half of them complained of hyposmia, while one-third of them had isolated hypo/ageusia or both the chemo-sensitive dysfunctions after 4 weeks from the disease recovery.

Even if the exact pathogenesis of these chemo-sensitive disorders has not yet been clarified, some authors have hypothesized that SARS-CoV-2 could infect cells through interactions between its spike protein and the angiotensin converting enzyme 2 protein receptor along with the cell surface transmembrane protease serine 2, both diffusely expressed on the surface of cells located in the oral cavity mucous membrane as well as in the nasal mucous of the olfactory bulb [65, 66]. It is possible that in the period of exposure to infection, the direct viral invasion or the virus-induced host inflammatory response interaction with these structures could lead to smell and taste alterations. Regarding ageusia, an additional mechanism postulated is the impairment of salivary sialic acid metabolism [58–60].

Taken together, the above-mentioned findings argue for olfactory and/or gustatory acute or subacute impairment being a specific if not pathognomonic clinical feature of COVID-19, involving an elevated number of patients even in very early stages of disease. Thus, hypo/anosmia and hypo/ageusia represent a valid criterion to self-isolate and to start the diagnostic iter for SARS-CoV-2 demonstration, particularly when they occur alongside other non-specific flu-like common symptoms such as fever, fatigue, myalgia, joint pain, and gastrointestinal discomfort.

## Encephalopathies

Encephalopathy is an acute alteration in brain function presenting a multitude of causes including, but not limited to, metabolic disorders, toxins, medications, withdrawal and inflammatory conditions, or a combination of predisposing factors. It can often manifest as a change in personality and behavior, cognition, and alertness (delirium), especially in elderly patients with underlying cognitive decline. Analyzing and comparing data about such a multifaceted spectrum is extremely difficult, because of the heterogeneous case definition, classification, and diagnostic criteria adopted [11, 12, 67].

Beyond the causes, encephalopathy is universally found as one of the most common neurological complications in hospitalized COVID-19 patients [11, 12, 16,

19], with a prevalence ranging from 2.3% to 6.8% [18, 68, 69]. Risk factors for developing encephalopathy include increased age and concurrent comorbidities, such as high body mass index, hypertension, and diabetes [70]. Once present, it confers increased morbidity and mortality, independently of the disease severity [70, 71] and it also increases the likelihood of intubation [70].

To recognize such a condition according to standardized criteria is crucial to allow robust investigation for the underlying mechanisms, causes, and specific prognostic value in COVID-19.

## CNS Inflammatory Syndromes

Central neuroinflammation includes several conditions, namely encephalitis, encephalomyelitis, and myelitis, generally caused by infections or immune-mediated responses. To diagnose such conditions, there must be objective evidence of inflammation, whether this is from CSF analysis or neuroimaging [8, 9, 11, 12].

### *Encephalitis*

Encephalitis is an inflammation of the brain parenchyma, early and frequently identified in COVID-19 patients even if without objective investigations [4]. Conversely, a large prospective observational study using strict definitions did not describe any cases of encephalitis or myelitis associated with SARS-CoV-2, and autopsy findings attributed changes to hypoxic-ischemic sequelae [11, 12, 72].

However, after the first documented case of encephalitis associated with SARS-CoV-2 detection in CSF in a patient with negative nasopharyngeal testing, there have been multiple reports about this link [3, 7, 73–75]. Still, there is need for further investigation to assess other potential pathogens and causes of encephalitis [76].

Evidence also shows that there is a wide variety of presentations of encephalitis, including post-infectious conditions such as acute disseminated encephalomyelitis, brainstem encephalitis, limbic encephalitis, and autoimmune encephalitis with specifically identified autoantibodies [74–79].

### *Encephalomyelitis and Myelitis*

Encephalomyelitis is widely documented, generally presenting as ADEM [80]. Isolated spinal cord inflammation has been documented in several adult case reports, but this presentation is more frequently in children combined with ADEM [81–83].

## PNS and Neuromuscular Alterations

### *Guillain-Barré Syndrome Spectrum*

GBS, a heterogeneous group of acute immune-mediated neuropathies, is known to be a possible consequence of multiple infectious pathogens, and SARS-CoV-2 has been postulated as a further culprit. There have been several large case-control studies that have shown an increased incidence of GBS in association with COVID-19 [84, 85].

The clinical features of GBS associated with COVID-19 are very similar to the usual disease presentation [86, 87]. A further systematic review undertook classifying the variants of GBS and found that almost two-third of them were acute inflammatory demyelinating polyradiculopathy [88].

However, recent findings [83] indicated GBS as not consequent to SARS-CoV-2. A large observational study from Singapore showed a decreasing trend in GBS hospitalization during COVID-19 pandemic [89]. Another epidemiological cohort study comparing COVID-19 and non-COVID-19 associated GBS found a similar lower incidence [90]. There were also no phenotypical differences between the two groups other than COVID-19 associated cases having a higher rate of intubation, but it is presumed to be related to pulmonary distress rather than to neurological causes. Both these studies argue this reduction is likely a result of decreased social contact and increased hygiene preventing spread of other pathogens that lead to GBS.

Therefore, current findings highlight the importance of screening for other pathogens in GBS presentations associated with SARS-CoV-2, especially because in many previous studies this process has not been performed [8, 9].

### *Other Neuropathies and Neuromuscular Disorders*

Aside from GBS and its variants, peripheral neuropathies have been described in a few isolated reports. Needham and colleagues, who followed up severe COVID-19 patients, found several cases of vasculitic-like mononeuritis multiplex [55, 56]. However, PNS should even be associated with critical illness or medical interventions.

Concerning critical illness polyneuromyopathy (CIPNM), there are several case reports and case series [91, 92]. It is intriguing the fact that several risk factors for developing CIPNM (age, comorbidities, hyperglycemia, sepsis, acute respiratory distress syndrome, steroids, and neurosedatory medications) are observed in severe COVID-19 [93, 94]. Prone position, frequently essential in patients with viral pneumonia, may also lead to neuropathy, particularly brachial plexopathy [92].

Myopathy, and in particular myositis, has been described in case studies and case series and it has been postulated as an autoimmune consequence given the evidence of concomitant autoimmune disease, acute necrotizing myositis, its response to immunosuppression, and of autoantibody development [95–99]. Myopathy was documented in 3.1% of patients with other neurological manifestations and it was associated with a longer ITU stay.

About myasthenia gravis (MG), there have been several documented cases of the development of antibody (Ab) positive MG after COVID-19 symptom onset [100–102], presenting with a latency ranging from several days to several weeks. Speculation for an immune-mediated etiology secondary to SARS-CoV-2 is prevalent; nonetheless, further studies are necessary to establish possible causation and neuropathogenesis of this observed correlation. As with other patients who are immunosuppressed, there has been concern about MG patients' susceptibility to COVID-19, mainly considering the risk of myasthenic crises and respiratory involvement. Observational data from small numbers of pre-existing MG patients who required hospitalization for SARS-CoV-2 infection, even if presenting very variable findings, globally showed high rates of ITU admission, risk of intubation, and death [101, 103, 104].

## Cerebrovascular Disorders

Multiple cerebrovascular complications have been associated with COVID-19, including ischemic stroke, intracranial hemorrhage (both intracerebral and subarachnoid hemorrhage), cerebral venous sinus thrombosis, and cerebral vasculitis. Evidence from large national and multinational studies has shown that ischemic stroke is the most common cerebrovascular complication, followed by hemorrhage and then by thrombosis [57, 105, 106]. Individuals most likely to suffer cerebrovascular complications are older, have cardiovascular risk factors, and have more severe COVID-19 [57, 105].

### *Ischemic Stroke*

Acute ischemic stroke (AIS) is one of the most common neurological complications of COVID-19. Prevalence across hospitalized COVID-19 patients in large observational and case-control studies is about 1.1–1.9%, but there is a significant variability across the literature [57, 68, 105, 107, 108]. Risk factors for the development of acute ischemic stroke are increased age, more severe disease, and known cardiovascular disease.

The most frequent neuroimaging features of AIS in COVID-19 are large vessel occlusion and multiple territorial infarct [109, 110], suggesting an embolic cause rather than a thrombotic one, even if investigations often reveal no sources justifying such a phenomenon. Pro-thrombotic and hypercoagulable states are often found in these patients, presenting frequently high D-dimer levels and concomitant venous thromboembolism [110, 111]. The pathophysiology behind the increase in AIS risk is likely multifactorial, but the most frequently postulated theory is that the systemic inflammatory response and the consequent cytokines storm could activate coagulation cascades and thrombin production through endothelial cell dysfunction [55, 56].

While the pathophysiology is still debated, evidence clearly shows that ischemic stroke in the context of COVID-19 increases mortality, results in greater disability, and reduces the chance of recovery when compared to non-COVID AIS [107, 112]. Given the case number globally, this will put a significant strain on long-term rehabilitation and health services. Given these data and regardless of its pathophysiology, the pro-thrombotic state caused by COVID-19 has led to the development of prophylactic anticoagulation guidelines, of course to be balanced with bleeding risk.

## *Intracranial Hemorrhage*

Intracranial hemorrhage (ICH) has been associated with COVID-19 with a prevalence ranging from 0.2% to 0.5%, with a mortality rate assessed to be about 44.7–48.6% [57, 105, 108, 113]. Risk factors for developing ICH were older age, more severe disease requiring mechanical ventilation, and concurrent anticoagulation therapy or documented coagulopathy [114, 115]; unsurprisingly, there is a significant risk of ICH in patients who underwent extracorporeal membrane oxygenation treatment [116].

In a large observational case series [117], acute hemorrhages were found in 4.5% of computed tomography (CT) and magnetic resonance imaging (MRI) scans in neurologically symptomatic patients within 2 weeks of SARS-CoV-2 detection. However, no hemorrhages were present at the development of acute altered mental state, suggesting that imaging should be reserved for focal neurological deficits.

Nevertheless, despite substantial documentation of ICH with COVID-19, there is evidence that this finding could be related to acute respiratory distress syndrome rather than to COVID-19 itself [118].

## *Cerebral Venous Sinus Thrombosis*

Cerebral venous sinus thrombosis (CVST) in association with COVID-19 has been well documented by Baldini and colleagues [119], estimating a cumulative prevalence of less than 0.1%; this linkage is corroborated by the frequent recurrence of coagulopathy sequelae and peripheral venous thromboembolic phenomena in SARS-CoV-2 infection. A further supportive finding is that COVID-19 patients have fewer CVST risk factors when compared to CVST in absence of SARS-CoV-2 infection [119–121].

Globally, CVST associated with COVID-19 typically affects older individuals and leads to a high mortality rate, ranging from 23.1% to 40%. However, data currently available are scarce, and further studies combined with growing evidence about CVST occurring post-vaccine administration [122] could allow a deeper understanding of a possible rare but severe COVID-19 associated complication.

## *Cerebral Vasculopathy*

Cerebral vasculitis and vasculopathy have been documented in two studies by radiological appearance [79, 123]. Thickening and enhancement of vessel walls on MRI scans have been discovered in another study including sixty-nine patients with neurological manifestations [124]; the same study did not find these abnormal MRI features in the twenty-five patients without SARS-CoV-2, suggesting a possible specific association.

These phenomena could be a consequence of the aforementioned pathways, systemic inflammation, and direct viral invasion of endothelial cells [51–53]. About the clinical impact of cerebral blood vessel disorders, they could be one of the contributing factors to the incidence of stroke in COVID-19 patients [125].

## Neuro-Covid Imaging

Despite the difficulties encountered carrying out radiological exams in relation to the need of infection control and to transport intubated or ventilated patients, neuroimaging findings of several studies conducted worldwide in COVID-19 patients documented a conspicuous involvement of the nervous system. A retrospective study conducted in March and April 2020, involving a cohort of 3000 COVID-19 patients in three hospitals in New York, showed that acute stroke (mainly AIS) was the most common finding in neuroimaging, seen in 92.5% of patients with abnormal brain scans, and present in 1.1% of hospitalized COVID-19 patients. In addition, due to the increased mortality found in these patients, acute stroke has doubtlessly represented a common strong prognostic marker of poor outcome in COVID-19 patients [126].

To date, scientific evidence from literature has revealed that central nervous system involvement is mainly characterized by acute and subacute cerebral infarcts, embracing large vessel occlusion (Fig. 18.2a–f), small vessel, and watershed stroke representing the most common findings followed by cerebral micro-hemorrhages (Fig. 18.2g–i), acute spontaneous intracerebral hemorrhages (Fig. 18.2j–l), and cerebral venous thrombosis (Fig. 18.2m–o). All these findings could be explained by the severe coagulopathy often present in COVID-19 [130]. It is plausible that cerebral micro-hemorrhages could be a late complication of critical-stage COVID-19 related to hypoxia and/or small vessel vasculopathy. Nevertheless, the underlying mechanism responsible for development of cerebral micro-bleeding is still uncertain.

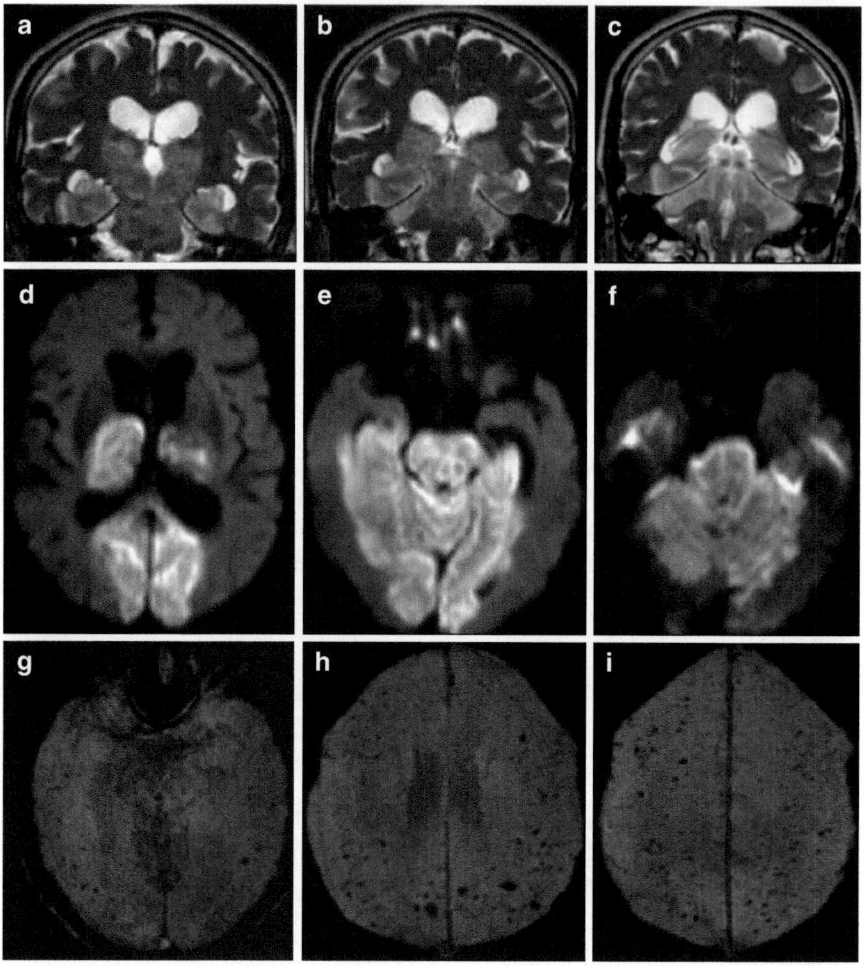


**Fig. 18.2** Most common neuroimaging findings in COVID-19 patients with CNS involvement. Brain MRI (**a–c**) coronal T2-weighted imaging, and (**d–f**) axial diffusion-weighted imaging (DWI) of acute infarct (large vessel occlusion) involving the basilar artery territories (brainstem, bilateral thalami, occipital and inferior temporal lobes, and cerebellum). (**g–i**) Brain MRI axial susceptibility weighted imaging (SWI) demonstrates numerous cerebral microbleeds in the temporal, frontal, and parietal lobes, predominantly located at the gray/white matter junction. (**j–l**) CT head without contrast reveals extensive pontine and midbrain hemorrhage with intraventricular extension involving the third and fourth ventricles and early hydrocephalus: axial image at the level of the pons (**j**), coronal image centered at largest diameter of intraparenchymal hematoma (**k**), and sagittal image showing hemorrhage extending to fourth and third ventricles (**l**). (**m–o**) Cerebral venous thrombosis: non-contrast brain CT asymmetric hyperdensity of the left of the left transverse sinus (dense vein sign; yellow arrow) (**m**), consistent with no associated parenchymal edema; magnetic resonance venography (MRV) confirms cerebral venous thrombosis in the left transverse sinus and shows hypoplasia in the sigmoid sinus and jugular bulb (yellow arrows) (**n**); MRV after 5 weeks shows recanalization of the small caliber left transverse sinus (yellow arrow) with persistent hypoplasia of sigmoid sinus and jugular bulb. (Figures and captions modified from (**a–f**) Khedr et al. [127], (**g–i**) Paterson et al. [110], (**j–l**) Flores et al. [128], (**m–o**) Khan et al. [129], and licensed under Creative Common License CC BY 4.0 (https://creativecommons.org/licenses/by/4.0/))

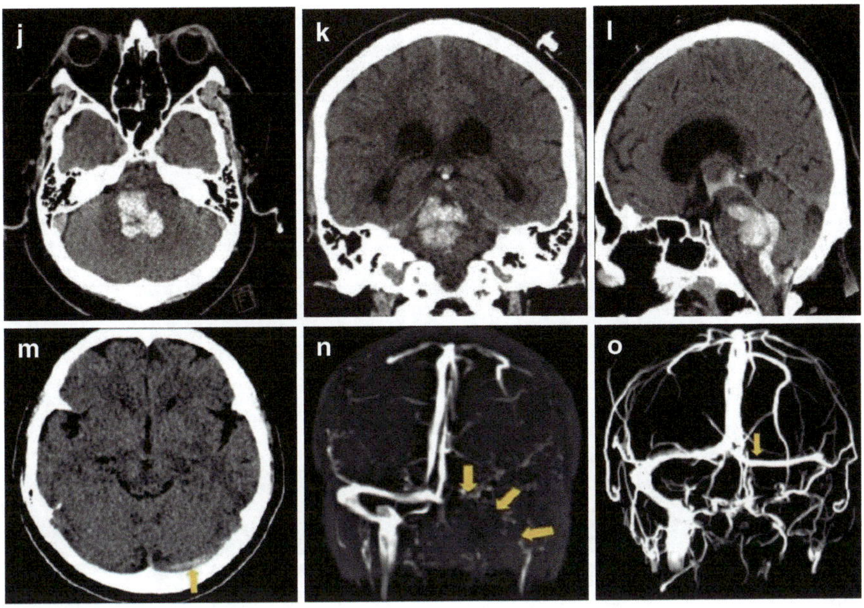


**Fig. 18.2** (continued)

A multicenter study [43] highlights eight main patterns of MRI alterations between abnormal scans of 37 COVID-19 patients with neurological symptoms. Signal abnormalities in the medial temporal lobe (Fig. 18.3) resulted as the most frequent (16 of 37, 43%), followed by white matter hyperintensities associated with micro-bleeding on fluid-attenuated inversion recovery (FLAIR) sequences (30%) and by extensive and isolated white matter micro-hemorrhages (24%). Furthermore, the same study confirmed the correlation between cerebral hemorrhage and worst prognosis.

ADEM neuroradiological findings have been detected in adults (Fig. 18.4), especially in elderly with previous severe infection [131]. However, the exact pathophysiology remains still unclear. Rare cases of post-infectious ADEM-like syndromes have been described in children [81], with patchy or confluent hyperintensities on T2-weighted scans in both gray and white matter, with or without reduced diffusion or enhancement. However, these pediatric patients were found to be positive for antibodies against the myelin oligodendrocyte glycoprotein (MOG) and the N-methyl-D-aspartate receptor (NMDAR). Given that neurological illnesses related to anti-MOG-Ab and anti-NMDAR-Ab can appear in post-viral illness, these cases raise the likelihood that COVID-19 could have an association with immune-mediated CNS pathology.

MRI findings in myelitis, both isolated (Fig. 18.5a) and in combination with brain abnormalities (Fig. 18.5b), were predominantly characterized by the involvement of central cord gray matter, presenting T2-weighted hyperintensities, like

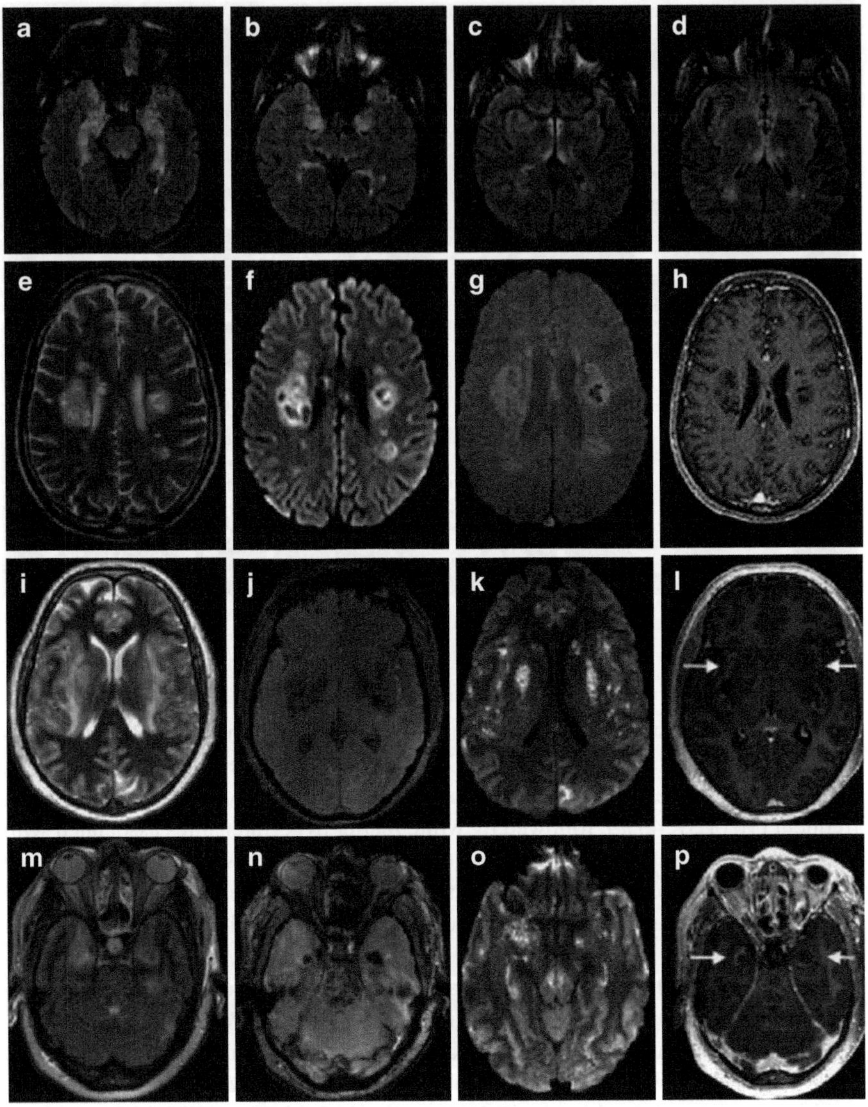


**Fig. 18.3** (**a**–**d**) Axial FLAIR images show bilateral hyperintensity in the mesial temporal lobes (**a** and **b**), hypothalamus (**c**) temporal lobes, and thalamus (**d**). (**e**–**h**) Axial T2-weighted (**e**), DWI (**f**), (SWI) (**g**), and post-contrast T1-weighted (**h**) images show multifocal clusters of lesions involving the deep white matter of both cerebral hemispheres, intralesional cyst-like areas of varied sizes, and some peripheral rims of restricted diffusion (**f**), some hemorrhagic changes (**g**), and T1 hypointense "black holes" without contrast enhancement (**h**). (**i**–**p**) Axial images at the level of the insula and basal ganglia (**i**–**l**) and at the level of the temporal lobes and upper pons (**m**–**p**). T2-weighted images (**I** and **m**), SWI images (**j** and **n**), DWI images (**k** and **o**), and contrast-enhanced images (**l** and **p**). There are extensive confluent areas of T2 hyperintensity (**i** and **m**), with hemorrhagic change on SWI imaging (**j** and **n**), restricted diffusion on DWI images (**k** and **o**), and peripheral contrast-enhancement (white arrows in **l** and **p**) in the insular region, basal ganglia, and left occipital lobe (**i**–**l**) as well as in the medial temporal lobes and upper pons (**m**–**p**). (Figure and caption modified from Paterson et al. [110] and licensed under Creative Common License CC BY 4.0 (https://creativecommons.org/licenses/by/4.0/))

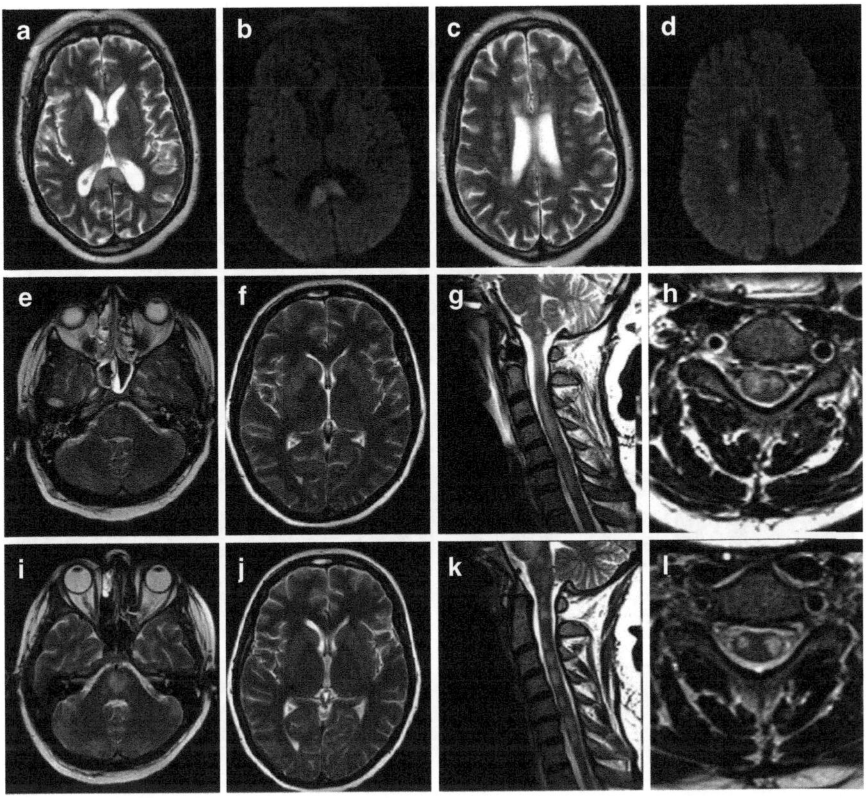


**Fig. 18.4** MRI images of two COVID-19 patients presenting ADEM. (**a**–**d**) Patient 1. Axial T2 (**a** and **c**) and DWI (**b** and **d**) images show multifocal lesions involving corpus callosum and corona radiata. (**e**–**l**) Patient 2. Axial T2-weighted images and sagittal T2-weighted of the spinal cord acquired on admission (**e**–**h**) and after 26 days (**i**–**l**). Axial T2-weighted images show multifocal hyperintense lesions in the brainstem (**e** and **i**), basal ganglia and supratentorial white matter (**f** and **j**). The pontomedullary hyperintensities have become more confluent (**i**) since admission (**e**). After 26 days, the signal abnormalities in the basal ganglia and the supratentorial white matter (**j**) are grossly similar to baseline (**f**). Sagittal and axial T2-weighted images show diffuse high T2-weighted signal intrinsic to the spinal cord at baseline (**g** and **h**). After 26 days, the cord edema has reduced, and the spinal cord lesions appear less confluent and more discrete (**k** and **l**). (Figure and caption modified from Paterson et al. [110] and licensed under Creative Common License CC BY 4.0 (https://creativecommons.org/licenses/by/4.0/))

other demyelinating myelopathies such as ADEM, neuromyelitis optica, anti-MOG-Ab associated encephalomyelitis, and idiopathic transverse myelitis. This pattern of spinal cord pathology resembled other few cases reported in children and adults with COVID-19 [134, 135]. MRI spinal nerve roots (Fig. 18.5c) and leptomeningeal

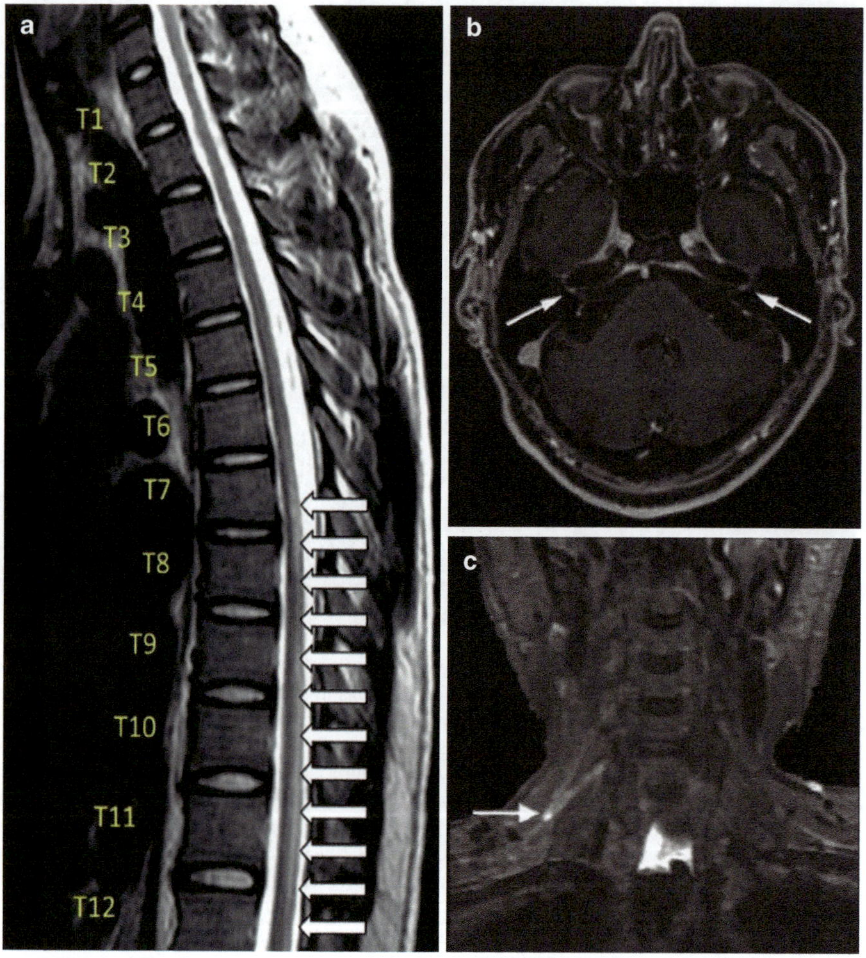


**Fig. 18.5** (**a**) MRI sagittal T2-weighted image of thoracic spine showing hyperintensity in the spinal cord (white arrows) from the seventh through the twelfth thoracic level suggestive of transverse myelitis. (**b**) Brain MRI axial T1-weighted fat-saturated post-contrast brain demonstrating bilateral facial nerve enhancement involving the labyrinthine segment (white arrows), tympanic segment, mastoid segment, and extracranial facial nerve. (**c**) MRI coronal short tau inversion recovery (STIR) image showing hyperintense signal abnormality of the upper trunk of the right brachial plexus (white arrow). (Figures and captions modified from (**a**) Durrani et al. [132], (**b**) Chan et al. [133], and (**c**) Paterson et al. [110] and licensed under Creative Common License CC BY 4.0 (https://creativecommons.org/licenses/by/4.0/))

enhancement have been observed even in GBS associated with COVID-19 [136]. However, this finding seems to be more common in classical GBS, as previously shown in a study conducted about Zika virus infected patients [137].

Imaging findings regarding the olfactory neuronal network involvement are mostly limited to case reports and series in patients affected by anosmia. Some works have shown MRI abnormalities in patients' olfactory bulbs (OB) [138]. Moreover, one neuroimaging study has reported increased T2-weighted MRI signal in the OB and in the bulbar tracts, with subtle contrast enhancement [139]. In addition, olfactory bulb atrophy after COVID-19 has also been described in patients with prolonged post-infectious anosmia, suggesting persistent OB damage [140]. Conversely, Shor and colleagues [141] have highlighted how the OB signal intensity could depend on the field strength applied, the imaging manufacturer, and the acquisition parameters adopted; moreover, OB abnormalities at MRI have been previously demonstrated even in non-COVID-19 patients with olfactory dysfunction [142].

Several studies investigated neuroimaging alterations occurring in long-COVID patients. One of them [143] has revealed a possible persistent disruption in microstructural and functional brain integrity in sixty previously hospitalized COVID-19 patients with neurological symptoms, even after a complete recovery from respiratory symptoms.

Fluorine-18 fluorodeoxyglucose positron emission tomography/computed tomography ($^{18}$F-FDG PET/CT) studies have shown intriguing new evidence in long-COVID patients, such as brain hypometabolism in bilateral rectal and orbital gyrus (including the olfactory gyrus), right temporal lobe (including amygdala and hippocampus), right thalamus, bilateral pons and medulla oblongata and bilateral cerebellum [144]. Another PET/CT study has showed reduced $^{18}$F-FDG metabolism in right para-hippocampal gyrus and thalamus [145].

Furthermore, Donegani and colleagues [146] have demonstrated a relative $^{18}$F-FDG hypometabolism in bilateral para-hippocampal, fusiform gyri and in left insula, and an involvement of bilateral longitudinal fasciculi in patients with isolated persistent hyposmia after recovery from COVID-19 (Fig. 18.6). These results suggest a persistent CNS involvement in COVID-19 long-haulers.

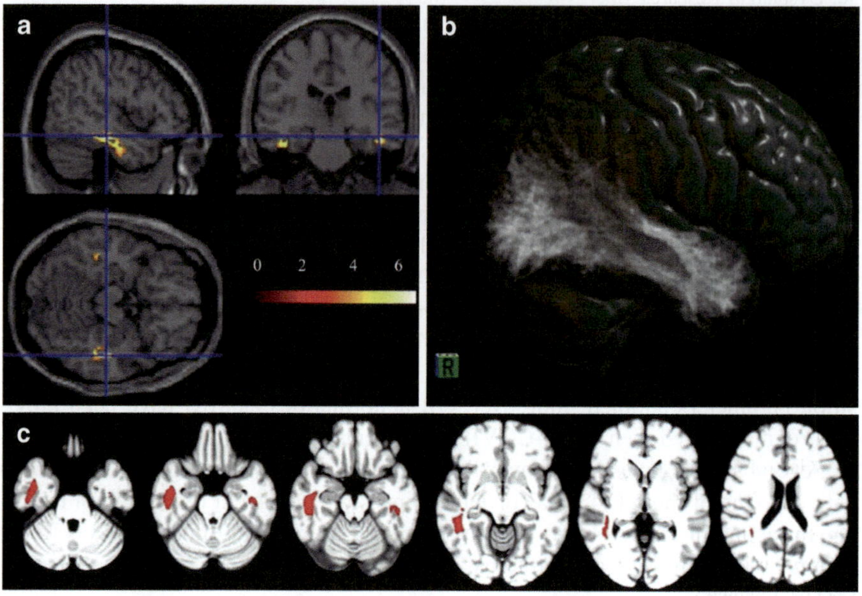


**Fig. 18.6** (**a**) Hypometabolism in patients still presenting with hyposmia during early recovery after SARS-CoV-2 infection was highlighted in para-hippocampal and fusiform gyri in both hemispheres (Brodmann area 20, 36, 37) and in the insula in the left hemisphere (Brodmann area 13). Height threshold of significance was set at $p < 0.05$ family-wise error-corrected at the cluster level. Regions of significant difference are shown color-graded in terms of Z values. (**b** and **c**) Structural connectivity of regions of hypometabolism in patients with olfactory dysfunction generated through the Brain Connectivity and Behaviour toolkit (http://www.toolkit.bcblab.com), which includes diffusion MRI data from healthy control subjects. (**a**) The connectome map indicated a significant probability of connection of the hyposmia cluster with the inferior longitudinal fasciculus. (**b**) Tractography results of the hyposmia cluster. (Figures and captions modified from Donegani et al. [146] and licensed under Creative Common License CC BY 4.0 (https://creativecommons.org/licenses/by/4.0/))

## Moving Forward

Despite prevalence of neurological complications being lower than respiratory symptoms, Neuro-COVID is still a significant negative prognostic factor, strongly impacting on clinical outcomes and mortality of COVID-19 patients. Looking at prior respiratory viruses, it is totally reliable that such a plethora of neurological manifestations could be associated with SARS-CoV-2 infection. The pathophysiology of these complications is likely multifaceted, including at least systemic cytokines passage across a disrupted blood–brain barrier, host immune-mediated reactions, spreading via infected endothelial cells, and direct viral neuroinvasion.

To date, almost all the aforementioned hypotheses seem to be simultaneously reasonable and questionable, confirming the well-established and loudly requested need for further standardized molecular, microbiological, radiological, and clinical research about neuro-COVID [147–149].

To gain such a target, a continuous and immediate data sharing is vital, and this goal can be achieved only through a worldwide, collaborative, and harmonized research engagement. Thanks to the efforts of several study groups, national and international research co-operations are being undertaken to answer this call, including the Global Consortium Study of Neurological Dysfunction in COVID-19 [68], the COVID-19 Neuro Databank-Biobank [150], the European Academy of Neurology Neuro-Covid Registry Consortium [151], the CoroNerve Studies Group [152], the Post-hospitalization COVID-19 study [153], and the upcoming Post-Acute Sequelae of SARS-CoV-2 infection Initiative, announced by the National Institute of Health [154].

Agreeing with the Lancet Neurology Editorial [155], our greatest hopes lie in a global neuro-COVID network, because "approaches need to be standardized, and case definitions should be used consistently across studies. With the aim to refine guidelines for the management of patients with COVID-19 and characterize its long-term neurological manifestations, large-scale and multidisciplinary collaborations will be essential." Until this objective will not be achieved, a global "collaboration to improve our knowledge of COVID-19, including its long-term neurological manifestations, must continue to be a high priority."

**Acknowledgments** All the authors are thankful to their teammates and collaborators. They also thank all health workers around the world who are dealing with this pandemic; all the authors express their deepest condolences and offer a heartfelt thanks to all colleagues fallen fighting against this invisible enemy, as well as to their families.

**Disclosure Statement** DW, RA, GKW, EP, IAI, and FL declare no conflict of interest and do not receive any financial aid. BDM is supported to conduct COVID-19 neuroscience research by the UKRI/MRC (MR/V03605X/1); for additional neurological inflammation research due to viral infection BDM is also supported by grants from the MRC/UKRI (MR/V007181//1), MRC (MR/T028750/1) and Wellcome (ISSF201902/3).

**Funding** This research received no external funding.

**Author Contributions** Conceptualization: DW, RA, FL, and BDM.; literature research, screening, and selection: DW, RA, GKW, EP, and IAI; original draft preparation: all authors; writing and editing: all authors.

All the authors have read and approved the definitive version of the manuscript.

## References


1. Cleret de Langavant L, Petit A, Nguyen QTR, Gendre T, Abdelhedi J, Djellaoui A, Seddik L, et al. Clinical description of the broad range of neurological presentations of COVID-19: a retrospective case series. Rev Neurol. 2021;177(3):275–82. https://doi.org/10.1016/j.neurol.2021.01.004.
2. Maury A, Lyoubi A, Peiffer-Smadja N, de Broucker T, Meppiel E. Neurological manifestations associated with SARS-CoV-2 and other coronaviruses: a narrative review for clinicians. Rev Neurol (Paris). 2021;177(1-2):51–64. https://doi.org/10.1016/j.neurol.2020.10.001.
3. Varatharaj A, Thomas N, Ellul MA, Davies NWS, Pollak TA, Tenorio EL, Sultan M, et al. Neurological and neuropsychiatric complications of COVID-19 in 153 patients: a UK-wide surveillance study. Lancet Psychiatry. 2020;7(10):875–82. https://doi.org/10.1016/S2215-0366(20)30287-X.
4. Pouga L. Encephalitic syndrome and anosmia in COVID-19: do these clinical presentations really reflect SARS-CoV-2 neurotropism? A theory based on the review of 25 COVID-19 cases. J Med Virol. 2021;93(1):550–8. https://doi.org/10.1002/jmv.26309.
5. Rogers JP, Watson C, Badenoch J, Cross B, Butler M, Song J, Hafeez D, et al. The neurology and neuropsychiatry of COVID-19: a systematic review and meta-analysis of the early literature reveals frequent CNS manifestations and key emerging narratives. J Neurol Neurosurg Psychiatry. 2021;92(9):932–41. https://doi.org/10.1101/2021.02.24.21252335.
6. Helms J, Kremer S, Merdji H, Schenck M, Severac F, Clere-Jehl R, Studer A, et al. Delirium and encephalopathy in severe COVID-19: a cohort analysis of ICU patients. Crit Care. 2020;24(1):491. https://doi.org/10.1186/s13054-020-03200-1.
7. Romero-Sánchez CM, Díaz-Maroto I, Fernández-Díaz E, Sánchez-Larsen Á, Layos-Romero A, García-García J, González E, et al. Neurologic manifestations in hospitalized patients with COVID-19: the ALBACOVID registry. Neurology. 2020;95(8):e1060–70. https://doi.org/10.1212/WNL.0000000000009937.
8. Ellul MA, Benjamin L, Singh B, Lant S, Michael BD, Easton A, Kneen R, Defres S, Sejvar J, Solomon T. Neurological associations of COVID-19. Lancet Neurol. 2020a;19(9):767–83. https://doi.org/10.1016/S1474-4422(20)30221-0.
9. Ellul M, Varatharaj A, Nicholson TR, Pollak TA, Thomas N, Easton A, Michael S. Zandi, et al. Defining causality in COVID-19 and neurological disorders. J Neurol Neurosurg Psychiatry. 2020b;91(8):811–2. https://doi.org/10.1136/jnnp-2020-323667.
10. Eskandar EN, Altschul DJ, de la Garza Ramos R, Cezayirli P, Unda SR, Benton J, Dardick J, et al. Neurologic syndromes predict higher in-hospital mortality in COVID-19. Neurology. 2021;96(11):e1527–38. https://doi.org/10.1212/wnl.0000000000011356.
11. Frontera JA, Balcer L, Galetta S. Author response: a prospective study of neurologic disorders in hospitalized patients with COVID-19 in New York City. Neurology. 2021a;96(11):549–50. https://doi.org/10.1212/wnl.0000000000011609.
12. Frontera JA, Sabadia S, Lalchan R, Fang T, Flusty B, Millar-Vernetti P, Snyder T, et al. A prospective study of neurologic disorders in hospitalized patients with COVID-19 in New York City. Neurology. 2021b;96(4):e575–86. https://doi.org/10.1212/WNL.0000000000010979.
13. Koh JS, De Silva DA, Quek AML, Chiew HJ, Tian Ming T, Seet CYH, Hoe RHM, et al. Neurology of COVID-19 in Singapore. J Neurol Sci. 2020;418:117118. https://doi.org/10.1016/j.jns.2020.117118.
14. Portela-Sánchez S, Sánchez-Soblechero A, Otalora PJM, López ÁR, Alonso GV, Palacios-Mendoza MA, Caramé CC, et al. Neurological complications of COVID-19 in hospitalized patients: the registry of a neurology department in the first wave of the pandemic. Eur J Neurol. 2021;28(10):3339–47. https://doi.org/10.1111/ene.14748.
15. Rifino N, Censori B, Agazzi E, Alimonti D, Bonito V, Camera G, Conti MZ, et al. Neurologic manifestations in 1760 COVID-19 patients admitted to papa Giovanni XXIII Hospital, Bergamo, Italy. J Neurol. 2020;268(7):2331–8. https://doi.org/10.1007/s00415-020-10251-5.

16. Brucki SMD, Corazza LA, de Queiroz AP, Barros MP, Tatsch JFS, Riso IL, Batista NA, et al. Neurological complications in COVID-19 patients from Latin America. Brain. 2020;144(3):e29. https://doi.org/10.1093/brain/awaa440.
17. Chuang DT, Aydemir S, Magda P, Thomas C, Zarnegar R. Neurological manifestations as primary presentation of COVID-19 in hospitalized patients. Acta Neurol Scand. 2021;143(5):569–74. https://doi.org/10.1111/ane.13399.
18. Dravid AN, Mane DN, Khan ZA. Neurological issues during severe COVID-19 in a tertiary level hospital in Western India. Neurosci Lett. 2021;749:135692. https://doi.org/10.1016/j.neulet.2021.135692.
19. Meppiel E, Peiffer-Smadja N, Maury A, Bekri I, Delorme C, Desestret V, Gorza L, et al. Neurologic manifestations associated with COVID-19: a multicentre registry. Clin Microbiol Infect. 2021;27(3):458–66. https://doi.org/10.1016/j.cmi.2020.11.005.
20. Benussi A, Pilotto A, Premi E, Libri I, Giunta M, Agosti C, Alberici A, et al. Clinical characteristics and outcomes of inpatients with neurologic disease and COVID-19 in Brescia, Lombardy, Italy. Neurology. 2020;95(7):e910–20. https://doi.org/10.1212/WNL.0000000000009848.
21. Taquet M, Geddes JR, Husain M, Luciano S, Harrison PJ. 6-month neurological and psychiatric outcomes in 236 379 survivors of COVID-19: a retrospective cohort study using electronic health records. Lancet Psychiatry. 2021;8(5):416–27. https://doi.org/10.1016/s2215-0366(21)00084-5.
22. Anderson WW, Mary Jaros R. Neurologic complications of Asian influenza. Neurology. 1958;8(7):568–70. https://doi.org/10.1212/wnl.8.7.568.
23. Farooq O, Faden HS, Cohen ME, Ramanathan M, Barrett H, Farkas MK, Langan TJ, Ann Yeh E. Neurologic complications of 2009 influenza - A H1N1 infection in children. J Child Neurol. 2012;27(4):431–8. https://doi.org/10.1177/0883073811417873.
24. Glaser CA, Winter K, DuBray K, Harriman K, Uyeki TM, Sejvar J, Gilliam S, Louie JK. A population-based study of neurologic manifestations of severe influenza A(H1N1)Pdm09 in California. Clin Infect Dis. 2012;55(4):514–20. https://doi.org/10.1093/cid/cis454.
25. Goenka A, Michael BD, Ledger E, Hart IJ, Absoud M, Chow G, Lilleker J, et al. Neurological manifestations of influenza infection in children and adults: results of a National British Surveillance Study. Clin Infect Dis. 2014;58(6):775–84. https://doi.org/10.1093/cid/cit922.
26. Ekstrand JJ. Neurologic complications of influenza. Semin Pediatr Neurol. 2012;19(3):96–100. https://doi.org/10.1016/j.spen.2012.02.004.
27. McEntire CRS, Song KW, McInnis RP, Rhee JY, Young M, Williams E, Leah L. Wibecan, et al. Neurologic manifestations of the World Health Organization's list of pandemic and epidemic diseases. Front Neurol. 2021;12:634827. https://doi.org/10.3389/fneur.2021.634827.
28. Van Den Tooren H, Ellul MA, Davies NWS, Easton A, Vincent A, Solomon T, Michael BD. Standing on the shoulders of giants: 100 years of neurology and epidemic infections. J Neurol Neurosurg Psychiatry. 2020;91(11):1129–31. https://doi.org/10.1136/jnnp-2020-324366.
29. Hung ECW, Chim SSC, Chan PKS, Tong YK, Ng EKO, Chiu RWK, Leung CB, Sung JJY, Tam JS, Dennis Lo YM. Detection of SARS coronavirus RNA in the cerebrospinal fluid of a patient with severe acute respiratory syndrome. Clin Chem. 2003;49(12):2108–9. https://doi.org/10.1373/clinchem.2003.025437.
30. Lau KK, Yu WC, Chu CM, Lau ST, Sheng B, Yuen KY. Possible central nervous system infection by SARS coronavirus. Emerg Infect Dis. 2004;10(2):342–4. https://doi.org/10.3201/eid1002.030638.
31. Xu J, Zhong S, Liu J, Li L, Li Y, Wu X, Li Z, et al. Detection of severe acute respiratory syndrome coronavirus in the brain: potential role of the chemokine Mig in pathogenesis. Clin Infect Dis. 2005;41(8):1089–96. https://doi.org/10.1086/444461.
32. Arabi YM, Harthi A, Hussein J, Bouchama A, Johani S, Hajeer AH, Saeed BT, et al. Severe neurologic syndrome associated with Middle East respiratory syndrome Corona virus (MERS-CoV). Infection. 2015;43(4):495–501. https://doi.org/10.1007/s15010-015-0720-y.

33. Kim JE, Heo JH, Kim HO, Song SH, Park SS, Park TH, Ahn JY, Kim MK, Choi JP. Neurological complications during treatment of Middle East respiratory syndrome. Journal of Clinical Neurology (Korea). 2017;13(3):227–33. https://doi.org/10.3988/jcn.2017.13.3.227.
34. Yeh EA, Collins A, Cohen ME, Duffner PK, Faden H. Detection of coronavirus in the central nervous system of a child with acute disseminated encephalomyelitis. Pediatrics. 2004;113(1 Pt 1):e73–6. https://doi.org/10.1542/peds.113.1.e73.
35. Sharma K, Tengsupakul S, Sanchez O, Phaltas R, Maertens P. Guillain-Barré syndrome with unilateral peripheral facial and bulbar palsy in a child: a case report. SAGE Open Med Case Rep. 2019;7:2050313X19838750. https://doi.org/10.1177/2050313X19838750.
36. Morfopoulou S, Brown JR, Graham Davies E, Anderson G, Virasami A, Qasim W, Wui K. Chong, et al. Human coronavirus OC43 associated with fatal encephalitis. N Engl J Med. 2016;375(5):497–8. https://doi.org/10.1056/nejmc1509458.
37. Nilsson A, Edner N, Albert J, Ternhag A. Fatal encephalitis associated with coronavirus OC43 in an immunocompromised child. Infect Dis. 2020;52(6):419–22. https://doi.org/10.1080/23744235.2020.1729403.
38. Hill AB. The environment and disease: association or causation? J R Soc Med. 2015;108(1):32–7. https://doi.org/10.1177/0141076814562718.
39. Alexopoulos H, Magira E, Bitzogli K, Kafasi N, Vlachoyiannopoulos P, Tzioufas A, Kotanidou A, Dalakas MC. Anti-SARS-CoV-2 antibodies in the CSF, blood-brain barrier dysfunction, and neurological outcome: studies in 8 stuporous and comatose patients. Neurol Neuroimmunol Neuroinflamm. 2020;7(6):e893. https://doi.org/10.1212/NXI.0000000000000893.
40. Buzhdygan TP, DeOre BJ, Baldwin-Leclair A, Bullock TA, McGary HM, Khan JA, Razmpour R, et al. The SARS-CoV-2 spike protein alters barrier function in 2D static and 3D microfluidic in-vitro models of the human blood–brain barrier. Neurobiol Dis. 2020;146:105131. https://doi.org/10.1016/j.nbd.2020.105131.
41. Reynolds JL, Mahajan SD. SARS-COV2 alters blood brain barrier integrity contributing to neuro-inflammation. J Neuroimmune Pharmacol. 2021;16(1):4–6. https://doi.org/10.1007/s11481-020-09975-y.
42. Kremer S, Lersy F, Anheim M, Merdji H, Schenck M, Oesterlé H, Bolognini F, et al. Neurologic and neuroimaging findings in patients with COVID-19: a retrospective multicenter study. Neurology. 2020a;95(13):e1868–82. https://doi.org/10.1212/WNL.0000000000010112.
43. Kremer S, Lersy F, De Sèze J, Ferré JC, Maamar A, Carsin-Nicol B, Collange O, et al. Brain MRI findings in severe COVID-19: a retrospective observational study. Radiology. 2020b;297(2):E242–51. https://doi.org/10.1148/RADIOL.2020202222.
44. Lou JJ, Movassaghi M, Gordy D, Olson MG, Zhang T, Khurana MS, Chen Z, et al. Neuropathology of COVID-19 (Neuro-COVID): clinicopathological update. Free Neuropathol. 2021;2:2. https://doi.org/10.17879/freeneuropathology-2021-2993.
45. Matschke J, Lütgehetmann M, Hagel C, Sperhake JP, Schröder AS, Edler C, Mushumba H, et al. Neuropathology of patients with COVID-19 in Germany: a post-mortem case series. Lancet Neurol. 2020;19(11):919–29. https://doi.org/10.1016/S1474-4422(20)30308-2.
46. Deigendesch N, Sironi L, Kutza M, Wischnewski S, Fuchs V, Hench J, Frank A, et al. Correlates of critical illness-related encephalopathy predominate postmortem COVID-19 neuropathology. Acta Neuropathol. 2020;140(4):583–6. https://doi.org/10.1007/s00401-020-02213-y.
47. Zubair AS, McAlpine LS, Gardin T, Farhadian S, Kuruvilla DE, Spudich S. Neuropathogenesis and neurologic manifestations of the coronaviruses in the age of coronavirus disease 2019: a review. JAMA Neurol. 2020;77(8):1018–27. https://doi.org/10.1001/jamaneurol.2020.2065.
48. Desforges M, Le Coupanec A, Brison É, Meessen-Pinard M, Talbot PJ. Neuroinvasive and neurotropic human respiratory coronaviruses: potential neurovirulent agents in humans. Adv Exp Med Biol. 2014;807:75–96. https://doi.org/10.1007/978-81-322-1777-0_6.
49. Li K, Wohlford-Lenane C, Perlman S, Zhao J, Jewell AK, Reznikov LR, Gibson-Corley KN, Meyerholz DK, McCray PB. Middle East respiratory syndrome coronavirus causes multiple organ damage and lethal disease in mice transgenic for human dipeptidyl peptidase 4. J Infect Dis. 2015;212(11):712–22. https://doi.org/10.1093/infdis/jiv499.

50. Netland J, Meyerholz DK, Moore S, Cassell M, Perlman S. Severe acute respiratory syndrome coronavirus infection causes neuronal death in the absence of encephalitis in mice transgenic for human ACE2. J Virol. 2008;82(15):7264–75. https://doi.org/10.1128/jvi.00737-08.
51. Paniz-Mondolfi A, Bryce C, Grimes Z, Gordon RE, Reidy J, Lednicky J, Sordillo EM, Fowkes M. Central nervous system involvement by severe acute respiratory syndrome Coronavirus-2 (SARS-CoV-2). J Med Virol. 2020;92(7):699–702. https://doi.org/10.1002/jmv.25915.
52. Song E, Zhang C, Israelow B, Lu-Culligan A, Prado AV, Skriabine S, Lu P, et al. Neuroinvasion of SARS-CoV-2 in human and mouse brain. J Exp Med. 2021;218(3):e20202135. https://doi.org/10.1084/JEM.20202135.
53. Varga Z, Flammer AJ, Steiger P, Haberecker M, Andermatt R, Zinkernagel AS, Mehra MR, Schuepbach RA, Ruschitzka F, Moch H. Endothelial cell infection and endotheliitis in COVID-19. Lancet. 2020;395(10234):1417–8. https://doi.org/10.1016/S0140-6736(20)30937-5.
54. Spiegel M, Schneider K, Weber F, Weidmann M, Hufert FT. Interaction of severe acute respiratory syndrome-associated coronavirus with dendritic cells. J Gen Virol. 2006;87(7):1953–60. https://doi.org/10.1099/vir.0.81624-0.
55. Needham EJ, Chou SHY, Coles AJ, Menon DK. Neurological implications of COVID-19 infections. Neurocrit Care. 2020a;32(3):667–71. https://doi.org/10.1007/s12028-020-00978-4.
56. Needham E, Newcombe V, Michell A, Thornton R, Grainger A, Anwar F, Warburton E, Menon D, Trivedi M, Sawcer S. Mononeuritis multiplex: an unexpectedly frequent feature of severe COVID-19. J Neurol. 2020b;268(8):2685–9. https://doi.org/10.1007/s00415-020-10321-8.
57. Li HF, Hao HJ, Chen XJ. Provisional case definitions for COVID-19-associated neurological disease. Lancet Neurol. 2020a;19(11):890–1. https://doi.org/10.1016/S1474-4422(20)30373-2.
58. Vaira LA, Salzano G, Deiana G, De Riu G. Anosmia and ageusia: common findings in COVID-19 patients. Laryngoscope. 2020a;130(7):1787. https://doi.org/10.1002/lary.28692.
59. Vaira LA, Hopkins C, Salzano G, Petrocelli M, Melis A, Cucurullo M, Ferrari M, et al. Olfactory and gustatory function impairment in COVID-19 patients: Italian objective multicenter-study. Head Neck. 2020b;42(7):1560–9. https://doi.org/10.1002/hed.26269.
60. Vaira LA, Salzano G, Fois AG, Piombino P, De Riu G. Potential pathogenesis of ageusia and anosmia in COVID-19 patients. Int Forum Allergy Rhinol. 2020c;10(9):1103–4. https://doi.org/10.1002/alr.22593.
61. Ibekwe TS, Fasunla AJ, Orimadegun AE. Systematic review and meta-analysis of smell and taste disorders in COVID-19. OTO Open. 2020;4(3):2473974X2095797. https://doi.org/10.1177/2473974x20957975.
62. Yan CH, Faraji F, Prajapati DP, Boone CE, DeConde AS. Association of chemosensory dysfunction and COVID-19 in patients presenting with influenza-like symptoms. Int Forum Allergy Rhinol. 2020;10(7):806–13. https://doi.org/10.1002/alr.22579.
63. Zhou P, Yang XL, Wang XG, Hu B, Zhang L, Zhang W, Si HR, et al. A pneumonia outbreak associated with a new coronavirus of probable bat origin. Nature. 2020;579(7798):270–3. https://doi.org/10.1038/s41586-020-2012-7.
64. Lechien JR, Chiesa-Estomba CM, De Siati DR, Horoi M, Le Bon SD, Rodriguez A, Dequanter D, et al. Olfactory and gustatory dysfunctions as a clinical presentation of mild-to-moderate forms of the coronavirus disease (COVID-19): A multicenter European study. Eur Arch Otorhinolaryngol. 2020;277(8):2251–61. https://doi.org/10.1007/s00405-020-05965-1.
65. Hoffmann M, Kleine-Weber H, Schroeder S, Krüger N, Herrler T, Erichsen S, Schiergens TS, et al. SARS-CoV-2 cell entry depends on ACE2 and TMPRSS2 and is blocked by a clinically proven protease inhibitor. Cell. 2020;181(2):271–280.e8. https://doi.org/10.1016/j.cell.2020.02.052.
66. Xia S, Liu M, Wang C, Xu W, Lan Q, Feng S, Qi F, et al. Inhibition of SARS-CoV-2 (previously 2019-NCoV) infection by a highly potent pan-coronavirus fusion inhibitor targeting its spike protein that harbors a high capacity to mediate membrane fusion. Cell Res. 2020;30(4):343–55. https://doi.org/10.1038/s41422-020-0305-x.

67. Slooter AJC, Otte WM, Devlin JW, Arora RC, Bleck TP, Claassen J, Matthew S. Duprey, et al. Updated nomenclature of delirium and acute encephalopathy: statement of ten societies. Intensive Care Med. 2020;46(5):1020–2. https://doi.org/10.1007/s00134-019-05907-4.
68. Frontera J, Mainali S, Fink EL, Robertson CL, Schober M, Ziai W, Menon D, et al. Global consortium study of neurological dysfunction in COVID-19 (GCS-NeuroCOVID): study design and rationale. Neurocrit Care. 2020;33(1):25–34. https://doi.org/10.1007/s12028-020-00995-3.
69. Nalleballe K, Onteddu SR, Sharma R, Dandu V, Brown A, Jasti M, Yadala S, et al. Spectrum of neuropsychiatric manifestations in COVID-19. Brain Behav Immun. 2020;88(August):71–4. https://doi.org/10.1016/j.bbi.2020.06.020.
70. Shah VA, Nalleballe K, Zaghlouleh ME, Onteddu S. Acute encephalopathy is associated with worse outcomes in COVID-19 patients. Brain Behav Immun Health. 2020;8:100136. https://doi.org/10.1016/j.bbih.2020.100136.
71. Liotta EM, Batra A, Clark JR, Shlobin NA, Hoffman SC, Orban ZS, Koralnik IJ. Frequent neurologic manifestations and encephalopathy-associated morbidity in Covid-19 patients. Ann Clin Transl Neurol. 2020;7(11):2221–30. https://doi.org/10.1002/acn3.51210.
72. Solomon IH, Normandin E, Bhattacharyya S, Mukerji SS, Keller K, Ali AS, Adams G, Hornick JL, Padera RF, Sabeti P. Neuropathological features of Covid-19. N Engl J Med. 2020;383(10):989–92. https://doi.org/10.1056/nejmc2019373.
73. Moriguchi T, Harii N, Goto J, Harada D, Sugawara H, Takamino J, Ueno M, et al. A first case of meningitis/encephalitis associated with SARS-Coronavirus-2. Int J Infect Dis. 2020;94(May):55–8. https://doi.org/10.1016/j.ijid.2020.03.062.
74. Pilotto A, Masciocchi S, Volonghi I, Crabbio M, Magni E, De Giuli V, Caprioli F, et al. Clinical presentation and outcomes of severe acute respiratory syndrome coronavirus 2-related encephalitis: the ENCOVID multicenter study. J Infect Dis. 2021;223(1):28–37. https://doi.org/10.1093/infdis/jiaa609.
75. Walton DWA, Thakur KT, Venkatesan A, Breen G, Solomon T, Michael BD. Encephalitis in a pandemic. Front Neurol. 2021;12:637586. https://doi.org/10.3389/fneur.2021.637586.
76. Huo L, Xu KL, Wang H. Clinical features of SARS-CoV-2-associated encephalitis and meningitis amid COVID-19 pandemic. World J Clin Cases. 2021;9(5):1058–78. https://doi.org/10.12998/wjcc.v9.i5.1058.
77. Franke C, Ferse C, Jakob K, Momsen Reincke S, Sanchez-Sendin E, Rocco A, Steinbrenner M, et al. High frequency of cerebrospinal fluid autoantibodies in COVID-19 patients with neurological symptoms. Brain Behav Immun. 2021;93(March):415–9. https://doi.org/10.1016/j.bbi.2020.12.022.
78. Khoo A, McLoughlin B, Cheema S, Weil RS, Lambert C, Manji H, Zandi MS, Morrow JM. Postinfectious brainstem encephalitis associated with SARS-CoV-2. J Neurol Neurosurg Psychiatry. 2020;91(9):1013–4. https://doi.org/10.1136/jnnp-2020-323816.
79. Pinto AA, Carroll LS, Nar V, Varatharaj A, Galea I. CNS inflammatory vasculopathy with antimyelin oligodendrocyte glycoprotein antibodies in COVID-19. Neurol Neuroimmunol Neuroinflamm. 2020;7(5):e813. https://doi.org/10.1212/NXI.0000000000000813.
80. Parsons T, Banks S, Bae C, Gelber J, Alahmadi H, Tichauer M. COVID-19-associated acute disseminated encephalomyelitis (ADEM). J Neurol. 2020;267(10):2799–802. https://doi.org/10.1007/s00415-020-09951-9.
81. Lindan CE, Mankad K, Ram D, Kociolek LK, Michelle Silvera V, Boddaert N, Stivaros SM, et al. Neuroimaging manifestations in children with SARS-CoV-2 infection: a multinational, multicentre collaborative study. Lancet Child Adolesc Health. 2021;5(3):167–77. https://doi.org/10.1016/S2352-4642(20)30362-X.
82. Sotoca J, Rodríguez-Álvarez Y. COVID-19-associated acute necrotizing myelitis. Neurol Neuroimmunol Neuroinflamm. 2020;7(5):e803. https://doi.org/10.1212/NXI.0000000000000803.
83. Zhao H, Shen D, Zhou H, Liu J, Chen S. Guillain-Barré syndrome associated with SARS-CoV-2 infection: causality or coincidence? Lancet Neurol. 2020;19(5):383–4. https://doi.org/10.1016/S1474-4422(20)30109-5.

84. Filosto M, Piccinelli SC, Gazzina S, Foresti C, Frigeni B, Servalli MC, Sessa M, et al. Guillain-Barré syndrome and COVID-19: an observational multicentre study from two Italian hotspot regions. J Neurol Neurosurg Psychiatry. 2020;92(7):751–6. https://doi.org/10.1136/jnnp-2020-324837.
85. Fragiel M, Miró Ò, Llorens P, Jiménez S, Piñera P, Burillo G, Martín A, et al. Incidence, clinical, risk factors and outcomes of Guillain-Barré in Covid-19. Ann Neurol. 2021;89(3):598–603. https://doi.org/10.1002/ana.25987.
86. Sansone P, Giaccari LG, Aurilio C, Coppolino F, Esposito V, Fiore M, Paladini A, Passavanti MB, Pota V, Pace MC. Post-infectious Guillain–Barré syndrome related to Sars-Cov-2 infection: a systematic review. Life (Basel). 2021;11(2):167. https://doi.org/10.3390/life11020167.
87. Zuberbühler P, Conti ME, Cejas LL, González FM, Bonardo P, Miquelini A, Halfon J, Martínez J, Gutiérrez MV, Reisin RC. Síndrome de Guillain-Barré Asociado a Infección Por COVID-19: Revisión de Casos Publicados. Rev Neurol. 2021;72(06):203. https://doi.org/10.33588/rn.7206.2020487.
88. Sriwastava S, Kataria S, Tandon M, Patel J, Patel R, Jowkar A, Daimee M, Bernitsas E, Jaiswal P, Lisak RP. Guillain Barré syndrome and its variants as a manifestation of COVID-19: a systemic review of case report and case series. J Neurol Sci. 2021;420:117263. https://doi.org/10.1016/j.jns.2020.117263.
89. Umapathi T, Er B, Koh JS, Goh YH, Chua L. Guillain-Barré syndrome decreases in Singapore during the COVID-19 pandemic. J Peripher Nerv Syst. 2021;26(2):235–6. https://doi.org/10.1111/jns.12439.
90. Keddie S, Pakpoor J, Mousele C, Pipis M, Machado PM, Foster M, Record CJ, et al. Epidemiological and cohort study finds no association between COVID-19 and Guillain-Barré syndrome. Brain. 2021;144(2):682–93. https://doi.org/10.1093/brain/awaa433.
91. Madia F, Merico B, Primiano G, Cutuli SL, De Pascale G, Servidei S. Acute Myopathic quadriplegia in patients with COVID-19 in the intensive care unit. Neurology. 2020;95(11):492–4. https://doi.org/10.1212/WNL.0000000000010280.
92. Nasuelli NA, Pettinaroli R, Godi L, Savoini C, De Marchi F, Mazzini L, Crimaldi F, Pagni A, Pompa CP, Colombo D. Critical illness neuro-myopathy (CINM) and focal Amyotrophy in intensive Care unit (ICU) patients with SARS-CoV-2: a case series. Neurol Sci. 2021;42(3):1119–21. https://doi.org/10.1007/s10072-020-04820-9.
93. McClafferty B, Umer I, Fye G, Kepko D, Kalayanamitra R, Shahid Z, Ramgobin D, et al. Approach to critical illness myopathy and polyneuropathy in the older SARS-CoV-2 patients. J Clin Neurosci. 2020;79:241–5. https://doi.org/10.1016/j.jocn.2020.07.058.
94. Shepherd S, Batra A, Lerner DP. Review of critical illness myopathy and neuropathy. Neurohospitalist. 2017;7(1):41–8. https://doi.org/10.1177/1941874416663279.
95. Dalakas MC. Guillain-Barré Syndrome: the first documented COVID-19-triggered autoimmune neurologic disease: more to come with myositis in the offing. Neurol Neuroimmunol Neuroinflamm. 2020a;7(5):e781. https://doi.org/10.1212/NXI.0000000000000781.
96. Dalakas MC. Inflammatory myopathies: update on diagnosis, pathogenesis and therapies, and COVID-19-related implications. Acta Myol. 2020b;39(4):289–301. https://doi.org/10.36185/2532-1900-032.
97. Paliwal VK, Garg RK, Gupta A, Tejan N. Neuromuscular presentations in patients with COVID-19. Neurol Sci. 2020;41(11):3039–56. https://doi.org/10.1007/s10072-020-04708-8.
98. Sacchi MC, Tamiazzo S, Lauritano EC, Bonometti R. Case report of COVID-19 in an elderly patient: could SARS-CoV2 trigger myositis? Eur Rev Med Pharmacol Sci. 2020;24(22):11960–3. https://doi.org/10.26355/eurrev_202011_23857.
99. Zhang H, Charmchi Z, Seidman RJ, Anziska Y, Velayudhan V, Perk J. COVID-19–associated myositis with severe proximal and bulbar weakness. Muscle Nerve. 2020;62(3):E57–60. https://doi.org/10.1002/mus.27003.
100. Assini A, Gandoglia I, Damato V, Rikani K, Evoli A, Del Sette M. Myasthenia gravis associated with anti-MuSK antibodies developed after SARS-CoV-2 infection. Eur J Neurol. 2021;28(10):3537–9. https://doi.org/10.1111/ene.14721.

101. Restivo DA, Centonze D, Alesina A, Marchese-Ragona R. Myasthenia gravis associated with SARS-CoV-2 infection. Ann Intern Med. 2020;173(12):1027–8. https://doi.org/10.7326/L20-0845.
102. Sriwastava S, Tandon M, Kataria S, Daimee M, Sultan S. New onset of ocular myasthenia gravis in a patient with COVID-19: a novel case report and literature review. J Neurol. 2020;268(8):2690–6. https://doi.org/10.1007/s00415-020-10263-1.
103. Camelo-Filho AE, Silva AMS, Estephan EP, Zambon AA, Mendonça RH, Souza PVS, Wladimir B.V.R. Pinto, et al. Myasthenia gravis and COVID-19: clinical characteristics and outcomes. Front Neurol. 2020;11:1053. https://doi.org/10.3389/fneur.2020.01053.
104. Muppidi S, Guptill JT, Jacob S, Li Y, Farrugia ME, Guidon AC, Tavee JO, et al. COVID-19-associated risks and effects in myasthenia gravis (CARE-MG). Lancet Neurol. 2020;19(12):970–1. https://doi.org/10.1016/S1474-4422(20)30413-0.
105. Li Y, Li M, Wang M, Zhou Y, Chang J, Xian Y, Wang D, Mao L, Jin H, Bo H. Acute cerebrovascular disease following COVID-19: A single center, retrospective, observational study. Stroke Vasc Neurol. 2020b;5(3):279–84. https://doi.org/10.1136/svn-2020-000431.
106. Shahjouei S, Naderi S, Li J, Khan A, Chaudhary D, Farahmand G, Male S, et al. Risk of stroke in hospitalized SARS-CoV-2 infected patients: a multinational study. EBioMedicine. 2020;59:102939. https://doi.org/10.1016/j.ebiom.2020.102939.
107. Qureshi AI, Baskett WI, Huang W, Shyu D, Myers D, Raju M, Lobanova I, et al. Acute ischemic stroke and COVID-19: an analysis of 27 676 patients. Stroke. 2021;52(3):905–12. https://doi.org/10.1161/STROKEAHA.120.031786.
108. Syahrul S, Maliga HA, Ilmawan M, Fahriani M, Mamada SS, Fajar JK, Frediansyah A, et al. Hemorrhagic and ischemic stroke in patients with coronavirus disease 2019: incidence, risk factors, and pathogenesis - a systematic review and meta-analysis. F1000Res. 2021;10:34. https://doi.org/10.12688/f1000research.42308.1.
109. Alam S, Dharia RN, Miller E, Rincon F, Tzeng DL, Bell RD. Coronavirus positive patients presenting with stroke-like symptoms. J Stroke Cerebrovasc Dis. 2021;30(4):105588. https://doi.org/10.1016/j.jstrokecerebrovasdis.2020.105588.
110. Paterson RW, Brown RL, Benjamin L, Nortley R, Wiethoff S, Bharucha T, Jayaseelan DL, et al. The emerging spectrum of COVID-19 neurology: clinical, radiological and laboratory findings. Brain. 2020;143(10):3104–20. https://doi.org/10.1093/brain/awaa240.
111. Beyrouti R, Adams ME, Benjamin L, Cohen H, Farmer SF, Goh YY, Humphries F, et al. Characteristics of Ischaemic stroke associated with COVID-19. J Neurol Neurosurg Psychiatry. 2020;91(8):889–91. https://doi.org/10.1136/jnnp-2020-323586.
112. Katsanos AH, Palaiodimou L, Zand R, Yaghi S, Kamel H, Navi BB, Turc G, et al. The impact of SARS-CoV-2 on stroke epidemiology and care: a meta-analysis. Ann Neurol. 2021;89(2):380–8. https://doi.org/10.1002/ana.25967.
113. Cheruiyot I, Sehmi P, Ominde B, Bundi P, Mislani M, Ngure B, Olabu B, Ogeng'o JA. Intracranial hemorrhage in coronavirus disease 2019 (COVID-19) patients. Neurol Sci. 2021;42(1):25–33. https://doi.org/10.1007/s10072-020-04870-z.
114. Altschul DJ, Unda SR, de La Garza Ramos R, Zampolin R, Benton J, Holland R, Fortunel A, Haranhalli N. Hemorrhagic presentations of COVID-19: risk factors for mortality. Clin Neurol Neurosurg. 2020;198(November):106112. https://doi.org/10.1016/j.clineuro.2020.106112.
115. Melmed KR, Cao M, Dogra S, Zhang R, Yaghi S, Lewis A, Jain R, et al. Risk factors for intracerebral hemorrhage in patients with COVID-19. J Thromb Thrombolysis. 2020;51(4):953–60. https://doi.org/10.1007/s11239-020-02288-0.
116. Masur J, Freeman CW, Mohan S. A double-edged sword: neurologic complications and mortality in extracorporeal membrane oxygenation therapy for COVID-19-related severe acute respiratory distress syndrome at a tertiary care center. Am J Neuroradiol. 2020;41(11):2009–11. https://doi.org/10.3174/ajnr.A6728.
117. Radmanesh A, Raz E, Zan E, Derman A, Kaminetzky M. Brain imaging utilization and findings in COVID-19: a single academic center experience in the epicenter of disease in the United States. Am J Neuroradiol. 2020;41(7):1179–83. https://doi.org/10.3174/AJNR.A6610.

118. Lang CN, Dettinger JS, Berchtold-Herz M, Utzolino S, Bemtgen X, Zotzmann V, Schmid B, et al. Intracerebral hemorrhage in COVID-19 patients with pulmonary failure: A propensity score-matched registry study. Neurocrit Care. 2021;34(3):739–47. https://doi.org/10.1007/s12028-021-01202-7.
119. Baldini T, Asioli GM, Romoli M, Dias MC, Schulte EC, Hauer L, De Sousa DA, Sellner J, Zini A. Cerebral venous thrombosis and severe acute respiratory syndrome Coronavirus-2 infection: a systematic review and meta-analysis. Eur J Neurol. 2021;28(10):3478–90. https://doi.org/10.1111/ene.14727.
120. Mowla A, Shakibajahromi B, Shahjouei S, Borhani-Haghighi A, Rahimian N, Baharvahdat H, Naderi S, et al. Cerebral venous sinus thrombosis associated with SARS-CoV-2; a multinational case series. J Neurol Sci. 2020;419:117183. https://doi.org/10.1016/j.jns.2020.117183.
121. Ostovan VR, Foroughi R, Rostami M, Almasi-Dooghaee M, Esmaili M, Bidaki AA, Behzadi Z, et al. Cerebral venous sinus thrombosis associated with COVID-19: a case series and literature review. J Neurol. 2021;268(10):3549–60. https://doi.org/10.1007/s00415-021-10450-8.
122. Ciccone A, Zanotti B. The importance of recognizing cerebral venous thrombosis following anti-COVID-19 vaccination. Eur J Intern Med. 2021;89:115–7. https://doi.org/10.1016/j.ejim.2021.05.006.
123. Hanafi R, Roger PA, Perin B, Kuchcinski G, Deleval N, Dallery F, Michel D, et al. COVID-19 neurologic complication with CNS vasculitis-like pattern. Am J Neuroradiol. 2020;41(8):1384–7. https://doi.org/10.3174/ajnr.A6651.
124. Lersy F, Anheim M, Willaume T, Chammas A, Brisset JC, Cotton F, Kremer S. Cerebral vasculitis of medium-sized vessels as a possible mechanism of brain damage in COVID-19 patients. J Neuroradiol. 2020;48(3):141–6. https://doi.org/10.1016/j.neurad.2020.11.004.
125. Elkhider H, Ibrahim F, Sharma R, Sheng S, Jasti M, Lotia M, Kapoor N, et al. COVID-19 and stroke, a case series and review of literature. Brain Behav Immun Health. 2020;9:100172. https://doi.org/10.1016/j.bbih.2020.100172.
126. Jain R, Young M, Dogra S, Kennedy H, Nguyen V, Jones S, Bilaloglu S, et al. COVID-19 related neuroimaging findings: A signal of thromboembolic complications and a strong prognostic marker of poor patient outcome. J Neurol Sci. 2020;414:116923. https://doi.org/10.1016/j.jns.2020.116923.
127. Khedr EM, Soliman RK, Abo-Elfetof N, Amin M, Mansour OY, Aly A, Zaki AF, Saber M. Clinical and radiological characteristics of acute cerebrovascular diseases among Egyptian patients with COVID-19 in upper Egypt. Front Neurol. 2021;12:635856. https://doi.org/10.3389/fneur.2021.635856.
128. Flores G, Kumar JI, Pressman E, Sack J, Alikhani P. Spontaneous brainstem hemorrhagic stroke in the setting of novel coronavirus disease 2019 - A case report. Cureus. 2020;12(10):e10809. https://doi.org/10.7759/cureus.10809.
129. Khan F, Sharma N, Ud Din M, Chetram R. Diagnostic and therapeutic challenges of cerebral venous thrombosis in SARS-CoV-2 infection: a case report and review of literature. Clin Pract. 2021;11(3):598–606. https://doi.org/10.3390/clinpract11030075.
130. Maas MB. Critical medical illness and the nervous system. Continuum (Minneap Minn). 2020;26(3):675–94. https://doi.org/10.1212/CON.0000000000000869.
131. Manzano GS, McEntire C, Martinez-Lage M, Mateen FJ, Hutto SK. Acute disseminated encephalomyelitis and acute hemorrhagic leukoencephalitis following COVID-19: systematic review and meta-synthesis. Neurol Neuroimmunol Neuroinflamm. 2021;8(6):e1080. https://doi.org/10.1212/NXI.0000000000001080.
132. Durrani M, Kucharski K, Smith Z, Fien S. Acute transverse myelitis secondary to severe acute respiratory syndrome coronavirus 2 (SARS-CoV-2): a case report. Clinical Pract Cases Emerg Med. 2020;4(3):344–8. https://doi.org/10.5811/cpcem.2020.6.48462.
133. Chan JL, Ebadi H, Sarna JR. Guillain-Barré syndrome with facial diplegia related to SARS-CoV-2 infection. J Can Sci Neurol. 2020;47(6):852–4. https://doi.org/10.1017/cjn.2020.106.
134. Kaur H, Mason JA, Bajracharya M, McGee J, Gunderson MD, Hart BL, Dehority W, et al. Transverse myelitis in a child with COVID-19. Pediatr Neurol. 2020;112(November):5–6. https://doi.org/10.1016/j.pediatrneurol.2020.07.017.

135. Munz M, Wessendorf S, Koretsis G, Tewald F, Baegi R, Krämer S, Geissler M, Reinhard M. Acute transverse myelitis after COVID-19 pneumonia. J Neurol. 2020;267(8):2196–7. https://doi.org/10.1007/s00415-020-09934-w.
136. Abu-Rumeileh S, Abdelhak A, Foschi M, Tumani H, Otto M. Guillain–Barré syndrome spectrum associated with COVID-19: an up-to-date systematic review of 73 cases. J Neurol. 2021;268(4):1133–70. https://doi.org/10.1007/s00415-020-10124-x.
137. Watrin L, Ghawché F, Larre P, Neau JP, Mathis S, Fournier E. Guillain-Barré syndrome (42 cases) occurring during a Zika virus outbreak in French Polynesia. Medicine (United States). 2016;95(14):e3257. https://doi.org/10.1097/MD.0000000000003257.
138. Aragão MFVV, Leal MC, Cartaxo Filho OQ, Fonseca TM, Valença MM. Anosmia in COVID-19 associated with injury to the olfactory bulbs evident on MRI. Am J Neuroradiol. 2020;41(9):1703–6. https://doi.org/10.3174/ajnr.A6675.
139. Klironomos S, Tzortzakakis A, Kits A, Öhberg C, Kollia E, Ahoromazdae A, Almqvist H, et al. Nervous system involvement in coronavirus disease 2019: results from a retrospective consecutive neuroimaging cohort. Radiology. 2020;297(3):E324–34. https://doi.org/10.1148/radiol.2020202791.
140. Moonis G, Filippi CG, Kirsch CFE, Mohan S, Stein EG, Hirsch JA, Mahajan A. The spectrum of neuroimaging findings on CT and MRI in adults with coronavirus disease (COVID-19). AJR Am J Roentgenol. 2020;217(4):959–74. https://doi.org/10.2214/ajr.20.24839.
141. Shor N, Chougar L, Pyatigorskaya N. MR imaging of the olfactory bulbs in patients with COVID-19 and anosmia: how to avoid misinterpretation. Am J Neuroradiol. 2021;42(3):E10–1. https://doi.org/10.3174/ajnr.a6921.
142. Chung MS, Choi WR, Jeong HY, Lee JH, Kim JH. MR imaging-based evaluations of olfactory bulb atrophy in patients with olfactory dysfunction. Am J Neuroradiol. 2018;39(3):532–7. https://doi.org/10.3174/ajnr.A5491.
143. Lu Y, Li X, Geng D, Mei N, Wu PY, Huang CC, Jia T, et al. Cerebral micro-structural changes in COVID-19 patients – an MRI-based 3-month follow-up study: A brief title: cerebral changes in COVID-19. EClinicalMedicine. 2020;25:100484. https://doi.org/10.1016/j.eclinm.2020.100484.
144. Guedj E, Campion JY, Dudouet P, Kaphan E, Bregeon F, Tissot-Dupont H, Guis S, et al. 18F-FDG brain PET hypometabolism in patients with long COVID. Eur J Nucl Med Mol Imaging. 2021;48(9):2823–33. https://doi.org/10.1007/s00259-021-05215-4.
145. Sollini M, Morbelli S, Ciccarelli M, Cecconi M, Aghemo A, Morelli P, Chiola S, Gelardi F, Chiti A. Long COVID hallmarks on [18F]FDG-PET/CT: a case-control study. Eur J Nucl Med Mol Imaging. 2021;48(10):3187–97. https://doi.org/10.1007/s00259-021-05294-3.
146. Donegani MI, Miceli A, Pardini M, Bauckneht M, Chiola S, Pennone M, Marini C, et al. Brain metabolic correlates of persistent olfactory dysfunction after SARS-Cov2 infection. Biomedicine. 2021;9(3):287. https://doi.org/10.3390/biomedicines9030287.
147. Leonardi M, Padovani A, McArthur JC. Neurological manifestations associated with COVID-19: A review and a call for action. J Neurol. 2020;267(6):1573–6. https://doi.org/10.1007/s00415-020-09896-z.
148. Román GC, Spencer PS, Reis J, Buguet A, Faris MEA, Katrak SM, Láinez M, et al. The neurology of COVID-19 revisited: A proposal from the environmental neurology specialty group of the World Federation of Neurology to Implement International Neurological Registries. J Neurol Sci. 2020;414:116884. https://doi.org/10.1016/j.jns.2020.116884.
149. Winkler AS, Knauss S, Schmutzhard E, Leonardi M, Padovani A, Abd-Allah F, Charway-Felli A, et al. A call for a global COVID-19 neuro research coalition. Lancet Neurol. 2020;19(6):482–4. https://doi.org/10.1016/S1474-4422(20)30150-2.
150. NYU Langone Health. 2021. https://med.nyu.edu/departments-institutes/population-health/divisions-sections-centers/biostatistics/research/neuro-databank-biobank.
151. ENERGY. 2020. https://www.ean.org/research/ean-neuro-covid-registry-energy.

152. CoroNerve. 2020. https://www.coronerve.com/#/.
153. PHOSP-COVID. 2020. https://www.phosp.org/.
154. NIH.2021.https://www.nih.gov/about-nih/who-we-are/nih-director/statements/nih-launches-new-initiative-study-long-covid.
155. The Lancet Neurology. Long COVID: understanding the neurological effects. Lancet Neurol. 2021;20(4):247. https://doi.org/10.1016/S1474-4422(21)00059-4.

# Chapter 19
# The Impact of COVID-19 on Surgical Disease

**Ali Elsaadi, Milos Buhavac, and Brittany K. Bankhead**

## COVID-19-Induced Hypercoagulability

The pro-inflammatory state due to COVID-19 causes immune-mediated thrombosis similar to that of sepsis. The hypoxic state associated with COVID-19 also causes transcription of hypoxia inducible factor which further activates platelets and plasma coagulation [1]. While these complications are more likely to be seen in the pulmonary circulation, other organs such as the kidney and spleen have also been affected by this pro-thrombotic state.

Examples of this hypercoagulability and its effect on surgical patients can be seen in numerous case reports published throughout the pandemic. One case report by Xu et al. describes a kidney-pancreas transplant recipient who developed an infarction in his transplanted kidney [2]. The patient received prophylactic anticoagulation during his hospitalization for COVID-19, which was discontinued upon discharge. Eight days after his discharge, he returned with left lower quadrant pain and was subsequently found to have a cortical hypodensity on imaging consistent with an infarction of the lower pole of the kidney [2]. In another case series by Dakay et al., three patients at their institution were found to have cerebral venous sinus thrombosis with concurrent COVID-19 infection. These patients had no obvious risk factors for a hypercoagulable state or cerebral venous sinus thrombosis [3]. One large study done by Goldberg-Stein et al. looked at CT scans of the abdomen and pelvis in 141 COVID positive patients. Of these 141 patients, 25 (17.7%) had a GI tract abnormality, and 14 (9.9%) had solid organ infarction or vascular thromboses. Of these 14 events, 4 were splenic infarcts, 4 were renal infarcts, 3 were deep

A. Elsaadi · M. Buhavac · B. K. Bankhead (✉)
Department of Surgery, Texas Tech University Health Sciences Center, Lubbock, TX, USA
e-mail: Ali.elsaadi@ttuhsc.edu; Milos.Buhavac@ttuhsc.edu; brittany.k.bankhead@ttuhsc.edu



S. Adibi et al. (eds.), *Frontiers of COVID-19*,
https://doi.org/10.1007/978-3-031-08045-6_19

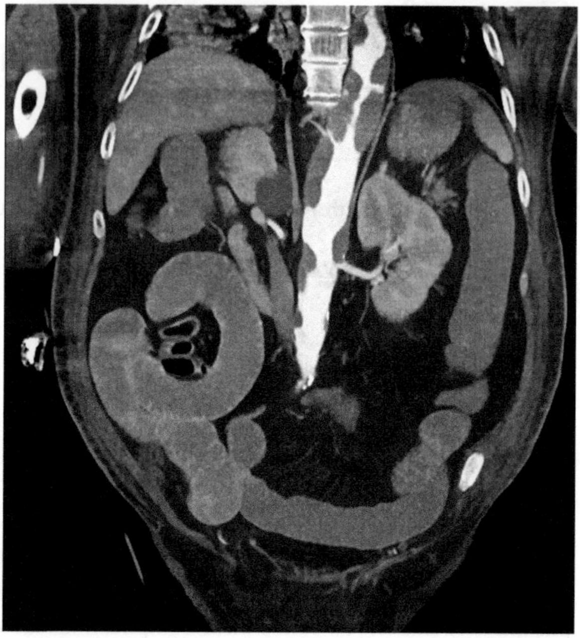

**Fig. 19.1** CT scan demonstrating severe aortic thrombosis in COVID patient. (de Roquetaillade C, Chousterman BG, Tomasoni D, Zeitouni M, Houdart E, Guedon A, Reiner P, Bordier R, Ga-yat E, Montalescot G, Metra M, Mebazaa A. Unusual arteri-al thrombotic events in Covid-19 patients. Int J Cardiol. 2021 Jan 15;323:281–284. https://doi.org/10.1016/j.ijcard.2020.08.103. Epub 2020 Sep 10. PMID: 32918938; PMCID: PMC7481127)

vein thromboses, and 3 peripheral-arterial occlusions [4]. In another study by de Roquetaillade et al., 20/209 (9.6%) of patients admitted with severe COVID-19 developed an acute thromboembolic event. These included 3 splenic infarcts, 9 coronary occlusions, 6 strokes, 3 ischemic limbs, and 2 aortic thromboses including 1 death (Fig. 19.1) [5].

To date, no data is available concerning sequelae of splenic infarcts in COVID patients such as rate of pseudoaneurysm formation, abscess, or need for surgery.

Intestinal malperfusion has been identified as another potential harmful byproduct of COVID-19 infection. In one case report by Azouz et al. a patient who initially presented with a stroke secondary to COVID developed abdominal pain 1 day later. CT angiography showed a free-floating thrombus within the aorta, as well as occlusion of the superior mesenteric artery, leading to intestinal ischemia [6]. In a larger study done by Etkin et al. looking at 43 COVID patients that developed thromboembolic disease, 2 of 43 had intestinal ischemia [7]. A single center study by Bellosta et al. suggests a solution to this issue. In their study, 17/20 patients with acute limb ischemia due to COVID underwent revascularization, of which 12 were successful. Patients with successful revascularization procedures were routinely on postoperative therapeutic heparin (0 vs 57%, $p = 0.042$). This suggests that therapeutic perioperative anticoagulation utilizing heparin may improve morbidity and mortality as well as increase the chances of limb salvage in COVID-19-induced acute limb ischemia [8].

## COVID-19-Induced Gastrointestinal Pathology

One prevailing theory for the mechanism behind digestive system involvement in COVID-19 suggests angiotensin converting enzyme 2 receptor, which the virus attaches to so it can infect cells, is expressed highly in the gastrointestinal (GI) system [9]. In a meta-analysis comprised of 29 studies performed by Mao et al. 15% of patients with COVID-19 had evidence of GI dysfunction. The most common symptoms were nausea/vomiting, diarrhea, or loss of appetite. A further 12 studies consisting of 1267 patients showed 19% of study patients had an abnormal elevation in liver function enzymes Interestingly, patients with GI involvement had a delay in diagnosis and a poorer disease course with an odd's ratio of 2.96 and 95% confidence interval of [1.17–7.48] [10].

Digestive surgical complications in COVID-19 patients also include intestinal perforation. In one case reported by De Nardi et al., a patient developed an intestinal perforation 14 days after the onset of symptoms which started February 17th, 2020. On day 5 of their hospitalization, the patient developed diarrhea and subsequent abdominal pain. Computed tomography (CT) scans done at that time showed large amounts of free air and the patient was emergently taken to the operating room. The intra-operative findings included profuse amount of free air, distension of the entire abdominal colon, and a minimal perforation on the anterolateral aspect. Neither obstruction of the distal colon nor distension of the small intestine was noted. A right colectomy with ileo-transverse anastomosis was performed [11]. Another case report from September of 2020 details a spontaneous rectal perforation in a patient with COVID-19. In this case, the patient presented to the emergency room (ER) mildly hypotensive with a distended abdomen, Blumberg's sign and a positive COVID-19 polymerase chain reaction (PCR). CT scan done showed perivisceral air indicative of a rectal perforation. In the discussion of this case, the predilection of COVID-19 for gastrointestinal angiotensin converting enzyme-2 receptor along with its propensity for causing thrombosis was the proposed causes for the perforation [12]. COVID-19-induced fistulas have also been seen and these sequelae can occur months after the initial infection. In one case report by Abbassi et al. a patient with COVID pneumonia 2 months prior presented to the hospital with a subacute obstruction and failure to thrive. Subsequent push enteroscopy revealed multiple jejuno-jejunal fistulas as well as a diffuse ulceration. On laparotomy, the patient was found to have a previous jejunal perforation which was the likely culprit for their issues [13].

## Tracheostomy in the COVID-19 Era

Tracheostomy placement has been identified as a high-risk procedure for providers and staff due to periprocedural aerosolization of viral particles. Aerosol-generating procedures were identified as a leading cause of viral transmission during the severe acute respiratory syndrome outbreak in 2003, with super-spreading events occurring throughout hospitals in Hong Kong, China, and Canada [14]. Patients with COVID-19 are sometimes on a ventilator for a disproportionally longer period of time before undergoing tracheostomy placement. Early in the pandemic, one guideline in the American Journal of Otolaryngology suggested a 21 day wait after intubation [15]. This may be due to the early high fraction of inspired oxygen (FiO2) requirements COVID-19 patients are having, making them poor candidates for an airway exchange, in addition to theoretical decreased viral load after a more extended period of time [15]. Another shift seen in tracheostomy placement practices involves the operating room. Due to the high-risk nature of this aerosolizing procedure, personnel had to be restricted. Current recommendations are to limit the number of providers and staff in the room to the bare minimum required to safely do a procedure or operation. While this varies among cases and patient acuity, this will usually consist of an attending and one senior resident or assistant, along with necessary nursing and anesthesia personnel. Only the anesthesia team should be in the room during intubation [14, 15].

## Impact on Elective and Non-Urgent Surgery

Due to initial shortage of personal protective equipment (PPE), many centers cancelled elective cases and only allowed emergent and urgent surgeries to take place. Naturally, certain subspecialties were hit harder than others. In one study by Bregman et al. looking at plastic surgery case volume, it was estimated that 286,327 cases and 1.2 billion dollars will be lost due to the pandemic (Fig. 19.2) [16].

These estimates were based on 94 days of shutting down elective practice with regard to the top 5 esthetic procedures performed by plastic surgeons. Unfortunately, these numbers may grossly underestimate the true financial impact experienced by this subspecialty.

Another subspecialty suffering financial losses during the pandemic included bariatric surgery. A study by Beglaibter et al. showed that of 53 bariatric surgeons in the country, 86% of them in the public sector had ceased to operate [17] due to mandates by the government. Of the surgeons who did still operate, cases would still be cancelled citing patients with pulmonary issues or those living in communities heavily affected by COVID-19 as the reason why [18]. In a larger survey of 169 bariatric surgeons, most preferred to postpone pre-operative endoscopies, defer postoperative visits to video chats and telemedicine, and others cancelled the procedure entirely [18].

Some subspecialties, including cardiac surgery, converted to staffing intensive care units. In a paper by Fudulu and Angelini, these authors discuss how some colleagues have taken on roles as critical care nurses or other intensive care unit positions that were needed. Often the only cardiac surgeries that were permissible

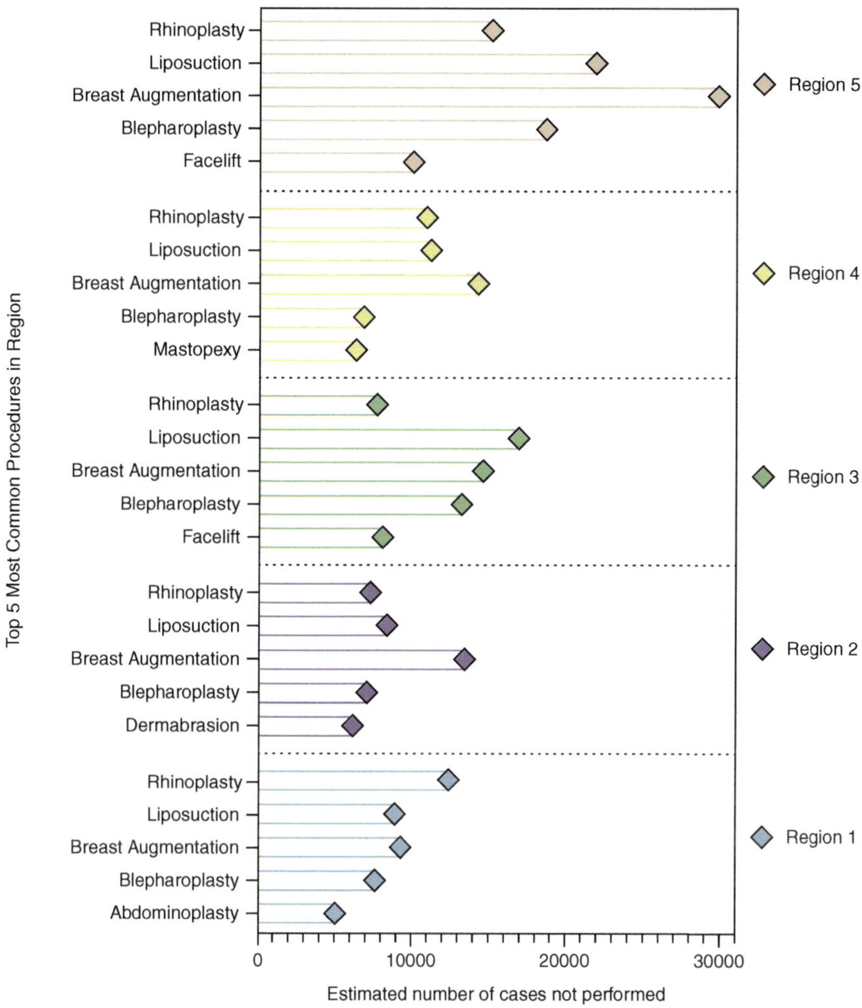


**Fig. 19.2** Regional estimates for lost case volume for the top five most common procedures if restrictions on cases extended from 3/19/20 to predicted date (94 days later) when invasive ventilation required for <0.5 patients. (Bregman DE, Cook T, Thorne C. Estimated National and Regional Impact of COVID-19 on Elective Case Volume in Aesthetic Plastic Surgery. Aesthet Surg J. 2021 Feb 12;41(3):358–369. https://doi.org/10.1093/asj/sjaa225. PMID: 32729892; PMCID: PMC7454284)

during the pandemic included aortic dissections, coronary bypass for vessel disease not amenable to percutaneous intervention, and valve surgery not amenable to transcatheter aortic valve replacement [19]. It was predicted that 28,404,603 operations would be cancelled or postponed during the 12-week peak of COVID-19. In the ensuing months, it was estimated this would require a 20% increase of operations for 45 weeks to make up for these missed cases (Fig. 19.3) [20].

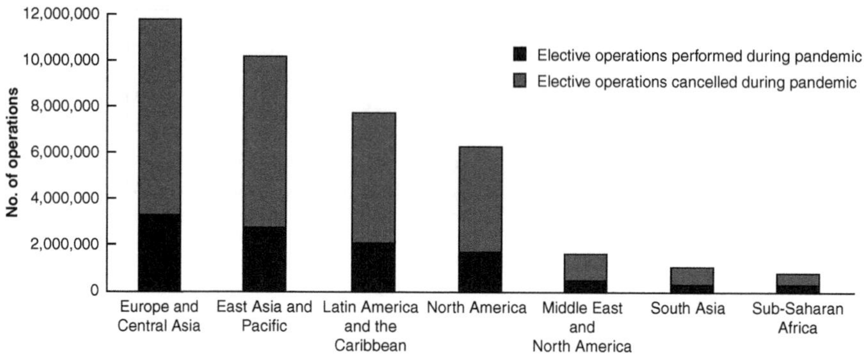


**Fig. 19.3** Best estimates for number of elective operations cancelled during the peak 12 weeks of disruption due to COVID-19, by geographical region. (COVIDSurg Collaborative. Elective surgery cancellations due to the COVID-19 pandemic: global predictive modelling to inform surgical recovery plans. Br J Surg. 2020 Oct;107(11):1440–1449. https://doi.org/10.1002/bjs.11746. Epub 2020 Jun 13. PMID: 32395848; PMCID: PMC7272903)

## Impact on Trauma/Acute Care Surgery

Of all the surgical subspecialties, the trauma and critical care team were involved in the care and management of COVID-19 patients the most. Due to their expertise in managing critically ill patients, they were often expected to continue with emergent general surgery cases in addition to managing and staffing COVID-19 patients in the surgical and medical intensive care units. Interestingly, even emergency services declined in the wake of the initial COVID-19 surge. A large study from Australia by Jacob et al. looked at trauma admissions during one of the peaks of COVID-19 (March/April 2020) and compared it to those same months from the prior 4 years. They found that there was a 23–34% decrease in the mean monthly average trauma admissions during March/April 2020 compared with previous 4 years. In addition, there was a 40–52% decrease and 13–29% decrease in admissions due to road traffic collisions and falls, respectively [21].

Another larger study by Berg et al. found similar results. Looking at 12,395 trauma patients across 88 centers during the first 5 months of 2020 compared to 2019, it was determined that trauma admissions decreased overall. Motor vehicle collision numbers decreased (1249 to 628), while penetrating trauma increased by 2.7% at a p value of 0.001, blunt trauma decreased by 3.1%, and head-injured patients presented with more severe traumatic brain injury based on injury severity score [22].

Penetrating trauma and traumatic brain injury trends were also demonstrated in a paper by Sherman et al. Looking at the US trauma registry from 2017 to 2019, 532 trauma activations were predicted to occur during the pandemic period from March 14th to May 14th 2020 based on linear trends. The actual number was only 372. There were also fewer blunt vs penetrating traumas, less motor vehicle collisions, and a higher number of gunshot wounds [23].

## Delays in Care Due to COVID-19

As hospitals became filled with patients afflicted with COVID, patients became more wary of going to a physician for regularly scheduled visits or minor concerns, including reductions in preventative screening—such as colonoscopy for colorectal cancers and mammograms for breast cancer. The UK national cancer screening programs—accounting for approximately 5% of all cancer diagnoses in the UK each year—further contributed to this reduction in screening [24]. While patients would still present for alarming symptoms such as rectal bleeding, vague cancer symptoms such as fatigue would go without a checkup because of the fear of contracting COVID-19 [24]. A study by Maringe et al. estimated the possible effects of this on breast, colorectal, lung, and esophageal cancer in the UK. After looking at over 90,000 patients with these cancers, they determined there would be a 7.9–9.6%, a 15.3–16.6%, 4.8–5.3%, and a 5.8–6.0% increase in deaths due to each of these tumors, respectively. This corresponds to over 3000 deaths in total attributable to delay in diagnosis [25].

Due to shortage in personal protective equipment, decreased hospital beds, and ventilators, non-emergent surgeries were delayed. Along with these factors, surgical oncologists have dealt with delays in diagnosis of cancer patients. The domino effect of this is that cancer surgeries were being postponed. This led to a set of recommendations for the delay of surgery by The Society of Surgical Oncology [26].

Hepatobiliary cancers with an indication for surgery followed by systemic chemotherapy would now be treated with neoadjuvant chemotherapy until the patient was no longer responding to therapy or was unable to tolerate the side effects. Breast cancer recommendations included delaying surgery for at least 3 months for atypia, prophylactic/risk-reducing surgery, reconstruction, and benign breast disease. In colorectal cancer, surgery was recommended to be postponed for all cancers in polyps, or otherwise early-stage disease [26].

With these delays, there was naturally an increase in mortality and morbidity for these patients. In a study by Larson and colleagues, the effects of a 3-month postponement of surgery for colon cancer were studied on 5-year survival. They found that patients who underwent surgery 1 month after diagnosis had a 25% mortality, while patients who underwent surgery at 4 months had a 37% mortality. In 2020, it was expected that there would be about 104,610 new cases of colon cancer in the USA. Using the estimates from earlier, this would amount to 30,965 deaths if delays of 4 or more months occur (Fig. 19.4) [27].

This effect carried over to other cancers as well. In a study by Mayne and colleagues, delays in surgery for certain stages of non-small cell lung cancer (IA2-IB adenocarcinoma and IB squamous cell carcinoma) led to an increase in mortality ($p$ value <0.004) [28].

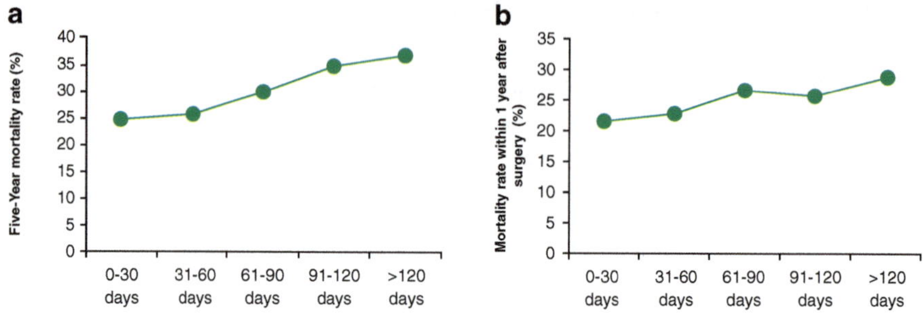


| | 0-30 days | 31-60 days | 61-90 days | 91-120 days | >120 days |
|---|---|---|---|---|---|
| **Dead** | 19,437 | 8458 | 1881 | 633 | 528 |
| **Alive** | 57,336 | 23,875 | 4281 | 1160 | 915 |
| **Total** | 76,773 | 32,333 | 6162 | 1739 | 1443 |
| **Exp.deaths[c]** | 20,922 | 25,106 | 25,106 | 29,290 | 30,965 |

| | 0-30 days | 31-60 days | 61-90 days | 91-120 days | >120 days |
|---|---|---|---|---|---|
| **<1 year[a]** | 4332 | 1947 | 509 | 164 | 155 |
| **>1 year[b]** | 15,105 | 6511 | 1372 | 469 | 373 |
| **Total** | 19,437 | 8458 | 1881 | 633 | 528 |
| **Exp.deaths[c]** | 4787 | 5005 | 5875 | 5657 | 6310 |

**Fig. 19.4** Risk of death within 5 years (**a**) and 1 year (**b**) after surgery according to the duration of the delay from diagnosis to surgery. Exp = expected. [a]Death within 1 year after surgery. [b]Death more than 1 year after surgery (the percentage presented is the number of deaths within 1 year divided by the number of deaths within 5 years). [c]The expected number of deaths according to the duration of delay between the diagnosis and surgery. The estimated total number of cases of stage I to III colon cancer in 2020 is 83,688 patients.[3] Of these patients, based on our previous study's results, 21,759 deaths (26%) would be expected within a 5-year follow-up. To calculate the predicted number of deaths for each delay in surgery period category, the assumption was given that all patients will have the surgery within this period of time (delay), and the estimated number of deaths was calculated based on the results (percentages) as shown in the figure. (Larson DW, Abd El Aziz MA, Mandrekar JN. How Many Lives Will Delay of Colon Cancer Surgery Cost During the COVID-19 Pandemic? An Analysis Based on the US National Cancer Database. Mayo Clin Proc. 2020 Aug;95(8):1805–1807. https://doi.org/10.1016/j.mayocp.2020.06.006. Epub 2020 Jun 15. PMID: 32753157; PMCID: PMC7294269)

## Perioperative Effects of COVID-19

When it comes to perioperative risk, most studies arrived at the same conclusion. Being COVID-19 positive increases your perioperative risk. In an international, prospective cohort study performed by the COVIDSURG Collaborative, it was noted that risks of postoperative morbidity and mortality are greatest if patients are operated within 6 weeks of diagnosis of COVID-19 infection (Fig. 19.5) [29]. In a study by Karayiannis et al. these types of patients were looked at in the setting of trauma requiring surgery. They found that for 484 patients, 30-day mortality was 1.9% in the postoperative period if they were COVID-19 negative. In COVID-19 positive patients, of which there were 27, mortality was 14.8% [30]. In a larger study involving 1569 patients, Clements and colleagues reported similar findings. In this case, 68 patients were found to have COVID-19 in the postoperative/perioperative period and their survival rate was 67.6% vs 95.8% compared to those without COVID-19 [31]. Unsurprisingly there was an increase in pulmonary complications post-op as well in COVID-19 patients. In a study done by the COVIDSURG Collaborative, 1128 patients diagnosed with COVID-19 7 days before or within 30 days after surgery were evaluated for mortality and pulmonary complications

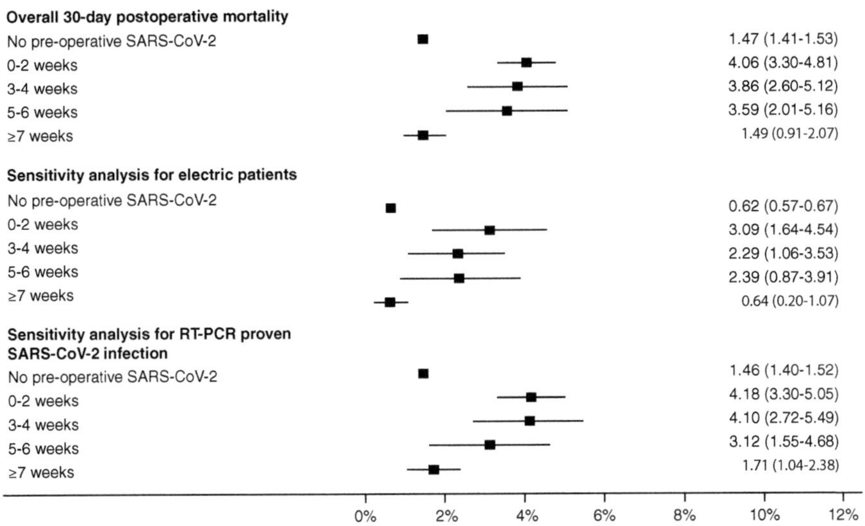


**Fig. 19.5** Overall adjusted 30-day postoperative mortality from main analysis and sensitivity analyses for patients having elective surgery and those patients with a reverse transcription polymerase chain reaction (RT-PCR) nasopharyngeal swab positive result for SARS-CoV-2. "No preoperative SARS-CoV-2" refers to patients without a diagnosis of SARS-CoV-2 infection. The time-periods relate to the timing of surgery following the diagnosis of SARS-CoV-2 infection. Sensitivity analysis for RT-PCR nasopharyngeal swab proven SARS-CoV-2 includes patients who either had RT-PCR nasopharyngeal swab proven SARS-CoV-2 or did not have a SARS-CoV-2 diagnosis. (COVIDSurg Collaborative; GlobalSurg Collaborative. Timing of surgery following SARS-CoV-2 infection: an international prospective cohort study. Anaesthesia. 2021 Jun;76(6):748–758. https://doi.org/10.1111/anae.15458. Epub 2021 Mar 9. PMID: 33690889; PMCID: PMC8206995)

from January first to March 31st of 2020. 30-day mortality was 23.8% (268 of 1128) and pulmonary complications occurred in 51.2% (577 of 1128) of patients (Fig. 19.5) [32].

While initial discussions between patient and surgeon may be to postpone surgery, this must be carefully balanced with the consequences of delaying care as outlined above.

## Future Considerations

Whether elective or emergent, COVID-19 has wide ranging implications for the practice of surgery. The various presentations including thrombotic events and gastrointestinal manifestations have added COVID-19 induced diseases to our differentials. If a patient previously had COVID-19, this now factors into determining their surgical risk due to the increase in perioperatively mortality with this virus. Delaying surgery due to this risk also has its own consequences and the backlog of cases accumulating from this may be something we can never overcome. While the strain on our healthcare system during this outbreak was evident, the sequelae of COVID-19 may present us with a whole new set of issues in the future.

## References


1. Schulman S. Coronavirus disease 2019, prothrombotic factors, and venous thromboembolism. Semin Thromb Hemost. 2020;46(7):772–6. https://doi.org/10.1055/s-0040-1710337; Epub 2020 May 11
2. Xu JJ, Samaha D, Mondhe S, Massicotte-Azarniouch D, Knoll G, Ruzicka M. Renal infarct in a COVID-19-positive kidney-pancreas transplant recipient. Am J Transplant. 2020;20(11):3221–4. https://doi.org/10.1111/ajt.16089; Epub 2020 Jun 24
3. Dakay K, Cooper J, Bloomfield J, Overby P, Mayer SA, Nuoman R, Sahni R, Gulko E, Kaur G, Santarelli J, Gandhi CD, Al-Mufti F. Cerebral venous sinus thrombosis in COVID-19 infection: a case series and review of the literature. J Stroke Cerebrovasc Dis. 2021;30(1):105434. https://doi.org/10.1016/j.jstrokecerebrovasdis.2020.105434; Epub 2020 Nov 6
4. Goldberg-Stein S, Fink A, Paroder V, Kobi M, Yee J, Chernyak V. Abdominopelvic CT findings in patients with novel coronavirus disease 2019 (COVID-19). Abdom Radiol (NY). 2020;45(9):2613–23. https://doi.org/10.1007/s00261-020-02669-2; Epub 2020 Aug 6
5. de Roquetaillade C, Chousterman BG, Tomasoni D, Zeitouni M, Houdart E, Guedon A, Reiner P, Bordier R, Gayat E, Montalescot G, Metra M, Mebazaa A. Unusual arterial thrombotic events in Covid-19 patients. Int J Cardiol. 2021;323:281–4. https://doi.org/10.1016/j.ijcard.2020.08.103; Epub 2020 Sep 10
6. Azouz E, Yang S, Monnier-Cholley L, Arrivé L. Systemic arterial thrombosis and acute mesenteric ischemia in a patient with COVID-19. Intensive Care Med. 2020;46(7):1464–5. https://doi.org/10.1007/s00134-020-06079-2; Epub 2020 May 18
7. Etkin Y, Conway AM, Silpe J, Qato K, Carroccio A, Manvar-Singh P, Giangola G, Deitch JS, Davila-Santini L, Schor JA, Singh K, Mussa FF, Landis GS. Acute arterial thromboembolism in patients with COVID-19 in the New York City area. Ann Vasc Surg. 2021;70:290–4. https://doi.org/10.1016/j.avsg.2020.08.085; Epub 2020 Aug 28
8. Bellosta R, Luzzani L, Natalini G, Pegorer MA, Attisani L, Cossu LG, Ferrandina C, Fossati A, Conti E, Bush RL, Piffaretti G. Acute limb ischemia in patients with COVID-19 pneumonia. J Vasc Surg. 2020;72(6):1864–72. https://doi.org/10.1016/j.jvs.2020.04.483; Epub 2020 Apr 29
9. Su S, Shen J, Zhu L, Qiu Y, He JS, Tan JY, Iacucci M, Ng SC, Ghosh S, Mao R, Liang J. Involvement of digestive system in COVID-19: manifestations, pathology, management and challenges. Ther Adv Gastroenterol. 2020 Jun;18(13):1756284820934626. https://doi.org/10.1177/1756284820934626.
10. Mao R, Qiu Y, He JS, Tan JY, Li XH, Liang J, Shen J, Zhu LR, Chen Y, Iacucci M, Ng SC, Ghosh S, Chen MH. Manifestations and prognosis of gastrointestinal and liver involvement in patients with COVID-19: a systematic review and meta-analysis. Lancet Gastroenterol Hepatol. 2020;5(7):667–78. https://doi.org/10.1016/S2468-1253(20)30126-6; Epub 2020 May 12. Erratum in: Lancet Gastroenterol Hepatol. 2020 Jul;5(7):e6
11. De Nardi P, Parolini DC, Ripa M, Racca S, Rosati R. Bowel perforation in a Covid-19 patient: case report. Int J Colorectal Dis. 2020;35(9):1797–800. https://doi.org/10.1007/s00384-020-03627-6; Epub 2020 May 27
12. Giuffrè M, Bozzato AM, Di Bella S, Occhipinti AA, Martingano P, Cavallaro MFM, Luzzati R, Monica F, Cova MA, Crocè LS. Spontaneous rectal perforation in a patient with SARS-CoV-2 infection. J Pers Med. 2020;10(4):157. https://doi.org/10.3390/jpm10040157.

13. Abbassi B, Deb A, Costilla V, Bankhead-Kendall B. Subacute enteritis two months after COVID-19 pneumonia with mucosal bleeding, perforation, and internal fistulas. Am Surg. 2021;1:31348211023461. https://doi.org/10.1177/00031348211023461; Epub ahead of print
14. McGrath BA, Brenner MJ, Warrillow SJ, Pandian V, Arora A, Cameron TS, Añon JM, Hernández Martínez G, Truog RD, Block SD, Lui GCY, McDonald C, Rassekh CH, Atkins J, Qiang L, Vergez S, Dulguerov P, Zenk J, Antonelli M, Pelosi P, Walsh BK, Ward E, Shang Y, Gasparini S, Donati A, Singer M, Openshaw PJM, Tolley N, Markel H, Feller-Kopman DJ. Tracheostomy in the COVID-19 era: global and multidisciplinary guidance. Lancet Respir Med. 2020;8(7):717–25. https://doi.org/10.1016/S2213-2600(20)30230-7; Epub 2020 May 15
15. Smith D, Montagne J, Raices M, Dietrich A, Bisso IC, Las Heras M, San Román JE, García Fornari G, Figari M. Tracheostomy in the intensive care unit: Guidelines during COVID-19 worldwide pandemic. Am J Otolaryngol. 2020;41(5):102578. https://doi.org/10.1016/j.amjoto.2020.102578; Epub 2020 Jun 1
16. Bregman DE, Cook T, Thorne C. Estimated national and regional impact of COVID-19 on elective case volume in aesthetic plastic surgery. Aesthet Surg J. 2021;41(3):358–69. https://doi.org/10.1093/asj/sjaa225.
17. Beglaibter N, Zelekha O, Keinan-Boker L, Sakran N, Mahajna A. Practices and attitudes of bariatric surgeons in Israel during the first phase of the COVID-19 pandemic. Isr J Health Policy Res. 2020;9(1):59. https://doi.org/10.1186/s13584-020-00420-2.
18. Lazaridis II, Kraljević M, Schneider R, Klasen JM, Schizas D, Peterli R, Kow L, Delko T, Collaborators. The impact of the COVID-19 pandemic on bariatric surgery: results from a worldwide survey. Obes Surg. 2020;30(11):4428–36. https://doi.org/10.1007/s11695-020-04830-8; Epub 2020 Jul 11
19. Fudulu DP, Angelini GD. Cardiac surgery in the time of the coronavirus. J Card Surg. 2020;35(6):1177–9. https://doi.org/10.1111/jocs.14580; Epub 2020 Apr 25
20. COVIDSurg Collaborative. Elective surgery cancellations due to the COVID-19 pandemic: global predictive modelling to inform surgical recovery plans. Br J Surg. 2020;107(11):1440–9. https://doi.org/10.1002/bjs.11746; Epub 2020 Jun 13
21. Jacob S, Mwagiru D, Thakur I, Moghadam A, Oh T, Hsu J. Impact of societal restrictions and lockdown on trauma admissions during the COVID-19 pandemic: a single-centre cross-sectional observational study. ANZ J Surg. 2020;90(11):2227–31. https://doi.org/10.1111/ans.16307; Epub 2020 Sep 29
22. Berg GM, Wyse RJ, Morse JL, Chipko J, Garland JM, Slivinski A, Lieser M, Biswas S, Carrick MM, Rhodes H, Acuna D, Watts DD, Wilson NY, Shen Y, Deas S, Fakhry SM. Decreased adult trauma admission volumes and changing injury patterns during the COVID-19 pandemic at 85 trauma centers in a multistate healthcare system. Trauma Surg Acute Care Open. 2021;6(1):e000642. https://doi.org/10.1136/tsaco-2020-000642.
23. Sherman WF, Khadra HS, Kale NN, Wu VJ, Gladden PB, Lee OC. How did the number and type of injuries in patients presenting to a regional level I trauma center change during the COVID-19 pandemic with a stay-at-home order? Clin Orthop Relat Res. 2021;479(2):266–75. https://doi.org/10.1097/CORR.0000000000001484.
24. Jones D, Neal RD, Duffy SRG, Scott SE, Whitaker KL, Brain K. Impact of the COVID-19 pandemic on the symptomatic diagnosis of cancer: the view from primary care. Lancet Oncol. 2020;21(6):748–50. https://doi.org/10.1016/S1470-2045(20)30242-4; Epub 2020 Apr 30
25. Maringe C, Spicer J, Morris M, Purushotham A, Nolte E, Sullivan R, Rachet B, Aggarwal A. The impact of the COVID-19 pandemic on cancer deaths due to delays in diagnosis in England, UK: a national, population-based, modelling study. Lancet Oncol. 2020;21(8):1023–34. https://doi.org/10.1016/S1470-2045(20)30388-0; Epub 2020 Jul 20. Erratum in: Lancet Oncol. 2021 Jan;22(1):e5
26. Bartlett DL, Howe JR, Chang G, Crago A, Hogg M, Karakousis G, Levine E, Maker A, Mamounas E, McGuire K, Merchant N, Shibata D, Sohn V, Solorzano C, Turaga K, White R, Yang A, Yoon S, Society of Surgical Oncology. Management of cancer surgery cases during

the COVID-19 pandemic: considerations. Ann Surg Oncol. 2020;27(6):1717–20. https://doi.org/10.1245/s10434-020-08461-2; Epub 2020 Apr 8
27. Larson DW, Abd El Aziz MA, Mandrekar JN. How many lives will delay of colon cancer surgery cost during the COVID-19 pandemic? An analysis based on the US National Cancer Database. Mayo Clin Proc. 2020;95(8):1805–7. https://doi.org/10.1016/j.mayocp.2020.06.006; Epub 2020 Jun 15
28. Mayne NR, Elser H, Darling AJ, Raman V, Liou D, Colson Y, D'Amico TA, Yang CJ. Estimating the impact of extended delay to surgery for stage I non-small-cell lung cancer on survival: lessons for the COVID-19 pandemic. Ann Surg. 2021;273(5):850–7. https://doi.org/10.1097/SLA.0000000000004811; Epub ahead of print
29. COVIDSurg Collaborative; GlobalSurg Collaborative. Timing of surgery following SARS-CoV-2 infection: an international prospective cohort study. Anaesthesia. 2021;76(6):748–58. https://doi.org/10.1111/anae.15458; Epub 2021 Mar 9
30. Karayiannis PN, Roberts V, Cassidy R, Mayne AIW, McAuley D, Milligan DJ, Diamond O. 30-day mortality following trauma and orthopaedic surgery during the peak of the COVID-19 pandemic: a multicentre regional analysis of 484 patients. Bone Jt Open. 2020;1(7):392–7. https://doi.org/10.1302/2633-1462.17.BJO-2020-0075.R1.
31. Clement ND, Hall AJ, Makaram NS, Robinson PG, Patton RFL, Moran M, Macpherson GJ, Duckworth AD, Jenkins PJ. IMPACT-restart: the influence of COVID-19 on postoperative mortality and risk factors associated with SARS-CoV-2 infection after orthopaedic and trauma surgery. Bone Joint J. 2020;102-B(12):1774–81. https://doi.org/10.1302/0301-620X.102B12.BJJ-2020-1395.R2; Epub 2020 Oct 21
32. COVIDSurg Collaborative. Mortality and pulmonary complications in patients undergoing surgery with perioperative SARS-CoV-2 infection: an international cohort study. Lancet. 2020;396(10243):27–38. https://doi.org/10.1016/S0140-6736(20)31182-X; Epub 2020 May 29. Erratum in: Lancet. 2020 Jun 9

# Part III
# Interventions and Treatments

# Chapter 20
# Pre-hospital Management of COVID-19: Looking for a Future Perspective

**Davide Salmi, Ingrid Andreea Ilie, Nadia Pagnoncelli, Greta Gandolfi, Marta Trucillo, Francesca Bertoldi, Luigino Ildebrando Manna, and Francesco Lanfranchi**

D. Salmi
Anesthesia and Intensive Care Unit, Biotechnology and Life Sciences Department, University of Insubria, Varese, Italy

I. A. Ilie
Department of Life Sciences and Biotechnology, School of Biology, University of Ferrara, Ferrara, Italy

N. Pagnoncelli
Psychiatry Unit, Department of Clinical and Experimental Sciences, University of Brescia, Brescia, Italy

G. Gandolfi
Anesthesia and Intensive Care Unit, Department of Clinical and Experimental Sciences, University of Brescia, Brescia, Italy

M. Trucillo
Department of Mental and Physical Health and Preventive Medicine, School of Medical Sciences, University of Campania Luigi Vanvitelli, Naples, Italy

F. Bertoldi · F. Lanfranchi (✉)
Department of Health Sciences (DISSAL), University of Genoa, Genoa, Italy
e-mail: flanfranchi@hotmail.com

L. I. Manna
General Practitioner, Brescia, Italy


S. Adibi et al. (eds.), *Frontiers of COVID-19*,
https://doi.org/10.1007/978-3-031-08045-6_20

## Introduction

After more than 1 year from the discovery of severe acute respiratory syndrome coronavirus-2 (SARS-CoV-2), it is still a major concern how to manage this pandemic without generating an important pressure on health care systems (HCSs). In fact, while findings about standardized in-hospital procedures are increasing, there is a lack of evidence about home care. Patients severely affected by novel coronavirus disease (COVID-19) need to receive proper treatment in hospital, but a different approach should be evaluated for categories at lower risk. Growing data about the multifaceted spectrum of long COVID syndrome [1, 2] lead to think at the pandemic as a long-term situation, imposing to look for sustainable future strategies. Numerous investigations illustrated the impact of the pandemic on health systems worldwide [3–7], highlighting the consequently reduced resources, drastic economic efforts, and increased discrepancies between country at different income levels. Moreover, several reports showed a decreasing number of hospital accesses and a rising severity presentation of patients affected by non-COVID acute emergencies, such as myocardial infarction [8, 9] and stroke [10–12].

Reducing pressures on HCSs is extremely important to guarantee a proper standard of care (SOC) for COVID-19 patients and for non-COVID ones, as well as for avoiding the concrete risk of health-workers burnout. The meta-analysis conducted by Phiri and co-authors [13] investigating health workers reported pooled prevalence of anxiety, depression, and post-traumatic stress disorder (PTSD) pair to 21.9% (95% CI, 18.7–25), to 23.4% (95% CI, 20.6–26.3), and to 25% (95% CI, 18.931.2), respectively. As observed in SARS and in Middle East respiratory syndrome (MERS) [14], persistent mental symptoms are common in COVID-19 patients after discharge [15–18] and their frequency resulted independent from the intensity of treatment received [16].

The aim of the present chapter (graphically summarized in Fig. 20.1) is to analyze data from meta-analyses or randomized clinical trials (RCTs) and to hypothesize their reproducibility in a pre-hospital setting according to the pathogenetic mechanisms of SARS-CoV-2 infection [19, 20].

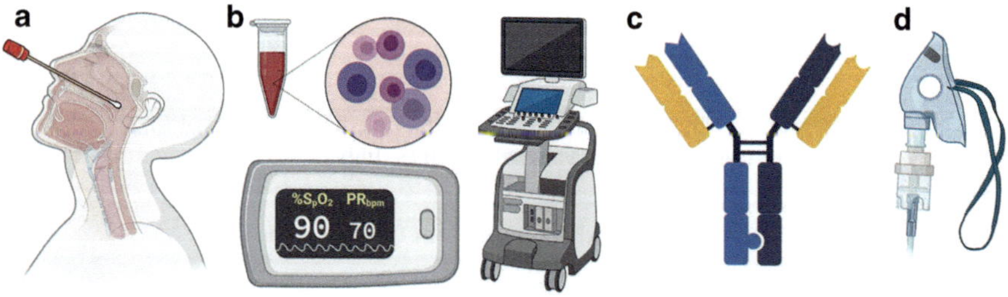


**Fig. 20.1** Graphical summary of pre-hospital interventions for COVID-19 patients' management. (**a**) Viral demonstration, (**b**) multidimensional assessment, (**c**) treatment, and (**d**) respiratory support. Created with BioRender.com

## SARS-CoV-2 Diagnosis

The certain diagnosis of SARS-CoV-2 infection is based on the demonstration of the causative pathogen in biological samples. Available techniques included naso-pharyngeal swab followed by viral ribonucleic acid (RNA) detection with real-time polymerase chain reaction (RT-PCR) or by identification of the spike protein; another option is to measure specific antibodies (Abs) serum levels.

The systematic review and meta-analysis conducted by Böger and co-authors [21], including sixteen studies for a cumulative number of 2297 patients, reported the sensitivity of RT-PCR methods in different biological samples. Namely, they found the following sensitivity values: 97.2% (95% CI: 90.3–99.7%) in sputum, 73.3% (95% CI: 68.1–78%) in nasopharyngeal aspirate or swab and throat swab, 62.3% (95% CI: 54.5–69.6%) in saliva, 24.1% (95% CI: 16.7–33.0%) in rectal stool or swab, 7.3% (95% CI: 4.1–11.7%) in plasma, and 0% (95% CI: 0.0–3.7%) in urine, respectively.

Pooled specificities and predictive were not estimated, because just two studies [22, 23] evaluated RT-PCR specificity in control groups, pair to 98.6% and 90% for throat swab and sputum samples, respectively, and to 100% when combined with the other samples. However, the best timing to perform RT-PCR and its effectiveness in pre-symptomatic patients are still unclear. The meta-analysis conducted by Mallett and colleagues [24] showed a high percentage of viral RNA detection from 0 to 4 days after clinical onset (Fig. 20.2). However, it is well known that the incubation time is very variable between different subjects, ranging from 4.5 to 6 days [25]. Identifying an optimal testing performance is complicated even more by the lack of standardized protocols for patients' recruitment and RT-PCR timing in different clinical trials [21].

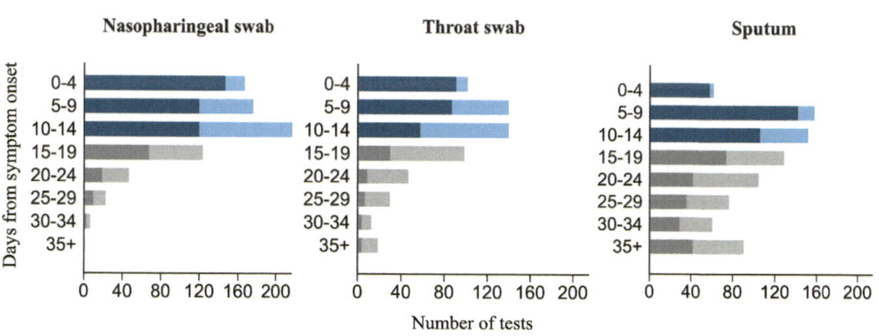


**Fig. 20.2** Number of positive and negative RT-PCR test results since symptom onset. Throat included throat and oropharyngeal. Each panel shows 5-day time periods since the onset of symptoms: 0–4 days, 5–9 days, 10–14 days, 15–19 days, 20–25 days, 26–30 days, 31–34 days, and 35 to max days. The number of positive RT-PCR tests is shown as dark blue bars and dark gray bars from 0 to 14 days and 15 to 40 days, respectively, and the number of negative RT-PCR results is shown similarly as light blue bars and light gray bars. Different colors are used before and after 15 days to indicate caution, as after 15 days testing is enriched in more severely ill participants. Figure and caption modified from Mallett et al. [24] and licensed under Creative Common License CC BY 4.0 (https://creativecommons.org/licenses/by/4.0/)

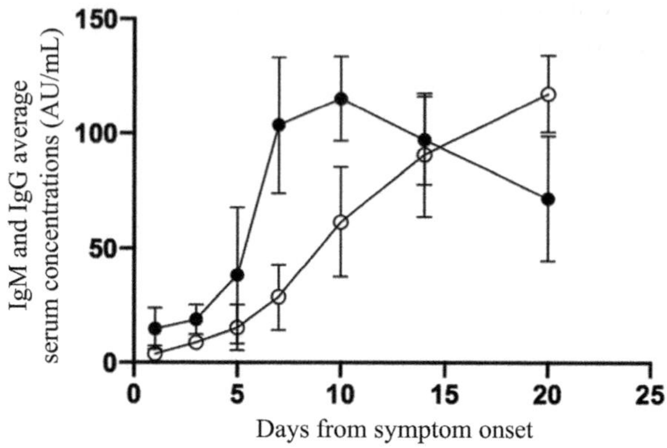


**Fig. 20.3** Kinetics of IgM (black) and IgG (white) antibodies against SARS-CoV-2 in continuously monitored patients with COVID-19 disease. Figure and caption modified from Qin et al. [29] and licensed under Creative Common License CC BY 4.0 (https://creativecommons.org/licenses/by/4.0/)

Meta-analysis data [26] reported extremely variable results about rapid antigen tests (RAT) accuracy, with sensitivity ranging from 28.9% (95% CI: 16.4–44.3%) and 98.3% (95% CI: 91.1–99.7%) and specificity from 92.4% (95% CI: 87.4–95.9%) and 100% (95% CI: 99.7–100%). However, RAT showed higher sensitivities when performed early after symptom onset [27] and it could be considered a potential useful method for pre-hospital assessment.

Abs sensitivity and specificity were higher when combining immunoglobulin of M and G type (IgM and IgG), reaching 84.5% (95% CI: 82.2–86.6%) and 91.6% (95% CI: 86–95.4%), respectively [21]. In the meta-analysis conducted by Zhang and colleagues [28], IgM and IgG showed pooled sensitivities of 74% (95% CI: 65–81%) and of 85% (95% CI: 79–90%), respectively, and pooled specificities of 99% (95% CI: 97–100%) and 99% (95% CI: 98–100%), respectively. However, the main limit of serological testing is the delay from symptom onset and Abs peak [29] (Fig. 20.3) and the consequent low-test accuracy in early stages (Lisboa [30]).

## Home Setting

Before evaluating the possibility to manage a COVID-19 patient at home, it is necessary to assess the domestic setting, considering even strict contacts. In accordance with the World Health Organization (WHO) recommendations [31], the home evaluation should be performed by a dedicated health worker. When suspecting a COVID-19 case, this figure should correctly and precisely instruct the household to perform correct hygiene measures [32, 33]. High-risk contacts should be isolated from the suspect or transferred to another location, with special regard to children.

Fever and flu-like symptoms should be frequently monitored [34]. Oxygenation could be easily determined by using pulse oximetry (PO), an effective method for the detection of hypoxic conditions [35] and for the evaluation of the risk of hospitalization [36]. Online free tools, such as the one provided by the Centers for Disease

Control and Prevention [37], could be helpful in clinical self-assessment. The most warning signs and symptoms are breathing difficulty, chest pain, confusion, motor impairment, and skin-color alteration. In these cases, patients should be informed about how to access hospital services [38].

## Multidimensional Assessment

### *Early Clinical Symptoms*

Between numerous clinical presentations associated with COVID-19 poor prognosis [39], only the most specific, independent, and typical ones were considered. Flu-like symptoms were of debatable value, considering their high frequency in COVID-19 [40]. According to the meta-analysis conducted by Li and co-authors [25], including 281,461 patients from 212 studies, acutely unmodifiable characteristics associated with disease severity appeared to be older age, male gender, and comorbidities, especially hypertension, diabetes, malignancies, and renal, pulmonary, or cardiac chronic affections. Comparing COVID-19 survivors with non-survivors, these differences were confirmed and resulted to be strongly associated with mortality.

The clinical presentations more frequently detected in severe COVID-19 compared to milder stages included chills, abdominal pain, and dizziness. Meta-regression results indicated abdominal pain as independently associated with disease severity. Even if it is difficult to find a rationale for this result, this finding was confirmed by a subsequent analogous work [41]. However, no presenting symptom seems to be associated with the mortality rate.

### *Laboratory Biomarkers*

PO is a bedside easily usable and cheap tool showing high prognostic value [35, 42], even in patients without clinical evidence of dyspnea and tachypnea [43].

According to the large study conducted by Li and colleagues [25], serum elevation of hepatic enzymes, urea, C reactive protein, and white blood cell and neutrophil counts resulted more frequent in severe patients; another remarkable feature was the reduction in circulating lymphocytes. However, meta-regression data confirmed only immunosuppression as associated with disease severity. Considering the mortality rate, these biochemical abnormalities were confirmed as independent predictors. In addition, the same study showed that raised levels of serum creatinine, lactate dehydrogenase, procalcitonin, and reduced concentrations of albumin were associated with a significantly higher risk of death.

Coagulation state is an early discovered [44] and well-known predictor of COVID-19 prognosis. Routine tests such as D-dimer levels [45, 46], fibrinogen concentrations [47], and platelet count alterations [48, 49] emerged as reliable prognostic indicators.

## *Imaging and Instrumental Tools*

Pulmonary involvement is a major criterion for bad prognosis [25] (Fig. 20.4). In fact, excluding systemic complications, pneumonia is the critical symptom occurring in severe disease stages [51]. According to systematic review and meta-analysis data [52], computed tomography (CT) imaging was the most sensitive and specific tool, showing values pair to 87.9% (95% CI: 84.6–90.6%) and to 80.0% (95% CI: 74.9–84.3%), respectively. Between the forty-one studies included for a cumulative number of 16,133 participants (with 8110 cases), only nine of them used specific staging scores, resulting in higher specificity values and in a parallel sensitivity decrease.

The analysis of nine studies about chest X-ray (CXR) (3694 participants with 2111 cases) and of five works regarding lung ultrasound (LUS) (211 cases between 446 participants) reported these methods being more sensitive (80.6%, 95% CI: 69.1–88.6% and 86.4%, 95% CI: 72.7–93.9%) than specific (71.5%, 95% CI: 59.8–80.8% and 54.6%, 95% CI: 35.3–72.6%). Assuming CT imaging as the gold standard, CXR appeared to be similar in both sensitivity and specificity [53], while LUS appeared comparable in sensitivity values [54]. Regarding the comparison between CXR and LUS, the first approach showed higher specificity, while the second one resulted in more sensitive [55]. According to Finance and co-authors [50], LUS was a valid tool for early diagnosis and outcome prediction (Fig. 20.5). Portable scanners could obtain similar results than the standard ones [56], leading to the necessity of further investigations focused on the effectiveness of bedside LUS.

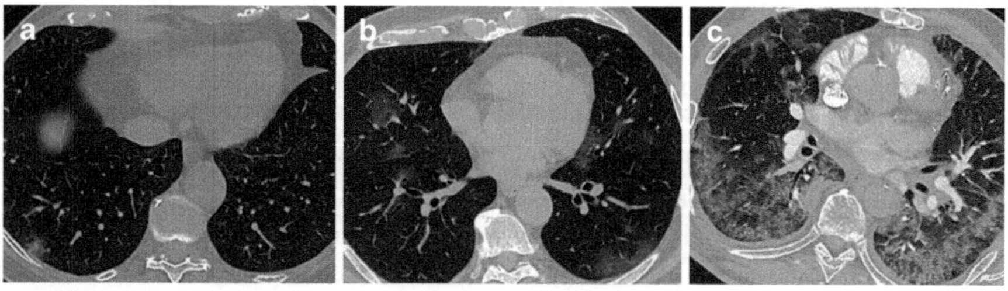


**Fig. 20.4** Low-dose non-contrast chest CT scans with 3D volumetric reconstruction in patients with proven COVID-19 infection. (**a**) Minimal lung involvement, (**b**) moderate lung involvement, and (**c**) severe lung involvement. (Figure and caption modified from Finance et al. [50] and licensed under Creative Common License CC BY 4.0 (https://creativecommons.org/licenses/by/4.0/))

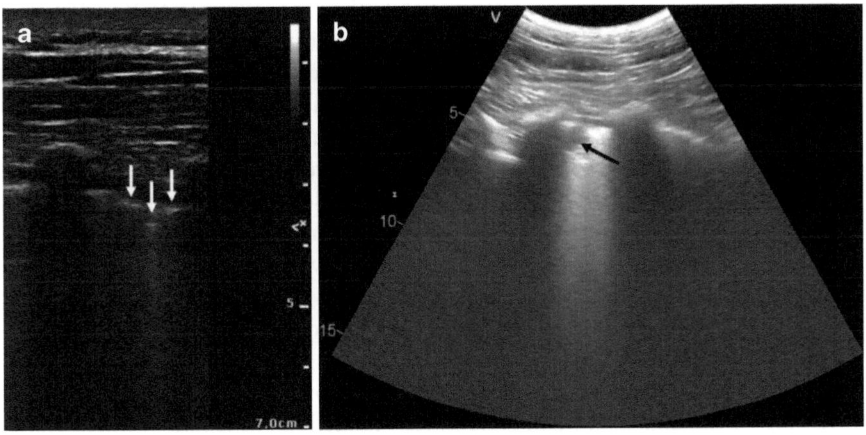


**Fig. 20.5** Lung ultrasound images in patients with proven COVID-19 infection. (**a**) Longitudinal scan with a high-frequency linear probe showing pleural line irregularities (white arrows). (**b**) Longitudinal scan with a low-frequency convex probe showing subpleural consolidation (black arrow). (Figure and caption modified from Finance et al. [50] and licensed under Creative Common License CC BY 4.0 (https://creativecommons.org/licenses/by/4.0/))

Beyond pulmonary assessment, portable ultrasound devices could be used for cardiac investigation [57], in order to identify heart comorbidities or complications independently suggestive for hospitalization [58]. In parallel, electrocardiography (EKG) should be easily performed in confirmed positive patients eligible for pharmacological treatment. In fact, several medications proposed as effective in COVID-19 could elongate QT interval. Even if subsequent findings led to reconsider the frequencies of drug-induced long-QT frequency [59, 60], it should be preferable to identify a baseline EKG reference.

## Pharmacological Interventions

In the present chapter, interventions easily available, cheap, safe, well-tolerated, and applicable at home were considered. Assuming that flu-like symptoms are not specific, their therapies were not discussed.

### *Monoclonal Antibodies*

Monoclonal antibodies (mAbs) resulted beneficial in non-hospitalized patients when administrated in the first days since symptom onset. Patients showed a faster reduction in the viral load and a lower rate of hospitalization and frequency of hospital accesses. However, data available are just provided by interim results concerning Sotrovimab [61], Bamlanivimab both in monotherapy [62] and in multidrug treatment [63], and the combination of Casirivimab and Imdevimab [64]. Among non-hospitalized patients with mild-to-moderate COVID-19, treatment with Bamlanivimab and Etesevimab was associated with a statistically significant reduction in SARS-CoV-2 viral load at day 11 when compared with placebo [63]. Bamlanivimab resulted effective in COVID-19 prevention after a follow-up of 8 weeks in exposed elderly [65]. However, this molecule could have reduced efficacy against some virus variants [66]. Regarding immunomodulatory antibodies, Tocilizumab appeared to be effective in association with SOC [67] in terms of mortality rate and discharging time (Fig. 20.6). This molecule appeared to reduce mechanical ventilation necessity and death [70, 71] in patients with pneumonia. The meta-analysis conducted by Tharmarajah and colleagues [72] concluded that interleukin-6 inhibition is associated with clinical improvement. However, other RCTs assessing Tocilizumab showed no significant reduction in the rate of intubation or death in patients with moderate or severe COVID-19 [73, 74]. For this reason, this molecule is recommended in addition with SOC just in severe or critical patients. Other immunomodulatory mAbs tested, such as Sarilumab [75] and Anakinra [76] did not show a beneficial effect.

To date, ongoing trial investigating mAbs did not report a strong rationale for a fast application in pre-symptomatic or very mild COVID-19 patients. Regarding the molecules demonstrated to be effective in early stages, currently available data are just provided by interim analysis, and it is necessary to wait for larger and definitive results.

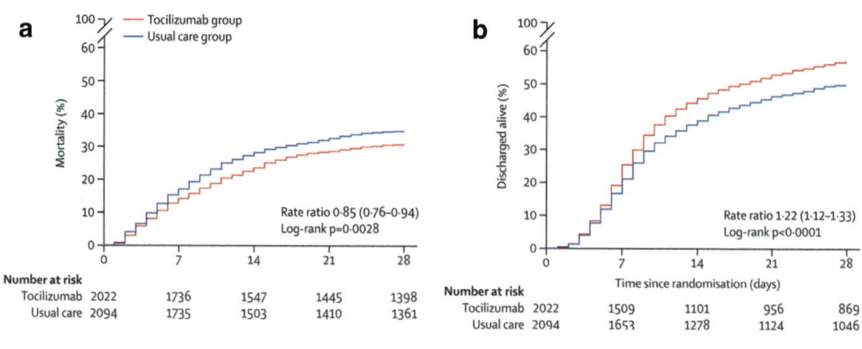


**Fig. 20.6** Effect of allocation to Tocilizumab on (**a**) 28-day mortality and (**b**) discharge from hospital within 28 days of randomization. (Figure and caption modified from The RECOVERY Collaborative Group [67] and licensed under Creative Common License CC BY 4.0 (https://creativecommons.org/licenses/by/4.0/))

## *Antiviral Agents*

The final report of the ACTT-1 study [77], including more than a thousand of hospitalized patients with evidence of lower respiratory tract infection, showed a reduction in recovery time in the intravenous Remdesivir harm. The same trial reported a lower rate of death (6.7% vs 11.9%), even if not statistically significant. Conversely, interim results from the WHO Solidarity Trial indicated no effectiveness on mortality and time to discharge [78], confirming previous data aimed to evaluate the clinical improvement rate [79] (Fig. 20.7a). In a big number of patients (1614 treated vs 3424 placebo), the combination of Lopinavir and Ritonavir did not show any efficacy neither in mortality (Fig. 20.7b), disease progression, and time to discharge [80], as previously detected in a smaller sample [81]. Favipiravir showed discordant benefits in studies investigating the viral shedding [82, 83]. Molnupiravir was announced as able to determine a faster RT-PCR negativity in two-hundred non-hospitalized patients [84], and its efficacy was demonstrated in pre-clinical studies [85, 86].

To date, antiviral agents assessed as a possible resource for SARS-CoV-2 treatment showed discordant proof of efficacy. Intravenous Remdesivir is not eligible for home administration and its effectiveness in early stages of disease remains unclear.

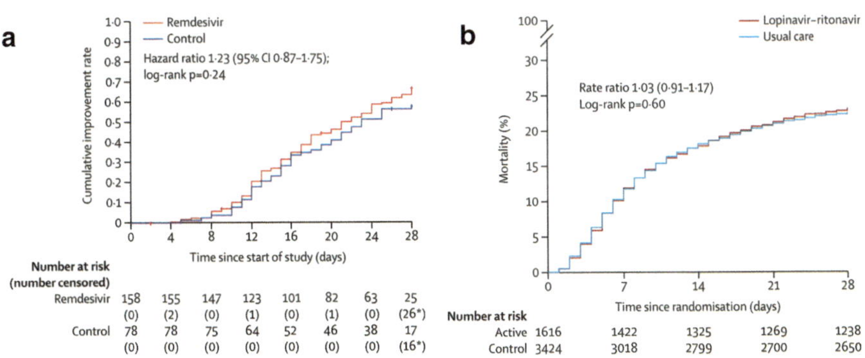


**Fig. 20.7** (**a**) Time to clinical improvement in the intention-to-treat population. Adjusted hazard ratio for randomization stratification was 1.25 (95% CI: 0.88–1.78). * Including deaths before day 28 as right censored at day 28, the number of patients without clinical improvement was still included in the number at risk. (**b**) Effect of allocation to Lopinavir-Ritonavir on 28-day mortality. (Figures and captions modified (**a**) from Wang et al. [79] and (**b**) from The RECOVERY Collaborative Group [80] and licensed under Creative Common License CC BY 4.0 (https://creativecommons.org/licenses/by/4.0/))

## *Corticosteroids*

Corticosteroids (CS), especially Dexamethasone, were tested in several RCTs, giving proof of high efficacy in patients with advanced pulmonary disease. The meta-analysis conducted by Pulakurthi and co-authors [87] confirmed that the rate of mortality and the necessity of mechanical ventilation were significantly lower in patients receiving CS when compared to SOC. No significant difference was detected regarding the frequency of adverse events and superinfections. However, no data justify an indiscriminate use of CS in COVID-19 patients, and this report is consistent with the pathogenesis of the viral infection itself. In fact, if Dexamethasone efficacy in critically ill patients requiring oxygen support was widely demonstrated [68, 88], its use in non-severe COVID-19 remains strongly not recommended [89].

The STOIC study [90] demonstrated a significant reduction in the number of hospital accesses and in clinical progression by early administration of inhaled Budesonide in adults with mild COVID-19. Inhaled CS are well-known, safe, and easily available and usable at home, making this result very interesting if confirmed in further larger studies.

## *Other Drugs*

Acetylsalicylic acid (ASA) was proposed as a possible therapy for COVID-19. A retrospective study [91] including 412 hospitalized patients reported lower rates of mechanical ventilation, admission to intensive care unit (ICU) and mortality in patients receiving ASA treatment. Conversely, the preprint paper from the RECOVERY Trial showed scarce benefits from ASA administration [69]. Thus, the role of ASA and the proper timing of its administration are still unclear.

Colchicine showed a decrease in the composite rate of hospitalization and death in treated outpatients compared to the placebo group in the COLCORONA trial [92], even if the difference is quite moderate (4.6% vs 6.0%). However, in the absence of pre-hospital SOC these results are not sufficient to confirm an effective role of Colchicine in COVID-19 therapy.

Most RCTs findings about hydroxychloroquine (HCQ), including the WHO Solidarity clinical trial for COVID-19 treatments [93], works conducted in mild patients [94] and in post-exposure subjects [95], did not find a significant positive effect. However, HCQ resulted effective against SARS-CoV-2 [96], and the very early administration of this drug in outpatients appeared to be associated with better outcomes in preliminary studies [97, 98]. This data suggested further prospective trials including subjects in very early phases of disease. In fact, if HCQ resulted ineffective in reducing the mortality rate [99, 100], it should be able to decrease the frequency of hospitalization [97]. Regarding safety and tolerability, the first evidence of higher HCQ-induced cardiac mortality was retracted [101], and subsequent findings about EKG alterations directly induced by the viral infection could lead to a re-evaluation of their frequency during HCQ therapy [59, 60].

The use of the antiparasitic agent Ivermectin was supported by pre-clinical results [102, 103] and limited findings in humans [104–106]. These benefits were not reported in mild COVID-19 patients recruited in a subsequent larger RCT [107], confirming results from Chaccour and colleagues [108]. Ivermectin showed a moderate effect on symptoms resolution and a discordant efficacy in duration of viral load and of positive RT-PCR testing [109].

The usefulness of antimicrobial therapy is a debated topic, especially because the definition of secondary bacterial infections in COVID-19 was not standardized between different studies [110]. In fact, the bacterial infection rate ranged from 6.9% [111] until 32% [112], with important differences depending on the stage of disease and the requirement of ventilation. Previous pre-clinical findings suggested antiviral and immunomodulatory effects of two antimicrobial molecules proposed in COVID-19 therapy, namely Azithromycin [113–117] and Doxycycline [118–121]. Both these molecules showed in vitro properties against SARS-CoV-2 [96, 122]. However, no clinical data supported their effectiveness in COVID-19 [123–125], even if their use in early phases of disease remains to be assessed.

It is clearly established that thromboembolic phenomena are as frequent as potentially severe in patients affected by SARS-CoV-2 [126–128]. Anticoagulation treatments showed benefits in hospitalized patients [129, 130], and the prophylactic dosage in non-severe stages of disease resulted effective and safe [130, 131]. Thus, in absence of contraindications, prophylactic heparin therapy should be tested in prospective clinical trial to be conducted in home settings.

Several vitamins and antioxidant agents were tested in addition to SOC, but results are discordant, and their real efficacy is still debated. RCTs about both vitamin C [132, 133] and vitamin D [134] showed no clinical benefits. Considering the differences in the SOCs they were addicted to, the discordant proof of effectiveness, the labile data about kinetics and bioavailability, and the not-specific mechanisms on which their action should be based on, it is not possible to express definitive conclusions about these molecules. However, the multifaceted benefits of vitamin and antioxidant supplements remain clear.

## Respiratory Support

Despite several proposed pathogenetic mechanism of SARS-CoV-2 infection, severe COVID-19 usually leads to atypical pneumonia [51]. Protocols for hypoxia treatment in COVID-19 patients are widely discussed, especially regarding the management of hospitalized patients in advanced stages of disease [135–140]. Conversely, data about hypoxia therapy and prevention are still lacking in outpatients, resulting in clinical-practice-based interventions more than in evidence-based ones.

## *Oxygen Therapy*

As summarized by Jiang and Wei [141], in-hospital ventilation options for COVID-19 pneumonia included oxygen nasal cannula and face mask oxygenation, high flow nasal oxygenation, non-invasive ventilation techniques (continuous positive airway pressure and helmet ventilation), and invasive mechanical ventilation. Between these procedures, just low-flow nasal cannula and mask oxygenation are applicable at home. However, no data driven SOC or guidelines about timing and duration of non-hospital oxygenation are available. For this reason, it could be useful to base the research on the different SARS-CoV-2 pulmonary damage mechanisms. In fact, as highlighted by Gattinoni and colleagues [142, 143], COVID-19 pneumonia could be classified in two main phenotypes (Fig. 20.8), namely L (type 1) and H (type 2). The first one occurred in early phases of disease with a relative higher frequency, and it showed a higher responsiveness to oxygen therapy. Increased fraction of inspired oxygen resulted quickly effective in early disease phases, with or without dyspnea. To reach this target, both nasal cannula and facial masks were easily usable at home. Aggressive ventilation approaches could be a concomitant cause of pulmonary damage [144] and they appeared to be linked to L-to-H phenotype shift [142], a pattern frequent in patients admitted to intensive care units (from 20% to 30%) and related to bad outcomes and to the need for SARS treatment. For this reason, when possible, it should be applied a gradual approach in patients requiring oxygen therapy, in order to minimize side effects and to avoid pulmonary stress.

Because of the lacking evidence about COVID-19 home ventilation, it is reasonable to evaluate procedures adopted for other pulmonary conditions such as chronic obstructive pulmonary disease (COPD). In fact, COPD is a well-known home-treated lung disorder, and its protocols could be effective for guiding other pulmonary conditions' management [145]. According to the 2020 Global

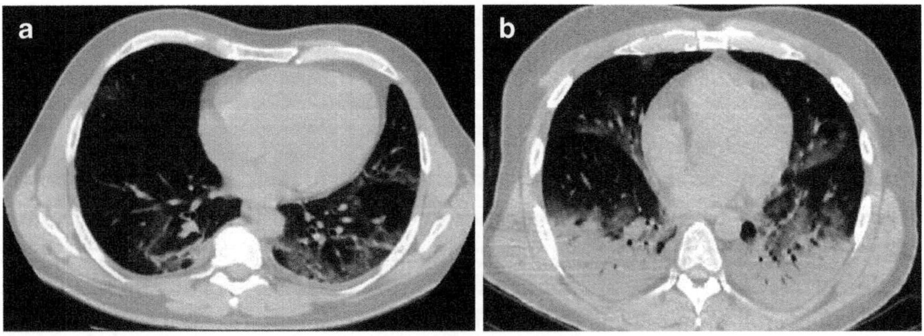


**Fig. 20.8** CT scans of (**a**) type 1 and (**b**) type 2 COVID-19 pneumonia. (Figure and caption modified from Gattinoni et al. [143] and licensed under Creative Common License CC BY 4.0 (https://creativecommons.org/licenses/by/4.0/))

Initiative for Chronic Obstructive Lung Diseases report [146], PO is a reliable marker of long-term oxygen therapy effectiveness. As well established for clinical monitoring of SARS-CoV-2 infection evolution, PO should be easily used even to guide the timing and the titration of oxygen support. Considering the availability and the effectiveness of these procedures, it is critically important to perform further trials to define peripheral oxygen targets specific for outpatients with COVID-19.

### *Prone Positioning and Pulmonary Rehabilitation*

As established by the PROSEVA study [147], prone positioning is a key feature in treatment of acute respiratory distress syndrome, and this finding was confirmed in several studies about COVID-19 respiratory syndrome [148–157]. Moreover, this intervention resulted effective and well-tolerated both in critically ill patients and in awake non-intubated ones [149]. Considering the benefits related to an early application of the prone positioning [147], it could be used in a home setting [152]. However, further studies are necessary to detect standardized interventions and their proper most effective timing of application [148, 149, 156, 157]. In parallel with in-hospital developed international guidelines [158] and ongoing RCTs such as the PRO-CARF trial [159], bedside clinical investigations should be performed to confirm prone positioning effectiveness in early phases of disease and to eventually standardize protocols.

The prevalence of respiratory sequelae in COVID-19 patients [2] is not surprising, considering data reported about SARS and MERS [14]. As expected, subjects recovering after hospitalization showed better respiratory outcomes when undergoing a pulmonary rehabilitation (PR) program [145, 160–163]. In some cases [164], the beneficial effect of PR resulted independent of the severity of the infection, suggesting this tool as potentially effective even in mild COVID-19. Despite the availability of guidelines and recommendations [145, 165], a SOC for bedside pulmonary rehabilitation is still missing. Thus, it is necessary to enlarge and to standardize home-based PR approaches, including telerehabilitation as proposed for COPD patients [166, 167].

## Future Perspectives

It is necessary to progressively shift COVID-19 patients management from hospital facilities to a pre-hospital or a home-based setting. Because of the lacking evidence about the effectiveness of outpatients' interventions, it is reasonable to focus our effort on the following pathogenetic knowledge. In fact, reliable results can be obtained only if adopting specific clinical, diagnostic, and therapeutic measures at the proper time. Retrospective studies could be of interest, but they are not sufficient [168], and prospective well-designed clinical trials are necessary.

Despite the daily large number of discharged or not hospitalized patients affected by COVID-19, data about standardized protocols dedicated to pre-hospital management are limited. Extensive international open-access data banks should be instituted and the realization of pre-hospital clinical prospective trials should be encouraged. An early routine and commonly shared approach is fundamental for dealing even with the wide spectrum of the long COVID syndrome. In fact, current evidence shows too many discrepancies in patients' baseline assessment and follow-up. This high heterogeneity does not allow the immediate possibility to organize multicenter interventions.

Furthermore, remote approaches should be enlarged and widely investigated in COVID-19 management. These techniques could improve the clinical assessment and follow-up of suspicious or confirmed patients, as well as the monitoring of treatment effectiveness and side effects.

Sharing the idea that "[…] preventing hospitalizations and the chronic sequelae of COVID-19 will not only save lives, but also will help restore medical systems and other institutions that are overburdened by the effects of the pandemic" [169], a global effort should be done as early as possible in order to restore the essential function of health care systems.

**Acknowledgments** All the authors are thankful to their teammates and collaborators. They also thank all health workers around the world who are dealing with this pandemic; all the authors express their deepest condolences and offer a heartfelt thanks to all colleagues fallen fighting against this invisible enemy, as well as to their families.

**Disclosure Statement** The authors declare no conflict of interests.

**Funding** This research received no external funding.

**Author Contributions** Conceptualization: DS, IAI, LIM, and FL; literature research, screening, and selection: DS, IAI, and NP; original draft preparation: DS, IAI, NP, and LIM; review: GG, MT, and FB; writing and editing: all authors.

All authors have read and approved the definitive version of the manuscript.

## References

1. Huang C, Huang L, Wang YY, Li X, Ren L, Xiaoying G, Kang L, et al. 6-month consequences of COVID-19 in patients discharged from hospital: a cohort study. Lancet. 2021;397(10270):220–32. https://doi.org/10.1016/S0140-6736(20)32656-8.
2. Olliaro PL. An integrated understanding of long-term sequelae after acute COVID-19. Lancet Respir Med. 2021;9(7):679–80. https://doi.org/10.1016/s2213-2600(21)00206-x.
3. Balser J, Ryu J, Hood M, Kaplan G, Perlin J, Siegel B. Care systems COVID-19 impact assessment: lessons learned and compelling needs. NAM Perspect. 2021;2021. https://doi.org/10.31478/202104d.

4. Blumenthal D, Fowler EJ, Abrams M, Collins SR. Covid-19 — implications for the health care system. N Engl J Med. 2020;383(15):1483–8. https://doi.org/10.1056/nejmsb2021088.
5. Kaye AD, Okeagu CN, Pham AD, Silva RA, Hurley JJ, Arron BL, Sarfraz N, et al. Economic impact of COVID-19 pandemic on healthcare facilities and systems: international perspectives. Best Pract Res Clin Anaesthesiol. 2020;35(3):293–306. https://doi.org/10.1016/j.bpa.2020.11.009.
6. Kuehn BM. Despite improvements, COVID-19's health care disruptions persist. JAMA. 2021;325(23):2335. https://doi.org/10.1001/jama.2021.9134.
7. Mercier G, Arquizan C, Roubille F. Understanding the effects of COVID-19 on health care and systems. Lancet Public Health. 2020;5(10):e524. https://doi.org/10.1016/S2468-2667(20)30213-9.
8. Pessoa-Amorim G, Camm CF, Gajendragadkar P, De Maria GL, Arsac C, Laroche C, Zamorano JL, et al. Admission of patients with STEMI since the outbreak of the COVID-19 pandemic: a survey by the European Society of Cardiology. Eur Heart J Qual Care Clin Outcomes. 2020;6(3):210–6. https://doi.org/10.1093/ehjqcco/qcaa046.
9. Primessnig U, Pieske BM, Sherif M. Increased mortality and worse cardiac outcome of acute myocardial infarction during the early COVID-19 pandemic. ESC Heart Fail. 2021;8(1):333–43. https://doi.org/10.1002/ehf2.13075.
10. Padmanabhan N, Natarajan I, Gunston R, Raseta M, Roffe C. Impact of COVID-19 on stroke admissions, treatments, and outcomes at a comprehensive stroke centre in the United Kingdom. Neurol Sci. 2021;42(1):15–20. https://doi.org/10.1007/s10072-020-04775-x.
11. Schirmer CM, Ringer AJ, Arthur AS, Binning MJ, Christopher Fox W, James RF, Levitt MR, et al. Delayed presentation of acute ischemic strokes during the COVID-19 crisis. J Neurointerv Surg. 2020;12(7):639–42. https://doi.org/10.1136/neurintsurg-2020-016299.
12. Wu Y, Chen F, Wang Z, Feng W, Liu Y, Wang Y, Song H. Reductions in hospital admissions and delays in acute stroke care during the pandemic of COVID-19. Front Neurol. 2020;11(November):584734. https://doi.org/10.3389/fneur.2020.584734.
13. Phiri P, Ramakrishnan R, Rathod S, Elliot K, Thayanandan T, Sandle N, Haque N, et al. An evaluation of the mental health impact of SARS-CoV-2 on patients, general public and healthcare professionals: a systematic review and meta-analysis. EClinicalMedicine. 2021;34:100806. https://doi.org/10.1016/j.eclinm.2021.100806.
14. Ahmed H, Patel K, Greenwood DC, Halpin S, Lewthwaite P, Salawu A, Eyre L, et al. Long-term clinical outcomes in survivors of Severe Acute Respiratory Syndrome (SARS) and Middle East Respiratory Syndrome (MERS) coronavirus outbreaks after hospitalisation or ICU admission: a systematic review and meta-analysis. J Rehabil Med. 2020;52(5):jrm00063. https://doi.org/10.2340/16501977-2694.
15. Mukaetova-Ladinska EB, Kronenberg G. Psychological and Neuropsychiatric Implications of COVID-19. Eur Arch Psychiatry Clin Neurosci. 2021;271(2):235–48. https://doi.org/10.1007/s00406-020-01210-2.
16. Naidu SB, Shah AJ, Saigal A, Smith C, Brill SE, Goldring J, Hurst JR, Jarvis H, Lipman M, Mandal S. The high mental health burden of 'Long COVID' and its association with on-going physical and respiratory symptoms in all adults discharged from hospital. Eur Respir J. 2021;57(6):2004364. https://doi.org/10.1183/13993003.04364-2020.
17. Sahoo S, Mehra A, Dua D, Suri V, Malhotra P, Yaddanapudi LN, Puri GD, Grover S. Psychological experience of patients admitted with SARS-CoV-2 infection. Asian J Psychiatr. 2020;54:102355. https://doi.org/10.1016/j.ajp.2020.102355.
18. Zandifar A, Badrfam R, Yazdani S, Seyed MA, Rahimi F, Ghasemi S, et al. Prevalence and severity of depression, anxiety, stress and perceived stress in hospitalized patients with COVID-19. J Diabetes Metab Disord. 2020;19:1431–8. https://doi.org/10.1007/s40200-020-00667-1/Published.
19. Cevik M, Kuppalli K, Kindrachuk J, Peiris M. Virology, transmission, and pathogenesis of SARS-CoV-2. BMJ. 2020;371:m3862. https://doi.org/10.1136/bmj.m3862.
20. Harrison AG, Lin T, Wang P. Mechanisms of SARS-CoV-2 transmission and pathogenesis. Trends Immunol. 2020;41(12):1100–15. https://doi.org/10.1016/j.it.2020.10.004.

21. Böger B, Fachi MM, Vilhena RO, Cobre AF, Tonin FS, Pontarolo R. Systematic review with meta-analysis of the accuracy of diagnostic tests for COVID-19. Am J Infect Control. 2021;49(1):21–9. https://doi.org/10.1016/j.ajic.2020.07.011.
22. Xie C, Jiang L, Huang G, Hong P, Gong B, Lin H, Ma S, et al. Comparison of different samples for 2019 novel coronavirus detection by nucleic acid amplification tests. Int J Infect Dis. 2020;93(April):264–7. https://doi.org/10.1016/j.ijid.2020.02.050.
23. Yu F, Yan L, Wang N, Yang S, Wang L, Tang Y, Gao G, et al. Quantitative detection and viral load analysis of SARS-CoV-2 in infected patients. Clin Infect Dis. 2020;71(15):793–8. https://doi.org/10.1093/cid/ciaa345.
24. Mallett S, Joy Allen A, Graziadio S, Taylor SA, Sakai NS, Green K, Suklan J, et al. At what times during infection is SARS-CoV-2 detectable and no longer detectable using RT-PCR-based tests? A systematic review of individual participant data. BMC Med. 2020;18(1):1–17. https://doi.org/10.1186/s12916-020-01810-8.
25. Li J, Huang DQ, Zou B, Yang H, Hui WZ, Rui F, Yee NTS, et al. Epidemiology of COVID-19: a systematic review and meta-analysis of clinical characteristics, risk factors, and outcomes. J Med Virol. 2021;93(3):1449–58. https://doi.org/10.1002/jmv.26424.
26. Hayer J, Kasapic D, Zemmrich C. Real-world clinical performance of commercial SARS-CoV-2 rapid antigen tests in suspected COVID-19: a systematic meta-analysis of available data as per November 20, 2020. Int J Infect Dis. 2021;108:592–602. https://doi.org/10.1016/j.ijid.2021.05.029.
27. Berger A, Nsoga MTN, Perez-Rodriguez FJ, Aad YA, Sattonnet-Roche P, Gayet-Ageron A, Jaksic C, et al. Diagnostic accuracy of two commercial SARSCoV- 2 antigen-detecting rapid tests at the point of care in community-based testing centers. PLoS One. 2021;16:e0248921. https://doi.org/10.1371/journal.pone.0248921.
28. Zhang ZL, Hou YL, Li DT, Li FZ. Diagnostic efficacy of anti-SARS-CoV-2 IgG/IgM test for COVID-19: a meta-analysis. J Med Virol. 2021;93(1):366–74. https://doi.org/10.1002/jmv.26211.
29. Qin X, Shen J, Dai E, Li H, Tang G, Zhang L, Hou X, et al. The seroprevalence and kinetics of IgM and IgG in the progression of COVID-19. BMC Immunol. 2021;22(1):1–7. https://doi.org/10.1186/s12865-021-00404-0.
30. Bastos L, Mayara GT, Abidi SK, Campbell JR, Haraoui LP, Johnston JC, Lan Z, et al. Diagnostic accuracy of serological tests for Covid-19: systematic review and meta-analysis. BMJ. 2020;370(July):2516. https://doi.org/10.1136/bmj.m2516.
31. WHO Interim Guidance. 2020. https://apps.who.int/iris/handle/10665/333782.
32. Donno DR, Grattagliano I, Rossi A, Aprile PL, Medea G, Lagolio E, Granata G, Petrosillo N, Cricelli C. How to treat COVID-19 patients at home in the Italian context: an expert opinion. Infect Dis Rep. 2021;13(1):251–8. https://doi.org/10.3390/idr13010028.
33. Luks AM, Swenson ER. Pulse oximetry for monitoring patients with COVID-19 at home potential pitfalls and practical guidance. Ann Am Thoracic Soc. 2020;17(9):1040–6. https://doi.org/10.1513/AnnalsATS.202005-418FR.
34. CDC Advice for Caregivers in Non-Healthcare Settings. 2021. https://www.cdc.gov/coronavirus/2019-ncov/if-you-are-sick/care-for-someone.html.
35. Jouffroy R, Jost D, Prunet B. Prehospital pulse oximetry: a red flag for early detection of silent hypoxemia in COVID-19 patients. Crit Care. 2020;24(1):313. https://doi.org/10.1186/s13054-020-03036-9.
36. Shah S, Majmudar K, Stein A, Gupta N, Suppes S, Karamanis M, Capannari J, Sethi S, Patte C. Novel use of home pulse oximetry monitoring in COVID-19 patients discharged from the emergency department identifies need for hospitalization. Acad Emerg Med. 2020;27(8):681–92. https://doi.org/10.1111/acem.14053.
37. CDC Self-Checker. 2021. https://www.cdc.gov/coronavirus/2019-ncov/symptoms-testing/symptoms.html.
38. NICE COVID-19 Rapid Guideline. 2021. https://www.nice.org.uk/guidance/ng191.
39. Izcovich A, Ragusa MA, Tortosa F, Marzio MAL, Agnoletti C, Bengolea A, Ceirano A, et al. Prognostic factors for severity and mortality in patients infected with COVID-19: a systematic review. PLoS One. 2020;15(11):e0241955. https://doi.org/10.1371/journal.pone.0241955.

40. Grant MC, Geoghegan L, Arbyn M, Mohammed Z, McGuinness L, Clarke EL, Wade RG. The prevalence of symptoms in 24,410 adults infected by the novel coronavirus (SARS-CoV-2; COVID-19): a systematic review and meta-analysis of 148 studies from 9 countries. PLoS One. 2020;15(6):e0234765. https://doi.org/10.1371/journal.pone.0234765.
41. He X, Cheng X, Feng X, Wan H, Chen S, Xiong M. Clinical symptom differences between mild and severe COVID-19 patients in China: a meta-analysis. Front Public Health. 2021;8:561264. https://doi.org/10.3389/fpubh.2020.561264.
42. Brouqui P, Amrane S, Million M, Cortaredona S, Parola P, Lagier JC, Raoult D. Asymptomatic hypoxia in COVID-19 is associated with poor outcome. Int J Infect Dis. 2021;102(January):233–8. https://doi.org/10.1016/j.ijid.2020.10.067.
43. Galwankar S, Paladino L, David G, Nanayakkara K, Somma S, Grover J, Stawicki S. Management algorithm for subclinical hypoxemia in coronavirus disease-2019 patients: intercepting the 'Silent Killer'. J Emerg Trauma Shock. 2020;13(2):110–3. https://doi.org/10.4103/JETS.JETS_72_20.
44. Arachchillage DRJ, Laffan M. Abnormal coagulation parameters are associated with poor prognosis in patients with novel coronavirus pneumonia. J Thromb Haemost. 2020;18(4):844–7. https://doi.org/10.1111/jth.14820.
45. Bansal A, Singh AD, Jain V, Aggarwal M, Gupta S, Padappayil RP, Nadeem M, et al. The association of D-dimers with mortality, intensive care unit admission or acute respiratory distress syndrome in patients hospitalized with coronavirus disease 2019 (COVID-19): a systematic review and meta-analysis. Heart Lung. 2021;50(1):9–12. https://doi.org/10.1016/j.hrtlng.2020.08.024.
46. Nugroho J, Wardhana A, Maghfirah I, Mulia EPB, Rachmi DA, Qurota M, A'yun, and Imanita Septianda. Relationship of D-dimer with severity and mortality in SARS-CoV-2 patients: a meta-analysis. Int J Lab Hematol. 2021a;43(1):110–5. https://doi.org/10.1111/ijlh.13336.
47. Nugroho J, Wardhana A, Mulia EP, Maghfirah I, Rachmi DA, A'Yun MQ, Septianda I. Elevated fibrinogen and fibrin degradation product are associated with poor outcome in COVID-19 patients: a meta-analysis. Clin Hemorheol Microcirc. 2021b;77(2):221–31. https://doi.org/10.3233/CH-200978.
48. Pranata R, Lim MA, Yonas E, Huang I, Nasution SA, Setiati S, Alwi I, Kuswardhani RAT. Thrombocytopenia as a prognostic marker in COVID-19 patients: diagnostic test accuracy meta-analysis. Epidemiol Infect. 2021;149:e40. https://doi.org/10.1017/S0950268821000236.
49. Zong X, Yajun G, Hongjian Y, Li Z, Wang Y. Thrombocytopenia is associated with Covid-19 severity and outcome: an updated meta-analysis of 5637 patients with multiple outcomes. Lab Med. 2021;52(1):10–5. https://doi.org/10.1093/LABMED/LMAA067.
50. Finance J, Zieleskewicz L, Habert P, Jacquier A, Parola P, Boussuges A, Bregeon F, Eldin C. Low dose chest CT and lung ultrasound for the diagnosis and management of COVID-19. J Clin Med. 2021;10(10):2196. https://doi.org/10.3390/jcm10102196.
51. Zhu N, Zhang D, Wang W, Li X, Yang B, Song J, Zhao X, et al. A novel coronavirus from patients with pneumonia in China, 2019. N Engl J Med. 2020;382(8):727–33. https://doi.org/10.1056/nejmoa2001017.
52. Islam N, Ebrahimzadeh S, Salameh J-P, Kazi S, Fabiano N, Lee T, Absi M, et al. Thoracic imaging tests for the diagnosis of COVID-19. Cochrane Database Syst Rev. 2021;3(3):CD013639. https://doi.org/10.1002/14651858.CD013639.pub4.
53. Borakati A, Perera A, Johnson J, Sood T. Diagnostic accuracy of X-ray versus CT in COVID-19: a propensity-matched database study. BMJ Open. 2020;10:42946. https://doi.org/10.1136/bmjopen-2020-042946.
54. Narinx N, Smismans A, Symons R, Frans J, Demeyere A, Gillis M. Feasibility of using point-of-care lung ultrasound for early triage of COVID-19 patients in the emergency room. Emerg Radiol. 2020;27(6):663–70. https://doi.org/10.1007/s10140-020-01849-3.
55. Pare JR, Camelo I, Mayo KC, Leo MM, Dugas JN, Nelson KP, Baker WE, Shareef F, Mitchell PM, Schechter-Perkins EM. Point-of-care lung ultrasound is more sensitive than chest radiograph for evaluation of COVID-19. West J Emerg Med. 2020;21(4):771–8. https://doi.org/10.5811/westjem.2020.5.47743.

56. Bennett D, De Vita E, Mezzasalma F, Lanzarone N, Cameli P, Bianchi F, Perillo F, et al. Portable pocket-sized ultrasound scanner for the evaluation of lung involvement in coronavirus disease 2019 patients. Ultrasound Med Biol. 2021;47(1):19–24. https://doi.org/10.1016/j.ultrasmedbio.2020.09.014.
57. Khanji MY, Ricci F, Patel RS, Chahal AA, Bhattacharyya S, Galusko V, Narula J, Ionescu A. Special article - the role of hand-held ultrasound for cardiopulmonary assessment during a pandemic. Prog Cardiovasc Dis. 2020;63(5):690–5. https://doi.org/10.1016/j.pcad.2020.07.003.
58. O'Hearn M, Liu J, Cudhea F, Micha R, Mozaffarian D. Coronavirus disease 2019 hospitalizations attributable to cardiometabolic conditions in the United States: a comparative risk assessment analysis. J Am Heart Assoc. 2021;10(5):1–27. https://doi.org/10.1161/JAHA.120.019259.
59. Anupama BK, Adhikari S, Chaudhuri D. Prolonged QT interval in a patient with coronavirus Disease-2019: beyond hydroxychloroquine and azithromycin. J Investig Med High Impact Case Rep. 2020;8:2324709620948407. https://doi.org/10.1177/2324709620948407.
60. Bessière F, Roccia H, Delinière A, Charrière R, Chevalier P, Argaud L, Cour M. Assessment of QT intervals in a case series of patients with coronavirus disease 2019 (COVID-19) infection treated with hydroxychloroquine alone or in combination with azithromycin in an intensive care unit. JAMA Cardiol. 2020;5(9):1067. https://doi.org/10.1001/jamacardio.2020.1787.
61. GSK Press Releases. 2021. https://www.gsk.com/en-gb/media/press-releases/gsk-and-vir-biotechnology-announce-submission-of-emergency-use-authorization-request-to-fda-for-vir-7831-for-the-early-treatment-of-covid-19/.
62. Chen P, Nirula A, Heller B, Gottlieb RL, Boscia J, Morris J, Huhn G, et al. SARS-CoV-2 neutralizing antibody LY-CoV555 in outpatients with Covid-19. N Engl J Med. 2021;384(3):229–37. https://doi.org/10.1056/nejmoa2029849.
63. Gottlieb RL, Nirula A, Chen P, Boscia J, Heller B, Morris J, Huhn G, et al. Effect of Bamlanivimab as monotherapy or in combination with Etesevimab on viral load in patients with mild to moderate COVID-19: a randomized clinical trial. JAMA. 2021;325(7):632–44. https://doi.org/10.1001/jama.2021.0202.
64. Weinreich DM, Sivapalasingam S, Norton T, Ali S, Gao H, Bhore R, Musser BJ, et al. REGN-COV2, a neutralizing antibody cocktail, in outpatients with Covid-19. N Engl J Med. 2021;384(3):238–51. https://doi.org/10.1056/nejmoa2035002.
65. Lilly BLAZE-2 Trial. 2021. https://investor.lilly.com/news-releases/news-release-details/lillys-neutralizing-antibody-bamlanivimab-ly-cov555-prevented.
66. Wang P, Nair MS, Liu L, Iketani S, Luo Y, Guo Y, Wang M, et al. Antibody resistance of SARS-CoV-2 variants B.1.351 and B.1.1.7. Nature. 2021;593(7857):130–5. https://doi.org/10.1038/s41586-021-03398-2.
67. The RECOVERY Collaborative Group. Tocilizumab in patients admitted to hospital with COVID-19 (RECOVERY): preliminary results of a randomised, controlled, open-label, platform trial. Lancet. 2021a;397(10285):1637–45. https://doi.org/10.1101/2021.02.11.21249258.
68. The RECOVERY Collaborative Group. Dexamethasone in hospitalized patients with Covid-19. N Engl J Med. 2021b;384(8):693–704. https://doi.org/10.1056/nejmoa2021436.
69. The RECOVERY Collaborative Group. Aspirin in patients admitted to hospital with COVID-19 (RECOVERY): a randomised, controlled, open-label, platform trial. Lancet. 2021c;399(10320):143–51. https://doi.org/10.1101/2021.06.08.21258132.
70. Salama C, Han J, Yau L, Reiss WG, Kramer B, Neidhart JD, Criner GJ, et al. Tocilizumab in patients hospitalized with Covid-19 pneumonia. N Engl J Med. 2021;384(1):20–30. https://doi.org/10.1056/nejmoa2030340.
71. The REMAP-CAP Investigators. Interleukin-6 receptor antagonists in critically ill patients with Covid-19. N Engl J Med. 2021;384(16):1491–502. https://doi.org/10.1056/nejmoa2100433.

72. Tharmarajah E, Buazon A, Patel V, Hannah JR, Adas M, Allen VB, Bechman K, et al. IL-6 inhibition in the treatment of COVID-19: a meta-analysis and meta-regression. J Infect. 2021;82(5):178–85. https://doi.org/10.1016/j.jinf.2021.03.008.
73. Rosas IO, Bräu N, Waters M, Go RC, Hunter BD, Bhagani S, Skiest D, et al. Tocilizumab in hospitalized patients with severe Covid-19 pneumonia. N Engl J Med. 2021;384(16):1503–16. https://doi.org/10.1056/nejmoa2028700.
74. Stone JH, Frigault MJ, Serling-Boyd NJ, Fernandes AD, Harvey L, Foulkes AS, Horick NK, et al. Efficacy of tocilizumab in patients hospitalized with Covid-19. N Engl J Med. 2020;383(24):2333–44. https://doi.org/10.1056/nejmoa2028836.
75. Lescure F-X, Honda H, Fowler RA, Lazar JS, Shi G, Wung P, Patel N, et al. Sarilumab in patients admitted to hospital with severe or critical COVID-19: a randomised, double-blind, placebo-controlled, phase 3 trial. Lancet Respir Med. 2021;9(5):522–54. https://doi.org/10.1016/s2213-2600(21)00099-0.
76. Mariette X, Hermine O, Resche-Rigon M, Porcher R, Ravaud P, Bureau S, Dougados M, et al. Effect of Anakinra versus usual care in adults in hospital with COVID-19 and mild-to-moderate pneumonia (CORIMUNO-ANA-1): a randomised controlled trial. Lancet Respir Med. 2021;9(3):295–304. https://doi.org/10.1016/S2213-2600(20)30556-7.
77. Beigel JH, Tomashek KM, Dodd LE, Mehta AK, Zingman BS, Kalil AC, Hohmann E, et al. Remdesivir for the treatment of Covid-19 — final report. N Engl J Med. 2020;383(19):1813–26. https://doi.org/10.1056/nejmoa2007764.
78. WHO Solidarity Trial Consortium. Repurposed antiviral drugs for Covid-19 — interim WHO solidarity trial results. N Engl J Med. 2021;384(6):497–511. https://doi.org/10.1056/nejmoa2023184.
79. Wang Y, Zhang D, Du G, Du R, Zhao J, Jin Y, Fu S, Gao L, Cheng Z, Lu Q, Hu Y, Luo G, Wang K, Lu Y, Li H, Wang S, Ruan S, Yang C, Mei C, Wang Y, et al. Remdesivir in adults with severe COVID-19: a randomised, double-blind, placebo-controlled, multicentre trial. Lancet. 2020;395(10236):1569–78. https://doi.org/10.1016/S0140-6736(20)31022-9.
80. The RECOVERY Collaborative Group. Lopinavir–ritonavir in patients admitted to hospital with COVID-19 (RECOVERY): a randomised, controlled, open-label, platform trial. Lancet. 2020;396(10259):1345–52. https://doi.org/10.1016/S0140-6736(20)32013-4.
81. Cao B, Wang Y, Wen D, Liu W, Wang J, Fan G, Ruan L, et al. A trial of Lopinavir–Ritonavir in adults hospitalized with severe Covid-19. N Engl J Med. 2020;382(19):1787–99. https://doi.org/10.1056/nejmoa2001282.
82. Ivashchenko AA, Dmitriev KA, Vostokova NV, Azarova VN, Blinow AA, Egorova AN, Gordeev IG, et al. AVIFAVIR for treatment of patients with moderate coronavirus disease 2019 (COVID-19): interim results of a phase II/III multicenter randomized clinical trial. Clin Infect Dis. 2020;73(3):531–4. https://doi.org/10.1093/cid/ciaa1176.
83. Udwadia ZF, Singh P, Barkate H, Patil S, Rangwala S, Pendse A, Kadam J, Wen W, Caracta CF, Tandon M. Efficacy and safety of Favipiravir, an oral RNA-dependent RNA polymerase inhibitor, in mild-to-moderate COVID-19: a randomized, comparative, open-label, multicenter, phase 3 clinical trial. Int J Infect Dis. 2021;103:62–71. https://doi.org/10.1016/j.ijid.2020.11.142.
84. Ridgeback Biotherapeutics and Merck. 2021. https://www.merck.com/news/ridgeback-biotherapeutics-and-merck-announce-preliminary-findings-from-a-phase-2a-trial-of-investigational-covid-19-therapeutic-molnupiravir/.
85. Cox RM, Wolf JD, Plemper RK. Therapeutically administered ribonucleoside analogue MK-4482/EIDD-2801 blocks SARS-CoV-2 transmission in ferrets. Nat Microbiol. 2021;6(1):11–8. https://doi.org/10.1038/s41564-020-00835-2.
86. Wahl A, Gralinski LE, Johnson CE, Yao W, Kovarova M, Dinnon KH, Liu H, et al. SARS-CoV-2 infection is effectively treated and prevented by EIDD-2801. Nature. 2021;591(7850):451–7. https://doi.org/10.1038/s41586-021-03312-w.

87. Pulakurthi YS, Pederson JM, Saravu K, Gupta N, Balasubramanian P, Kamrowski S, Schmidt M, et al. Corticosteroid therapy for COVID-19: a systematic review and meta-analysis of randomized controlled trials. Medicine. 2021;100(20):e25719. https://doi.org/10.1097/MD.0000000000025719.
88. Sterne JAC, Murthy S, Diaz JV, Slutsky AS, Villar J, Angus DC, Annane D, et al. Association between administration of systemic corticosteroids and mortality among critically ill patients with COVID-19: a meta-analysis. JAMA. 2020;324(13):1330–41. https://doi.org/10.1001/jama.2020.17023.
89. WHO Corticosteroids for COVID-19. 2021. https://www.who.int/publications/i/item/WHO-2019-nCoV-Corticosteroids-2020.1.
90. Ramakrishnan S, Nicolau DV, Langford B, Mahdi M, Jeffers H, Mwasuku C, Krassowska K, et al. Inhaled budesonide in the treatment of early COVID-19 (STOIC): a phase 2, open-label, randomised controlled trial. Lancet Respir Med. 2021;9(7):763–72. https://doi.org/10.1016/s2213-2600(21)00160-0.
91. Chow JH, Khanna AK, Kethireddy S, Yamane D, Levine A, Jackson AM, McCurdy MT, et al. Aspirin use is associated with decreased mechanical ventilation, intensive care unit admission, and in-hospital mortality in hospitalized patients with coronavirus disease 2019. Anesth Analg. 2021;132(4):930–41. https://doi.org/10.1213/ANE.0000000000005292.
92. Tardif J-C, Bouabdallaoui N, L'allier PL, Gaudet D, Shah B, Pillinger MH, Lopez-Sendon J, et al. Efficacy of colchicine in non-hospitalized patients with COVID-19. MedRxiv. 2021. 2021.01.26.21250494. https://doi.org/10.1101/2021.01.26.21250494.
93. WHO News. 2020. https://www.who.int/news/item/04-07-2020-who-discontinues-hydroxychloroquine-and-lopinavir-ritonavir-treatment-arms-for-covid-19.
94. Skipper CP, Pastick KA, Engen NW, Bangdiwala AS, Abassi M, Lofgren SM, Williams DA, et al. Hydroxychloroquine in nonhospitalized adults with early COVID-19: a randomized trial. Ann Intern Med. 2020;173(8):623–31. https://doi.org/10.7326/M20-4207.
95. Boulware DR, Pullen MF, Bangdiwala AS, Pastick KA, Lofgren SM, Okafor EC, Skipper CP, et al. A randomized trial of hydroxychloroquine as postexposure prophylaxis for Covid-19. N Engl J Med. 2020;383(6):517–25. https://doi.org/10.1056/nejmoa2016638.
96. Andreani J, Le Bideau M, Duflot I, Jardot P, Rolland C, Boxberger M, Wurtz N, et al. In vitro testing of combined hydroxychloroquine and azithromycin on SARS-CoV-2 shows synergistic effect. Microb Pathog. 2020;145:104228. https://doi.org/10.1016/j.micpath.2020.104228.
97. Ip A, Ahn J, Zhou Y, Goy AH, Hansen E, Pecora AL, Sinclaire BA, et al. Hydroxychloroquine in the treatment of outpatients with mildly symptomatic COVID-19: a multi-center observational study. BMC Infect Dis. 2021;21(1):1–12. https://doi.org/10.1186/s12879-021-05773-w.
98. Ladapo JA, McKinnon JE, McCullough PA, Risch HA. Randomized controlled trials of early ambulatory hydroxychloroquine in the prevention of COVID-19 infection, hospitalization, and death: meta-analysis. MedRxiv. 2020; 2020.09.30.20204693. https://doi.org/10.1101/2020.09.30.20204693.
99. Axfors C, Schmitt AM, Janiaud P, van't Hooft J, Abd-Elsalam S, Abdo EF, Abella BS, et al. Mortality outcomes with hydroxychloroquine and chloroquine in COVID-19 from an international collaborative meta-analysis of randomized trials. Nat Commun. 2021;12(1):1–13. https://doi.org/10.1038/s41467-021-22446-z.
100. Fiolet T, Guihur A, Rebeaud ME, Mulot M, Peiffer-Smadja N, Mahamat-Saleh Y. Effect of hydroxychloroquine with or without azithromycin on the mortality of coronavirus disease 2019 (COVID-19) patients: a systematic review and meta-analysis. Clin Microbiol Infect. 2021;27(1):19–27. https://doi.org/10.1016/j.cmi.2020.08.022.
101. Mehra MR, Desai SS, Ruschitzka F, Patel AN. RETRACTED: hydroxychloroquine or chloroquine with or without a macrolide for treatment of COVID-19: a multinational registry analysis. Lancet. 2020. https://doi.org/10.1016/S0140-6736(20)31180-6.
102. Arévalo AP, Pagotto R, Pórfido JL, Daghero H, Segovia M, Yamasaki K, Varela B, et al. Ivermectin reduces in vivo coronavirus infection in a mouse experimental model. Sci Rep. 2021;11(1):7132. https://doi.org/10.1038/s41598-021-86679-0.

103. Caly L, Druce JD, Catton MG, Jans DA, Wagstaff KM. The FDA-approved drug Ivermectin inhibits the replication of SARS-CoV-2 in vitro. Antivir Res. 2020;178(June):104787. https://doi.org/10.1016/j.antiviral.2020.104787.
104. Ahmed S, Karim MM, Ross AG, Hossain MS, Clemens JD, Sumiya MK, Phru CS, et al. A five-Day course of Ivermectin for the treatment of COVID-19 may reduce the duration of illness. Int J Infect Dis. 2021;103(February):214–6. https://doi.org/10.1016/j.ijid.2020.11.191.
105. Krolewiecki A, Lifschitz A, Moragas M, Travacio M, Valentini R, Alonso DF, Solari R, et al. Antiviral effect of high-dose Ivermectin in adults with COVID-19: a pilot randomised, controlled, open label, multicentre trial. SSRN Electron J. 2020. https://doi.org/10.2139/ssrn.3714649.
106. Rajter JC, Sherman MS, Fatteh N, Vogel F, Sacks J, Rajter JJ. Use of Ivermectin is associated with lower mortality in hospitalized patients with coronavirus disease 2019: the Ivermectin in COVID nineteen study. Chest. 2021;159(1):85–92. https://doi.org/10.1016/j.chest.2020.10.009.
107. López-Medina E, López P, Hurtado IC, Dávalos DM, Ramirez O, Martínez E, Díazgranados JA, et al. Effect of Ivermectin on time to resolution of symptoms among adults with mild COVID-19: a randomized clinical trial. JAMA. 2021;325(14):1426–35. https://doi.org/10.1001/jama.2021.3071.
108. Chaccour C, Casellas A, Matteo AB-D, Pineda I, Fernandez-Montero A, Ruiz-Castillo P, Richardson MA, et al. The effect of early treatment with Ivermectin on viral load, symptoms and humoral response in patients with non-severe COVID-19: a pilot, double-blind, placebo-controlled, randomized clinical trial. EClinicalMedicine. 2021;32:100720. https://doi.org/10.1016/j.eclinm.2020.100720.
109. Biber, Asaf, Michal Mandelboim, Geva Harmelin, Dana Lev, Li Ram, Amit Shaham, Ital Nemet, Limor Kliker, Oran Erster, and Eli Schwartz. Favorable outcome on viral load and culture viability using Ivermectin in early treatment of non-hospitalized patients with mild COVID-19-a double-blind, randomized Placebo-2 controlled trial. 2021. MedRxiv, 2021.05.31.21258081. https://doi.org/10.1101/2021.05.31.21258081.
110. Feldman C, Anderson R. The role of co-infections and secondary infections in patients with COVID-19. Pneumonia (Nathan). 2021;13(1):5. https://doi.org/10.1186/s41479-021-00083-w.
111. Langford BJ, So M, Raybardhan S, Leung V, Westwood D, MacFadden DR, Jean PR, Soucy, and Nick Daneman. Bacterial co-infection and secondary infection in patients with COVID-19: a living rapid review and meta-analysis. Clin Microbiol Infect. 2020;26(12):1622–9. https://doi.org/10.1016/j.cmi.2020.07.016.
112. Clancy CJ, Schwartz IS, Kula B, Hong M, Nguyen. Bacterial superinfections among persons with coronavirus disease 2019: a comprehensive review of data from postmortem studies. Open Forum Infect Dis. 2021;8(3):ofab065. https://doi.org/10.1093/ofid/ofab065.
113. Beigelman A, Isaacson-Schmid M, Sajol G, Baty J, Rodriguez OM, Leege E, Lyons K, et al. Randomized trial to evaluate Azithromycin's effects on serum and upper airway IL-8 levels and recurrent wheezing in infants with respiratory syncytial virus bronchiolitis. J Allergy Clin Immunol. 2015;135(5):1171–1178.e1. https://doi.org/10.1016/j.jaci.2014.10.001.
114. Li C, Shulong Z, Deng YQ, Li D, Parvatiyar K, Quanquin N, Shang J, et al. Azithromycin protects against Zika virus infection by upregulating virus-induced type I and III interferon responses. Antimicrob Agents Chemother. 2019;63(12):e00394-19. https://doi.org/10.1128/AAC.00394-19.
115. Mosquera RA, De Jesus-Rojas W, Stark JM, Yadav A, Jon CK, Atkins CL, Samuels CL, et al. Role of prophylactic azithromycin to reduce airway inflammation and mortality in a RSV mouse infection model. Pediatr Pulmonol. 2018;53(5):567–74. https://doi.org/10.1002/ppul.23956.
116. Retallack H, Di Lullo E, Arias C, Knopp KA, Laurie MT, Sandoval-Espinosa C, Mancia Leon WR, et al. Zika virus cell tropism in the developing human brain and inhibition by

azithromycin. Proc Natl Acad Sci U S A. 2016;113(50):14408–13. https://doi.org/10.1073/pnas.1618029113.
117. Tran DH, Sugamata R, Hirose T, Suzuki S, Noguchi Y, Sugawara A, Ito F, et al. Azithromycin, a 15-membered macrolide antibiotic, inhibits influenza A(H1N1)Pdm09 virus infection by interfering with virus internalization process. J Antibiot. 2019;72(10):759–68. https://doi.org/10.1038/s41429-019-0204-x.
118. Castro JZ, Fredeking T. Doxycycline modify the cytokine storm in patients with dengue and dengue hemorrhagic fever. Int J Infect Dis. 2010;14(March):e44. https://doi.org/10.1016/j.ijid.2010.02.1586.
119. Rothan HA, Bahrani H, Mohamed Z, Teoh TC, Shankar EM, Rahman NA, Yusof R. A combination of doxycycline and ribavirin alleviated chikungunya infection. PLoS One. 2015;10(5):e0126360. https://doi.org/10.1371/journal.pone.0126360.
120. Rothan HA, Mohamed Z, Paydar M, Rahman NA, Yusof R. Inhibitory effect of doxycycline against dengue virus replication in vitro. Arch Virol. 2014;159(4):711–8. https://doi.org/10.1007/s00705-013-1880-7.
121. Sturtz FG. Antimurine retroviral effect of doxycycline. Methods Find Exp Clin Pharmacol. 1998;20(8):643–7. https://doi.org/10.1358/mf.1998.20.8.487489.
122. Gendrot M, Andreani J, Jardot P, Hutter S, Delandre O, Boxberger M, Mosnier J, et al. In vitro antiviral activity of doxycycline against SARS-CoV-2. Molecules. 2020;25(21):5064. https://doi.org/10.3390/molecules25215064.
123. Butler CC, Dorward J, Ly Mee Y, Gbinigie O, Hayward G, Saville BR, Van Hecke O, et al. Azithromycin for community treatment of suspected COVID-19 in people at increased risk of an adverse clinical course in the UK (PRINCIPLE): a randomised, controlled, open-label, adaptive platform trial. Lancet. 2021;397(10279):1063–74. https://doi.org/10.1016/S0140-6736(21)00461-X.
124. Furtado RHM, Berwanger O, Fonseca HA, Corrêa TD, Ferraz LR, Lapa MG, Zampieri FG, et al. Azithromycin in addition to standard of care versus standard of care alone in the treatment of patients admitted to the hospital with severe COVID-19 in Brazil (COALITION II): a randomised clinical trial. Lancet. 2020;396(10256):959–67. https://doi.org/10.1016/S0140-6736(20)31862-6.
125. Rosenberg ES, Dufort EM, Udo T, Wilberschied LA, Kumar J, Tesoriero J, Weinberg P, et al. Association of treatment with hydroxychloroquine or azithromycin with in-hospital mortality in patients with COVID-19 in New York state. JAMA. 2020;323(24):2493–502. https://doi.org/10.1001/jama.2020.8630.
126. Boonyawat K, Chantrathammachart P, Numthavej P, Nanthatanti N, Phusanti S, Phuphuakrat A, Niparuck P, Angchaisuksiri P. Incidence of thromboembolism in patients with COVID-19: a systematic review and meta-analysis. Thromb J. 2020;18(1):1–12. https://doi.org/10.1186/s12959-020-00248-5.
127. Kunutsor SK, Laukkanen JA. Incidence of venous and arterial thromboembolic complications in COVID-19: a systematic review and meta-analysis. Thromb Res. 2020;196:27–30. https://doi.org/10.1016/j.thromres.2020.08.022.
128. Malas MB, Naazie IN, Elsayed N, Mathlouthi A, Marmor R, Clary B. Thromboembolism risk of COVID-19 is high and associated with a higher risk of mortality: a systematic review and meta-analysis. EClinicalMedicine. 2020;29:100639. https://doi.org/10.1016/j.eclinm.2020.100639.
129. McBane RD, Torres Roldan VD, Niven AS, Pruthi RK, Franco PM, Linderbaum JA, Casanegra AI, et al. Anticoagulation in COVID-19: a systematic review, meta-analysis, and rapid guidance from Mayo Clinic. Mayo Clin Proc. 2020;95(11):2467–86. https://doi.org/10.1016/j.mayocp.2020.08.030.
130. Parisi R, Costanzo S, Di Castelnuovo A, De Gaetano G, Donati MB, Iacoviello L. Different anticoagulant regimens, mortality, and bleeding in hospitalized patients with COVID-19: a systematic review and an updated meta-analysis. Semin Thromb Hemost. 2021;47(4):372–91. https://doi.org/10.1055/s-0041-1726034.

131. Rentsch CT, Beckman JA, Tomlinson L, Gellad WF, Alcorn C, Kidwai-Khan F, Skanderson M, et al. Early initiation of prophylactic anticoagulation for prevention of coronavirus disease 2019 mortality in patients admitted to hospital in the United States: cohort study. BMJ. 2021;372:n311. https://doi.org/10.1136/bmj.n311.
132. JamaliMoghadamSiahkali S, Zarezade B, Koolaji S, SeyedAlinaghi SA, Zendehdel A, Tabarestani M, Moghadam ES, et al. Safety and effectiveness of high-dose vitamin C in patients with COVID-19: a randomized open-label clinical trial. Eur J Med Res. 2021;26(1):20. https://doi.org/10.1186/s40001-021-00490-1.
133. Thomas S, Patel D, Bittel B, Wolski K, Wang Q, Kumar A, Il'Giovine ZJ, et al. Effect of high-dose zinc and ascorbic acid supplementation vs usual care on symptom length and reduction among ambulatory patients with SARS-CoV-2 infection: the COVID A to Z randomized clinical trial. JAMA Netw Open. 2021;4(2):e210369. https://doi.org/10.1001/jamanetworkopen.2021.0369.
134. Murai IH, Fernandes AL, Sales LP, Pinto AJ, Goessler KF, Duran CSC, Silva CBR, et al. Effect of a single high dose of vitamin D3on hospital length of stay in patients with moderate to severe COVID-19: a randomized clinical trial. JAMA. 2021;325(11):1053–60. https://doi.org/10.1001/jama.2020.26848.
135. Chalmers JD, Crichton ML, Goeminne PC, Cao B, Humbert M, Shteinberg M, Antoniou KM, et al. Management of hospitalised adults with coronavirus disease 2019 (COVID-19): a European Respiratory Society living guideline. Eur Respir J. 2021;57(4):2100048. https://doi.org/10.1183/13993003.00048-2021.
136. Gorman E, Connolly B, Couper K, Perkins GD, McAuley DF. Non-invasive respiratory support strategies in COVID-19. Lancet Respir Med. 2021;9(6):553–6. https://doi.org/10.1016/S2213-2600(21)00168-5.
137. Grieco DL, Menga LS, Cesarano M, Rosà T, Spadaro S, Bitondo MM, Montomoli J, et al. Effect of helmet noninvasive ventilation vs high-flow nasal oxygen on days free of respiratory support in patients with COVID-19 and moderate to severe hypoxemic respiratory failure: the HENIVOT randomized clinical trial. JAMA. 2021;325(17):1731–43. https://doi.org/10.1001/jama.2021.4682.
138. Mellado-Artigas R, Ferreyro BL, Angriman F, Hernández-Sanz M, Arruti E, Torres A, Villar J, et al. High-flow nasal oxygen in patients with COVID-19-associated acute respiratory failure. Crit Care. 2021;25(1):1–10. https://doi.org/10.1186/s13054-021-03469-w.
139. Voshaar T, Stais P, Köhler D, Dellweg D. Conservative management of COVID-19 associated hypoxaemia. ERJ Open Res. 2021;7(1):00026–2021. https://doi.org/10.1183/23120541.00026-2021.
140. Young PJ. Effect of oxygen therapy on mortality in the ICU. N Engl J Med. 2021;384(14):1361–3. https://doi.org/10.1056/nejme2101538.
141. Jiang B, Wei H. Oxygen therapy strategies and techniques to treat hypoxia in COVID-19 patients. Eur Rev Med Pharmacol Sci. 2020;24(19):10239–46. https://doi.org/10.26355/eurrev_202010_23248.
142. Gattinoni L, Chiumello D, Caironi P, Busana M, Romitti F, Brazzi L, Camporota L, Gattinoni L. COVID-19 pneumonia: different respiratory treatment for different phenotypes? Intensive Care Med. 2020a;46(6):1099–102. https://doi.org/10.1007/s00134-020-06033-2.
143. Gattinoni L, Chiumello D, Rossi S. COVID-19 pneumonia: ARDS or not? Crit Care. 2020b;24(1):154. https://doi.org/10.1186/s13054-020-02880-z.
144. Brochard L, Slutsky A, Pesenti A. Mechanical ventilation to minimize progression of lung injury in acute respiratory failure. Am J Respir Crit Care Med. 2017;195(4):438–42. https://doi.org/10.1164/rccm.201605-1081CP.
145. Yang L-L, Yang T. Pulmonary rehabilitation for patients with coronavirus disease 2019 (COVID-19). Chro Dis Transl Med. 2020;6(2):79–86. https://doi.org/10.1016/j.cdtm.2020.05.002.
146. 2020 GOLD Report. 2020. https://goldcopd.org/gold-reports/.

147. Guérin C, Reignier J, Richard J-C, Beuret P, Gacouin A, Boulain T, Mercier E, et al. Prone positioning in severe acute respiratory distress syndrome. N Engl J Med. 2013;368(23):2159–68. https://doi.org/10.1056/NEJMoa1214103.
148. Chad T, Sampson C. Prone positioning in conscious patients on medical wards: a review of the evidence and its relevance to patients with COVID-19 Infection. Clin Med (Lond). 2020;20(4):e97. https://doi.org/10.7861/CLINMED.2020-0179.
149. Coppo A, Bellani G, Winterton D, Di Pierro M, Soria A, Faverio P, Cairo M, et al. Feasibility and physiological effects of prone positioning in non-intubated patients with acute respiratory failure due to COVID-19 (PRON-COVID): a prospective cohort study. Lancet Respir Med. 2020;8(8):765–74. https://doi.org/10.1016/S2213-2600(20)30268-X.
150. Ding L, Wang L, Ma W, He H. Efficacy and safety of early prone positioning combined with HFNC or NIV in moderate to severe ARDS: a multi-center prospective cohort study. Crit Care. 2020;24(1):28. https://doi.org/10.1186/s13054-020-2738-5.
151. Ng Z, Tay WC, Ho CHB. Awake prone positioning for non-intubated oxygen dependent COVID-19 pneumonia patients. Eur Respir J. 2020;56(1):2001198. https://doi.org/10.1183/13993003.01198-2020.
152. Paul V, Patel S, Royse M, Odish M, Malhotra A, Koenig S. Proning in non-intubated (PINI) in times of COVID-19: case series and a review. J Intensive Care Med. 2020;35(8):818–24. https://doi.org/10.1177/0885066620934801.
153. Pb S, Mittal S, Madan K, Mohan A, Tiwari P, Hadda V, Pandey RM, Guleria R. Awake prone positioning in non-intubated patients for the management of hypoxemia in COVID-19: a systematic review and meta-analysis. Monaldi Arch Chest Dis. 2021;91 (2). https://doi.org/10.4081/monaldi.2021.1623.
154. Reddy P, Mallikarjuna AS, Afroz A, Billah B, Lim ZJ, Zubarev A, Blecher G, et al. Prone positioning of nonintubated patients with coronavirus disease 2019-a systematic review and meta-analysis. Crit Care Med. 2021;49(10):e1001–14. https://doi.org/10.1097/CCM.0000000000005086.
155. Qadri SK, Ng P, Toh TSW, Loh SW, Tan HL, Lin CB, Fan E, Lee JH. Critically ill patients with COVID-19: a narrative review on prone position. Pulm Ther. 2020;6(2):233–46. https://doi.org/10.1007/s41030-020-00135-4.
156. Raoof S, Nava S, Carpati C, Hill NS. High-flow, noninvasive ventilation and awake (nonintubation) proning in patients with coronavirus disease 2019 with respiratory failure. Chest. 2020;158(5):1992–2002. https://doi.org/10.1016/j.chest.2020.07.013.
157. Touchon F, Trigui Y, Prud'homme E, Lefebvre L, Giraud A, Dols A-M, Martinez S, et al. Awake prone positioning for hypoxaemic respiratory failure: past, COVID-19 and perspectives. Eur Respir Rev. 2021;30(160):210022. https://doi.org/10.1183/16000617.0022-2021.
158. Bamford P, Bentley A, Dean J, Whitmore D, Wilson-Baig N. ICS guidance for prone positioning of the conscious COVID patient 2020. 2020.
159. Ibarra-Estrada M, Marín-Rosales M, García-Salcido R, Aguirre-Díaz SA, Vargas-Obieta A, Chávez-Peña Q, López-Pulgarín JA, Mijangos-Méndez JC, Aguirre-Avalos G. Prone positioning in non-intubated patients with COVID-19 associated acute respiratory failure, the PRO-CARF trial: a structured summary of a study protocol for a randomised controlled trial. Trials. 2020;21(1):940. https://doi.org/10.1186/s13063-020-04882-2.
160. Chikhanie Y, Al D, Veale M, Schoeffler J, Pépin L, Verges S, Hérengt F. Effectiveness of pulmonary rehabilitation in COVID-19 respiratory failure patients post-ICU. Respir Physiol Neurobiol. 2021;287:103639. https://doi.org/10.1016/j.resp.2021.103639.
161. Goodwin VA, Allan L, Bethel A, Cowley A, Cross JL, Day J, Drummond A, et al. Rehabilitation to enable recovery from COVID-19: a rapid systematic review. Physiotherapy. 2021;111:4–22. https://doi.org/10.1016/j.physio.2021.01.007.
162. Santana AV, Fontana AD, Pitta F. Pulmonary rehabilitation after COVID-19. J Bras Pneumol. 2021;47(1):e20210034. https://doi.org/10.36416/1806-3756/e20210034.
163. Zampogna E, Paneroni M, Belli S, Aliani M, Gandolfo A, Visca D, Bellanti MT, Ambrosino N, Vitacca M. Pulmonary rehabilitation in patients recovering from COVID-19. Respiration. 2021;100(5):1–7. https://doi.org/10.1159/000514387.

164. Gloeckl R, Leitl D, Jarosch I, Schneeberger T, Nell C, Stenzel N, Vogelmeier CF, et al. Early view benefits of pulmonary rehabilitation in COVID-19-a prospective observational cohort study figure benefits of pulmonary rehabilitation in COVID-19-a prospective observational cohort study. ERJ Open Res. 2021. https://doi.org/10.1183/23120541.00108-2021.
165. Agostini F, Mangone M, Ruiu P, Paolucci T, Santilli V, Bernetti A. Rehabilitation settings during and after COVID-19: an overview of recommendations. J Rehabil Med. 2021;53(1):jrm00141. https://doi.org/10.2340/16501977-2776.
166. Lundell S, Holmner Å, Rehn B, Nyberg A, Wadell K. Telehealthcare in COPD: a systematic review and meta-analysis on physical outcomes and dyspnea. Respir Med. 2015;109(1):11–26. https://doi.org/10.1016/j.rmed.2014.10.008.
167. Tsutsui M, Gerayeli F, Sin DD. Pulmonary rehabilitation in a post-Covid-19 world: telerehabilitation as a new standard in patients with Copd. Int J Chron Obstruct Pulmon Dis. 2021;16:379–91. https://doi.org/10.2147/COPD.S263031.
168. Suter F, Consolaro E, Pedroni S, Moroni C, Pastò E, Paganini MV, Pravettoni G, et al. A simple, home-therapy algorithm to prevent hospitalisation for COVID-19 patients: a retrospective observational matched-cohort study. EClinicalMedicine. 2021;37:100941. https://doi.org/10.1016/j.eclinm.2021.100941.
169. Kim PS, Read SW, Fauci AS. Therapy for early COVID-19: a critical need. JAMA. 2020;324(21):2149–50. https://doi.org/10.1001/jama.2020.22813.

# Chapter 21
# Biotechnological Strategies in the Intervention and Treatment of COVID-19

**Norma P. Silva-Beltrán, Ana P. Balderrama-Carmona, Juan-Carlos Gálvez-Ruíz, Marcelo A. Umsza-Guez, and Eduardo Ruiz Bustos**

## Introduction

SARS-CoV-2 exhibits a rapid human-to-human spreading via the respiratory tract and is responsible for a syndrome known as coronavirus disease of 2019 (COVID-19) [1]. Since its discovery, COVID-19 has become a pandemic outbreak with more than 228.981 million people tested positive for the virus, and more than 4.6 million deaths around the world by mid-September 2021 [2]. In this sense, this spread still requires deceleration mechanisms that include pharmacological and immunological approaches, not only to treat infected patients, but also to prevent future infections or, at least, serious manifestations of the disease.

In order to establish intervention and treatment strategies, laboratories worldwide strengthen their efforts to fully understand SARS-CoV-2, causative agent of the COVID-19, as well as its interactions with the host, resulting in over 140

N. P. Silva-Beltrán (✉)
Departamento de Ciencias de la Salud, Universidad de Sonora,
Ciudad Obregón, Sonora, Mexico
e-mail: norma.silva@unison.mx

A. P. Balderrama-Carmona
Departamento de Ciencias Químico Biológicas y Agropecuarias, Unidad Regional Sur,
Universidad de Sonora, Navojoa, Sonora, Mexico
e-mail: paola.balderrama@unison.mx

J.-C. Gálvez-Ruíz · E. R. Bustos
Departamento de Ciencias Químico Biológicas, Universidad de Sonora,
Hermosillo, Sonora, Mexico
e-mail: juan.galvez@unison.mx; eduardo.ruiz@unison.mx

M. A. Umsza-Guez
Departamento de Biotecnologia, Universidade Federal da Bahia, Salvador, Brazil
e-mail: marcelo.umsza@ufba.br



S. Adibi et al. (eds.), *Frontiers of COVID-19*,
https://doi.org/10.1007/978-3-031-08045-6_21

thousand publications around the world, including those related with biotechnological alternatives for the disease's treatment and prevention, with some examples shown in Fig. 21.1. These studies include those with current drugs, mainly antivirals, in order to determine their effect against COVID-19, as well as other medications and strategies used to treat signs and symptoms associated with this viral agent; due to the lack of specific anti-coronavirus antivirals, the reuse of currently available drugs used to treat unrelated diseases but capable of inhibiting the viral replication of SARS-CoV-2 and thus reducing the symptoms and complications of the disease has been the main focus to find a source of potential antiviral therapy. However, reuse has had some mixed results, which are shown in this chapter.

Undoubtedly, research has centered onto the design of an immunological approach to develop a vaccine against this pathogen using different platforms, such as modified viral mRNA, the use of different viral vectors and inactivated virus. This to such extent that different vaccines are being applied worldwide in order to reduce the infection's impact on the population, with overall promising results. However, work is still necessary to determine the extent of the protection induced by the immunoprophylactic agents, as well as the median and long-term effects and the support actions required by the population, in order to maximize the positive impact of the vaccines in the reduction of the impact of SARS-Cov-2 and its variants.

Another approach that is being undertaken for the treatment of the disease is the use of monoclonal antibodies and natural products and/or their components, which are studied either to potentiate the effect of the drug used or to reduce the side effects associated with the vaccine. The substances used in these last studies include some vitamins, plant extracts, and propolis or component(s) extracted from them.

The purpose of this chapter is to summarize the main studies and advances within the context of the above-mentioned biotechnological approaches that have risen since the onset of the COVID-19 pandemic.

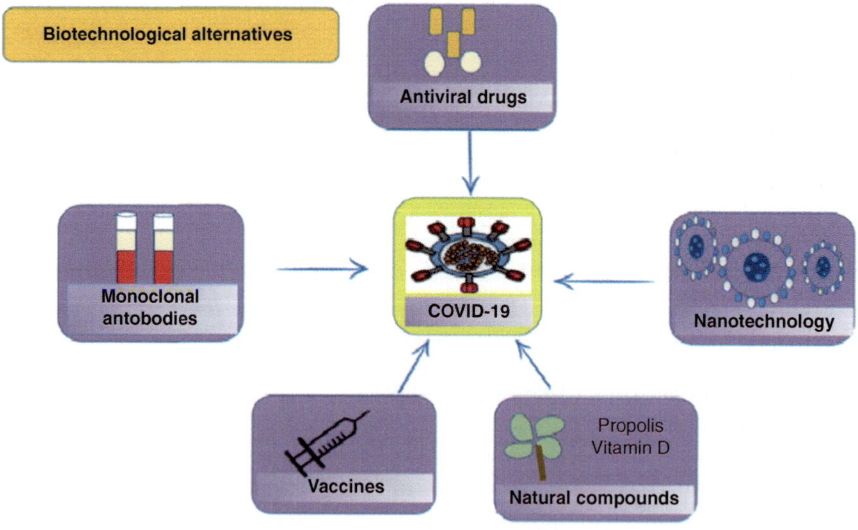


**Fig. 21.1** Biotechnological strategies studied by the scientific community to eliminate and control SARS-CoV-2 infection

## Repurposing of Known Drugs Against COVID-19

Much effort has been set to find a drug, currently available, cost-effective, and safe enough to prevent the SARS-CoV-2 from entering cells, eliminate its replication or, if the person is already infected, minimize infection-related adverse effects. Scientists have focused on studying known broad-spectrum drugs (mainly antiviral), including in silico studies of non-antiviral drugs that could repurpose or reposition in the fight against this disease. These studies have set the bases to synthesize potentially effective new compounds, considering the structure–activity relationship, efficacy which should be tested in further studies.

The SARS-CoV-2 genome sequencing, the identification of the proteins involved in the mechanism of action, both virus and host, and the cumulated understanding about related viruses increase the possibility to succeed in the race for a protective or curative therapy. In this sense, computational chemistry is a valuable tool for an efficient drug discovery, design, or development, by applying the basic principles of medicinal chemistry, target identification, lead identification, and lead optimization. The elucidation of many viral druggable proteins crystal structure has allowed through computational techniques, to quickly study hundreds of thousands of drugs. Computational simulations, molecular docking, high throughput screening, deep docking, molecular dynamics, bioinformatics-based homology modeling, structure-assisted drug design, among others, have allowed the determination of binding energy, stability, and dynamic behavior of the target–drug interaction. The most used druggable targets for in silico studies are proteins related to the entry, replication, and release of SARS-CoV-2, including the receptor-binding domain of the Spike protein (RBD), 3CL protease (Mpro), angiotensin-converting enzyme-2 (ACE-2), transmembrane serine protease-2 (TMPRS2), RNA-dependent RNA polymerase (RdRp). Some potentially effective known drugs with good physicochemical and pharmacokinetic properties identified are shown in Fig. 21.2.

In the same sense, using artificial intelligence and network medicine led to the proposal that Mefuparib may have more potent antiviral activity than remdesivir. Also, Toremifene shows to block the interaction of the virus with the Spike protein and ACE2, a fact supporting the observed antiviral activity shown in vitro assays [3].

Although computational studies give a very close idea of the drugs behavior against a pathogen, they cannot fully predict what may happen in vivo since other conditions will affect the outcome, resulting in vitro and in vivo studies essential to confirm whether the predicted properties of the compounds hold. In this regard, many of the drugs determined as candidates at the computational level were tested in vitro using different cell lines related to tissues that are potentially infected by the SARS-Cov-2 virus, showing only a few drugs a promising antiviral activity, from over ten thousand drugs. These include, amodiaquine, acitretin, apilimod, astemizole, clofazimine, chlorpromazine, hanfangchin A, imatinib, mefloquine, MLN-3897, and β-D-N4-hydroxycytidine-5′-isopropyl ester (Molnupiravir) [4–6].

The in vitro analysis focuses on their efficacy to stop the advance of the disease and the adverse events that may occur due to the interaction with other drugs that patients are being medicated with. Only some repurposed drugs have advanced into clinical trials to determine their effectiveness in reducing viral load, the severity of

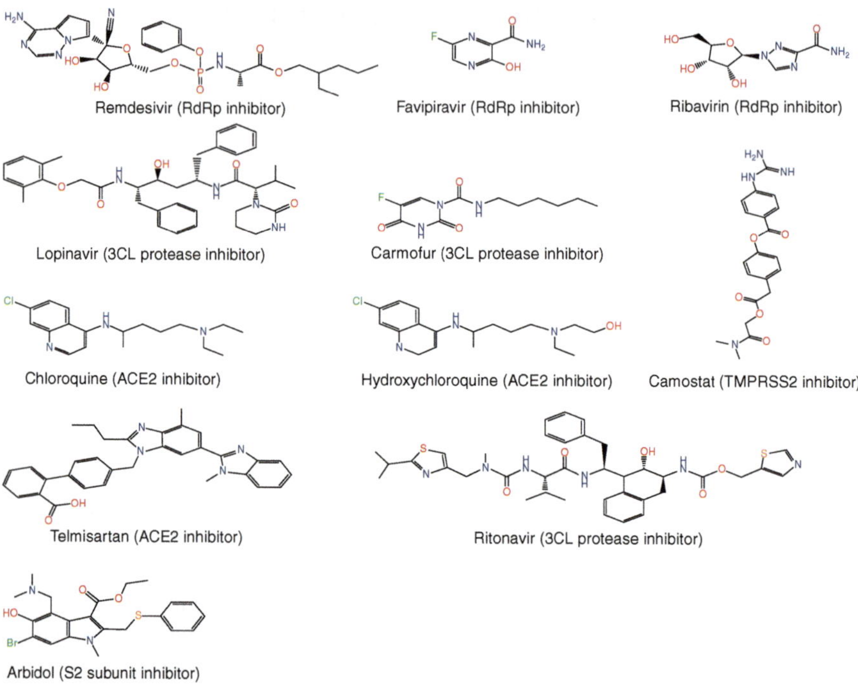


**Fig. 21.2** Some known drugs computationally detected as potential treatment against SARS-CoV-2. The target is named in pare

symptoms, hospitalization time, and mortality. Thus, very few drugs have been used worldwide to treat the disease until now. The earlier clinical trials tested some known drugs such as arbidol (umifenovir), chloroquine, darunavir, favipiravir, fingolimod, hydroxychloroquine, lopinavir, methylprednisolone, molnupiravir, oseltamivir, pirfenidone, PB28, remdesivir, ritonavir, thalidomide, vitamin C [7].

Because of the urgent need for a drug that could be used for the treatment at different stages of disease severity, the FDA, based on available evidence from clinical trials, has given emergency authorization for the use of certain drugs against COVID-19. However, studies using more patients and conditions have shown that the utility was not as expected, and the authorization was revoked. An example of this is chloroquine and hydroxychloroquine, drugs used in China as treatment against COVID-19. In an in vitro study, these drugs showed anti-SARS-CoV-2 activity, and in a small clinical trial, the patients needed less time to recover. However, shortly after the emergency authorization, the FDA emitted a pharmacovigilance memorandum due to adverse events related to these drugs [8]. This exemplifies the importance of balancing the need for a drug against the disease, with the quality and quantity of the results. Studies should encompass the most significant number of participants to represent all variables that could influence drug outcomes in patients., including age, general health status, pre-existing diseases, and infection duration.

Those and other parameters were employed during the clinical trials conducted with the drug remdesivir. Remdesivir is another repurposed drug that received the

FDA authorization for emergency use in severely ill patients. This drug blocks the virus replication by competing for viral ATP and then incorporated as a false nucleoside into the new viral RNA chain, interrupting the RNA synthesis and viral replication. Remdesivir is an inhibitor of RNA-directed viral RNA polymerase (RpRd). In addition, in vitro studies also consider its therapeutic target, nsp8 and nsp12 proteins of the RpRd of MERS-CoV [9, 10]. Remdesivir reduces the recovery time by 4–5 days for clinical improvement in hospitalized patients (average age 65) with severe disease and mortality of 3% [11]. It also prevents the progression of the disease to a more severe or acute level reducing the number of days with supplementary oxygen in patients (average age 58) with lower respiratory tract infections [12]. Some adverse events observed during the administration of remdesivir include rectal hemorrhages, diarrhea, and liver damages. Furthermore, remdesivir is not currently available for oral administration, and thus, the intravenous application requires patient's hospitalization [9]. By late October 2020, FDA formally approved the use of remdesivir in all hospitalized patients older than 12 years and 40 kg weight, regardless of the severity of the disease [13]. However, by the end of 2020, the WHO warned that improvement shown by this drug was slight in terms of hospitalization time, ventilation, or mortality [14] (WHO Solidarity trial consortium, 2020). The use of remdesivir remains controversial; however, it is the only drug approved by FDA for COVID-19 treatment. During the pandemic, several remdesivir-resistant SARS-CoV-2 strains have appeared [15]. Two phase 2/3 trials in hospitalized and non-hospitalized patients using doses of Molnupiravir twice a day for 5 days indicate that this drug showed any clinical benefit in the hospitalized patient. However, it showed to be a promising treatment for the non-hospitalized patient, and this trial advances to phase 3 [16].

Another repurposed drug inhibitor of SARS-CoV-2 RdRp is favipiravir, used in Russia, Turkey, China, Chile, and other countries to treat COVID-19 patients. Favipiravir showed promising results in phase III clinical trial conducted in 156 patients without severe pneumonia by reducing the recovery time from the disease [17]. However, there is evidence that Favipiravir increases plasma uric acid levels in patients that use this drug [18]. Analysis of results obtained from clinical trials using this drug suggests that it does not reduce mortality in patients with mild to moderate disease but could help patients in the initial stage of hospitalization [19, 20].

In order to improve the effect of some drugs that in individual therapy have not been as effective as expected, some therapies have been used combining two or more drugs considering the potential synergism. An illustration of this drug combination is that of lopinavir/ ritonavir. In vitro, lopinavir is a much more active selective protease inhibitor than ritonavir. However, in vivo, this is not the case since cytochrome P-450 enzymes inactivate it. The combination with ritonavir is crucial because this drug inhibits the cytochrome responsible for the inactivation of lopinavir, thus preventing lopinavir from avoiding or decreasing metabolic inactivation. Frequently, drugs are used to stimulate or mimic the immune system to support it in the defense against the virus and avoid further damage to the body's tissues. For example, a clinical trial in 80 patients showed that the combination of favipiravir with interferon (IFN)-α generated a better patient response and led to better viral clearance than a combination of lopinavir, ritonavir, and IFN-α [21]. The combination of ribavirin, interferon beta-1b, and lopinavir-ritonavir reduced viral load, time to symptom relief, and hospitalization in adult patients participating in phase II clinical trial [22]. The use of interferons to promote the recuperation of patients with COVID-19 is being explored in some clinical trials, having promising preliminary results. For instance, a clinical trial is ongoing with an inhaled form of interferon (SNG001), which reduces the risk of severe COVID-19 disease [23]. Artificial intelligence techniques, such as a network-based methodology, had made it possible to find a combination of drugs potentially effective against COVID-19, such as dactinomycin-sirolimus, melatonin-mercaptopurine, emodin-toremifene, and toremifene-melatonin. A combinatorial therapy using toremifene-melatonin has been tested in patients at early stages of the disease [3].

While most efforts have been directed at finding drugs that target viral proteins, consideration has also been given to the use of specific host therapeutic targets that are known to be used by SARS-CoV-2 to enter cells and replicate. Many known drugs that can block these host proteins and prevent infection have been identified through in vitro studies. These include clemastine, cloperastine, haloperidol, chloroquine, hydroxychloroquine, progesterone, siramesine, ternatine-4, zotatifine, PB28, PD-144418, and PS3061 [24]. The most used have been chloroquine and hydroxychloroquine that block angiotensin-converting enzyme-2 (ACE-2). Recently, plitidepsin, a drug used to treat multiple myeloma, has attracted attention due to promising preclinical results. The drug showed more potent anti-SARS-CoV-2 activity, in vitro, than remdesivir, low cytotoxicity, and reduced viral replication in mouse models. The drug works by blocking the eEF1A protein present in human cells and is used by SARS-CoV-2 to infect the cells; it is currently in phase II/III clinical study [25, 26]. It is crucial to keep in mind that this drug should be intravenously administrated and could limit its use in non-hospitalized patients. Even though drugs such as hydroxychloroquine, plitidepsin, and camostat can be highly active agents against SARS-CoV-2, caution must be applied since the targeting of host proteins such as ACE-2, eEF1A, and TMPRSS2 often leads to adverse effects such as cytotoxicity problems, making their use questionable.

To deal with the inflammatory response developed in patients with COVID-19 causing multiple organ failure, dexamethasone, prednisone, methylprednisolone, or hydrocortisone has been used as a treatment for hospitalized patients with mechanical ventilators or oxygen (NIH 2021; WHO REACT-Working Group, 2020). FDA authorized the emergency use of Baricitinib in combination with remdesivir to treat hospitalized patients (adults and pediatrics of 2 years and older) who require supplemental oxygen, invasive mechanical ventilator, or extracorporeal membrane oxygenation [27]. This combination of drugs reduces mortality, and the effect is more pronounced in patients receiving non-invasive mechanical ventilation [28]. In addition, the NIH recommends using Baricitinib in combination with remdesivir to reduce inflammation in hospitalized patients if corticosteroids cannot be used [29]. Fluvoxamine [30], colchicine [31], and EXO-CD24 [32] have shown some promising results to stop the inflammation in a patient with COVID-19, and some clinical trials are undergoing.

The repurposing or repositing of available drugs has had some mixed results. Some administered drugs have improved the recovery of COVID-19, Fig. 21.3, patients but others severely affect them, with even dangerous cardiovascular

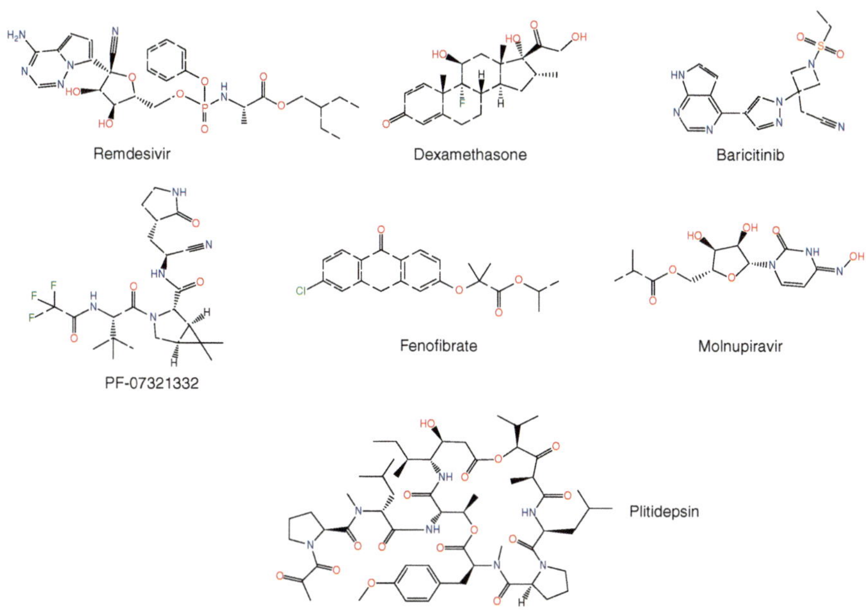


**Fig. 21.3** Approved, or promising, drugs against SARS-CoV-2

complications, which prompted the World Health Organization to suspend some ongoing clinical trials. It should be kept in mind that the same drug may not be the most effective to manage the disease from the first symptoms to the most severe stages that lead to hospitalization. In addition, the comorbidities that the patient may have could restrict the use of certain substances due to adverse events that may occur due to the interaction between drugs.

The presence of virus variants represents a new challenge since the effectiveness of a particular drug could vary and, in the worst case, cease to be effective because of the alteration in the target–drug interaction derived from the mutations. However, some advances in the knowledge of viral molecular biology, and the identification of main potential antiviral targets, seem to encourage the generation of future specific therapeutics agents capable of inhibiting virus entry to the host cell. Those with protease activity, and antiviral ARN replication, alone or in combinations, are the most eligible drugs to improve pharmacological effectivity and reduce the risk of selecting resistant variants.

## First COVID-19 Vaccines: Efficacy and Clinical Symptoms After Application

The advancement of an effective vaccine that is developed on a large scale, in its initial stage is very important and requires a very wide diffusion and logistics for its application in the general population, especially in the initial stages when the availability of the vaccine is still limited. Vaccines must generate a robust immune response. Currently, various vaccine platforms have been designed, this section describes the main platforms used to develop vaccines against COVID-19. Figure 21.4 shows the percent efficacy of the core mRNA vaccines.

## *Vaccines from Modified Viral mRNA*

Vaccines based RNA are the ones that have attracted the most attention due to their revolutionary techniques. By mid-2021, researchers were developing seven vaccines that use this technology (BNT162, mRNA-1273, CVnCoV, LNP-nCoVsaRNA,

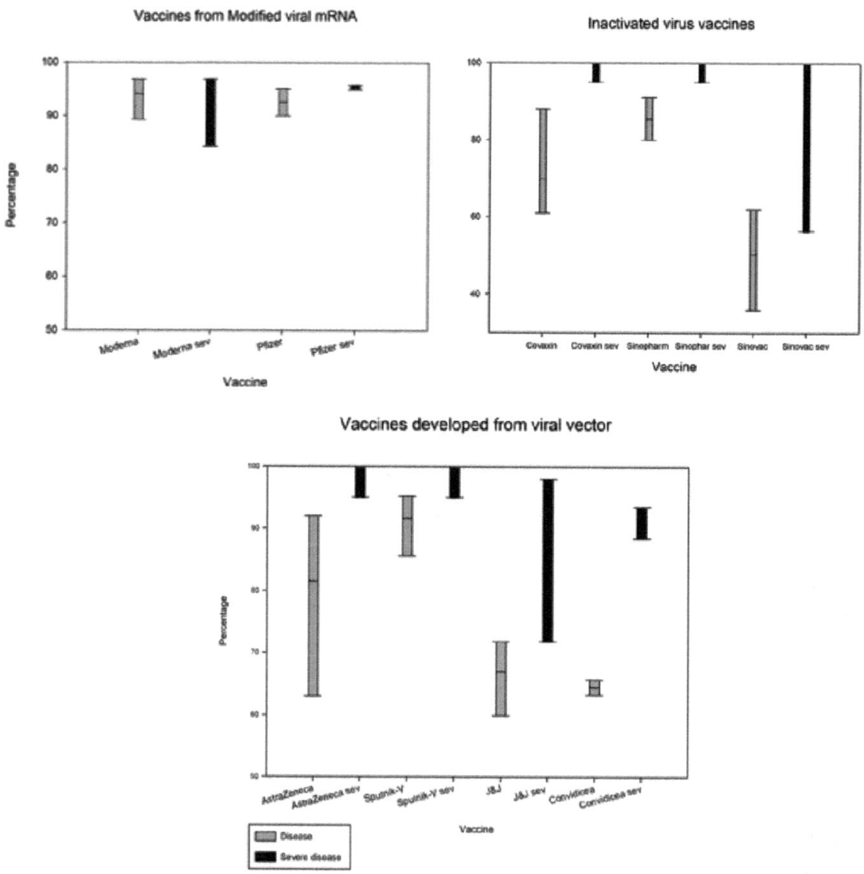


**Fig. 21.4** Vaccine efficacy percentage (95% CI) for COVID-19 disease and severe disease per vaccine platform

ARCT-021, mRNA Vaccine by PLA/Walvax Biotech/Abogen Biosciences).

However, two mRNA COVID-19 vaccines are authorized for their use Pfizer and Moderna.

Tozinameran (BNT162b2) mRNA COVID-19 vaccine developed for the fusion of the American company Pfizer and the German pharmaceutical BioNTech shows the efficacy of 95.3% (94.9–95.7) against infection and 96.7% (96.0–97.3) for severe or critical disease both results in two doses (0.3 mL each) 3 weeks apart all age groups (≥16 years). It is approved in Argentina, Australia, Bahrain, Canada, Chile, Costa Rica, Ecuador, Hong Kong, Iraq, Israel, Jordan, Kuwait, Malaysia, Mexico, Oman, Panama, the Philippines, Qatar, Saudi Arabia, Singapore, South Korea, the United Arab Emirates, and administered in Europa and the USA [33, 34].

The National Institute of Allergy and Infectious Disease and the American pharmaceutical Moderna developed Moderna (mRNA-1273 vaccine). Grants the user of 94.1% (89.3–96.8) protection against COVID-19 illness and severe diseases after administering two doses in the same arm, in a volume of 0.5 mL containing 100 μg given 28 days apart [35–37]. The distribution of Moderna vaccine includes the USA, the European Commission, Japan, Canada, Switzerland, Israel, and Singapore.

## *Vaccines Developed from a Viral Vector*

Oxford University and AstraZeneca Company developed the adenoviral vector vaccine ChAdOx1 nCoV-19 (AZD1222). In India, this vaccine is called Covishield. The vaccine shows an 82.4% (62.7–91.7) efficacy against SARS-CoV-2 after two doses (0.5 mL) separately with 4 to 12 weeks [38] and 100% efficacy against severe disease [39]. In non-EU countries, including Argentina, Bangladesh, Brazil, the Dominican Republic, El Salvador, India, Malaysia, Mexico, Nepal, Vietnam, Pakistan, the Philippines, Sri Lanka, and Taiwan, this vaccine was approved.

Adenovirus (rAd)-based Sputnik V (Gamelaya GamCovidVac), also known as Gam-COVID-Vac, is the Russian vaccine that uses a heterologous recombinant adenovirus approach using adenovirus 26 (Ad26) and adenovirus 5 (Ad5) as vector. It shows the efficacy of 91.6% (85.6–95.2) and 100% for severe disease in two doses (0.5 mL per dose); approved in Algeria, Bolivia, Serbia, Czech Republic, Turkey, the Palestinian territories and distributed in India, Uzbekistan, Mexico, Nepal, and Egypt [40].

Ad26.COV2. S developed for The American multinational corporation Janssen of Johnson & Johnson has an efficacy of 66.3% (59.9–71.8) against symptomatic COVID-19 and 93% (71–98) against hospitalization in a single dose of 0.5 mL [33, 41]. Ad5-nCoV Convidicea viral vector vaccine for COVID-19 developed by the China company CanSino Biologics and Wuhan Institute of Biological Products show 91% efficacy in preventing severe disease and 65.7% efficacy in preventing moderate symptoms of COVID-19 in a single dose; Pakistan, Mexico, Chile, Argentina, and Russia approved the vaccine. Figure 21.4 shows the different efficacy of the platforms.

## *Inactivated Virus Vaccines*

The Chinese vaccine made from the inactivated virus is Coronavac, developed by Sinovac Biotech, that demonstrated an efficacy of 50.7% (36.0–62.0) 14 days after the second dose (3 μg in 0.5 mL) and of 100% (56.4–100) against severe COVID-19 [42]. In many low- and middle-income countries Sinovac is at present the principal COVID-19 vaccine [43]. In addition, BBIBP-CorV developed for the Chinese pharmaceutical company Sinopharm reached 90% (88–91) efficacy against COVID-19 infection in two-dose immunization with two μg/dose. However, the world health organization (WHO) reports that protection against severe disease is a moderate level of confidence [14]. On the other hand India developed covaxin BBV152, a whole-virion inactivated vaccine developed by Bharat Biotech, shown 78% (61–88) efficacy after a two-dose regimen delivered 28 days have 100% of efficacy against severe COVID-19 disease [44].

## *Anaphylactic Reactions and Thrombotic Events*

Since December 2020, anaphylactic responses after administering the Pfizer-BioNTech vaccine have been reported [45]; later, similar reactions occurred with the Moderna vaccine [2]. Although the primary adverse effects reported in clinical trials for COVID-19 mRNA vaccines are pain, swelling, redness at the application site, fever, fatigue, headache, chills, and vomiting [36, 46], these did not contemplate risk for allergies. Universal vaccination reduces the economic costs and provides the best health results [37], mainly since anaphylactic reactions to vaccinations are infrequent, occurring at a rate of about one per million to 30 per 100,000 vaccinations [45]. However, risk stratification is necessary because the reactions presented are not unique to allergies and may be due to other immune-mediated phenomena [47]. Therefore, the main recommendations for administering the vaccines are 30 minutes of observation for persons with mild allergy history, those who suffer from anaphylaxis, allergic to another type of vaccines, mastocytosis, severe acute illness, or women in pregnancy/breastfeeding. Only in persons with a history of allergy to any vaccine component (e.g., PEG, polysorbate) is the vaccination not recommended [46, 48].

Oxford-AstraZeneca vaccine was temporally suspended in March 2021 in several European countries due to blood clot events and death reports. The case report by D'Agostino et al. [49] discloses that the only temporal factor associated with disseminated intravascular coagulation in a woman was the Oxford-AstraZeneca vaccine administration. Nevertheless, epidemiologists conclude that benefits outweigh the population's risk, and multiple causative factors for blood clots events were untested and undetermined [50, 51].

## *Variants*

Viruses constantly change through mutation and appear in new variants. Many variants of the virus have been documented during the pandemic. The top variants reported are the following B.1.1.7 (first detected in the UK), B.1.351 (first detected in South Africa), P.1 (detected in Manaus, Brazil), B.1.526 (identified in New York), B.1.427, and B.1.429 (first identified in California). AstraZeneca reports a 74.6% of efficacy for the B.1.1.7 variant for the approved vaccines. Conversely, Johnson & Johnson reports efficacy of 57% for the B.1.3.5.1 variant, and Novavax declares an efficacy of 85.6% for B.1.1.7 and 60% for B1.3.5.1 variants [1].

To date, 2.8 billion covid vaccines have been administrated 2.8 billion COVID-19 vaccines, and about 40.8 million are now administered per day worldwide. However, vaccination coverage varies significantly by region and country's income level. For example, more than 30% of people in North America and 28% of people in Europe are fully vaccinated, compared to about 11% in South America and 8% in Asia. On the other hand, less than 1% of the population of africa is vaccinated [52]. This lack of vaccines in low-income countries could cause second and third waves where poor hospital care would generate even more deaths from the pandemic.

## Neutralizing Monoclonal Antibodies for COVID-19 Treatment and Prophylaxis

The estimated production and distribution of COVID-19 vaccines worldwide is to take from 1 to 2 years approximately [53]. An alternative that has recently gained interest is passive immunization with neutralizing monoclonal antibodies, been this technology was previously used to treat several viral infections and autoimmune conditions. The monoclonal antibodies are molecules derived from B cells in plasma of recovering COVID-19 convalescent patients developed in a laboratory and designed as an imitator of the body's natural immune system response; then are cloned to mass-produce neutralizing monoclonal antibodies to target different epitopes of SARS2 spike glycoprotein, blocking the viral attachment and entry into human cells as can be seen in Fig. 21.5 [54–56].

Monoclonal antibodies therapy is recommended for patients recently diagnosed with COVID-19 who do not have severe symptoms but do have some risk factors [53], as well as those with preexposure or postexposure such as the unvaccinated or recently vaccinated people [57], vulnerable populations, and high-risk patients including those older than 65 years, with a suppressed immune system, or with certain medical conditions including obesity. Monoclonal antibodies provide another path for the prevention of COVID-19, can produce direct protection from

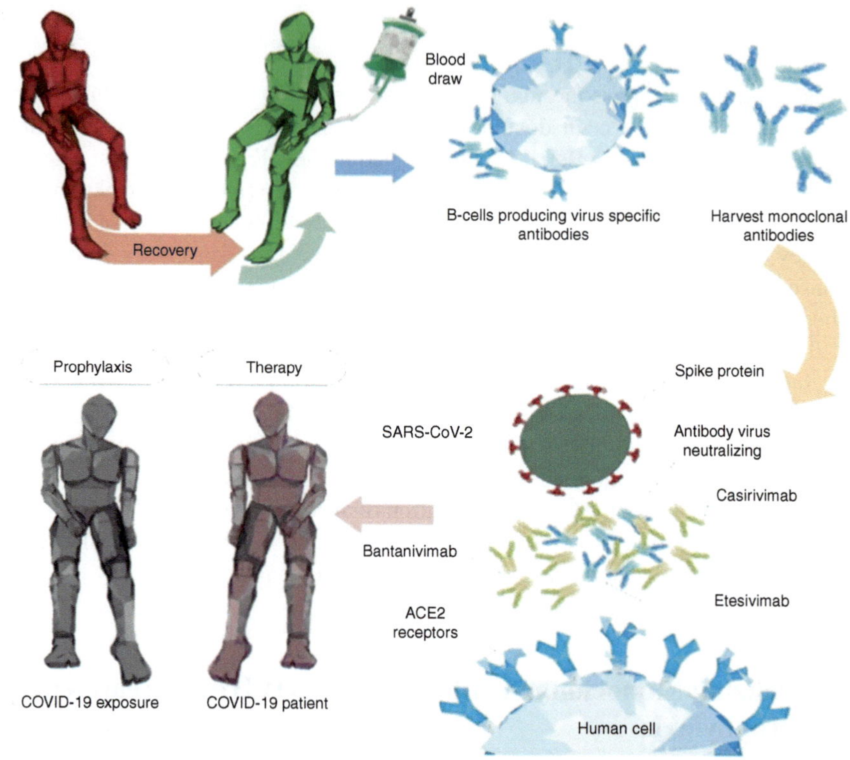


**Fig. 21.5** Monoclonal antibodies produced from B cells of recovered COVID-19 patients attach to the spike protein blocking the viral invasion. Bamlanivimab plus etesevimab and casirivimab-imdevimab are drugs developed from monoclonal antibodies, being tested in patients as a COVID-19 therapy or prophylactic treatment

infection. Inclusive with the new variants of the SARS-CoV-2 monoclonal antibodies have been shown to be effective against the B.1.1.7 variant. However, mutations in the virus can cause variations in the spike protein that could inhibit the efficacy of monoclonal antibodies [56]. For the treatment, the intravenous infusion must be given as soon as possible within 10 days for outpatients who develop symptoms and have comorbid illness conditions with high risks for adverse outcomes [54, 56]. Therapeutic trials will include the treatment of SARS-CoV-2 infected patients with varying degrees of disease. To block the progression of the disease, the patient can receive an intravenous infusion of a monoclonal antibody, showing antiviral activity with treatment in early intervention for medical assistance and avoiding the devastating impact of the virus [16, 53–55].

The FDA has authorized products developed with monoclonal antibodies like casirivimab-imdevimab, sotrovimab, basiliximabvimab, etesevimab, and bamlanivimab (Autrizan Amlanivimab, LY-CoV555) for emergency use against COVID-19. Therapeutic trials will include the treatment of SARS-CoV-2-infected patients with varying degrees of disease. To block the progression of the disease, the patient can receive an intravenous infusion of a monoclonal antibody, showing antiviral activity with treatment in early intervention for medical assistance and avoiding the devastating impact of the virus [58]. Casirivimab-imdevimab (REGEN-COV2) is a two recombinant human immunoglobulin G1 monoclonal antibodies formulation; developed by Regeneron Pharmaceuticals, Inc. [59]. Sotrovimab (Xevudy VIR-7831, GSK4182136) is an investigational human neutralizing dual-action monoclonal antibody development by GlaxoSmithKline and Vir Biotechnology, Inc. [60]. All these monoclonal antibody drugs attach to the spike protein suppressing the ACE2 receptor blocking the viral attachment and entry into the human to stop the spread of the virus, Fig. 21.5. This blockage prevents SARS-CoV-2 infection. These medications are recommended for adults and adolescents at high risk for severe COVID-19 and for patients with mild to moderate COVID-19 disease. These products are not authorized in patients who are hospitalized for COVID-19, who require oxygen therapy, or who need an increase in baseline oxygen flow rate due to COVID-19 [16, 57–60].

Monotherapy patients receiving bamlanivimab show higher rates of COVID-19-related hospitalization compared with patients receiving casirivimab-imdevimab treatment [61]. It is possible that this difference may be due to an increase in SARS-CoV-2 viral variants that are resistant to bamlanivimab alone, due to the failure in the treatment FDA revoked the emergency use of bamlanivimab in April of 2021 [58]. For these reasons Eli Lilly as a result of the collaborative efforts of the Institute of Microbiology of the Chinese Academy of Science developed later etesevimab, both monoclonal antibody compounds bamlanivimab plus etesevimab demonstrate a better mean reduction neutralizing monoclonal antibodies compounds bamlanivimab plus etesevimab demonstrate a better mean reduction in the viral load [16, 62]. Some patients could show experience either an allergic or nonallergic infusion-related reaction [56]. The only clinical complication observed with casirivimab-imdevimab was secondary bacterial pneumonia in one patient, which was successfully treated with a 7-day course of antibiotic therapy [59]. Other consequences of the administration of monoclonal antibodies are flushing, itching, shortness of breath, or low blood pressure [56]. Nevertheless, the benefits of neutralizing monoclonal antibodies significantly reduce hospitalizations and mortality, without posing significant risks based on case or control studies.

## Natural Products in the Treatment Against COVID-19

Several natural products (bioactive compounds, animal products (propolis), vitamins, and others) are promising antivirals against COVID-19. In addition, recent in vitro or silico reports have proposed natural substances against SARS-CoV-2. However, no drugs have been approved as specific antiviral therapy for coronavirus disease so far. Nevertheless, due to the urgency of an effective antiviral treatment against the infection, health specialists have been exploring a wide range of products that could be safely administered. This context includes herbal formulations, most of which are considered safe due to their long history of use; however, there are reports of toxicity due to misidentification or overdose [63]. In that sense, the use of approved natural substances is recommended. Nevertheless, there is already some evidence from clinical cases that study or demonstrate the effectiveness of natural compounds for the COVID-19 treatment.

## *Bioactive Substances and Vitamins in the Treatment of COVID-19*

There are more than 6597 clinical trials registered on ClinicalTrials.gov looking for effective interventions for COVID-19 infection (https://www.clinicaltrials.Gov/ accessed September 20, 2021). In these studies, the components of natural origin are being evaluated and the interventions indicating the doses of the drugs or natural compounds administered to the participants either as a prophylactic or therapeutic treatment in case of positive COVID-19 patients. Figure 21.6 shows the countries conducting studies with the approved natural components studied; it also shows the number of participants in these studies and the stages of clinical trials. Likewise, it can be observed that food supplements such as vitamins D and C are being studied, for the most part, followed by colchicine and the phenolic compound quercetin.

The oral consumption of the FDA approved quercetin has high availability and low toxicity. In vitro studies evaluated its effect (and derivatives); inhibits the

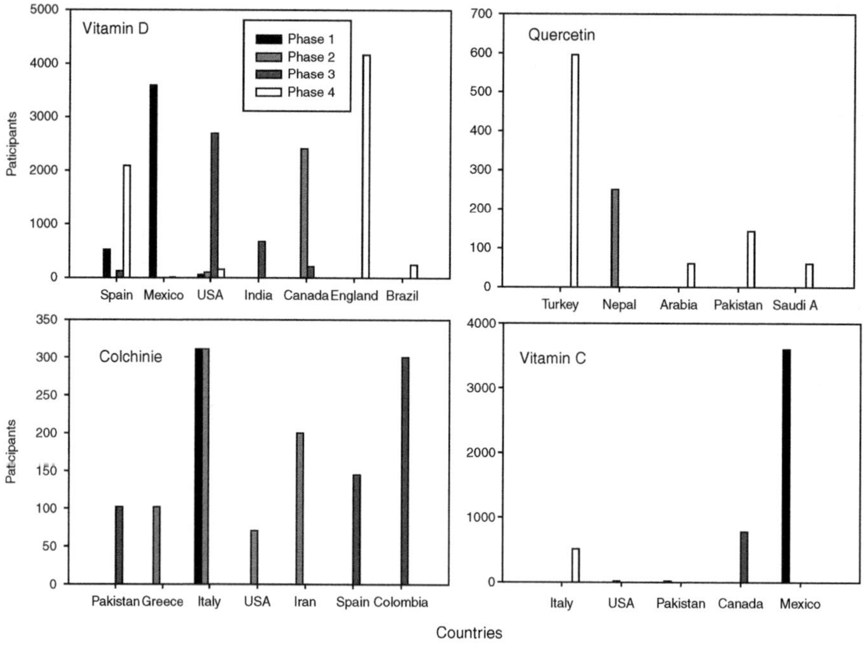


**Fig. 21.6** Intervention studies against COVID-19 were carried out in the world. Information is analyzed in the database of ClinicalTrials.gov

SARS-CoV-1 and MERS-CoV main protease, and the cellular unfolded protein response (UPR) modulation-anti-coronavirus effects have also been found to inhibit the protease of chymotrypsin type 3 ($3CL^{pro}$) which is essential for the replication of the coronavirus [64]. Willianson and Keremy [65] have proposed nasal application of quercetin against the initial infection process of the viral spike protein SARS-CoV-2. However, oral administration of even high doses of quercetin, either as a drug in pure form or in food, has low plasma concentrations.

Colchicine is a traditional anti-inflammatory obtained from the *Colchicum autumnale* plant; it inhibits chemotaxis and neutrophil activity in response to vascular injury, reduces the production of active interleukin-1β and neutrophil-platelet interaction and aggregation [66]. Studies in COVID patients using colchicine show that participants improved statistically significantly reduces cytokine levels as well as the activation of macrophages, neutrophils, and the inflammasome. However, they note that these findings should be interpreted cautiously [67].

Several studies suggest that vitamin D may mediate processes that regulate immunity, supporting antiviral activity and modulating inflammatory responses by reducing the receptive capacity of ACE2 [68]. As shown in Fig. 21.5 several countries are studying the administration of this supplement, England has the highest number of participants in clinical trials, followed by Mexico and the United States of America (USA), and studies carried out in this country have shown that vitamin D deficiency is strongly associated with an increased risk of disease COVID-19.

To date, only one study conducted in Brazil by the group Murai et al. [69] has reported results and observed that high doses of vitamin D3 did not significantly reduce hospital stay in patients with moderate to high COVID-19 infection. Conversely, Mexico has recently completed its study with 41 healthy participants who were administered vitamin D, and their serum levels of the vitamin were measured for 6 months but have not yet reported results.

Vitamin C is a powerful antioxidant that reduces oxidative stress by protecting tissues, in addition to promoting immune functions in the body, causing modulation of cytokines and promoting the production of interferon-α, this property has been used to treat COVID-19 [70]. Ongoing studies are mainly applying this compound intravenously in patients with hypoxia. Fowler et al. [71] show the effects in the treatment of sepsis and acute respiratory tract, indicating the administration of ~15 g/day of vitamin C IV for 4 days with significant benefits in the patient. However, a recent replication carried out in its last study published in the JAMA journal shows that intravenous vitamin C in high doses can alter blood sugar levels and lead to inappropriate use of insulin. They recommend that vitamin C levels in plasma do not exceed approximately 250 μmol to avoid interference in devices https://jamanetwork.com/journals/jama/article-abstract/2761635.

Conversely, other natural compounds such as cannabinoids are being studied in clinical trials; for example, in the USA study with 200,000 patients with the administration of medicinal cannabis is being initiated, and the doses will also be following state laws. Brazil is conducting a similar study and is in phase 2 with 100 positive SARS CoV-2 patients given a daily dose of cannabinoids of 300 mg/day for 14 days. Likewise, regarding plant extracts evaluation, Canada has a study with 480 patients administering one capsule (520 mg) of Açaí Palm Berry extract every 8 h, for 30 days. In China, berberine hydrochloride extract is administered 0.3 g, three times a day by oral or daily tube feeding, until day 14 of the study. In addition, prophylactic studies are being carried out in Pakistan, with more than 1000 participants supplying natural honey mixed with *Nigella Sativa* extract [72].

## *Propolis: A New Alternative Against COVID-19—Cases of Reports*

Propolis (produced by bees) and its extract (usually ethanolic) are known to have positive effects in the treatment of various diseases due to their pharmacological activity complex mixture of substances, in which more than 300 chemical moieties have already been identified, among which the compounds with biological activities [73, 74]. The pharmacological with biological activities [73, 74], including antiviral [75, 76]. In silico, in vitro and in vivo studies show propolis as a promising source for SARS-CoV-2 inhibitor compounds [77]. Rapiri et al. [78] proposed investigating clinical trials to add propolis to antivirals and vaccines in order to reduce the use of medications and side effects. Thus, propolis could be used as a prophylactic or even as a therapeutic in the prevention of SARS-CoV-2, due to its biological properties including production of pro-inflammatory cytokines, p21-activated kinases (PAKs), inhibition of the angiotensin-converting enzyme (ACE), generation of reactive oxygen species production of type I IFN by virus-infected cells, antibody production (humoral immunity), and cell-mediated immunity, which can be increased by propolis.

## *The Use of Propolis: Clinical Cases*

Clinical research using propolis/propolis extract against coronavirus is scarce, most of the research is still in silico studies. Clinical studies referring to the safety (absence of acute toxicity) of the use of propolis extracts (ingestion of 375 mg/day for 5 days of Standardized Propolis Extract (EPP -AF®)) were carried out by Berreta et al. [79].

A recent clinical study, referring to the use of green propolis extract EPP-AF® (standardized green propolis extract) in the treatment of COVID-19 has been carried out by Silveira et al. [80]. The researchers evaluated 124 patients hospitalized with COVID-19, divided into 3 groups: control (without propolis), 40 patients who received 400 mg/day of EPP-AF®, and 42 who received 800 mg/day of EPP-AF®. The researchers found that there was a reduction in post-hospitalization time in the two groups that used propolis compared to the control group of 7 days versus 12 days (400 mg/day of EPP-AF®) and a median of 6 days versus 12 days (800 mg/

day of EPP-AF®). Propolis administration did not significantly affect the need for oxygenation supplementation. In the group that received 800 mg/day of propolis EPP-AF®, there was a lower rate of acute kidney injury than in the controls (4.8 vs 23.8%), and none of the patients treated with propolis (both concentrations) had their treatment stopped due to adverse events. Fiorini et al. [81] reported the first case indicating the therapeutic potential of propolis in SARS-CoV-2 infection observed with the administration of green propolis extracts (EPP-AFs, Apis Flora Indl. Coml. Ltda, Ribeirão Preto, Brazil) up to dose of 45 drops three times a day for 14 days. The patient showed improvement in clinical condition after 12 days with a negative RT-PCR test result.

Currently, there are ongoing studies [72] that use propolis or propolis combined with another natural compound for COVID-19 treatments. Likewise, many efforts are being made by the scientific community to identify the possible therapeutic benefits of propolis against SARS-CoV-2 infection [75, 79, 82].

## Concluding Remarks

The pandemic caused by COVID-19, there is still no adequate control of the pandemic, and prophylactic and therapeutic strategies are still being sought. Most of the reuse drugs that have been used to treat SARS-CoV-2 infection have shown a limited effect and some produce adverse consequences such as cardiovascular problems or bleeding, which have led to the suspension of drug administration. A combination of nucleoside drugs that directly target the viral target in combination with anti-inflammatory drugs appears to be the most promising alternative, as they show a reduction in hospitalization time and the severity of symptoms associated with COVID-19 infection. In addition to this, there are experimental drugs. The development of drugs using neutralizing monoclonal antibodies benefits unvaccinated people with high-risk comorbidities for preventing and treating COVID-19 infection. Although current vaccines have shown an efficiency greater than 90%, recent results in their application to the general population have also shown adverse results and in some cases have led to the temporary suspension in countries of America and Europe, therefore, the use of natural products (vitamins, natural compounds, propolis). Approved by the FDA, they have been used as a complementary biotechnology strategy for the treatment of this infection; however, more clinical trials are still required to adequately support their use. Therefore, regardless of the success of these current interventions, it is important to remain alert to viral genetic changes that could modify the serotype, as well as drug-targeting viral enzymes, resulting in the emergence of resistant strains. Likewise, we must consider the rapid genetic variation that SARS-Cov-2 has been developing, which has given rise to various waves of contagion in the world. Therefore, we must bear in mind that all biotechnological strategies must be reinforced with sanitary measures and timely diagnosis of the infection to stop the impact that COVID-19 has on the population.

## References


1. Mahase E. Coronavirus covid-19 has killed more people than SARS and MERS combined, despite lower case fatality rate. BMJ. 2020;368:m641. Available from:. https://doi.org/10.1136/bmj.m641.
2. Vaccines for COVID-19 | CDC [Internet]. [cited 2021 Sep 22]. https://www.cdc.gov/coronavirus/2019-ncov/vaccines/index.html
3. Zhou Y, Wang F, Tang J, Nussinov R, Cheng F. Artificial intelligence in COVID-19 drug repurposing. Lancet Digit Health. 2020;2(12):e667–76. https://doi.org/10.1016/S2589-7500(20)30192-8.
4. Riva L, Yuan S, Yin X, Martin-Sancho L, Matsunaga N, Burgstaller-Muehlbacher S, et al. A large-scale drug repositioning survey for SARS-CoV-2 antivirals. bioRxiv [Internet]. 2020 [cited 2021 Sep 22];2020.04.16.044016. https://www.biorxiv.org/content/10.1101/2020.04.16.044016v1
5. Sheahan T, Sims A, Zhou S, Graham R, Pruijssers A, Agostini M, et al. An orally bioavailable broad-spectrum antiviral inhibits SARS-CoV-2 in human airway epithelial cell cultures and multiple coronaviruses in mice. Sci Transl Med. 2020;12(541):eabb5883. https://doi.org/10.1126/scitranslmed.abb5883.
6. Weston S, Coleman CM, Haupt R, Logue J, Matthews K, Li Y, et al. Broad anti-coronavirus activity of Food and Drug Administration-approved drugs against SARS-CoV-2 *in vitro* and SARS-CoV *in vivo*. J Virol. 2020;94(21):e01218–20.
7. SGV R, Santos WC. Clinical trials on drug repositioning for COVID-19 treatment. Rev Panam Salud Publica. 2020;44:e40. https://doi.org/10.26633/RPSP.2020.40.
8. Gupta A, Malviya A. Chloroquine and hydroxychloroquine for COVID-19: time to close the chapter. Postgrad Med J. 2020;97(1152):676–7. https://doi.org/10.1136/postgradmedj-2020-138585.
9. Elmi A, S Al Jawad Sayem, Ahmed M, Mohamed F. Natural compounds from Djiboutian medicinal plants as inhibitors of COVID-19 by in silico investigations. 2020. https://chemrxiv.org/engage/chemrxiv/article-details/60c74b5b4c89191f7ead3421
10. Reina J. Remdesivir, the antiviral hope against SARS-CoV-2. Rev Esp Quimioter. 2020;33(3):176–9. https://doi.org/10.37201/req/098.2020.
11. Wang Y, Zhang L, Sang L, Ye F, Ruan S, Zhong B, et al. Kinetics of viral load and antibody response in relation to COVID-19 severity. J Clin Invest. 2020;130(10):5235–44.
12. Beigel J, Tomashek K, Dodd L, Mehta A, Zingman B, Kalil A, et al. Remdesivir for the treatment of Covid-19 - final report. N Engl J Med. 2020;383(19):1813–26. https://doi.org/10.1056/NEJMoa2007764.
13. Emergency Use Authorization | FDA [Internet]. [cited 2021 Sept 22]. https://www.fda.gov/emergency-preparedness-and-response/mcm-legal-regulatory-and-policy-framework/emergency-use-authorization
14. WHO Solidarity Trial Consortium, Pan H, Peto R, Karim QA, Alejandria M, Henao-Restrepo AM, et al. Repurposed antiviral drugs for COVID-19 –interim WHO SOLIDARITY trial results. N Engl J Med. 2021;384(6):497–511. https://doi.org/10.1056/NEJMoa2023184.
15. Shannon A, Le N, Selisko B, Eydoux C, Alvarez K, Guillemot J, et al. Remdesivir and SARS-CoV-2: structural requirements at both nsp12 RdRp and nsp14 exonuclease active-sites. Antiviral Res. 2020;178:104793. https://doi.org/10.1016/j.antiviral.2020.104793.
16. Nathan R, Shawa I, De La Torre I, Pustizzi JM, Haustrup N, Patel DR, et al. A narrative review of the clinical practicalities of Bamlanivimab and Etesevimab antibody therapies for SARS-CoV-2. Infect Dis Ther. 2021;10(4):1933–47. https://doi.org/10.1007/s40121-021-00515-6.
17. Anti-influenza drug Avigan® Tablet Meets Primary Endpoint in Phase III Clinical Trial in Japan for COVID-19 patients | Fujifilm [Japan] [Internet]. [cited 2021 Sep 22]. https://www.fujifilm.com/jp/en/news/hq/5451
18. ISP, Instituto de Salud Pública M de S. ISP autoriza solicitud de importación del medicamento Avifavir para su uso controlado. 2020. http://www.ispch.cl/noticia/30300

19. Hassanipour S, Arab-Zozani M, Amani B, Heidarzad F, Fathalipour M, Martinez-de-Hoyo R. The efficacy and safety of Favipiravir in treatment of COVID-19: A systematic review and meta-analysis of clinical trials. Sci Rep. 2021;11(1):11022. https://doi.org/10.1038/s41598-021-90551-6.
20. Efficacy of Favipiravir in treatment of mild & moderate COVID-19 infection in Nepal - Full Text View - ClinicalTrials.gov [Internet]. [cited 2021 Sept 29]. https://clinicaltrials.gov/ct2/show/NCT04694612
21. Cai Q, Yang M, Liu D, Chen J, Shu D, Xia J, et al. Experimental treatment with Favipiravir for COVID-19: an open-label control study. Engineering (Beijing). 2020;6(10):1192–8. https://doi.org/10.1016/j.eng.2020.03.007.
22. Hung I, Lung K, Tso E, Liu R, Chung T, Chu M, et al. Triple combination of interferon beta-1b, lopinavir-ritonavir, and ribavirin in the treatment of patients admitted to hospital with COVID-19: an open-label, randomised, phase 2 trial. Lancet. 2020;395(10238):1695–704. https://doi.org/10.1016/S0140-6736(20)31042-4.
23. Monk PD, Marsden RJ, Tear VJ, Brookes J, Batten TN, Mankowski M, et al. Safety and efficacy of inhaled nebulised interferon beta-1a (SNG001) for treatment of SARS-CoV-2 infection: a randomised, double-blind, placebo-controlled, phase 2 trial. Lancet Respir Med. 2021;9(2):196–206.
24. Gordon DE, Jang GM, Bouhaddou M, Xu J, Obernier K, White KM, et al. A SARS-CoV-2 protein interaction map reveals targets for drug repurposing. Nature. 2020;583(7816):459–68. https://doi.org/10.1038/s41586-020-2286-9.
25. White KM, Rosales R, Yildiz S, Kehrer T, Miorin L, Moreno E, et al. Plitidepsin has potent preclinical efficacy against SARS-CoV-2 by targeting the host protein eEF1A. Science. 2021;371(6532):926–31. https://doi.org/10.1126/science.abf4058.
26. Proof of concept study to evaluate the safety profile of Plitidepsin in patients with COVID-19 - Full Text View - ClinicalTrials.gov [Internet]. [cited 2021 Sept 29]. https://clinicaltrials.gov/ct2/show/NCT04382066
27. FDA Registration Services for Food, Drug, Medical Device and Cosmetics I FDAbasics [Internet]. [cited 2021 Sep 27]. https://www.fdabasics.com/our-service/fda-registration-services/?https://www.fdabasics.com/our-service/fda-registration-services/&gclid=Cj0KCQjw18WKBhCUARIsAFiW7JxQoRnvned7vSDki6fX6kkKoLR2W2JdeZYpPeIt89G2DOfM2p6HbRYaApc8EALw_wcB
28. Lilly and Incyte announce results from the Phase 3 COV-BARRIER study of baricitinib in hospitalized COVID-19 patients [Internet]. [cited 2021 Sep 27]. https://www.prnewswire.com/news-releases/lilly-and-incyte-announce-results-from-the-phase-3-cov-barrier-study-of-baricitinib-in-hospitalized-covid-19-patients-301264421.html
29. Hospitalized adults: therapeutic management I COVID-19 treatment guidelines [Internet]. [cited 2021 Sept 29]. https://www.covid19treatmentguidelines.nih.gov/management/clinical-management/hospitalized-adults%2D%2Dtherapeutic-management/
30. Fluvoxamine for Early Treatment of Covid-19 (Stop Covid 2) - Full Text View - ClinicalTrials.gov [Internet]. [cited 2021 Sept 29]. https://clinicaltrials.gov/ct2/show/NCT04668950
31. Double blind randomized clinical trial of use of colchicine added to standard treatment in hospitalized with Covid-19 - Full Text View - ClinicalTrials.gov [Internet]. [cited 2021 Sept 29]. https://clinicaltrials.gov/ct2/show/NCT04997551
32. A phase II randomized, double-blind, placebo-controlled study to evaluate the safety and efficacy of exosomes overexpressing CD24 to prevent clinical deterioration in patients with moderate or severe COVID-19 infection - Full Text View - ClinicalTrials.gov [Internet]. [cited 2021 Sept 29]. https://clinicaltrials.gov/ct2/show/NCT04969172
33. Doroftei B, Ciobica A, Ilie O, Maftei R, Ilea C. Mini-review discussing the reliability and efficiency of COVID-19 vaccines. Diagnostics (Basel). 2021;11(4):579. https://doi.org/10.3390/diagnostics11040579.
34. Haas EJ, Angulo FJ, McLaughlin JM, Anis E, Singer SR, Khan F, et al. Impact and effectiveness of mRNA BNT162b2 vaccine against SARS-CoV-2 infections and COVID-19 cases,

hospitalisations, and deaths following a nationwide vaccination campaign in Israel: an observational study using national surveillance data. Lancet. 2021;397(10287):1819–29. https://doi.org/10.1016/S0140-6736(21)00947-8.
35. Živković S, Gruener G, Narayanaswami P. Doctor-should i get the COVID-19 vaccine? Infection and immunization in individuals with neuromuscular disorders. Muscle Nerve. 2021;63(3):294–303. https://doi.org/10.1002/mus.27179.
36. Meo S, Bukhari I, Akram J, Meo A, Klonoff D. COVID-19 vaccines: comparison of biological, pharmacological characteristics and adverse effects of Pfizer/BioNTech and Moderna vaccines. Eur Rev Med Pharmacol Sci. 2021;25(3):1663–79. https://doi.org/10.26355/eurrev_202102_24877.
37. Shaker M, Abrams E, Greenhawt M. A cost-effectiveness evaluation of hospitalizations, fatalities, and economic outcomes associated with universal versus anaphylaxis risk-stratified COVID-19 vaccination strategies. J Allergy Clin Immunol Pract. 2021;9(7):2658–2668.e3. https://doi.org/10.1016/j.jaip.2021.02.054.
38. Voysey M, Clemens SAC, Madhi SA, Weckx LY, Folegatti PM, Aley PK, et al. Safety and efficacy of the ChAdOx1 nCoV-19 vaccine (AZD1222) against SARS-CoV-2: an interim analysis of four randomised controlled trials in Brazil, South Africa, and the UK. Lancet. 2021;397(10269):99–111. https://doi.org/10.1016/S0140-6736(20)32661-1.
39. Pramod S, Govindan D, Ramasubramani P, Kar SS, Aggarwal R, JIPMER vaccine effectiveness study group. Effectiveness of Covishield vaccine in preventing Covid-19 -- A test-negative case-control study. Vaccine. 2021;40(24):3294–7. https://doi.org/10.1016/j.vaccine.2022.02.014.
40. Logunov DY, Dolzhikova IV, Shcheblyakov DV, Tukhvatulin AI, Zubkova OV, Dzharullaeva AS, et al. Safety and efficacy of an rAd26 and rAd5 vector-based heterologous prime-boost COVID-19 vaccine: an interim analysis of a randomised controlled phase 3 trial in Russia. Lancet. 2021;397(10275):671–81. https://doi.org/10.1016/S0140-6736(21)00234-8.
41. Olliaro P, Torreele E, Vaillant M. COVID-19 vaccine efficacy and effectiveness—the elephant (not) in the room. Lancet Microbe. 2021;2(7):e279–80. https://doi.org/10.1016/S2666-5247(21)00069-0.
42. Palacios R, Batista AP, Albuquerque CSN, Patiño EG, Joane do Prado Santos, Tilli Reis Pessoa Conde M, et al. Efficacy and safety of a COVID-19 inactivated vaccine in healthcare professionals in Brazil: the PROFISCOV study. SSRN Electron J. 2021. https://papers.ssrn.com/abstract=3822780
43. Lloyd-Sherlock P, Muljono P, Ebrahim S. Ageism in Indonesia's national covid-19 vaccination programme. BMJ. 2021;372:n299. https://doi.org/10.1136/bmj.n299.
44. Merck and Ridgeback biotherapeutics provide update on progress of clinical development program for Molnupiravir, an investigational oral therapeutic for the treatment of mild-to-moderate COVID-19 | Business Wire [Internet]. [cited 2021 Sept 27]. https://www.businesswire.com/news/home/20210415005258/en/Merck-and-Ridgeback-Biotherapeutics-Provide-Update-on-Progress-of-Clinical-Development-Program-for-Molnupiravir-an-Investigational-Oral-Thera peutic-for-the-Treatment-of-Mild-to-Moderate-COVID-19
45. Klimek L, Novak N, Hamelmann E, Werfel T, Wagenmann M, Taube C, et al. Severe allergic reactions after COVID-19 vaccination with the Pfizer/BioNTech vaccine in Great Britain and USA: Position statement of the German Allergy Societies: Medical Association of German Allergologists (AeDA), German Society for Allergology and Clinical Immunology (DGAKI) and Society for Pediatric Allergology and Environmental Medicine (GPA). Allergo J Int. 2021;30(2):51–5. https://doi.org/10.1007/s40629-020-00160-4.
46. CDC COVID-19 Response Team, Food and Drug Administration. Allergic reactions including anaphylaxis after receipt of the first dose of Moderna COVID-19 vaccine — United States, December 21, 2020–January 10, 2021. Morb Mortal Wkly Rep. 2021;70(4):125. https://doi.org/10.15585/mmwr.mm7004e1.
47. Greenhawt G, Abrams E, Oppenheimer J, Vander Leek T, Mack D, Singer A, et al. The COVID-19 pandemic in 2021: avoiding overdiagnosis of anaphylaxis risk while safely vacci-

nating the world. J allergy Clin Immunol Pract. 2021;9(4):1438–41. https://doi.org/10.1016/j.jaip.2021.01.022.
48. Ortega Rodríguez N, Audícana Berasategui M, de la Hoz Caballer B, Valero Santiago A. The century of mRNA vaccines: COVID-19 vaccines and allergy. J Investig Allergol Clin Immunol. 2021;31(1):89–91. https://doi.org/10.18176/jiaci.0665.
49. D'Agostino V, Caranci F, Negro A, Piscitelli V, Tuccillo B, Fasano F, et al. A rare case of cerebral venous thrombosis and disseminated intravascular coagulation temporally associated to the COVID-19 vaccine administration. J Pers Med. 2021;11(4):285. https://doi.org/10.3390/jpm11040285.
50. Tobaiqy M, Elkout H, MacLure K. Analysis of thrombotic adverse reactions of COVID-19 AstraZeneca vaccine reported to EudraVigilance Database. Vaccines2021 9(4):393. https://doi.org/10.3390/vaccines9040393
51. Wise J. Covid-19: European countries suspend use of Oxford-AstraZeneca vaccine after reports of blood clots. BMJ. 2021;372:n699. https://doi.org/10.1136/bmj.n699.
52. Mathieu E, Ritchie H, Ortiz-Ospina E, Roser M, Hasell J, Appel C, et al. A global database of COVID-19 vaccinations. Nat Hum Behav. 2021;5(7):947–53. https://doi.org/10.1038/s41562-021-01122-8.
53. Jaworski J. Neutralizing monoclonal antibodies for COVID-19 treatment and prevention. Biomed J. 2021;44(1):7–17. https://doi.org/10.1016/j.bj.2020.11.011.
54. Pallotta A, Kim C, Gordon S, Kim A. Monoclonal antibodies for treating COVID-19. Cleve Clin J Med. 2021. https://doi.org/10.3949/ccjm.88a.ccc074
55. Marovich M, Mascola JR, Cohen MS. Monoclonal antibodies for prevention and treatment of COVID-19. JAMA. 2020;324(2):131–2. https://doi.org/10.1001/jama.2020.10245.
56. Lloyd E, Gandhi T, Petty L. Monoclonal antibodies for COVID-19. JAMA. 2021;325(10):1015. https://doi.org/10.1001/jama.2021.1225.
57. Taylor PC, Adams AC, Hufford MM, de la Torre I, Winthrop K, Gottlieb RL. Neutralizing monoclonal antibodies for treatment of COVID-19. Nat Rev Immunol. 2021;21(6):382–93. https://doi.org/10.1038/s41577-021-00542-x.
58. Tuccori M, Convertino I, Ferraro S, Valdiserra G, Cappello E, Fini E, et al. An overview of the preclinical discovery and development of bamlanivimab for the treatment of novel coronavirus infection (COVID-19): reasons for limited clinical use and lessons for the future. Expert Opin Drug Discov. 2021;16(12):1403–14.
59. Weinreich DM, Sivapalasingam S, Norton T, Ali S, Gao H, Bhore R, et al. REGN-COV2, a neutralizing antibody cocktail, in outpatients with Covid-19. N Engl J Med. 2021;384(3):238–51.
60. Aschenbrenner DS. Monoclonal antibodies receive EUA to treat mild to moderate COVID-19. Am J Nurs. 2021;121(2):26.
61. Hurt A, Wheatley A. Neutralizing antibody therapeutics for COVID-19. Viruses. 2021;13(4):628. https://doi.org/10.3390/v13040628.
62. Dougan M, Nirula A, Azizad M, Mocherla B, Gottlieb RL, Chen P, et al. Bamlanivimab plus Etesevimab in mild or moderate Covid-19. N Engl J Med. 2021;385(15):1382–92. https://doi.org/10.1056/NEJMoa2102685.
63. Lutoti S, Okwany P, Ajayi CO, Oloro J. Formulation and standardization of herbal medicinal products: a review of formulation considerations, quality control and safety of herbal products. J Pharm Drug Res. 2020;3(3):373–81.
64. Polansky H, Lori G. Coronavirus disease 2019 (COVID-19): first indication of efficacy of Gene-Eden-VIR/Novirin in SARS-CoV-2 infection. Int J Antimicrob Agents. 2020;55(6):105971.
65. Williamson G, Kerimi A. Testing of natural products in clinical trials targeting the SARS-CoV-2 (Covid-19) viral spike protein-angiotensin converting enzyme-2 (ACE2) interaction. Biochem Pharmacol. 2020;178:114123. https://doi.org/10.1016/j.bcp.2020.114123.
66. Leung Y, Yao Hui L, Kraus V. Colchicine--Update on mechanisms of action and therapeutic uses. Semin Arthritis Rheum. 2015;45(3):341–50. https://doi.org/10.1016/j.semarthrit.2015.06.013.
67. Deftereos SG, Giannopoulos G, Vrachatis DA, Siasos GD, Giotaki SG, Gargalianos P, et al. Effect of Colchicine vs Standard Care on Cardiac and Inflammatory Biomarkers and Clinical

Outcomes in Patients Hospitalized With Coronavirus Disease 2019: The GRECCO-19 Randomized Clinical Trial. JAMA Netw Open. 2020;3(6):e2013136. https://doi.org/10.1001/jamanetworkopen.2020.13136.
68. Manson J, Bassuk S. Commentary. Eliminating vitamin D deficiency during the COVID-19 pandemic: a call to action. Metabolism. 2020;112:154322. https://doi.org/10.1016/j.metabol.2020.154322.
69. Murai I, Fernandes A, Sales L, Pinto A, Goessler K, Duran C, et al. Effect of a single high dose of vitamin D3 on hospital length of stay in patients with moderate to severe COVID-19: a randomized clinical trial. JAMA. 2021;325(11):1053–60. https://doi.org/10.1001/jama.2020.26848.
70. Carr A. A new clinical trial to test high-dose vitamin C in patients with COVID-19. Crit Care. 2020;24(1):133. https://doi.org/10.1186/s13054-020-02851-4.
71. Fowler A, Fisher B, Kashiouris M. Vitamin C for sepsis and acute respiratory failure-reply. JAMA. 2020;323(8):792–3. https://doi.org/10.1001/jama.2019.21987.
72. ClinicalTrials.gov [Internet]. [cited 2021 Sep 29]. https://www.clinicaltrials.gov/
73. Devequi-Nunes D, Machado BAS, Barreto G d A, Silva JR, da Silva DF, da JLC R, et al. Chemical characterization and biological activity of six different extracts of propolis through conventional methods and supercritical extraction. PLoS One. 2018;13(12):e0207676. https://doi.org/10.1371/journal.pone.0207676.
74. Bankova VS, de Castro SL, Marcucci MC. Propolis: recent advances in chemistry and plant origin. Apidologie. 2000;31(1):3–15. https://doi.org/10.1051/apido:2000102.
75. Bachevski D, Damevska K, Simeonovski V, Dimova M. Back to the basics: propolis and COVID-19. Dermatol Ther. 2020;33(4):e13780. https://doi.org/10.1111/dth.13780.
76. Santos L, Fonseca M, Sokolonski A, Deegan K, Araújo R, Umsza-Guez M, et al. Propolis: types, composition, biological activities, and veterinary product patent prospecting. J Sci Food Agric. 2020;100(4):1369–82. https://doi.org/10.1002/jsfa.10024.
77. Guler H, Tatar G, Yildiz O, Belduz A, Kolayli S. Investigation of potential inhibitor properties of ethanolic propolis extracts against ACE-II receptors for COVID-19 treatment by molecular docking study. Arch Microbiol. 2021;203(6):3557–64. https://doi.org/10.1007/s00203-021-02351-1.
78. Ripari N, Sartori AA, da Silva Honorio M, Conte FL, Tasca KI, Santiago KB, et al. Propolis antiviral and immunomodulatory activity: a review and perspectives for COVID-19 treatment. J Pharm Pharmacol. 2021;73(3):281–99. https://doi.org/10.1093/jpp/rgaa067.
79. Berretta AA, Silveira MAD, Cóndor Capcha JM, De Jong D. Propolis and its potential against SARS-CoV-2 infection mechanisms and COVID-19 disease: running title: Propolis against SARS-CoV-2 infection and COVID-19. Biomed Pharmacother. 2020;131:110622.
80. Silveira M, Teles F, Berretta A, Sanches T, Rodrigues C, Seguro A, et al. Effects of Brazilian green propolis on proteinuria and renal function in patients with chronic kidney disease: a randomized, double-blind, placebo-controlled trial. BMC Nephrol. 2019;20(1):140. https://doi.org/10.1186/s12882-019-1337-7.
81. Fiorini AC, Scorza CA, de Almeida A-CG, Fonseca MCM, Finsterer J, Fonseca FLA, et al. Antiviral activity of Brazilian Green Propolis extract against SARS-CoV-2 (Severe Acute Respiratory Syndrome - Coronavirus 2) infection: case report and review. Clinics. 2021;76:1–4. https://doi.org/10.6061/clinics/2021/e2357.
82. Scorza C, Gonçalves V, Scorza F, Fiorini A, de Almeida A, Fonseca M, et al. Propolis and coronavirus disease 2019 (COVID-19): lessons from nature. Complement Ther Clin Pract. 2020;41:101227. https://doi.org/10.1016/j.ctcp.2020.101227.

# Chapter 22
# Vitamin D: A Potential Prophylactic and Therapeutic Agent against COVID-19

**Zaki A. Sherif**

## Introduction

The dilemma for academic and clinical researchers is whether vitamin D has any role against COVID-19. This essential micronutrient is considered an important factor in immune homeostasis. Vitamin D deficiency or insufficiency is associated with suboptimal health across the spectrum. In the current coronavirus pandemic, the contribution of vitamin D deficiency to respiratory infections, inflammation, progressive disease, and cardiovascular dysregulation is not universally accepted. The novel coronavirus, which causes COVID-19 (Coronavirus Disease of 2019) and identified as Severe Acute Respiratory Syndrome Coronavirus-2 (SARS-CoV-2), has globally killed more people than SARS-CoV-1 (10%) and Middle East Respiratory Syndrome Coronavirus (MERS-CoV, 34%) combined, despite lower case fatality rate of 2% [1]. As of September 30, 2021, the global estimate of infections is about 3% (233,479,934) and 4,777,581 deaths linked to SARS-CoV-2, according to the latest data from the Johns Hopkins University tracking dashboard [2]. Although cases have been documented across virtually all demographics, patients over 60 years old and those with comorbidities experienced the highest mortality rate [3–7]. The coronavirus incidence was declared a global pandemic on March 11, 2020 by the World Health Organization (WHO). In the USA, which is the leading country in infection and mortality rates, approximately 43,370,976 people have been infected, with a death toll of over 695,523 [2]. It seems that distribution of cases and deaths across the globe are unequal, with most African

Z. A. Sherif (✉)
Department of Biochemistry & Molecular Biology, Howard University College of Medicine, Washington, DC, USA
e-mail: Zaki.sherif@howard.edu


S. Adibi et al. (eds.), *Frontiers of COVID-19*,
https://doi.org/10.1007/978-3-031-08045-6_22

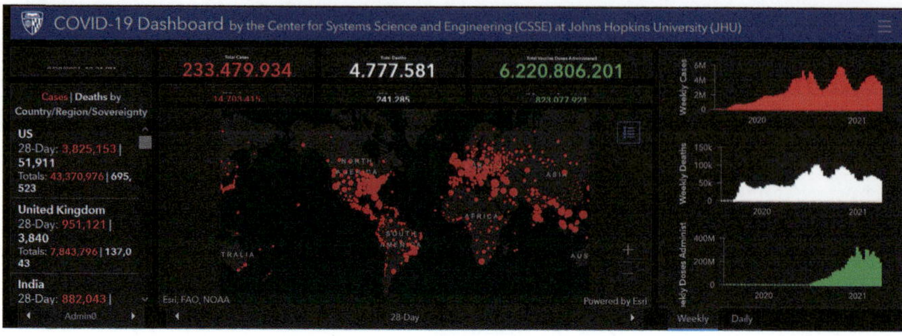


**Fig. 22.1** Global map tracking COVID-19 cases, deaths, and vaccinations [2]

countries being spared the worst of the pandemics as vividly demonstrated on the updated Global pandemic map dated September 29, 2021 [2] (Fig. 22.1) (https://coronavirus.jhu.edu/map.html).

For over a year, avoiding transmission of the virus and prevention of the disease were only possible by donning personal protective equipment (PPE), keeping personal hygiene, social distancing, and wide-scale lockdowns by governments worldwide. Those exposed to the virus or infected by it had to quarantine and isolate themselves for about two weeks during the mild and moderate phases of COVID-19. However, those exhibiting severe symptoms including persistent high fever and shortness of breath (dyspnea) had to be hospitalized with supplemental oxygen, or under critical situations, admitted to intensive care units (ICUs), intubated, and placed on ventilators where most of the early victims of the virus perished [8]. It is probable that the main vehicles or vectors for the widespread transmission of the virus among people in the local community and beyond were asymptomatic individuals who were not aware of their infection.

## *SARS-CoV-2 and COVID-19*

SARS-CoV-2 belongs to Coronaviruses (CoVs) family called Coronaviridae, which are a group of highly diverse, enveloped, positive-sense viruses, with single-stranded RNA genomes ranging from 26 to 32 kilobases in length [9]. All coronaviruses, which have been known to exist since the 1960s, share similarities in the organizational structure and expression of their genome, which consists of 16 nonstructural proteins (nsp1 through nsp16), encoded by open reading frame (ORF) 1a/b at the 5′ end, trimeric structural protein, spike (S), envelope (E), membrane (M), and nucleocapsid (N), which are encoded by other ORFs at the 3′ end. There are four genera in CoVs: alpha-CoV (group 1), beta-CoV (group 2), gamma-CoV (group 3), and delta-CoV (group 4) [10, 11]. These viruses vary broadly from benevolent infections like seasonal flu caused by rhinoviruses and influenza A or B to lethal infections like COVID-19 caused by the emerging SARS-CoV-2. The COVID-19 pandemic has demonstrated that a significant number of infected subjects remain asymptomatic or experience only mild symptoms (e.g., fever, cough, dyspnea, myalgia, fatigue, or intermittent diarrhea). However, there are many others that develop moderate to severe disease, exemplified by interstitial pneumonia that can progress to acute respiratory distress syndrome (ARDS) and result in death from critical respiratory failure or other complications [12, 13].

The outcome of SARS-CoV-2 infection may also depend on the degree of imbalance in the host immune system [14–16]. The immune system is divided into two types: innate (i.e., general) or nonspecific, and adaptive (i.e., specialized) or specific immunity. In the primary immune response against pathogenic antigens, the natural exertion will have a positive effect against infection, facilitating viral clearance. However, the hypothesis with respect to SARS-CoV-2 is that the secondary immune response, in a segment of the population, may be exaggerated and challenge tissue architectural integrity and perturb physiological homeostasis, which may lead to multiple organ failure, ARDS, and death [16]. Older age and the presence of major comorbidities (e.g., chronic obstructive pulmonary disease, chronic cardiovascular disease, chronic renal disease, diabetes mellitus, hypertension, obesity, and other endocrine disorders) may exacerbate the COVID-19 condition and lead to fatality due to elevated cytokine levels or other inflammatory markers virally driven by hyperinflammation, known as "cytokine storm" [4, 6, 7, 17, 18].

Despite rigorous attempts to curtail SARS-CoV-2 infection, transmission, and its adverse effects on the human body, even after seventeen months of this pandemic, there has been little progress in treatment options for almost a year until the vaccines came to the rescue. In the early stages of the pandemic, one persistent challenge in curtailing the course of the disease has been the absence of experimental evidence to support effective pharmacologic interventions to prevent or treat COVID-19. The early hospitalized victims of this megapandemic were subjected to varied levels of treatment regimen consisting of individual off-label drugs or a combination of FDA-approved (i.e., under Emergency Authorization Use) antiviral drugs like remdesivir; antimalarial drugs like hydroxychloroquine; corticosteroids such as dexamethasone; monoclonal antibody infusions; convalescent plasma; and/or a cocktail of minerals like zinc, vitamins C and D [19–23].

## *Vitamin D, Its Various Forms, and Functions*

Vitamin D is a fat-soluble vitamin that is stored in the liver and serves as a steroid hormone. There are several forms and metabolites of vitamin D. The two major forms are vitamin $D_2$ (ergocalciferol), which is synthesized by fungi such as mushrooms, and vitamin $D_3$ (cholecalciferol), which is naturally made by the body in response to sunlight. The chemical formulas and structures of vitamin $D_2$ and vitamin $D_3$ are shown in Fig. 22.2.

Both vitamins $D_2$ and $D_3$, which undergo an identical metabolic process, can be used for supplementation. However, a meta-analysis of randomized controlled trials

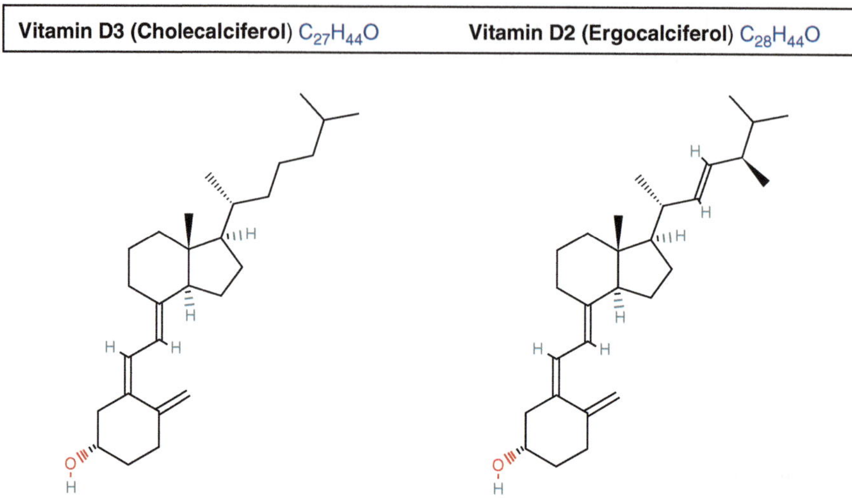


**Fig. 22.2** The structures of the two major forms of vitamin D in foods and dietary supplements. (Image Credit: https://pubchem.ncbi.nlm.nih.gov)

(RCTs) indicates that vitamin $D_3$ is more efficacious at raising serum 25-hydroxyvitamin D [25(OH)D] concentrations than vitamin $D_2$ and may be a better choice for supplementation [24]. This essential micronutrient is considered an important factor in immune homeostasis particularly due to vitamin D receptor (VDR) and Cytochrome P450 Family 27 Subfamily B Member 1 (CYP27B1) expression in most of the immune cells. As an essential nutrient, vitamin D has various roles in the body including the development, function, and maintenance of healthy bones and teeth through the regulation of mineral homeostasis of the skeleton by promoting calcium and phosphorus absorption in the gut system [25]. Almost every cell in our body has a receptor for VDR, which is a member of the nuclear receptor/steroid hormone superfamily that also includes receptors for thyroid and steroid hormones as well as retinoids [26]. Vitamin D is also essential for immune system function and cardiovascular homeostasis, and can help protect against cancer [27–30]. Unfortunately, subclinical vitamin D deficiency is more prevalent and is linked to the occurrence of rickets in children, and osteomalacia (bone-softening) and osteoporosis (bone fracturing) in adults [31]. Nevertheless, additional research is required to examine the metabolic pathways involved in oral and intramuscular administration of vitamin D and the effects across age, sex, and ethnicity, which this review was unable to verify.

The sunlight source of vitamin D is ultraviolet B (UVB) radiation, which activates a photochemical reaction in the plasma membrane of epidermal keratinocytes and dermal fibroblasts in the skin, producing an unstable 7-dehydrocholesterol, which forms pre-vitamin $D_3$, which upon thermal isomerization produces a stable form of vitamin $D_3$ (cholecalciferol). The photosynthesized vitamin $D_3$ binds to vitamin D binding protein (VBP) and is converted in the liver by 25-hydroxylase (aka CYP2R1) to form a biologically inactive 25-hydroxyvitamin $D_3$ (aka 25-hydroxychlecalceferol or calcidiol or calcifediol), through the action of cytochrome P450 enzymes [32]. The 25-hydroxycholecalciferol [25(OH)$D_3$] is the storage form of vitamin D. In the kidney, 25(OH)$D_3$ undergoes further hydroxylation at the C-1α or C-24 positions by the enzyme 1α-hydroxylase (aka CYP27B1) to produce 1,25-dihydroxyvitamin D [1α,25(OH)2$D_3$] or [1,25$(OH)_2$D]), the active hormonal form in the body and the ligand for a transcription factor, the vitamin D receptor (VDR), as shown in Fig. 22.3.

The conversion of calcidiol to calcitriol (1,25-dihydroxycholecalciferol) mainly occurs in the kidney. But this conversion also occurs in the different cells and tissues of the immune system such as the lymph nodes, alveolar macrophages as well as the alveoli cells [33]. If so, vitamin D may be activated in the alveoli, the sac-like cells responsible for gas exchange between oxygen and carbon dioxide. These are the same cells that bacteria as well as viruses such as the influenza and coronavirus invade in our lungs. It is therefore possible that our lungs exert a natural ability to fight off respiratory infections.

The natural dietary sources of vitamin D include fatty fish like salmon, sardines, mackerel, and herring. Fortified products such as milk and cereals that are designed to reduce rickets in young children and osteomalacia in adults, also contain a small amount of vitamin D. The term vitamin D insufficiency has been used to describe low levels of serum 25-hydroxyvitamin D (aka calcidiol and abbreviated as [25(OH) D],) that may be associated with an increased risk of death in adults from cardiovascular diseases, cognitive impairment [34], chronic kidney disease [35] and cancer [36]. Mega doses from foods or supplements can be toxic. There is no international consensus on the right amount of vitamin D to supplement the diet since people can obtain the daily required dose both from sunlight and dietary sources. However,

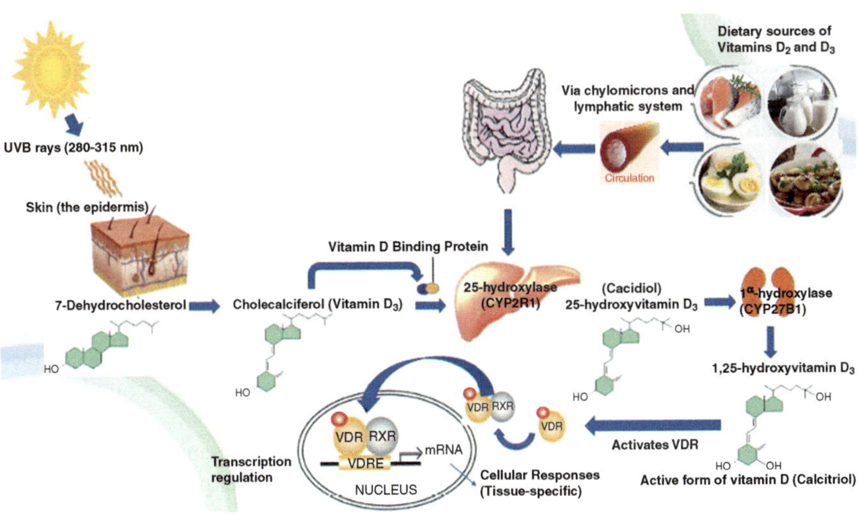


**Fig. 22.3** The biosynthesis of 1,25-hydroxyvitamin $D_3$

**Table 22.1** Serum 25-Hydroxyvitamin D [25(OH)D] Concentrations

| Status | Serum 25-hydroxyvitamin D [25(OH)D]) ng/ml | Serum 25-hydroxyvitamin D [25(OH)D]) nmol/L |
|---|---|---|
| Normal levels | Above 20 | Above 50 |
| Vitamin D insufficiency | 12 to 20 | 30 to 50 |
| Vitamin D deficiency | Less than 12 | Less than 30 |
| Adverse effects | Above 50 | Above 125 |

[a]Serum concentrations of 25(OH)D. are reported in both nanomoles per liter (nmol/L) and nanograms per milliliter (ng/mL). One nmol/L = 0.4 ng/ml, and 1 ng/ml = 2.5 nmol/L

there is a standard range of serum concentrations of 25(OH)D from deficient to adverse levels published by the Institute of Medicine, Food and Nutrition Board (https://www.ncbi.nlm.nih.gov/books/NBK56070/) [37] (see Table 22.1).

The chief source of Vitamin $D_3$ is sunlight and not food. About 50% to 90% of vitamin D is absorbed through the skin via sunlight while the rest comes from the diet [38]. Twenty minutes of sunshine daily with over 40% of skin exposed is required to prevent vitamin D deficiency [39, 40]. Effective sun exposure is decreased in individuals who use sunscreens consistently. It is important to note that in humans, sunlight exposure is the primary determinant of vitamin D level mainly in northern latitudes from November to March, when there are insufficient UVB rays to produce vitamin D, whose status has become of a major health concern since 2009 when U.S. population trend health study declared that 75% of U.S. teenagers and adults were deficient in vitamin D [41, 42]. This is also particularly true, as ecological studies report, for human populations in countries (with some exceptions) that lie at the 35 degrees north latitude, above which humans receive insufficient sunlight for vitamin D adequacy during winter [43, 44]. For comparison, 40 degrees north latitude runs through the middle of the United States.

The cutaneous production of the vitamin involves several factors including geography. Humans first evolved in Africa near the equator where the sun's rays directly hit the earth most of the year, and for our ancestors who received adequate vitamin D, their sole protection from the damaging effects of UVB radiation came from melanin in their dark skin. However, as more humans moved away from the equator, their skins lightened to efficiently absorb vitamin D because of reduced direct sunshine. This is because during the winter months, the earth tilts away from the sun, causing less rays reaching the earth. Darker-skinned people will absorb less UVB light, leading to less vitamin D production. Therefore, the distribution of 25(OH)D concentrations presented in Table 22.1 may need to be elevated for dark-skinned people as demonstrated by a study that examined similar 25(OH)D serum levels by race and ethnicity (Fig. 22.4).

It is known that at higher latitudes, people with more melanin content in their skin tend to have lower blood levels of vitamin D even after exposure to sunlight. A recent article speculates that this vitamin D deficiency significantly linked to the disproportionately high COVID-19 cases and deaths among US Black and Latino populations [46].

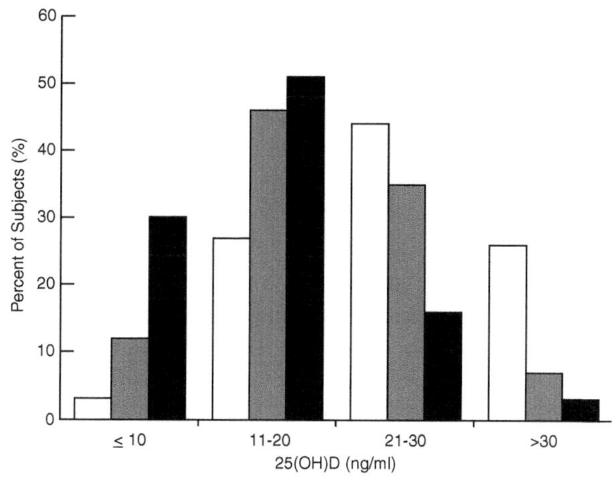


**Fig. 22.4** Distribution of 25(OH)D concentrations by race and ethnicity. White bars indicate white participants ($N = 4309$), gray bars indicate Mexican American participants ($N = 2025$), and black bars indicate black participants ($N = 2081$) [45]

The aging process. also leads to less efficient production of vitamin D, which is common in older people. Vitamin $D_3$, which is converted to the active form of vitamin D, 1,25-dihydroxycholecalciferol (aka calcitriol), has many important roles in the body including signaling the intestine to absorb calcium into the bloodstream to avoid breaking down bones to enhance calcium levels in the blood; to reduce bone fractures in the elderly by preventing muscle deterioration. Lower vitamin D intake orally is more prevalent in the elderly population [47]. Recently reported cases of elevated COVID-19 cases occurred in Italy and Spain, two countries with high prevalence of vitamin D deficiency, which is associated with obesity, hypertension, diabetes, and ethnicity—features also common in COVID-19 patients [44].

## The Role of Vitamin D in Respiratory Infections and COVID-19: A Case for Its Prophylactic Effect

Although, vitamin D testing has drastically increased recently, the relevance and widespread vitamin D deficiency are still under debate [48]. Some researchers even dismiss vitamin D's role more as an associative than a causal factor in acute and chronic disease. On the other hand, a low vitamin D status is emerging as a public health concern worldwide, and several studies from basic science to clinical applications have highlighted a strong association with chronic diseases, as well as acute conditions. Moreover, the large amount of observational data currently available are also supported by pathophysiological links of vitamin D with energy homeostasis, as well as regulation of the immune and endocrine systems [49]. Furthermore, more recent reports indicate that vitamin D plays a protective role in reducing the risk and the severity of respiratory tract infections (RTIs) caused not only by seasonal viruses such as the human influenza A and B but also by the beta coronavirus family members SARS-CoV-1, Middle East Respiratory Syndrome (MERS), and SARS-CoV-2

[41, 42, 50–53]. The beneficial effects of vitamin D on the musculoskeletal system and the pleiotropic extraskeletal effects of this vitamin are increasingly being recognized and acknowledged [54–56]. Latest clinical reports also reveal that vitamin D deficiency contributes to ARDS because of SARS-CoV-2 infection, and that case-fatality rates increase concomitantly with age and viral load [57, 58]. The postulation here is that vitamin D status may be important in determining the severity of the immune response to SARS-CoV-2 infection [59]. Vitamin D appears to enhance the capability of the immune system to inhibit pulmonary inflammatory responses while bolstering innate defense mechanisms against respiratory pathogens including SARS. There are population-based studies currently underway that show signs of an association between circulating vitamin D levels and lung function.

In a recent Italian study, COVID-19 patients with severe symptoms exhibited significantly lower 25-hydroxy vitamin D [25(OH)D] levels (less than 18.2 ng/ml) than mildly symptomatic COVID-19 patients (30.3 ng/ml) and non–SARS-CoV-2-infected controls (25.4 ng/ml) [60]. Furthermore, even though no direct correlation can be made, 25(OH)D and interleukin-6 (IL-6) levels were significantly lower in mild and nonsymptomatic patients, but higher in critically symptomatic COVID-19 patients admitted to intensive care Unit (ICU) compared to those not requiring ICU admission. These results, the authors concluded, suggest, at least in this Italian cohort, that low 25(OH)D (calcidiol) levels were inversely correlated with high IL-6 levels and can independently predict the severity and mortality of COVID-19 [60].

Additional published report of vitamin's role in reducing COVID-19 cases studied twenty European countries for average vitamin D levels, COVID-19 cases, and COVID-19 mortality and found that there is an inverse relationship between vitamin D levels and COVID-19 cases, and between vitamin D levels and mortality per million population [50]. Racial/ethnic differences also exist in the USA with important implications for known health disparities regarding African American adults who have the highest prevalence rate of vitamin D deficiency followed by Hispanic adults [61]. The coronavirus pandemic of 2019, which has disproportionally affected Blacks and Hispanics, has revealed additional risk factors for vitamin D deficiency that included obesity, lack of college education, and lack of daily milk consumption [62]. COVID-19 risk increased among Black individuals with vitamin D level less than 40 ng/mL compared with those with 40 ng/ml or greater and decreased with increasing levels among individuals with levels greater than 30 ng/ml [63]. In the National Health and Nutrition Examination Survey (NHANES) in which there were 8415 participants (25% Black and 24% Mexican American), there were racial differences in the relationship between vitamin D, bone mineral density, and parathyroid hormone [45]. Calcidiol [25-hydroxycalciferol] can be considered as a supplement for patients with fat malabsorption or severe liver disease.

Vitamin D signaling is dependent on the availability and turnover of the active Vitamin D receptor (VDR) ligand, 1,25-dihydroxycholecalciferol and on the efficiency of VDR transactivation. Activating and inactivating metabolizing-p450 enzymes, are responsible for ligand availability based on substrate production in the skin and of nutritional intake of precursors. The presence of active hormone depends on the delivery of substrate and activating and inactivating enzymes. The critical enzyme 1-alpha-hydroxylase, for example, is upregulated in the kidney by low calcium intake and parathyroid hormone, but it is downregulated by proinflammatory signal transduction as demonstrated by patients with kidney disease (nephrotic syndrome) who lose vitamin $D_3$ [64]. Lately, it has also been evident that many modifiers of Vitamin D signaling are targets of disease patterns in the form of inherited and acquired syndromes. This is further evidence that vitamin D signaling is modulated at multiple levels and is more complex than mere mechanistic ligand–receptor–DNA interaction [32, 65].

## *Can Vitamin D Deficiency Increase the Susceptibility to COVID-19?*

COVID-19 can be described as an acute virally induced respiratory illness with a potentially severe outcome. A landmark 2017 meta-analysis published in the *British Medical Journal* assessing vitamin D supplementation to prevent acute respiratory tract infections in 11,321 non–COVID-19 subjects across 25 eligible randomized controlled trials (RCT) showed that vitamin D supplementation decreased mortality by reducing the risk of acute respiratory illnesses [66]. Recent studies have provided further evidence for the role of vitamin D as an immune function regulator especially with respect to the innate immune response against infectious agents. The vitamin D receptor (VDR) is expressed in various myeloid and lymphoid lineages of human cells and vitamin D may bolster the increased expression of antimicrobial peptides such as cathelicidin (hCAP-18), which is known to counteract the effects of respiratory tract pathogens in monocytes and neutrophils [67] Therefore, vitamin D deficiency may lead to suboptimal immune responses toward bacterial and viral infections such as SARS-CoV-2.

There was a study of 25-hydroxyvitamin D concentrations in 107 hospitalized patients with PCR for SARS-CoV-2 infection in Switzerland [68]. The investigators analyzed the vitamin D level of people with positive and negative PCR tests for SARS-CoV-2. The SARS-CoV-2–negative subjects had a higher vitamin D level than those with a positive test. Although these results were statistically significant, this negative correlation does not lend itself for a conclusive evidence that vitamin D deficiency is a causative effect for SARS-CoV-2 infection. This fact was highlighted in a small study where nine healthy nonsmoking individuals received an infusion of *E. coli*–derived endotoxin, a lipopolysaccharide (LPS), to induce systemic inflammation, which resulted in a significant reduction in plasma 25-hydroxyvitamin D [25-(OH) D] levels [69]. These findings suggest that confounders like LPS that cause systemic inflammation may be the culprit that lowers circulating 25(OH)D from its baseline levels in humans.

There are, however, several large population studies and relatively smaller ones that point to the association of low preexisting plasma 25-(OH)D level with increased risk of COVID-19 infection and positivity rates across ethnicities, age groups, hospitalization settings, and geographical locations [70–73]. But these were mainly observational studies, which need to be confirmed with a large prospective, randomized placebo-controlled clinical trials. In the meantime, a pilot randomized clinical study assessing the requirements for admission to the intensive care unit (ICU) in patients hospitalized with COVID-19 (treated or not with calcifediol [25(OH)$D_3$] revealed that only 2% of the intervention group receiving daily regimen of calcifediol was placed in the ICU as opposed to 50% of the placebo group, again suggesting that the therapeutic effect of vitamin D was beneficial in keeping patients away from the extreme outcomes of the disease.

There is also a casual association between vitamin D and BMI and older age. There is more than twofold decline in cutaneous pre-vitamin $D_3$ level in older adults ranging in age from 77–82 [74]. In an observational study, it was shown that obese patients exhibited a reduced bioavailability of cutaneously synthesized cholecalciferol (Vitamin $D_3$), possibly due to the concentration of most of the vitamin in adipose tissues where it is stored and less circulation in the blood [75–77]. Another observational but prospective study involving about 10,000 adult (50–75 years old) patients followed for 15 years in Germany to assess their vitamin D deficiency (less than 30 nmol/L) and insufficiency (30 to 50 nmol/L) and compared them to sufficient vitamin D status (greater than 50 nmol/L) for mortality from respiratory diseases prior to the COVID-19 pandemic reveals in their death certificates that those with above 50 nmol/L survived longer than those with less than 30 nmol/L [78]. This large study confirmed, after adjusting for several variables, the independent association of vitamin D sufficiency with reduction in respiratory mortality in this German cohort.

A growing number of contemporary reports support a prophylactic role for vitamin D in abating the risk/severity of respiratory tract infections (RTIs), especially in the context of influenza and COVID-19 [41, 42, 50, 52, 53]. On the interventional side, a frequently cited landmark meta-analysis paper that compiled data from 11,321 subjects in 25 randomized placebo-controlled trials (2009–2016), which examined the effect of vitamin D supplementation in preventing acute respiratory tract infections in a pre-COVID-19 pandemic era, concluded that there was "a major indication for vitamin D supplementation in the prevention of acute respiratory tract infections" [66]. Another randomized trial of vitamin D supplementation was conducted in Japan to prevent influenza A in 334 school children. The children were given 1200 IU/day of vitamin $D_3$ versus placebo. The endpoint was influenza A antigen testing by nasal swab. The results showed that the students with the vitamin D supplementation had an influenza A incidence of 10.8% compared to 18.6% in the placebo group with an absolute risk reduction (ARR) of 7.8% indicating a low NNT (number needed to treat) of 13 suggesting the potency of the supplementation even in school children to reduce infection with the flu [79]. The most recent meta-analysis study [80] that examined the link between vitamin D supplementation and prevention of acute respiratory tract infections (ARTIs) in an updated version of the 2017 meta-analysis [66] confirmed that vitamin D supplementation was safe and overall reduced the risk of ARTI by administration of daily doses of 400–1000 IU for up to 12 months compared with placebo, although the risk reduction was small but significant [80]. The relevance of both the observational and interventional findings of these studies to COVID-19 is not known and requires further investigation. These interventional studies confirmed the data that was generated from other observational studies with respect to vitamin D's role in reducing general ARTIs.

## *Immunophenotype of COVID-19 and Vitamin D Deficiency*

Vitamin D modulates immune responses and may prevent the release of pro-inflammatory cytokines. The immunophenotype and biochemical data between COVID-19 and vitamin D deficiency are surprisingly very similar and may be indicative of the cytokine storm syndrome (see Table 22.2).

The status of interferon gamma and T helper1 was detected late in disease (i.e., COVID-19) progression [97, 98]. These common immunophenotypes between vitamin D and ARTIs also extend to seasonal viruses such as rhinoviruses, influenza viruses, and other coronaviruses. However, hypercoagulability seems to be the exclusive characteristic of COVID-19. This was demonstrated in a small number of autopsies of patients with COVID-19 who had a ninefold increase in pulmonary blood clots (alveolar capillary microthrombi) when compared to non–COVID-19 autopsies of patients who died from acute respiratory distress syndrome (ARDS) secondary to influenza A(H1N1) infection, and uninfected control lungs [85]. Therefore, vitamin D can prevent the development of oxidative stress and multiple organ damage by reducing inflammatory cytokines in many tissues and protecting

**Table 22.2** The immune phenotypes of COVID-19 and vitamin D deficiency

| | COVID-19 | Vitamin D deficiency | References |
|---|---|---|---|
| ACE-2 expression | ↓ | ↓ | Aygun [81], Hanff et al. [82] |
| Coagulability | ↑ | ↑ | Aygun [81], Quesada-Gomez et al. [83], Somasundaram et al. [84], Ackermann et al. [85] |
| Cathelicidins | ↓ | ↓ | Jiang et al. [86], Hansdottir et al. [87] |
| C-reactive protein (CRP) | ↑ | ↑ | Mehta et al. [15], Demir et al. [88] |
| D-dimer | ↑ | ↑ | Mehta et al. [15], Demir et al. [88] |
| Interleuken-6 (IL-6) | ↑ | ↑ | Aygun [81], Palmer et al. [89] |
| Interferon-gamma (*IFN-γ*) | ↑ | ↑ | Conti et al. [90], Huang et al. [91] |
| Th1 adaptive response | ↑ | ↑ | Ardizzone et al. [92], Schleithoff et al. [93], Cantorna and Mahon [94], Aygun [81], Conti et al. [90] |
| TNF-α | ↑ | ↑ | Conti et al. [90], Huang et al. [91], Chen et al. [95], Peterson and Heffernan [96] |

Note: ACE-2 (angiotensin-converting enzyme 2); Th1 (T helper1); TNF (tumor necrosis factor). The arrows indicate the fall (↓) and rise (↑) of immune phenotypes affected by COVID-19 and vitamin D deficiency against symptoms of the COVID-19 infection, especially by increasing the level of ACE-2 in the lungs. Furthermore, a new study showed that human recombinant soluble ACE-2 treatment may significantly suppress early stages of SARS-CoV-2 infections [99]. ACE-2 is the key SARS receptor that plays a protective role in SARS-mediated ARDS [81, 100, 101]. This is further supported by the decrease observed in COVID-19 PCR positivity in people with higher levels of vitamin D [68, 88, 102, 103]. Even among COVID-19–positive patients, those with vitamin D levels of >30 ng/ml had significantly lower D-dimer and C-reactive protein (CRP) levels as well as shorter hospital stays [88]. This does not necessarily suggest association or causation between vitamin D and ARTIs but gives credence to the postulation that vitamin D deficiency plays a role in COVID-19 development and severity leading to progressive respiratory failure as the primary cause of death in Covid-19 patients. Vitamin D plays a positive role against respiratory infections. Furthermore, its deficiency is associated with COVID-19 positivity and severity of disease [88]. There is no international consensus on a single optimal vitamin D dosage that is acceptable by all organizations, scientists, or doctors around the world.

## Management of Vitamin D Deficiency for a Therapeutic Effect

The global epidemic status of vitamin D deficiency is reflected by about 1 billion people who reportedly have vitamin D deficiency, while 50% have vitamin D insufficiency [104]. In the United States, the prevalence of patients with vitamin D deficiency is highest (50–60%) in the elderly, obese patients, nursing home residents, and hospitalized patients, all common features of developed nations [105, 106]. Interestingly, the prevalence of vitamin D deficiency is 35% higher in obese individuals regardless of latitude and age [107]. Moreover, in the United States, 47% of African American infants and 56% of European American infants have vitamin D deficiency [108]. Therefore, the dosage required to treat vitamin D deficiency depends largely on the degree of the shortage and underlying risk factors. For non–dark-skinned people, supplementation could start with a robust 8-week schedule of vitamin $D_3$ either at 6000 IU daily or 50,000 IU weekly [109]. Once the serum 25-hydroxyvitamin D level exceeds 30 ng/ml, a maintenance daily dose of 1000–2000 IU is recommended. For dark-skinned people and high-risk adults with vitamin D deficiency (African Americans, Hispanics, obese, taking certain medications, malabsorption syndrome), a higher initial dose of vitamin $D_3$ at 10,000 IU daily may be needed. Once serum 25-hydroxyvitamin D level exceeds 30 ng/ml, 3000–6000 IU/day maintenance dose is recommended [40]. Children who have vitamin D deficiency may require 2000 IU/day of vitamin $D_3$ or 50,000 IU of vitamin $D_3$ once weekly for 6 weeks [40]. Once the serum 25(OH)D level is stable above 30 ng/ml or 50 nmol/L, 1000 IU/day maintenance regimen may be administered.

Similarly in England, an examination of the primary care records of 17,421,033 revealed that the major risk factors among the 10,926 who died of COVID-19 were being male, older age as well as comorbidities such as diabetes, obesity, and ethnicity with Black and South Asians being at higher risk than Whites [110]. These are the same risks exhibited by vitamin D deficiency: older age, obesity—and its associated metabolic syndrome—and dark-skinned people, suggesting that vitamin D may play a role in COVID-19 susceptibility. In another study that demonstrates the therapeutic agency of vitamin D, a meta-analysis of 18 randomized controlled trials (RCTs) with over 57,000 participants found that intake of daily doses of vitamin D supplements drastically reduced total mortality rates [111]. In the Women's Health Initiative, the combined supplementation of calcium and vitamin D reduced the risk of total cancer including breast and colorectal cancer particularly in postmenopausal women [112, 113]. In a meta-analysis study from three randomized controlled trials, vitamin D supplementation was found to reduce the rate of COPD exacerbations in patients with vitamin D levels below 25 nmol/L [114]. It also possible that all these positive effects of vitamin D levels may be indicative of comorbidities that may themselves impact COVID outcomes.

## *Regulation of Thrombotic Complications by Vitamin D—A Therapeutic Model?*

Over-reactive inflammatory response leading to hypercoagulability has been the leading characteristic of disease severity in COVID-19 patients and marked with poor prognosis [115]. In the ICUs, severe cases of COVID-19 were exhibiting intravascular hypercoagulability sometimes accompanied by pulmonary embolism and/or deep vein thrombosis. Microthrombi in lungs and in other organs with marked inflammatory changes were common in the autopsy reports of COVID-19 patients. At the advent of the pandemic when treatment options were not available and dire conditions pervaded hospital wards, vitamin D supplementation was recommended by many clinicians across the globe to improve clinical symptoms of COVID-19 patients, mainly due to its immunomodulatory roles on immune cells. In addition, vitamin D is known to regulate a variety of thrombotic pathways directly or indirectly. It was even proposed that vitamin D supplementation would mitigate the risk of ARDS and play a role in reducing coagulation abnormalities in critically ill COVID-19 patients [115]. There are currently several randomized placebo control clinical trials investigating the efficacy of vitamin D supplementation in abating the risk of COVID-19 infection and reducing the risk of coagulopathy by measuring circulating D-dimer and fibrinogen levels in COVID-19 patients [116]. The first line of defense against viral infections and subsequent inflammation is the innate immune system followed by an adaptive immunity that eventually activates the coagulation pathway. Scanning electron micrographs of microvascular corrosion in the COVID-19-damaged lung show substantial architectural distortion and loss of a clearly visible vessel hierarchy in the alveolar plexus [85]. Activation of coagulation, in turn, markedly affects the inflammatory activity [117]. Extensive cross talk between the two systems is associated with the formation of microvascular thrombi often leading to organ dysfunction in severe sepsis [85, 118]. Similar alteration in the lungs of COVID-19 patients can be seen in Fig. 22.5 [119].

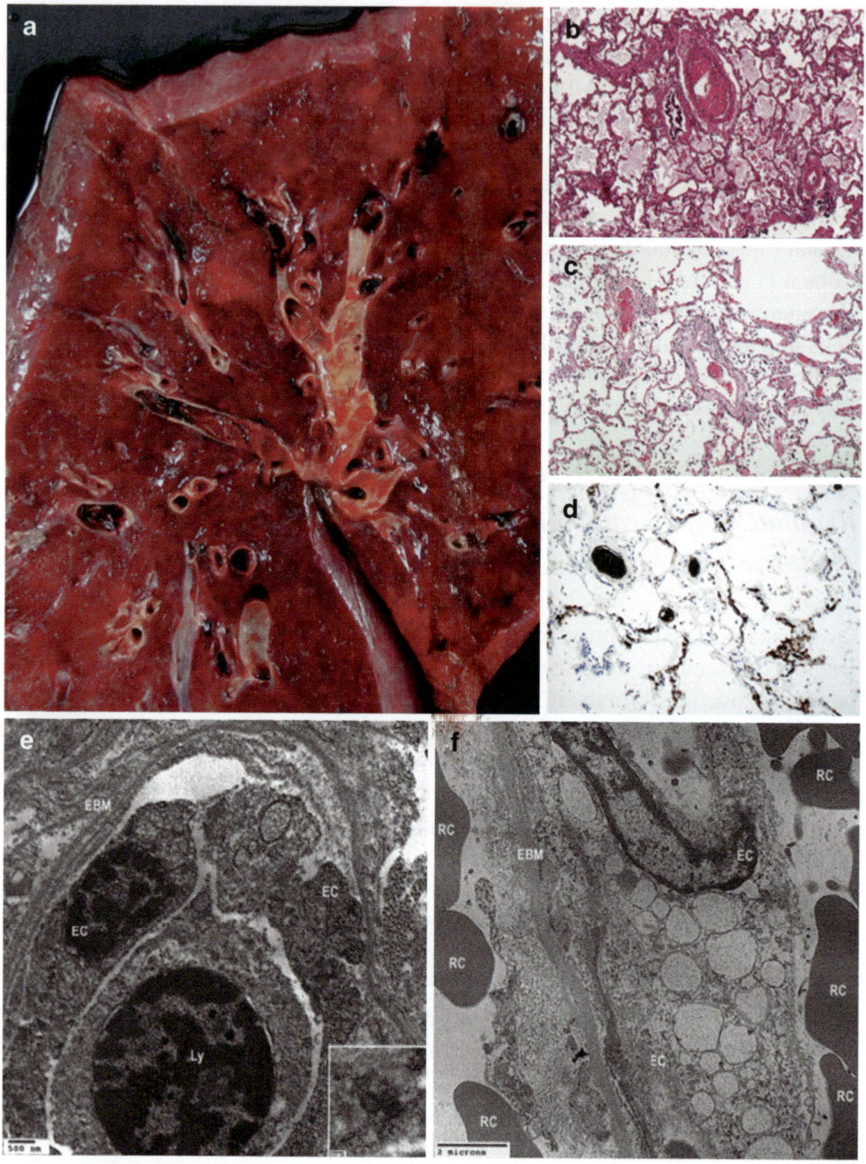


**Fig. 22.5** Vascular injury in the lung of COVID-19 patient. (**a**) A gross image showing multiple thrombi. (**b**) Along with large thrombi, smaller caliber arteries showing fibrin thrombi. (**c**) Thrombi in small arteries, including precapillary channels). (**d**) In some cases, thrombi were predominantly composed of platelets, and were also seen in the capillary bed. (**e**) The endothelial basement membrane was diffusely reduplicated. At higher magnification some putative viral particles were evident in endothelial cell cytoplasm. (**f**) Endothelial cells were swollen and showed numerous instances of cytoplasmic vacuolization. EC endothelial cell; EBM endothelial basement membrane; Ly lymphocyte; RC red cell (a—gross photograph, Hematoxylin and eosin b, c, ×100, CD61 diaminobenzidine immunohistochemistry, ×100, e–f transmission electron microscopy e × 12,000, inset ×70,000, f × 6000). (Adapted from Borczuk et al. [119])

The protective role of vitamin D as a ligand using VDR against COVID-19 disease severity has been ascribed to its impact on the immune system. The circulating vitamin D becomes a barrier to the production of inflammatory cytokines and actively blocks the proliferation of proinflammatory cells, necessary for the pathogenesis of inflammatory diseases. Furthermore, vitamin D improves the ratio of angiotensin-converting enzyme 2 (ACE-2) to ACE and consequently decreases the level of angiotensin II level by hydrolyzing the enzyme [43]. The ACE-2 receptor is expressed in multiple cells and tissues of the body including type II alveolar cells of the lungs, esophagus, upper and stratified epithelial cells, absorptive enterocytes from the ileum and colon, kidney proximal tubule cells, myocardial cells, bladder urothelial cells, and epithelial cells of the oral mucosa [120, 121]. Therefore, a reduction in ACE-2 expression during COVID-19 might be a greater risk of ARDS, acute lung inflammation, cardiac fibrosis, chronic kidney disease, and cardiovascular diseases including hypertension and heart failure [122]. The low ACE-2 expression in older people and men may be associated with high incidence of COVID-19 infection [81]. It is also known that vitamin D and its partner molecules also have a substantial effect on coagulation pathways lessening thrombosis [123]. Altogether these positive effects bode well for vitamin D supplementation in reducing the risk and adverse effects of acute lung injury associated with COVID-19.

## *Vitamin D and the Inflammatory Response*

Vitamin D can activate the cellular innate immunity. The link between vitamin D deficiency and COVID-19 may have been established via the inflammatory response pathway. 1-alpha-hydroxylase (CYP27B1), the key enzyme involved in the conversion of vitamin D to its active form, 1,25-dihydroxyvitamin $D_3$, and VDR are both expressed in dendritic cells (DC), macrophages, and T lymphocytes. These immune cells are implicated in mediating key immune/inflammatory response, which determines the biological basis for the role of vitamin D in inflammatory diseases [124]. CYP27B1 and VDR are upregulated during the activation of the toll-like receptor (TLR1/2) heterodimer in macrophages, thus resulting in the induction of the antimicrobial peptide cathelicidin, which can act against nonenveloped and enveloped viruses such as SARS-CoV-2 [125].

To block an overactive immune response, both forms of vitamin D—25(OH)D and $1,25(OH)_2D$—counteract LPS-induced p38 signaling to deactivate cytokine (IL-6 and TNF $\alpha$) production in monocytes/macrophages [126]. The 1,25(OH)2D active form of vitamin D can reduce MCP-1 and IL-6 expression by obstructing the activation of NF-$\kappa$B in macrophages [127]. Additionally, vitamin D naturally alleviates endoplasmic reticulum stress caused by COVID-19 and interferon (IFN)-$\gamma$-activated macrophages [128, 129]. The active form of vitamin D [$1,25(OH)_2D$] impedes the maturation and differentiation of human antigen presenting dendritic cells in a VDR-dependent manner causing the induction of T-regulatory cells. $1,25(OH)_2D$ can also block the production of proinflammatory cytokines such as

IFNγ, IL-17, and IL-21, elevate the production of the anti-inflammatory cytokine, IL-10, and help maintain tight junctions and gap junctions usually disrupted by pathogens such as bacteria and viruses [130–132].

## *The Positive Role of Vitamin D in COVID-19 Complications*

One of the hallmarks of COVID-19 is coagulopathy. Vitamin D and its metabolites have emerged as effective anticoagulants because of their ability to regulate the various pro- and anti-thrombotic agents involved in the coagulation cascade. Vitamin D is known to upregulate thrombomodulin (TM) and downregulate the antigen expression and mRNA levels of prothrombotic factor (TF) that initiates the activation of coagulation [133]. Ohsawa and colleagues also showed similar regulatory effects on TF and TM using synthetic vitamin D analogs mediated through VDR, and they suggested these synthetic analogs could be used as readily available therapeutic agents under controlled conditions [134]. Other similar studies have shown that adding calcitriol ($1,25(OH)_2D_3$) and paricalcitol ($19\text{-nor-}1,25\text{-}(OH)_2D_2$) reduces the activity of TF and TNF-α-induced expression in vascular smooth muscle cells. The mechanism by which reduction in these cytokines is accomplished is through the downregulation of PAR-2 expression and NF-κB signaling in which VDR plays a significant part [135]. A cascade of the activities that control the thrombotic regulation pathway also upregulates the tissue factor pathway inhibitor (TFPI) expression and restoration of VDR level. Topaloglu et al. also investigated the relationship between TFPI and vitamin D (serum $25(OH)D_3$) level and found a significant positive correlation between the two [136]. There are many clinical trials that have investigated the relationship (i.e., correlation) between vitamin D deficiency and thrombosis and have provided their conclusive comments (Table 22.3) [115].

Further studies on the effect of suboptimal levels of 25(OH)D and thrombosis were reported in patients with idiopathic lower-extremity deep vein thrombosis (DVT) [138], as well as in patients with ischemic stroke [141]. A rise in thrombosis in patients from Switzerland was counteracted by a high-dose of cholecalciferol (vitamin $D_3$) supplementation in patients in Switzerland [137]; and a similar high-dose of $1,25(OH)_2D_3$ regimen administered to cancer patients as reported by Beer et al. in a placebo-controlled randomized trial [140]. Lindqvist et al. [139] also investigated a potential correlation between routine sun exposures and occurrence of venous thromboembolism (VTE) by following a cohort of 40,000 women for a decade (Table 22.1). They reported a 30% reduction in the risk of VTE in the women with sun exposure compared to women without routine sunlight exposure. The latest evidence of vitamin D's constructive role comes from the UK in which the electronic health record of two hospital cohorts was retrospectively examined [142]. The study, which involved 80, 670 patients, revealed that lower vitamin D levels (serum 25-hydroxyvitamin D lower than 25 nmol/L (10 ng/ml) were correlated with hospitalization with COVID-19. Similar studies also examined the incidence of VTE in COVID-19 patients and concluded that the adverse effects of the

**Table 22.3** Clinical trials correlating vitamin D deficiency with elevated risk of thrombosis [115] [a]

| Study | Sample size | Clinical feature/ coagulation parameter | Findings | Conclusions |
|---|---|---|---|---|
| Blondon et al. [137], Martinez-Moreno et al. [135] | 48 | Prothrombotic profile | Vitamin D supplementation resulted in decrease in thrombin generation | Severe vitamin D deficiency might be associated with a potentially reversible prothrombotic profile |
| Wu et al. [141], Ohsawa et al. [134] | 180 | DVT in patients with history of ischemic stroke | Serum vitamin D levels were significantly lower in the DVT group than in the non-DVT group | Low vitamin D level is independent predictor of DVT |
| Khademvatani et al. [138], Koyama et al. [133] | 275 | DVT | 68.3% population in DVT group was vitamin D deficient | Vitamin D deficiency is associated with idiopathic lower-extremity DVT |
| Lindqvist et al. [139], Khademvatani et al. [138] | 40,000 | VTE | Women with greater exposure of sun have 30% lower risk of having VTE | Greater exposure of sunlight improves vitamin D status of a person resulting in the enhancement of anticoagulant property |
| Beer et al. [140], Topaloglu et al. [136] | 250 | Thrombosis in cancer patients | Events of thrombosis was only 2 in patients given calcitriol compared to 11 in placebo-treated control | High dose of vitamin D reduced thrombosis in cancer patients |

[a]Adapted from Sengupta et al. with slight modification [115]

overactive immune response (“cytokine storm”) and the subsequently induced hypoxia cause an increase induction in COVID-19-associated coagulopathy in ICU patients [143, 144]. The current standard of care for COVID-19 patients includes administering anticoagulants to prevent the potential occurrence of thrombosis. However, gastrointestinal bleeding has been one of the main concerns of clinicians [145]. Supplementing the anticoagulant therapy with vitamin D could offer one option to address the bleeding disorders in patients receiving anticoagulant therapy. Other investigators are promoting vitamin D as an adjuvant therapy for patients that receive anticoagulants [146]. Currently, there are no pharmacological or therapeutic antiviral agents administered to tackle the underlying SARS-CoV-2 infection that is causing hypercoagulability and the hyperactive inflammatory responses.

There are several large-scale randomized and prospective clinical trials that are underway in assessing and validating a direct relationship between vitamin D deficiency and elevated risk of thrombosis [147]. These studies will shed light on the direct role of vitamin D in offsetting the risk of coagulopathy and the “cytokine storm” that lead to severe disease and death in COVID-19 patients.

## Conclusions and Future Perspectives

This chapter has presented extensive yet not exhaustive data that indicate that one of the risk factors for severe acute respiratory syndrome coronavirus 2 (SARS-CoV-2) infection is vitamin D deficiency. It is apparent that more robust and large-scale double-blinded randomized placebo-controlled clinical trial will be necessary to conclusively demonstrate that vitamin D supplementation must be part of the prevention and treatment regimen to mitigate the deleterious impact of SARS-CoV-2 infection and COVID-19-associated coagulopathy. The further exploration of the efficacy of vitamin D supplementation in reducing COVID-19 severity and mortality will be very helpful not only for newly infected patients but also the post-acute sequela of SARS-CoV-2 long haulers.

## References

1. Mahase E. Coronavirus covid-19 has killed more people than SARS and MERS combined, despite lower case fatality rate. BMJ. 2020;368:m641.
2. Dong E, Du H, Gardner L. An interactive web-based dashboard to track COVID-19 in real time. Lancet Infect Dis. 2020;20(5):533–4.
3. Chan JF, Yuan S, Kok KH, To KK, Chu H, Yang J, Xing F, Liu J, Yip CC, Poon RW, Tsoi HW, Lo SK, Chan KH, Poon VK, Chan WM, Ip JD, Cai JP, Cheng VC, Chen H, Hui CK, Yuen KY. A familial cluster of pneumonia associated with the 2019 novel coronavirus indicating person-to-person transmission: a study of a family cluster. Lancet (London, England). 2020;395(10223):514–23.
4. Guan WJ, Ni ZY, Hu Y, Liang WH, Ou CQ, He JX, Liu L, Shan H, Lei CL, Hui DSC, Du B, Li LJ, Zeng G, Yuen KY, Chen RC, Tang CL, Wang T, Chen PY, Xiang J, Li SY, Wang JL, Liang ZJ, Peng YX, Wei L, Liu Y, Hu YH, Peng P, Wang JM, Liu JY, Chen Z, Li G, Zheng ZJ, Qiu SQ, Luo J, Ye CJ, Zhu SY, Zhong NS, China Medical Treatment Expert Group for COVID-19. Clinical characteristics of coronavirus disease 2019 in China. N Engl J Med. 2020;382(18):1708–20.
5. Lai CC, Shih TP, Ko WC, Tang HJ, Hsueh PR. Severe acute respiratory syndrome coronavirus 2 (SARS-CoV-2) and coronavirus disease-2019 (COVID-19): the epidemic and the challenges. Int J Antimicrob Agents. 2020;55(3):105924.
6. Wu C, Chen X, Cai Y, Xia J, Zhou X, Xu S, Huang H, Zhang L, Zhou X, Du C, Zhang Y, Song J, Wang S, Chao Y, Yang Z, Xu J, Zhou X, Chen D, Xiong W, Xu L, Zhou F, Jiang J, Bai C, Zheng J, Song Y. Risk factors associated with acute respiratory distress syndrome and death in patients with coronavirus disease 2019 pneumonia in Wuhan, China. JAMA Intern Med. 2020;180(7):934–43.
7. Zhou Y, Zhang Z, Tian J, Xiong S. Risk factors associated with disease progression in a cohort of patients infected with the 2019 novel coronavirus. Ann Palliat Med. 2020;9(2):428–36.
8. Elezkurtaj S, Greuel S, Ihlow J, Michaelis EG, Bischoff P, Kunze CA, Sinn BV, Gerhold M, Hauptmann K, Ingold-Heppner B, Miller F, Herbst H, Corman VM, Martin H, Radbruch H, Heppner FL, Horst D. Causes of death and comorbidities in hospitalized patients with COVID-19. Sci Rep. 2021;11(1):4263–5.
9. Su S, Wong G, Shi W, Liu J, Lai ACK, Zhou J, Liu W, Bi Y, Gao GF. Epidemiology, genetic recombination, and pathogenesis of coronaviruses. Trends Microbiol. 2016;24(6):490–502.
10. Coronaviridae Study Group of the International Committee on Taxonomy of Viruses. The species severe acute respiratory syndrome-related coronavirus: classifying 2019-nCoV and naming it SARS-CoV-2. Nat Microbiol. 2020;5(4):536–44.

11. Langereis MA, Van Vliet AL, Boot W, De Groot RJ. Attachment of mouse hepatitis virus to O-acetylated sialic acid is mediated by hemagglutinin-esterase and not by the spike protein. J Virol. 2010;84(17):8970–4.
12. Gibson PG, Qin L, Puah SH. COVID-19 acute respiratory distress syndrome (ARDS): clinical features and differences from typical pre-COVID-19 ARDS. Med J Aust. 2020;213(2):54–56.e1.
13. Li X, Ma X. Acute respiratory failure in COVID-19: is it "typical" ARDS? Crit Care. 2020;24(1):198–9.
14. McGonagle D, Sharif K, O'Regan A, Bridgewood C. The role of cytokines including Interleukin-6 in COVID-19 induced pneumonia and macrophage activation syndrome-like disease. Autoimmun Rev. 2020;19(6):102537.
15. Mehta P, McAuley DF, Brown M, Sanchez E, Tattersall RS, Manson JJ, HLH Across Speciality Collaboration, UK. COVID-19: consider cytokine storm syndromes and immunosuppression. Lancet. 2020;395(10229):1033–4.
16. Sarzi-Puttini P, Giorgi V, Sirotti S, Marotto D, Ardizzone S, Rizzardini G, Antinori S, Galli M. COVID-19, cytokines and immunosuppression: what can we learn from severe acute respiratory syndrome? Clin Exp Rheumatol. 2020;38(2):337–42.
17. Saghazadeh A, Rezaei N. Immune-epidemiological parameters of the novel coronavirus - a perspective. Expert Rev Clin Immunol. 2020;16(5):465–70.
18. Sanchez-Ramirez DC, Mackey D. Underlying respiratory diseases, specifically COPD, and smoking are associated with severe COVID-19 outcomes: A systematic review and meta-analysis. Respir Med. 2020;171:106096.
19. Alexander J, Tinkov A, Strand TA, Alehagen U, Skalny A, Aaseth J. Early nutritional interventions with zinc, selenium and vitamin D for raising anti-viral resistance against progressive COVID-19. Nutrients. 2020;12(8):2358. https://doi.org/10.3390/nu12082358.
20. He M, Wang C, Xu L, Zhang H, Liu Y, Zhao Y, He S, Zhang Y, Yang H, Liu Y, Miao M, Chen Z, Pang L. Epidemiological and clinical characteristics of 35 children with COVID-19 in Beijing, China. Pediatr Investig. 2020;4(4):230–5.
21. Kim PS, Read SW, Fauci AS. Therapy for early COVID-19: A critical need. JAMA. 2020;324(21):2149–50.
22. Ridruejo E, Soza A. The liver in times of COVID-19: what hepatologists should know. Ann Hepatol. 2020;19(4):353–8.
23. Yang X, Yu Y, Xu J, Shu H, Xia J, Liu H, Wu Y, Zhang L, Yu Z, Fang M, Yu T, Wang Y, Pan S, Zou X, Yuan S, Shang Y. Clinical course and outcomes of critically ill patients with SARS-CoV-2 pneumonia in Wuhan, China: a single-centered, retrospective, observational study. Lancet Respir Med. 2020;8(5):475–81.
24. Tripkovic L, Lambert H, Hart K, Smith CP, Bucca G, Penson S, Chope G, Hypponen E, Berry J, Vieth R, Lanham-New S. Comparison of vitamin D2 and vitamin D3 supplementation in raising serum 25-hydroxyvitamin D status: a systematic review and meta-analysis. Am J Clin Nutr. 2012;95(6):1357–64.
25. Biondi P, Pepe J, Biamonte F, Occhiuto M, Parisi M, Demofonti C, Baffa V, Minisola S, Cipriani C. Oral calcidiol is a good form of vitamin D supplementation. Clin Cases Miner Bone Metab. 2017;14(2):207–8.
26. Aranda A, Pascual A. Nuclear hormone receptors and gene expression. Physiol Rev. 2001;81(3):1269–304.
27. Cannell JJ, Vieth R, Umhau JC, Holick MF, Grant WB, Madronich S, Garland CF, Giovannucci E. Epidemic influenza and vitamin D. Epidemiol Infect. 2006;134(6):1129–40.
28. Dobnig H, Pilz S, Scharnagl H, Renner W, Seelhorst U, Wellnitz B, Kinkeldei J, Boehm BO, Weihrauch G, Maerz W. Independent association of low serum 25-hydroxyvitamin d and 1,25-dihydroxyvitamin d levels with all-cause and cardiovascular mortality. Arch Intern Med. 2008;168(12):1340–9.
29. Garland CF, Comstock GW, Garland FC, Helsing KJ, Shaw EK, Gorham ED. Serum 25-hydroxyvitamin D and colon cancer: eight-year prospective study. Lancet (London, England). 1989;2(8673):1176–8.

30. Laaksi I, Ruohola JP, Tuohimaa P, Auvinen A, Haataja R, Pihlajamaki H, Ylikomi T. An association of serum vitamin D concentrations < 40 nmol/L with acute respiratory tract infection in young Finnish men. Am J Clin Nutr. 2007;86(3):714–7.
31. Chang SW, Lee HC. Vitamin D and health - the missing vitamin in humans. Pediatr Neonatol. 2019;60(3):237–44.
32. Ebert R, Schutze N, Adamski J, Jakob F. Vitamin D signaling is modulated on multiple levels in health and disease. Mol Cell Endocrinol. 2006;248(1–2):149–59.
33. Kirby AC, Coles MC, Kaye PM. Alveolar macrophages transport pathogens to lung draining lymph nodes. J Immunol. 2009;183(3):1983–9.
34. Sultan S, Taimuri U, Basnan SA, Ai-Orabi WK, Awadallah A, Almowald F, Hazazi A. Low vitamin D and its association with cognitive impairment and dementia. J Aging Res. 2020;2020:6097820.
35. Franca Gois PH, Wolley M, Ranganathan D, Seguro AC. Vitamin D deficiency in chronic kidney disease: recent evidence and controversies. Int J Environ Res Public Health. 2018;15(8):1773. https://doi.org/10.3390/ijerph15081773.
36. Edlich R, Mason SS, Chase ME, Fisher AL, Gubler K, Long WB, Giesy JD, Foley ML. Scientific documentation of the relationship of vitamin D deficiency and the development of cancer. J Environ Pathol Toxicol Oncol. 2009;28(2):133–41.
37. Amrein K, Scherkl M, Hoffmann M, Neuwersch-Sommeregger S, Kostenberger M, Tmava Berisha A, Martucci G, Pilz S, Malle O. Vitamin D deficiency 2.0: an update on the current status worldwide. Eur J Clin Nutr. 2020;74(11):1498–513.
38. Holick MF. McCollum Award Lecture, 1994: vitamin D--new horizons for the 21st century. Am J Clin Nutr. 1994;60(4):619–30.
39. Naeem Z. Vitamin d deficiency- an ignored epidemic. Int J Health ScI (Qassim). 2010;4(1):V–VI.
40. Sizar O, Khare S, Goyal A, Bansal P, Givler A. Vitamin D deficiency. StatPearls. Treasure Island, FL: StatPearls Publishing LLC; 2021.
41. Ginde AA, Liu MC, Camargo CA. Demographic differences and trends of vitamin D insufficiency in the US population, 1988-2004. Arch Intern Med. 2009a;169(6):626–32.
42. Ginde AA, Mansbach JM, Camargo CA. Association between serum 25-hydroxyvitamin D level and upper respiratory tract infection in the third National Health and nutrition examination survey. Arch Intern Med. 2009b;169(4):384–90.
43. Rhodes JM, Subramanian S, Laird E, Griffin G, Kenny RA. Perspective: vitamin D deficiency and COVID-19 severity - plausibly linked by latitude, ethnicity, impacts on cytokines, ACE2 and thrombosis. J Intern Med. 2021;289(1):97–115.
44. Rhodes JM, Subramanian S, Laird E, Kenny RA. Editorial: low population mortality from COVID-19 in countries south of latitude 35 degrees North supports vitamin D as a factor determining severity. Aliment Pharmacol Ther. 2020;51(12):1434–7.
45. Gutierrez OM, Farwell WR, Kermah D, Taylor EN. Racial differences in the relationship between vitamin D, bone mineral density, and parathyroid hormone in the National Health and nutrition examination survey. Osteoporos Int. 2011;22(6):1745–53.
46. Campbell P, Young MW, Lee RC. Vitamin D clinical pharmacology: relevance to COVID-19 pathogenesis. J Natl Med Assoc. 2021;113(2):208–11.
47. Czernichow S, Fan T, Nocea G, Sen SS. Calcium and vitamin D intake by postmenopausal women with osteoporosis in France. Curr Med Res Opin. 2010;26(7):1667–74.
48. Zhang Y, Fang F, Tang J, Jia L, Feng Y, Xu P, Faramand A. Association between vitamin D supplementation and mortality: systematic review and meta-analysis. BMJ. 2019;366:l4673.
49. Bouillon R, Carmeliet G, Lieben L, Watanabe M, Perino A, Auwerx J, Schoonjans K, Verstuyf A. Vitamin D and energy homeostasis: of mice and men. Nat Rev Endocrinol. 2014;10(2):79–87.
50. Ilie PC, Stefanescu S, Smith L. The role of vitamin D in the prevention of coronavirus disease 2019 infection and mortality. Aging Clin Exp Res. 2020;32(7):1195–8.

51. Munshi R, Hussein MH, Toraih EA, Elshazli RM, Jardak C, Sultana N, Youssef MR, Omar M, Attia AS, Fawzy MS, Killackey M, Kandil E, Duchesne J. Vitamin D insufficiency as a potential culprit in critical COVID-19 patients. J Med Virol. 2021;93(2):733–40.
52. Panagiotou G, Tee SA, Ihsan Y, Athar W, Marchitelli G, Kelly D, Boot CS, Stock N, Macfarlane J, Martineau AR, Burns G, Quinton R. Low serum 25-hydroxyvitamin D (25[OH]D) levels in patients hospitalized with COVID-19 are associated with greater disease severity. Clin Endocrinol. 2020;93(4):508–11.
53. Science M, Maguire JL, Russell ML, Smieja M, Walter SD, Loeb M. Low serum 25-hydroxyvitamin D level and risk of upper respiratory tract infection in children and adolescents. Clin Infect Dis. 2013;57(3):392–7.
54. Crescioli C. Vitamin D restores skeletal muscle cell remodeling and myogenic program: potential impact on human health. Int J Mol Sci. 2021;22(4):1760. https://doi.org/10.3390/ijms22041760.
55. Grant WB, Holick MF. Benefits and requirements of vitamin D for optimal health: a review. Altern Med Rev. 2005;10(2):94–111.
56. Wintermeyer E, Ihle C, Ehnert S, Stockle U, Ochs G, De Zwart P, Flesch I, Bahrs C, Nussler AK. Crucial role of vitamin D in the musculoskeletal system. Nutrients. 2016;8(6):319. https://doi.org/10.3390/nu8060319.
57. Dancer RC, Parekh D, Lax S, D'Souza V, Zheng S, Bassford CR, Park D, Bartis DG, Mahida R, Turner AM, Sapey E, Wei W, Naidu B, Stewart PM, Fraser WD, Christopher KB, Cooper MS, Gao F, Sansom DM, Martineau AR, Perkins GD, Thickett DR. Vitamin D deficiency contributes directly to the acute respiratory distress syndrome (ARDS). Thorax. 2015;70(7):617–24.
58. Vyas N, Kurian SJ, Bagchi D, Manu MK, Saravu K, Unnikrishnan MK, Mukhopadhyay C, Rao M, Miraj SS. Vitamin D in prevention and treatment of COVID-19: current perspective and future prospects. J Am Coll Nutr. 2020;40:632–45.
59. Zwart SR, Smith SM. Vitamin D and COVID-19: lessons from spaceflight analogs. J Nutr. 2020;150(10):2624–7.
60. Campi I, Gennari L, Merlotti D, Mingiano C, Frosali A, Giovanelli L, Torlasco C, Pengo MF, Heilbron F, Soranna D, Zambon A, Di Stefano M, Aresta C, Bonomi M, Cangiano B, Favero V, Fatti L, Perego GB, Chiodini I, Parati G, Persani L. Vitamin D and COVID-19 severity and related mortality: a prospective study in Italy. BMC Infect Dis. 2021;21(1):566–7.
61. Parva NR, Tadepalli S, Singh P, Qian A, Joshi R, Kandala H, Nookala VK, Cheriyath P. Prevalence of vitamin D deficiency and associated risk factors in the US population (2011-2012). Cureus. 2018;10(6):e2741.
62. Forrest KY, Stuhldreher WL. Prevalence and correlates of vitamin D deficiency in US adults. Nutrition research (New York, NY). 2011;31(1):48–54.
63. Meltzer DO, Best TJ, Zhang H, Vokes T, Arora VM, Solway J. Association of vitamin D Levels, race/ethnicity, and clinical characteristics with COVID-19 test results. JAMA Netw Open. 2021;4(3):e214117.
64. Selewski DT, Chen A, Shatat IF, Pais P, Greenbaum LA, Geier P, Nelson RD, Kiessling SG, Brophy PD, Quiroga A, Seifert ME, Straatmann CE, Mahan JD, Ferris ME, Troost JP, Gipson DS. Vitamin D in incident nephrotic syndrome: a Midwest pediatric nephrology consortium study. Pediatr Nephrol. 2016;31(3):465–72.
65. Gilani SJ, Bin-Jumah M, Nadeem MS, Kazmi I. Vitamin D attenuates COVID-19 complications via modulation of proinflammatory cytokines, antiviral proteins, and autophagy. Expert Rev Anti-Infect Ther. 2021;20(2):231–41.
66. Martineau AR, Jolliffe DA, Hooper RL, Greenberg L, Aloia JF, Bergman P, Dubnov-Raz G, Esposito S, Ganmaa D, Ginde AA, Goodall EC, Grant CC, Griffiths CJ, Janssens W, Laaksi I, Manaseki-Holland S, Mauger D, Murdoch DR, Neale R, Rees JR, Simpson S, Stelmach I, Kumar GT, Urashima M, Camargo CA. Vitamin D supplementation to prevent acute respiratory tract infections: systematic review and meta-analysis of individual participant data. BMJ. 2017;356:i6583.

67. Gombart AF. The vitamin D-antimicrobial peptide pathway and its role in protection against infection. Future Microbiol. 2009;4(9):1151–65.
68. D'Avolio A, Avataneo V, Manca A, Cusato J, De Nicolo A, Lucchini R, Keller F, Cantu M. 25-Hydroxyvitamin D concentrations are lower in patients with positive PCR for SARS-CoV-2. Nutrients. 2020;12(5):1359. https://doi.org/10.3390/nu12051359.
69. Smolders J, Geven C, Pickkers P, Kox M. Letter to the editor: vitamin D deficiency in COVID-19: mixing up cause and consequence. Metab Clin Exp. 2021;115:154434.
70. Baktash V, Hosack T, Patel N, Shah S, Kandiah P, Van Den Abbeele K, Mandal AKJ, Missouris CG. Vitamin D status and outcomes for hospitalised older patients with COVID-19. Postgrad Med J. 2021;97(1149):442–7.
71. Kaufman HW, Niles JK, Kroll MH, Bi C, Holick MF. SARS-CoV-2 positivity rates associated with circulating 25-hydroxyvitamin D levels. PLoS One. 2020;15(9):e0239252.
72. Merzon E, Tworowski D, Gorohovski A, Vinker S, Golan Cohen A, Green I, Frenkel-Morgenstern M. Low plasma 25(OH) vitamin D level is associated with increased risk of COVID-19 infection: an Israeli population-based study. FEBS J. 2020;287(17):3693–702.
73. Radujkovic A, Hippchen T, Tiwari-Heckler S, Dreher S, Boxberger M, Merle U. Vitamin D deficiency and outcome of COVID-19 patients. Nutrients. 2020;12(9):2757. https://doi.org/10.3390/nu12092757.
74. Maclaughlin J, Holick MF. Aging decreases the capacity of human skin to produce vitamin D3. J Clin Invest. 1985;76(4):1536–8.
75. Belancic A, Kresovic A, Racki V. Potential pathophysiological mechanisms leading to increased COVID-19 susceptibility and severity in obesity. Obes Med. 2020;19:100259.
76. Dickerson RN, Holmes WL, Maish GO, Croce MA, Minard G. Obesity attenuates serum 25-hydroxyvitamin D response to cholecalciferol therapy in critically ill patients. Nutrition (Burbank, Los Angeles County, Calif). 2019;63-64:120–5.
77. Wortsman J, Matsuoka LY, Chen TC, Lu Z, Holick MF. Decreased bioavailability of vitamin D in obesity. Am J Clin Nutr. 2000;72(3):690–3.
78. Brenner H, Holleczek B, Schottker B. Vitamin D insufficiency and deficiency and mortality from respiratory diseases in a cohort of older adults: potential for limiting the death toll during and beyond the COVID-19 pandemic? Nutrients. 2020;12(8):2488. https://doi.org/10.3390/nu12082488.
79. Urashima M, Segawa T, Okazaki M, Kurihara M, Wada Y, Ida H. Randomized trial of vitamin D supplementation to prevent seasonal influenza A in schoolchildren. Am J Clin Nutr. 2010;91(5):1255–60.
80. Jolliffe DA, Camargo CA, Sluyter JD, Aglipay M, Aloia JF, Ganmaa D, Bergman P, Bischoff-Ferrari HA, Borzutzky A, Damsgaard CT, Dubnov-Raz G, Esposito S, Gilham C, Ginde AA, Golan-Tripto I, Goodall EC, Grant CC, Griffiths CJ, Hibbs AM, Janssens W, Khadilkar AV, Laaksi I, Lee MT, Loeb M, Maguire JL, Majak P, Mauger DT, Manaseki-Holland S, Murdoch DR, Nakashima A, Neale RE, Pham H, Rake C, Rees JR, Rosendahl J, Scragg R, Shah D, Shimizu Y, Simpson-Yap S, Trilok-Kumar G, Urashima M, Martineau AR. Vitamin D supplementation to prevent acute respiratory infections: a systematic review and meta-analysis of aggregate data from randomised controlled trials. Lancet Diabetes Endocrinol. 2021;9(5):276–92.
81. Aygun H. Vitamin D can prevent COVID-19 infection-induced multiple organ damage. Naunyn Schmiedeberg's Arch Pharmacol. 2020;393(7):1157–60.
82. Hanff TC, Harhay MO, Brown TS, Cohen JB, Mohareb AM. Is there an association between COVID-19 mortality and the renin-angiotensin system? A call for epidemiologic investigations. Clin Infect Dis. 2020;71(15):870–4.
83. Quesada-Gomez JM, Entrenas-Castillo M, Bouillon R. Vitamin D receptor stimulation to reduce acute respiratory distress syndrome (ARDS) in patients with coronavirus SARS-CoV-2 infections: revised Ms SBMB 2020_166. J Steroid Biochem Mol Biol. 2020;202:105719.
84. Somasundaram NP, Ranathunga I, Ratnasamy V, Wijewickrama PSA, Dissanayake HA, Yogendranathan N, Gamage KKK, De Silva NL, Sumanatilleke M, Katulanda P, Grossman

AB. The impact of SARS-Cov-2 virus infection on the endocrine system. J Endocr Soc. 2020;4(8):bvaa082.
85. Ackermann M, Verleden SE, Kuehnel M, Haverich A, Welte T, Laenger F, Vanstapel A, Werlein C, Stark H, Tzankov A, Li WW, Li VW, Mentzer SJ, Jonigk D. Pulmonary vascular endothelialitis, thrombosis, and angiogenesis in Covid-19. N Engl J Med. 2020;383(2):120–8.
86. Jiang JS, Chou HC, Chen CM. Cathelicidin attenuates hyperoxia-induced lung injury by inhibiting oxidative stress in newborn rats. Free Radic Biol Med. 2020;150:23–9.
87. Hansdottir S, Monick MM, Hinde SL, Lovan N, Look DC, Hunninghake GW. Respiratory epithelial cells convert inactive vitamin D to its active form: potential effects on host defense. J Immunol. 2008;181(10):7090–9.
88. Demir M, Demir F, Aygun H. Vitamin D deficiency is associated with COVID-19 positivity and severity of the disease. J Med Virol. 2021;93(5):2992–9.
89. Palmer MT, Lee YK, Maynard CL, Oliver JR, Bikle DD, Jetten AM, Weaver CT. Lineage-specific effects of 1,25-dihydroxyvitamin D(3) on the development of effector CD4 T cells. J Biol Chem. 2011;286(2):997–1004.
90. Conti P, Ronconi G, Caraffa A, Gallenga CE, Ross R, Frydas I, Kritas SK. Induction of pro-inflammatory cytokines (IL-1 and IL-6) and lung inflammation by Coronavirus-19 (COVI-19 or SARS-CoV-2): anti-inflammatory strategies. J Biol Regul Homeost Agents. 2020;34(2):327–31.
91. Huang C, Wang Y, Li X, Ren L, Zhao J, Hu Y, Zhang L, Fan G, Xu J, Gu X, Cheng Z, Yu T, Xia J, Wei Y, Wu W, Xie X, Yin W, Li H, Liu M, Xiao Y, Gao H, Guo L, Xie J, Wang G, Jiang R, Gao Z, Jin Q, Wang J, Cao B. Clinical features of patients infected with 2019 novel coronavirus in Wuhan, China. Lancet (London, England). 2020;395(10223):497–506.
92. Ardizzone S, Cassinotti A, Trabattoni D, Manzionna G, Rainone V, Bevilacqua M, Massari A, Manes G, Maconi G, Clerici M, Bianchi Porro G. Immunomodulatory effects of 1,25-dihydroxyvitamin D3 on TH1/TH2 cytokines in inflammatory bowel disease: an in vitro study. Int J Immunopathol Pharmacol. 2009;22(1):63–71.
93. Schleithoff SS, Zittermann A, Tenderich G, Berthold HK, Stehle P, Koerfer R. Vitamin D supplementation improves cytokine profiles in patients with congestive heart failure: a double-blind, randomized, placebo-controlled trial. Am J Clin Nutr. 2006;83(4):754–9.
94. Cantorna MT, Mahon BD. D-hormone and the immune system. J Rheumatol Suppl. 2005;76:11–20.
95. Chen N, Zhou M, Dong X, Qu J, Gong F, Han Y, Qiu Y, Wang J, Liu Y, Wei Y, Xia J, Yu T, Zhang X, Zhang L. Epidemiological and clinical characteristics of 99 cases of 2019 novel coronavirus pneumonia in Wuhan, China: a descriptive study. Lancet (London, England). 2020;395(10223):507–13.
96. Peterson CA, Heffernan ME. Serum tumor necrosis factor-alpha concentrations are negatively correlated with serum 25(OH)D concentrations in healthy women. J Inflamm (Lond). 2008;5:10.
97. Chen Z, John Wherry E. T cell responses in patients with COVID-19. Nat Rev Immunol. 2020;20(9):529–36.
98. Coperchini F, Chiovato L, Croce L, Magri F, Rotondi M. The cytokine storm in COVID-19: an overview of the involvement of the chemokine/chemokine-receptor system. Cytokine Growth Factor Rev. 2020;53:25–32.
99. Monteil V, Kwon H, Prado P, Hagelkruys A, Wimmer RA, Stahl M, Leopoldi A, Garreta E, Hurtado Del Pozo C, Prosper F, Romero JP, Wirnsberger G, Zhang H, Slutsky AS, Conder R, Montserrat N, Mirazimi A, Penninger JM. Inhibition of SARS-CoV-2 infections in engineered human tissues using clinical-grade soluble human ACE2. Cell. 2020;181(4):905–913.e7.
100. Imai Y, Kuba K, Penninger JM. Angiotensin-converting enzyme 2 in acute respiratory distress syndrome. Cell Mol Life Sci. 2007;64(15):2006–12.
101. Kuba K, Imai Y, Penninger JM. Multiple functions of angiotensin-converting enzyme 2 and its relevance in cardiovascular diseases. Circ J. 2013;77(2):301–8.

102. Meltzer DO, Best TJ, Zhang H, Vokes T, Arora V, Solway J. Association of vitamin D status and other clinical characteristics with COVID-19 test results. JAMA Netw Open. 2020;3(9):e2019722.
103. Teshome A, Adane A, Girma B, Mekonnen ZA. The impact of vitamin D level on COVID-19 infection: systematic review and meta-analysis. Front Public Health. 2021;9:624559.
104. Nair R, Maseeh A. Vitamin D: the "sunshine" vitamin. J Pharmacol Pharmacother. 2012;3(2):118–26.
105. Elliott ME, Binkley NC, Carnes M, Zimmerman DR, Petersen K, Knapp K, Behlke JM, Ahmann N, Kieser MA. Fracture risks for women in long-term care: high prevalence of calcaneal osteoporosis and hypovitaminosis D. Pharmacotherapy. 2003;23(6):702–10.
106. Kennel KA, Drake MT, Hurley DL. Vitamin D deficiency in adults: when to test and how to treat. Mayo Clin Proc. 2010;85(8):752–8.
107. Pereira-Santos M, Costa PR, Assis AM, Santos CA, Santos DB. Obesity and vitamin D deficiency: a systematic review and meta-analysis. Obes Rev. 2015;16(4):341–9.
108. PALACIOS C, GONZALEZ L. Is vitamin D deficiency a major global public health problem? J Steroid Biochem Mol Biol. 2014;144 Pt A:138–45.
109. Holick MF, Binkley NC, Bischoff-Ferrari HA, Gordon CM, Hanley DA, Heaney RP, Murad MH, Weaver CM, Endocrine Society. Evaluation, treatment, and prevention of vitamin D deficiency: an Endocrine Society clinical practice guideline. J Clin Endocrinol Metab. 2011;96(7):1911–30.
110. Williamson EJ, Walker AJ, Bhaskaran K, Bacon S, Bates C, Morton CE, Curtis HJ, Mehrkar A, Evans D, Inglesby P, Cockburn J, McDonald HI, Mackenna B, Tomlinson L, Douglas IJ, Rentsch CT, Mathur R, Wong AYS, Grieve R, Harrison D, Forbes H, Schultze A, Croker R, Parry J, Hester F, Harper S, Perera R, Evans SJW, Smeeth L, Goldacre B. Factors associated with COVID-19-related death using OpenSAFELY. Nature. 2020;584(7821):430–6.
111. Autier P, Gandini S. Vitamin D supplementation and total mortality: a meta-analysis of randomized controlled trials. Arch Intern Med. 2007;167(16):1730–7.
112. Bolland MJ, Grey A, Gamble GD, Reid IR. Calcium and vitamin D supplements and health outcomes: a reanalysis of the Women's Health Initiative (WHI) limited-access data set. Am J Clin Nutr. 2011;94(4):1144–9.
113. Lappe JM, Travers-Gustafson D, Davies KM, Recker RR, Heaney RP. Vitamin D and calcium supplementation reduces cancer risk: results of a randomized trial. Am J Clin Nutr. 2007;85(6):1586–91.
114. Jolliffe DA, Greenberg L, Hooper RL, Mathyssen C, Rafiq R, De Jongh RT, Camargo CA, Griffiths CJ, Janssens W, Martineau AR. Vitamin D to prevent exacerbations of COPD: systematic review and meta-analysis of individual participant data from randomised controlled trials. Thorax. 2019;74(4):337–45.
115. Sengupta T, Majumder R, Majumder S. Role of vitamin D in treating COVID-19-associated coagulopathy: problems and perspectives. Mol Cell Biochem. 2021;476(6):2421–7.
116. Tang N, Li D, Wang X, Sun Z. Abnormal coagulation parameters are associated with poor prognosis in patients with novel coronavirus pneumonia. J Thromb Haemost. 2020;18(4):844–7.
117. Levi M, Van Der Poll T. Inflammation and coagulation. Crit Care Med. 2010;38(2 Suppl):26.
118. Levi M, Keller TT, Van Gorp E, Ten Cate H. Infection and inflammation and the coagulation system. Cardiovasc Res. 2003;60(1):26–39.
119. Borczuk AC, Salvatore SP, Seshan SV, Patel SS, Bussel JB, Mostyka M, Elsoukkary S, He B, Del Vecchio C, Fortarezza F, Pezzuto F, Navalesi P, Crisanti A, Fowkes ME, Bryce CH, Calabrese F, Beasley MB. COVID-19 pulmonary pathology: a multi-institutional autopsy cohort from Italy and New York City. Mod Pathol. 2020;33(11):2156–68.
120. Xu H, Zhong L, Deng J, Peng J, Dan H, Zeng X, Li T, Chen Q. High expression of ACE2 receptor of 2019-nCoV on the epithelial cells of oral mucosa. Int J Oral Sci. 2020;12(1):8–x.
121. Zou X, Chen K, Zou J, Han P, Hao J, Han Z. Single-cell RNA-seq data analysis on the receptor ACE2 expression reveals the potential risk of different human organs vulnerable to 2019-nCoV infection. Front Med. 2020;14(2):185–92.

122. Tikellis C, Thomas MC. Angiotensin-converting enzyme 2 (ACE2) is a key modulator of the renin angiotensin system in health and disease. Int J Pept. 2012;2012:256294.
123. Mohammad S, Mishra A, Ashraf MZ. Emerging role of vitamin D and its associated molecules in pathways related to pathogenesis of thrombosis. Biomol Ther. 2019;9(11):649. https://doi.org/10.3390/biom9110649.
124. Burt LA, Billington EO, Rose MS, Raymond DA, Hanley DA, Boyd SK. Effect of high-dose vitamin D supplementation on volumetric bone density and bone strength: a randomized clinical trial. JAMA. 2019;322(8):736–45.
125. Ahmed A, Siman-Tov G, Hall G, Bhalla N, Narayanan A. Human antimicrobial peptides as therapeutics for viral infections. Viruses. 2019;11(8):704. https://doi.org/10.3390/v11080704.
126. ZHANG Y, LEUNG DY, RICHERS BN, LIU Y, REMIGIO LK, RICHES DW, GOLEVA E. Vitamin D inhibits monocyte/macrophage proinflammatory cytokine production by targeting MAPK phosphatase-1. J Immunol. 2012;188(5):2127–35.
127. Sanchez-Nino MD, Bozic M, Cordoba-Lanus E, Valcheva P, Gracia O, Ibarz M, Fernandez E, Navarro-Gonzalez JF, Ortiz A, Valdivielso JM. Beyond proteinuria: VDR activation reduces renal inflammation in experimental diabetic nephropathy. Am J Physiol Renal Physiol. 2012;302(6):647.
128. Helming L, Bose J, Ehrchen J, Schiebe S, Frahm T, Geffers R, Probst-Kepper M, Balling R, Lengeling A. 1alpha,25-Dihydroxyvitamin D3 is a potent suppressor of interferon gamma-mediated macrophage activation. Blood. 2005;106(13):4351–8.
129. Riek AE, Oh J, Sprague JE, Timpson A, De Las Fuentes L, Bernal-Mizrachi L, Schechtman KB, Bernal-Mizrachi C. Vitamin D suppression of endoplasmic reticulum stress promotes an antiatherogenic monocyte/macrophage phenotype in type 2 diabetic patients. J Biol Chem. 2012;287(46):38482–94.
130. Grant WB, Lahore H, Mcdonnell SL, Baggerly CA, French CB, Aliano JL, Bhattoa HP. Evidence that vitamin D supplementation could reduce risk of influenza and COVID-19 infections and deaths. Nutrients. 2020;12(4):988. https://doi.org/10.3390/nu12040988.
131. Heine G, Niesner U, Chang HD, Steinmeyer A, Zugel U, Zuberbier T, Radbruch A, Worm M. 1,25-dihydroxyvitamin D(3) promotes IL-10 production in human B cells. Eur J Immunol. 2008;38(8):2210–8.
132. Jeffery LE, Burke F, Mura M, Zheng Y, Qureshi OS, Hewison M, Walker LS, Lammas DA, Raza K, Sansom DM. 1,25-Dihydroxyvitamin D3 and IL-2 combine to inhibit T cell production of inflammatory cytokines and promote development of regulatory T cells expressing CTLA-4 and FoxP3. J Immunol. 2009;183(9):5458–67.
133. Koyama T, Shibakura M, Ohsawa M, Kamiyama R, Hirosawa S. Anticoagulant effects of 1alpha,25-dihydroxyvitamin D3 on human myelogenous leukemia cells and monocytes. Blood. 1998;92(1):160–7.
134. Ohsawa M, Koyama T, Yamamoto K, Hirosawa S, Kamei S, Kamiyama R. 1alpha,25-dihydroxyvitamin D(3) and its potent synthetic analogs downregulate tissue factor and upregulate thrombomodulin expression in monocytic cells, counteracting the effects of tumor necrosis factor and oxidized LDL. Circulation. 2000;102(23):2867–72.
135. Martinez-Moreno JM, Herencia C, Montes De Oca A, Munoz-Castaneda JR, Rodriguez-Ortiz ME, Diaz-Tocados JM, Peralbo-Santaella E, Camargo A, Canalejo A, Rodriguez M, Velasco-Gimena F, Almaden Y. Vitamin D modulates tissue factor and protease-activated receptor 2 expression in vascular smooth muscle cells. FASEB J. 2016;30(3):1367–76.
136. Topaloglu O, Arslan MS, Karakose M, Ucan B, Ginis Z, Cakir E, Akkaymak ET, Sahin M, Ozbek M, Cakal E, Delibasi T. Is there any association between thrombosis and tissue factor pathway inhibitor levels in patients with vitamin D deficiency? Clin Appl Thromb Hemost. 2015;21(5):428–33.
137. Blondon M, Biver E, Braillard O, Righini M, Fontana P, Casini A. Thrombin generation and fibrin clot structure after vitamin D supplementation. Endocr Connect. 2019;8(11):1447–54.

138. Khademvatani K, Seyyed-Mohammadzad MH, Akbari M, Rezaei Y, Eskandari R, Rostamzadeh A. The relationship between vitamin D status and idiopathic lower-extremity deep vein thrombosis. Int J Gen Med. 2014;7:303–9.
139. Lindqvist PG, Epstein E, Olsson H. Does an active sun exposure habit lower the risk of venous thrombotic events? A D-lightful hypothesis. J Thromb Haemost. 2009;7(4):605–10.
140. Beer TM, Venner PM, Ryan CW, Petrylak DP, Chatta G, Dean Ruether J, Chi KN, Curd JG, Deloughery TG. High dose calcitriol may reduce thrombosis in cancer patients. Br J Haematol. 2006;135(3):392–4.
141. Wu WX, He DR. Low Vitamin D Levels Are Associated With the Development of Deep Venous Thromboembolic Events in Patients With Ischemic Stroke. Clin Appl Thromb Hemost. 2018;24(9_suppl):69S–75S. https://doi.org/10.1177/1076029618786574. Epub 2018 Jul 22. PMID: 30033760;PMCID: PMC6714856.
142. Jude EB, Ling SF, Allcock R, Yeap BXY, Pappachan JM. Vitamin D deficiency is associated with higher hospitalisation risk from COVID-19: a retrospective case-control study. J Clin Endocrinol Metab. 2021;106(11):e4708–15.
143. Jose RJ, Manuel A. COVID-19 cytokine storm: the interplay between inflammation and coagulation. Lancet Respir Med. 2020;8(6):e46–7.
144. Lodigiani C, Iapichino G, Carenzo L, Cecconi M, Ferrazzi P, Sebastian T, Kucher N, Studt JD, Sacco C, Bertuzzi A, Sandri MT, Barco S, Humanitas COVID-19 Task Force. Venous and arterial thromboembolic complications in COVID-19 patients admitted to an academic hospital in Milan, Italy. Thromb Res. 2020;191:9–14.
145. Connors JM, Levy JH. COVID-19 and its implications for thrombosis and anticoagulation. Blood. 2020;135(23):2033–40.
146. Hejazi ME, Modarresi-Ghazani F, Hamishehkar H, Mesgari-Abbasi M, Dousti S, Entezari-Maleki T. The effect of treatment of vitamin D deficiency on the level of P-selectin and hs-CRP in patients with thromboembolism: A pilot randomized clinical trial. J Clin Pharmacol. 2017;57(1):40–7.
147. STOICHITOIU LE, PINTE L, BALEA MI, NEDELCU V, BADEA C, BAICUS C. Anticoagulant protein S in COVID-19: low activity, and associated with outcome. Rom J Intern Med. 2020;58(4):251–8.

# Part IV
# Current Trends and Future Directions

# Chapter 23
# Rational Repurposing of Drugs, Clinical Trial Candidates, and Natural Products for SARS-CoV-2 Therapy

**Sakshi Piplani, Puneet Singh, David A. Winkler, and Nikolai Petrovsky**

**Objective**
To describe how drug repurposing can identify therapies for SARS-CoV-2 that can be used in short time frames.

## The COVID-19 Pandemic and the Urgent Need for Effective Drug Treatments

SAR-CoV-2 is a novel virus whose origin and mode of entry to human population remains unknown [1] Coronaviruses are a family of positive-sense single-stranded RNA viruses approximately 26–32 kb in length that cause disease across diverse mammalian species. The first coronaviruses causing human disease were identified in the 1960s when it was recognized that other types of virus could cause similar upper respiratory tract symptoms to those of common cold viruses [2]. Subsequent

S. Piplani · N. Petrovsky
College of Medicine and Public Health, Flinders University, Bedford Park, SA, Australia

Vaxine Pty Ltd, Warradale, SA, Australia
e-mail: sakshi.piplani@flinders.edu.au; nikolai.petrovsky@flinders.edu.au

P. Singh
Vaxine Pty Ltd, Warradale, SA, Australia

D. A. Winkler (✉)
Department of Biochemistry and Chemistry, La Trobe Institute for Molecular Science, La Trobe University, Melbourne, VIC, Australia

Monash Institute of Pharmaceutical Sciences, Monash University, Parkville, VIC, Australia

School of Pharmacy, University of Nottingham, Nottingham, UK
e-mail: d.winkler@latrobe.edu.au


S. Adibi et al. (eds.), *Frontiers of COVID-19*,
https://doi.org/10.1007/978-3-031-08045-6_23

electron microscope characterization revealed that these viruses shared similar morphology, a crown-shaped (corona) spike protein, the unique feature giving these viruses their name [3]. Over 20 types of coronaviruses have now been identified.

Three coronaviruses have been responsible for human outbreaks over the last 20 years: severe acute respiratory syndrome coronavirus (SARS-CoV) in 2002; Middle East respiratory syndrome-related coronavirus (MERS-CoV) in 2012; and severe acute respiratory syndrome coronavirus-2 (SARS-CoV-2) in 2019. The SARS-CoV outbreak infected over 8000 people in 29 countries until controlled by quarantine measures [4, 5]. MERS-CoV has caused periodic zoonotic outbreaks in more than 2500 people in 27 countries. While it is currently under control, MERS continues to pose a major pandemic threat [6].

The COVID-19 pandemic is still an ongoing global health crisis with no end in sight. The failure to implement early, strict quarantine measures when the outbreak first began has allowed the virus to spread rapidly across the world. It is now an endemic infection in most countries, making it very difficult or impossible to eradicate by normal quarantine and social isolation practices. While several highly effective vaccines have been developed and have received emergency use authorization, they may not end the pandemic as it will take several years to immunize most of the world's population and achieve herd immunity. Additionally, vaccine hesitancy and antivaccination sentiment, fueled by misinformation on social media and public fear of very rare vaccination side effects, has stalled the vaccination effort in many countries. The pandemic is rapidly becoming a pandemic of the unvaccinated. The dominant product of SARS-CoV-2 mutation and adaptation to human hosts, the delta strain, is capable of being passed on my fully vaccinated individuals. A further threat to vaccine effectiveness is the likely emergence of vaccine-resistant SARS-CoV-2 strains. Hence while vaccines remain vitally important, effective drugs are also essential to treat many millions of patients before vaccines finally bring the pandemic under control.

Symptoms of coronavirus infection include sore throat, loss of smell, fever, dry cough, shortness of breath, headache, muscle aches, fatigue, and diarrhea, progressing to respiratory and multiorgan failure, thrombosis, neurological dysfunction, and ultimately death in the more severe cases [7]. Lung histology in fatal cases revealed marked diffuse alveolar damage, inflammatory cell infiltrate, bronchial epithelial denudation, loss of cilia, and squamous metaplasia [7]. Deaths resulted from respiratory, heart, and/or liver failure with the highest fatality rates being in the elderly or individuals with comorbidities such as diabetes or cardiovascular disease. Infected individuals recovering from coronavirus infections may become susceptible to reinfection due to waning immunity [8, 9]. In fact, some with waning immunity may be at risk of even more severe disease if reinfected with coronavirus [10]. SARS-CoV-1 reinfection studies showed that, although immune animals cleared lung virus much faster than naïve animals, the incidence and severity of lung inflammation were not reduced [11]. This suggests that CoV illness severity is not only dictated by viral load but is also influenced by host factors. It is also now clear that, even for patients who recover from COVID-19, some will experience long-term damage and symptoms known as "long COVID."

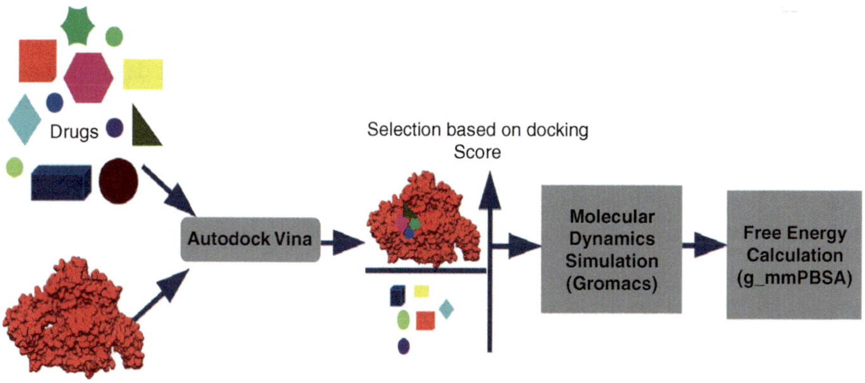


**Fig. 23.1** Flow chart for computational drug repurposing for COVID-19

Clearly, in a pandemic situation, time is of the essence and traditional drug discovery methods are much too slow to help patients as new drugs take on average 10–15 years to reach the clinic. Thus, for very rapid development of COVID-19 drugs, it is only feasible to usevn repurposed existing drugs or approved natural products that are already registered or have at least been assessed for safety in previous human trials. Computational screening algorithms have improved dramatically over recent years, as has the computational power available through cloud-accessible high-performance computing (HPC) services. Computational approaches are now sufficiently accurate to be used to rapidly screen drug libraries to identify potential drug candidates with activity against SARS-CoV-2. Hence computational methods can complement or substitute for more time consuming and expensive lab-based screening assays. In these computational screening approaches, specific virus protein targets are selected, their structures determined, key areas of the protein critical to its function identified, and docking algorithms used to screen drug libraries for potential binding to the critical functional site of the viral protein. The drugs with the highest docking score to each viral protein target are then subjected to molecular dynamic simulations to improve the binding pose in the protein and determine the binding strength (Fig. 23.1). The final ranked list of drugs with the best binding strength for each target viral protein can then be compiled. This process is then be repeated for each viral protein target and can even be run again for mutated viral proteins to counteract the development of resistance to a particular drug.

## Rationale for, and Examples of, Successful Drug Repurposing

Nearly all drugs, even those purposefully designed for a specific molecular target, exhibit polypharmacy. This means they modulate other off-target pathways as well as having their desired therapeutic effect. Consequently, drug repurposing is a useful, general strategy [12] catalyzed by important, serendipitous discoveries of blockbuster drugs. For example, minoxidil (Rogaine®) was originally developed as an ulcer drug, then registered as an antihypertensive, and subsequently and unexpectedly found to have hair growth properties. Similarly, sildenafil (Viagra®) was first developed as a cardiovascular agent and then serendipitously found to be effective against erectile dysfunction [13]. Drug repurposing to discover new therapies for stroke [14], infectious diseases [15], neglected tropical diseases [16], cancer [17–19], metabolic diseases [20], and neurological disorders [21] has been reviewed recently.

### *Computational Repurposing of Drugs*

Given the estimated US$1–2 billion cost and timescale of ~15 years to develop a new drug from scratch, it is clearly infeasible to do this for COVID-19 therapies. Registered drugs, clinically trials candidates, and approved natural products have been through regulatory processes and their pharmacokinetics and toxicology are known, providing scope for rapid deployment if they can be repurposed for use against SARS-CoV-2. Repurposing can be done using relatively time consuming and expensive in vitro high-throughput screening campaigns or by in silico virtual screening. The latter is much faster than the experimental approach and many studies have already reported the application of this approach to discovery of useful drug treatments for COVID-19.

The vast majority of in silico virtual screening studies use molecular docking algorithms such as AutoDock Vina (the most used open-source docking package) to predict the binding poses and energies of repurposing candidates from databases such as DrugBank, which contains ~12,000 known drugs. It has been shown recently that simulating the interactions of the most promising hits from docking calculations with target proteins using molecular dynamics (MD) results in more reliable predictions [22]. The most reliable published repurposing studies have used this combined approach. As many candidate drugs can be large and flexible, ligand entropy is an important but often overlooked contribution to the free energy of binding between drugs and protein targets in SARS-CoV-2 [23]. Consequently, the accuracy of the computational ranking of candidate drugs for repurposing can be quite variable. Recent papers have critically reviewed the literature on computational docking directed toward identifying potential new treatments for COVID-19 [24–27].

## SARS-CoV-2 Molecular Targets Used for Repurposing

To determine which viral proteins should be prioritized for drug screening, it is first important to understand the key features of SARS-CoV-2. Most pathogenic coronaviruses to date have had a zoonotic origin, with bats being natural reservoirs and the viruses being transmitted to humans through intermediate host species. The intermediate hosts for SARS-CoV and MERS-CoV are believed to be palm civets [28] and dromedary camels [29], respectively while the origin and intermediate host for SARS-CoV-2 remains unknown. SARS-CoV-2 genome shares a homology of almost 79% with SARS-CoV, but a similarity with MERS-CoV of only 50% [30]. Structurally, coronaviruses consist primarily of the same proteins, namely, (i) nucleocapsid, (ii) spike, (iii) envelope, and (iv) membrane proteins, plus additional accessory proteins [31]. The distinctive spike (S) protein, from which coronavirus derives its name, mediates attachment and viral entry into host cells, making it an attractive target for vaccines [32]. SARS-CoV and SARS-CoV-2 both employ angiotensin-converting enzyme-2 (ACE2) as a cell entry receptor, binding it through their spike proteins. In contrast, MERS-CoV uses dipeptidyl peptidase 4 (DPP4). The SARS-CoV-2 spike protein has a 10–20-fold higher binding affinity with human ACE-2 than does the SARS-CoV spike protein [33]. Transmembrane serine protease 2 (TMPRSS2) has been shown to be essential for cell entry for SARS-CoV, MERS-CoV, and SARS-CoV-2 as it primes the spike protein after receptor binding and allows for fusion of viral and cellular membrane [30, 34]. The expression levels and distribution of these receptors varies between cells and tissues in the body, which can influence disease pathology [35].

The SARS-CoV-2 genome encodes 29 proteins, many of which, especially the spike and the 16 nonstructural proteins (NSPs), are potential antiviral drug targets (Fig. 23.2) [36].

## *Spike*

In terms of human immune response and vaccine design, the most important features of SARS-CoV-2 are its S protein and a functional polybasic cleavage site at the S1–S2 boundary. The S monomer consists of a fusion peptide, two heptad repeats, an intracellular domain, an N-terminal domain, two subdomains, and a transmembrane region. The angiotensin converting enzyme 2 (ACE2) is the main receptor for the SARS-CoV-2 S protein, as it is for SARS-CoV. Binding to ACE2 is the critical initiating event for infection, although recent work has also identified a potential role for neuropilin 1. ACE2 is relatively ubiquitous in humans, existing in cell membranes in the lungs, arteries, heart, kidney, and intestines. It consists of an N-terminal peptidase M2 domain and a C-terminal collectrin renal amino acid transporter domain.

## *NSP3 (Papain-Like Protease) and NSP5 (3C-like Protease)*

The two proteases (PL pro and 3CL pro) are essential for virus replication. These enzymes cleave the PP1A and PP1AB polyproteins into functional components. 3-chymotrypsin-like protease (3CLpro, aka main protease, $M^{pro}$) catalytically

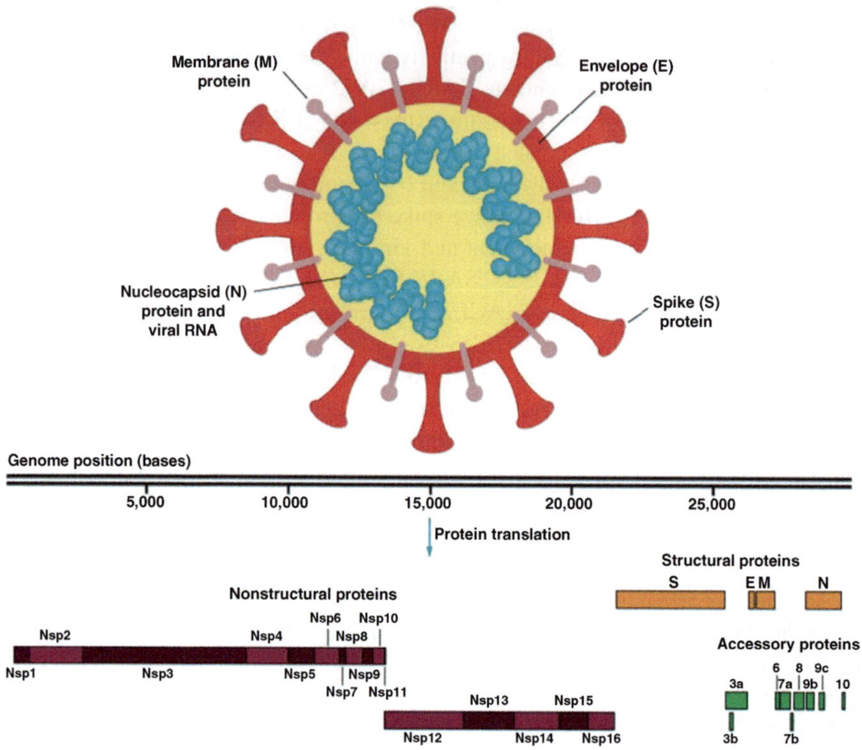


**Fig. 23.2** Virus entry and replicative cycle. $M^{pro}$ produces nonstructural proteins (NSPs) that are essential for assembly of the viral replication transcription complex needed for RNA synthesis. Used with permission from Katsnelson [37]

self-cleaves a peptide bond between a glutamine at position P1 and a small amino acid (serine, alanine, or glycine) at position P1'. This protease corresponds to non-structural protein 5 (nsp5), the main protease in coronaviruses. 3CL protease is crucial to the processing of the coronavirus replicase polyprotein (P0C6U8), cleaving it at 11 conserved sites. It employs a cys-his catalytic dyad in its active site where the cysteine sulfur is the nucleophile, and the histidine imidazole ring is a general base. $M^{pro}$ is a conserved drug target present in all *Coronavirinae*. SARS-CoV-2 $M^{pro}$ does not have a human homolog, reducing the risk of drugs inhibiting it exhibiting side effects [38]. Very recent research has shown that strong $M^{pro}$ inhibitors can substantially reduce SARS-CoV-2 virus titres, reduce weight loss and improve survival in mice, [39] making $M^{pro}$ a promising drug target for structure-based drug discovery.

## *NSP7, NSP8 and NSP12 (RNA-Dependent RNA Polymerase, RdRp)*

NSP7 and NSP8 are peptide cofactors that form a heterodimer that complexes with NSP12 and an NSP8 monomer to form the RNA polymerase that copies viral RNA. The complex with an NSP7–NSP8 heterodimer and an NSP8 monomer is essential to confer processivity of NSP12.

## *NSP13 Helicase*

The SARS-CoV-2 helicase (NSP13) has been much less studied than the above targets but has considerable potential for the discovery of drugs against, not only SARS-CoV-2, but other existing and emerging coronaviruses. It contains 601 amino acids, is part of the superfamily 1B, and is highly conserved in all coronaviruses. Helicases can have either 3′–5′ (SF1A subfamily) or 5′–3'(SF1B subfamily) translocation polarity, defined as the direction (characterized as 5′ → 3′ or 3′ → 5′) of helicase movement on the DNA/RNA single-strand along which it is moving. The SARS-CoV-2 helicase is a critical enzyme for viral replication as unwinds duplex RNA, initiating the first step of the RNA cap synthesis that is essential to protect to the virus from innate immune attack, stabilize it, and ensure its translation.

## *NSP14 (3′ to 5′ Endonuclease, N7-Methyltransferase)*

The guanine-N7-methyltransferase activity introduces the 5-cap of the virus. The γ-phosphate of the 5′ end of nascent mRNA is removed by the RNA triphosphatase (NSP13), a GMP moiety from a covalent enzyme-GMP intermediate is transferred to the resulting mRNA with a diphosphate end. Subsequnetly, the GpppA cap is methylated with S-adenosyl-methionine, which is catalyzed by the guanine-N7-methyltransferase (NSP14) to yield the cap-0 structure, and 2′-*O*-methylation by NSP16 of adenine gives the cap-1 structure.

## *NSP15 (endoRNAse)*

NSP15 of is an endoribonuclease that cleaves RNA at uridylates in the 3′-position to form a 2′ to 3′ cyclic phosphodiester product. It specifically targets and degrades the viral polyuridine sequences to prevent the host immune sensing system from detecting the virus.

### *NSP16 (2′-O-Ribose-Methyltransferase)*

The viral RNA has a 5′-cap, which protects it from mRNA degradation by 5′-exoribonucleases, promotes mRNA translation, and prevents the viral RNA from being recognized by innate immunity mechanisms. The RNA cap is an N7-methylated guanine nucleotide connected through a 5′–5′ triphosphate bridge to the first transcribed nucleotide (adenine). NSP16 methylates the 2′-hydroxy group of adenine using S-adenosylmethionine as the methyl sources.

## Computational Methods for Virtual Screening

### *Protein Structure Preparation and Grid Preparation*

All SARS-CoV-2 experimental crystal structures are archived in the Research Collaboratory for Structural Biology (http://www.rcsb.org) and are freely available. Protein structures must be curated and prepared prior to computational studies. Nonessential and nonbridging water molecules should be removed prior to molecular docking studies; in our case this was done using the UCSF Chimera package (https://www.cgl.ucsf.edu/chimera/). Docking packages frequently provide software tools to assist with preparing the protein and small molecule ligand structures. As we were using the widely known and robust AutoDock suite of docking algorithms, we used the accompanying AutoDock Tools (ADT) software to prepare the required files for use with AutoDock Vina. This assigns hydrogen to polar atoms, calculates Gasteiger partial charges on atoms in the protein structure, and converts the protein structure from the RCSB .pdb file format to .pdbqt format required by the AutoDock packages.

### *Drug and Clinical Trials Databases for Screening*

Fortunately, there are a several very large, small molecule databases available. For example, the ChEMBL database contains structures and biological data for 2.1 million small molecules. For drug and natural product repurposing studies an appropriate subset of molecules is available for download from the DrugBank [40] and CHEMBL database (FDA approved) [41]. For our in silico screening studies, a total of 8773 and 13,308 drugs were retrieved from DrugBank and CHEMBL database, respectively. The drugs were downloaded in .sdf file format that is accepted by most modeling software, and converted to AutoDock .pdbqt format using Raccoon (http://autodock.scripps.edu/resources/raccoon) [42].

## *Molecular Docking*

There are a wide range of public domain and proprietary software packages available for molecular docking. Each has their strengths and weaknesses as reviewed recently by Weng et al. and Kitchen et al. [43, 44]. We used the AutoDock Vina package (version 1.1.3) to dock small molecule ligand structures against protein structures. AutoDock Vina employs gradient-based conformational search and an energy-based empirical scoring function that includes an approximate correction for ligand conformational entropy. AutoDock Vina is also flexible, easily scripted, extensively validated in many published studies with a variety of proteins and ligands and takes advantage of large multi-CPU or -GPU machines to run calculations in parallel. The code has also been employed very successfully to dock millions of small molecule drug candidates into a series of protein targets to discover new potent drug leads. The package includes useful scripts for generating modified .pdb files required for grid calculations and for setting up the grid calculations around each protein automatically. The software requires the removal of hydrogens, addition of polar hydrogens, setting of the correct atom types, and calculation of atom charges compatible with the AutoGrid code. The algorithm generates a grid around each protein and calculates the interaction energy of a probe atom at each grid position outside and within internal cavities of the protein. The grid resolution was set to 1 Å, the maximum number of binding modes to output was fixed at 10, and the exhaustiveness level (controlling the number of independent runs performed) was set at 8 for the studies summarized below. Docking employed a genetic algorithm to optimize the binding conformations of the ligands during docking to the SARS-CoV-2 target protein site. Drugs were docked individually to the active sites of the three SARS-CoV-2 enzymes, with the grid coordinates (grid centre) and grid boxes of appropriate sizes generated. The top scoring compounds from docking studies were identified and subjected to molecular dynamic simulation. We analyzed the docked structures using UCSF Chimera [45] and LigPlot+ software [46] to illustrate hydrogen-bond and hydrophobic interactions. A total of fifty top compounds selected from each of the Drugbank and CHEMBL compounds by the molecular docking study and molecular dynamics simulations were conducted on these to obtain more accurate docking poses and binding free energies.

## *Molecular Dynamics Simulation and Binding Free Energy Estimation*

The structures of the top scoring docked compounds for each protein target were minimized with the CHARMm force field. Ligand topology files were prepared by Swissparam (http://www.swissparam.ch/) [47] and minimized in Gromacs2020 (http://www.gromacs.org/) [48]. Docked complexes of ligands and target

SARS-CoV-2 proteins were used as starting geometries for MD simulations. The simulations were carried out using the GPU accelerated version of the program with the CHARMm force field I and periodic boundary conditions in ORACLE server. Docked complexes were immersed in a truncated octahedral box of TIP3P water molecules. The solvated box was further neutralized with $Na^+$ or $Cl^-$ counter ions using the tleap program. Particle Mesh Ewald (PME) was employed to calculate the long-range electrostatic interactions. The cutoff distance for the long-range van der Waals (VDW) energy term was 12.0 Å. The whole system was minimized without any constraints. The above steps applied 2500 cycles of steepest descent minimization followed by 5000 cycles of conjugate gradient minimization. After system optimization, the MD simulations was initiated by gradually heating each system in the NVT ensemble from 0 to 300 K for 50 ps using a Langevin thermostat with a coupling coefficient of 1.0/ps and with a force constant of 2.0 kcal/mol Å$^2$ on the complex. Finally, a production run of 20 ns of MD simulation was performed under a constant temperature of 300 K in the NPT ensemble with periodic boundary conditions for each system. During the MD procedure, the SHAKE algorithm was applied to constrain all covalent bonds involving hydrogen atoms. The time step was set to 2 fs. The structural stability of the complex was monitored by the RMSD and RMSF values of the backbone atoms of the entire protein. Calculations were also performed for up to 100 ns on few compounds to ensure that 20 ns is sufficiently long for simulation convergence. Duplicate production runs starting with different random seeds were also performed to allow estimates of binding energy uncertainties to be obtained.

The binding free energies of the protein–protein complexes were evaluated in two ways. The traditional method is to calculate the energies of solvated SARS-CoV-2 proteins and small molecule ligands and that of the bound complex and derive the binding energy by subtraction.

$$\Delta G(\text{binding,aq.}) = \Delta G(\text{complex,aq.}) - (\Delta G(\text{protein,aq.}) + \Delta G(\text{ligand,aq.}) \quad (1)$$

We also calculated binding energies using the molecular mechanics Poisson Boltzmann surface area (MM/PBSA) tool in GROMACS that is derived from the nonbonded interaction energies of the complex. The method is also widely used method for binding free energy calculations. The MMPBSA calculations were conducted by GMXPBSA 2.160, a suite of Bash/Perl scripts for streamlining MM/PBSA calculations on structural ensembles derived from GROMACS trajectories and to automatically calculating binding free energies for protein–protein or ligand–protein complexes. GMXPBSA 2.1 calculates diverse MM/PBSA energy contributions from molecular mechanics (MM) and electrostatic contributions to solvation (PB) and nonpolar contributions to solvation (SA). This tool combines the capability of MD simulations (GROMACS) and the Poisson–Boltzmann equation (APBS) for calculating solvation energy [49]. The g_mmpbsa tool in GROMACS was used after molecular dynamics simulations, the output files obtained were used to post-process binding free energies by the single-trajectory MMPBSA method. In the current study we considered 100 frames at equal distance taken from the 20 ns trajectory files.

Specifically, for a noncovalent binding interaction in the aqueous phase the binding free energy, $\Delta G$ (bind,aq), is as follows.

$$\Delta G(\text{bind,aqu}) = \Delta G(\text{bind,vac}) + \Delta G(\text{bind,solv}) \tag{2}$$

where $\Delta G$ (bind, vac) is the binding free energy in vacuum, and $\Delta G$ (bind, solv) is the solvation free energy change upon binding.

$$\Delta G(\text{bind,solv}) = \Delta G(\text{R:L,solv}) - \Delta G(\text{R,solv}) - \Delta G(\text{L,solv}) \tag{3}$$

where $\Delta G$ (R:L, solv), $\Delta G$ (R, solv), and $\Delta G$ (L, solv) are solvation free energies of complex, receptor, and ligand, respectively.

Guterres and Im showed how substantial improvement in protein–ligand docking results could be achieved using high-throughput MD simulations [22]. As with our studies, they also employed AutoDock Vina for docking, followed by MD simulation using CHARMM. The MD parameters they advocated were very similar to those used in our study. Over 56 protein targets of 7 different protein classes docked with 560 ligands they demonstrated a 22% improvement in the area under receiver operating characteristics curve, from 0.68 using AutoDock Vina alone to 0.83 when the Vina results were refined by MD.

## Examples of Virtual Screening—Results, Validation, Leads

Of the 19 proteins encoded in the viral genome, the most promising and viable targets for structure-based drug design are the SARS-CoV-2 main protease (3CLpro or $M^{pro}$), RNA-dependent RNA polymerase (RdRp) and helicase enzymes. The following three case studies exemplify the computational repurposing approach we used to shortlist drugs and natural products for clinical use against COVID-19.

### *Main Protease ($M^{pro}$)*

We used AutoDock Vina and MD simulation to calculate binding poses and energies for repurposed drugs binding to the viral main protease $M^{pro}$ (3CLpro) [50]. This study identified 84 promising compounds for treating SARS-CoV-2 infections. The top hits consisted of a mixture of antiviral agents, natural products, and drugs developed for other disease applications. These included: bemcentinib, an inhibitor of the kinase domain of AXL receptor (Fig. 23.3); montelukast, a leukotriene receptor antagonist used for asthma therapy; ergotamine and mergocriptine, ergot

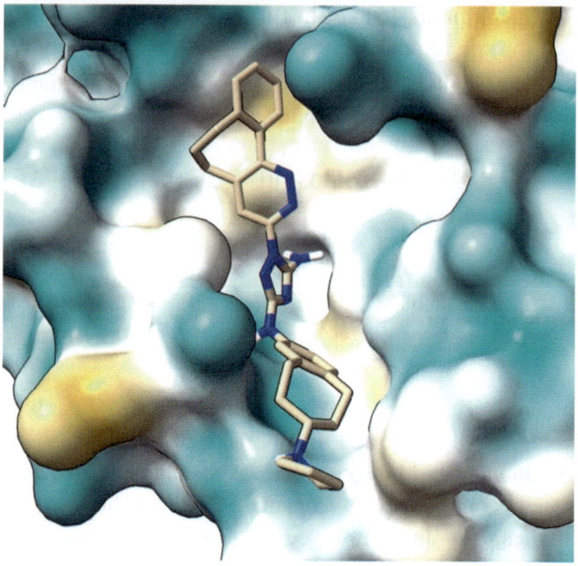

**Fig. 23.3** Hydrophobic protein surface representation of bemcentinib bound to pocket of $M^{pro}$ protein

compounds with α-1 selective adrenergic and dopamine receptor agonist activities; and remdesivir and several other antiviral agents.

The prognostic value of our computational approach was demonstrated by the fact that it identified a diverse range of drugs that have been shown to inhibit SARS-CoV-2 in vitro, or at a minimum had been reported as $M^{pro}$ hits in other computational screening studies. For example, the antiviral agents we identified using this approach, simeprevir, sofosbuvir, lopinavir, ritonavir, and remdesivir are being tested in clinical trials against SARS-CoV-2. These drugs have also been shown in in vitro assays to bind to $M^{pro}$ and have also been identified in other virtual screening studies. Drugs with greater novelty in our top 10 list, bemcentinib, PC786, montelukast, ergotamine, and mergocriptine, had binding affinities similar to the antiviral drugs. In some cases, they have been shown to have in vitro activity against SARS-CoV-2. Of the 80 drugs in our computational repurposing short list, at least 25% have confirmed in vitro or in vivo efficacy. This high success rate validates our virtual screening approach for identifying compounds with potentially useful activity against SARS-CoV-2 and, by analogy, other coronaviruses. We identified 28 drugs with high predicted binding energies to $M^{pro}$ that have not yet been screened for SARS-CoV-2 activity. These would be worthy of further consideration for testing.

## *RNA-Dependent RNA Polymerase (RdRp)*

The RNA-dependent RNA polymerase (RdRp) is another promising target for SARS-CoV-2 drug development. Again, we combined robust Vina docking to RdRP with MD simulations of the top 80 docking hits to yield a list of the most promising

RdRP inhibitors [51, 52]. Top hits included known antiviral drugs, paritaprevir, beclabuvir, remdesivir, voxilaprevir, setrobuvir, galidesvir, elbasvir, ciluprevir, faldaprevir, and tegobuvir. However, natural products and/or their synthetic analogs were also well represented in the top 20 hits, namely, ivermectin, digoxin, silibinin, rapamycin, novobiocin, eribulin, and ergotamine. These natural products are used to treat a diverse range of conditions including infections, cancers, cardiac insufficiency, liver damage, and circulatory issues. Almost all drugs in the top 20 hits have relatively large, complex structures and substantial ligand flexibility due to the large active site in RdRp. The literature revealed that more than 30% of our predicted RdRp inhibitors have reported in vitro activity or had been predicted by other modelling groups to have activity. The novel hits revealed by our screen can now be tested for activity in RdRp inhibition assays. These agents could also be quickly assessed in COVID-19 trials, as their safety and pharmacokinetics is already well understood.

### *Helicase*

We used the same computational virtual screening approach using AutoDock Vina and MD simulation in tandem to calculate binding poses and energies for repurposed drugs binding to the SARS-CoV-2 helicase. The top twenty molecules with the highest predicted binding affinity to the helicase could largely be characterized as having one or more hydrophobic aromatic moieties, separated by a linker from another polycyclic moiety containing hydrogen bond donors or acceptors. The molecules come from diverse drug classes, with antiviral agents making up 25% of the hits. Antihistamines and antipsychotics were also well represented. The tightest binding drugs included the natural products hesperidin (citrus flavanone glycoside) and rutin (flavonol glycoside); the antipsychotics pimozide, fluspirilene, and sertindole; the antihistamines fexofenadine and astemizole; and conivaptan (vasopressin inhibitor), aprepitant (NK1 antagonist), manidipine (Ca channel blocker, antihypertensive), aminoquinuride (trypanocidal agent), antrafenine (analgesic anti-inflammatory), epirubicin (anticancer intercalator), and dicoumarol (anticoagulant, potentially also useful for combatting clotting disorders induced by SARS-CoV-2). Again, more than 30% of the drugs in our computational screen short list have confirmed in vitro activity or are in clinical trials. These agents could be quickly assessed in COVID-19 trials, as their safety and pharmacokinetics is already well understood.

## Summary and Perspective

The results of the current drug repurposing study can robustly identify potential candidate drugs for testing and use in the current pandemic. We present a rational computational paradigm for identifying therapeutic agents for future viral pandemics and for identifying new therapies for other, important, nonviral diseases. Computational drug repurposing is extremely rapid, and by focusing on already approved drugs, provides a rationale for immediate use of the top hits in human trials. There are also opportunities to extend these methods to identify drugs that have pan-coronavirus activity by running similar computational screens on a large variety of different coronaviruses. The method has identified several repurposed drugs that inhibit two or more viral target protein, opening the way for developing multi-target drugs that viruses are less likely to develop resistance to. We predict that, increasingly, drug discovery will move from the wet lab to in silico, providing these enormous advantages in terms of time and cost. In silico approaches are particularly beneficial for rapidly screening for drugs active against pandemic viruses but clearly having much broader utility than this. Artificial intelligence and machine learning methods are also making rapid inroads into the drug repurposing field, recently reviewed generally [53, 54], and for COVID-19 treatment [55–57].

## References

1. Abdelrahman Z, Li M, Wang X. Comparative review of SARS-CoV-2, SARS-CoV, MERS-CoV, and influenza A respiratory viruses. Front Immunol. 2020;11:2309.
2. Kapikian AZ. The coronaviruses. Devel Biol Standard. 1975;28:42–64.
3. Almeida JD, Tyrrell DA. The morphology of three previously uncharacterized human respiratory viruses that grow in organ culture. J Gen Virol. 1967;1(2):175–8.
4. Drosten C, Gunther S, Preiser W, van der Werf S, Brodt HR, Becker S, et al. Identification of a novel coronavirus in patients with severe acute respiratory syndrome. N Engl J Med. 2003;348(20):1967–76.
5. Rota PA, Oberste MS, Monroe SS, Nix WA, Campagnoli R, Icenogle JP, et al. Characterization of a novel coronavirus associated with severe acute respiratory syndrome. Science. 2003;300(5624):1394–9.
6. Mubarak A, Alturaiki W, Hemida MG. Middle east respiratory syndrome coronavirus (MERS-CoV): infection, immunological response, and vaccine development. J Immunol Res. 2019;2019:6491738.
7. Zhu Z, Lian X, Su X, Wu W, Marraro GA, Zeng Y. From SARS and MERS to COVID-19: a brief summary and comparison of severe acute respiratory infections caused by three highly pathogenic human coronaviruses. Respir Res. 2020;21(1):1–14.
8. Callow KA, Parry HF, Sergeant M, Tyrrell DA. The time course of the immune response to experimental coronavirus infection of man. Epidemiol Infect. 1990;105(2):435–46.
9. Tang F, Quan Y, Xin ZT, Wrammert J, Ma MJ, Lv H, et al. Lack of peripheral memory B cell responses in recovered patients with severe acute respiratory syndrome: a six-year follow-up study. J Immunol. 2011;186(12):7264–8.
10. Wang SF, Tseng SP, Yen CH, Yang JY, Tsao CH, Shen CW, et al. Antibody-dependent SARS coronavirus infection is mediated by antibodies against spike proteins. Biochem Biophys Res Commun. 2014;451(2):208–14.
11. Clay C, Donart N, Fomukong N, Knight JB, Lei W, Price L, et al. Primary severe acute respiratory syndrome coronavirus infection limits replication but not lung inflammation upon homologous rechallenge. J Virol. 2012;86(8):4234–44.
12. Cavalla, D.; Oerton, E.; Bender, A., 1.02 - Drug Repurposing Review. In Comprehensive Medicinal Chemistry III, Chackalamannil, S.; Rotella, D.; Ward, S. E., Eds. Elsevier: Oxford, 2017;11–47.

13. Ban TA. The role of serendipity in drug discovery. Dialogues Clin Neurosci. 2006;8(3):335–44.
14. Fagan SC. Drug repurposing for drug development in stroke. Rev Neurol Dis. 2010;7(Suppl 1):S3–6.
15. Law GL, Tisoncik-Go J, Korth MJ, Katze MG. Drug repurposing: a better approach for infectious disease drug discovery? Curr Opin Immunol. 2013;25(5):588–92.
16. Klug DM, Gelb MH, Pollastri MP. Repurposing strategies for tropical disease drug discovery. Bioorg Med Chem Lett. 2016;26(11):2569–76.
17. Kale VP, Habib H, Chitren R, Patel M, Pramanik KC, Jonnalagadda SC, et al. Old drugs, new uses: drug repurposing in hematological malignancies. Semin Cancer Biol. 2021;68:242–8.
18. Khachigian LM. Repurposing drugs for skin cancer. Curr Med Chem. 2020;27(42):7214–21.
19. Spugnini EP, Fais S. Drug repurposing for anticancer therapies. A lesson from proton pump inhibitors. Expert Opin Ther Pat. 2020;30(1):15–25.
20. Finsterer J, Frank M. Repurposed drugs in metabolic disorders. Curr Top Med Chem. 2013;13(18):2386–94.
21. Shakkour Z, Habashy KJ, Berro M, Takkoush S, Abdelhady S, Koleilat N, et al. Drug repurposing in neurological disorders: implications for neurotherapy in traumatic brain injury. Neuroscientist. 2021;27(6):620–49.
22. Guterres H, Im W. Improving protein-ligand docking results with high-throughput molecular dynamics simulations. J Chem Inf Mod. 2020;60(4):2189–98.
23. Winkler DA. Ligand entropy is hard but should not be ignored. J Chem Inf Mod. 2020;60(10):4421–3.
24. Muratov E, Brown N, Fourches D, Kozakov D, Medina-Franco JL, Merz K, et al. Best practices of data modeling and rigorous computational approaches to enable drug discovery against COVID-19. Chem Soc Rev. 2021;50:9121–51.
25. Wang X, Guan Y. COVID-19 drug repurposing: A review of computational screening methods, clinical trials, and protein interaction assays. Med Res Rev. 2021;41(1):5–28.
26. Park K. A review of computational drug repurposing. Transl Clin Pharmacol. 2019;27(2):59–63.
27. Sadeghi SS, Keyvanpour MR. Computational drug repurposing: classification of the research opportunities and challenges. Curr Comput Aided Drug Des. 2020;16(4):354–64.
28. Guan Y, Zheng B, He Y, Liu X, Zhuang Z, Cheung C, et al. Isolation and characterization of viruses related to the SARS coronavirus from animals in southern China. Science. 2003;302(5643):276–8.
29. Chu DK, Poon LL, Gomaa MM, Shehata MM, Perera RA, Zeid DA, et al. MERS coronaviruses in dromedary camels, Egypt. Emerg Infect Dis. 2014;20(6):1049.
30. Hoffmann M, Kleine-Weber H, Schroeder S, Krüger N, Herrler T, Erichsen S, et al. SARS-CoV-2 cell entry depends on ACE2 and TMPRSS2 and is blocked by a clinically proven protease inhibitor. Cell. 2020;52(5):731–3.
31. V'kovski P, Kratzel A, Steiner S, Stalder H, Thiel V. Coronavirus biology and replication: implications for SARS-CoV-2. Nat Rev Microbiol. 2020:1–16.
32. Li F. Structure, function, and evolution of coronavirus spike proteins. Annu Rev Virol. 2016;3:237–61.
33. Wrapp D, Wang N, Corbett KS, Goldsmith JA, Hsieh C-L, Abiona O, et al. Cryo-EM structure of the 2019-nCoV spike in the prefusion conformation. Science. 2020;367(6483):1260–3.
34. Iwata-Yoshikawa N, Uda A, Suzuki T, Tsunetsugu-Yokota Y, Sato Y, Morikawa S, et al. Effects of toll-like receptor stimulation on eosinophilic infiltration in lungs of BALB/c mice immunized with UV-inactivated severe acute respiratory syndrome-related coronavirus vaccine. J Virol. 2014;88(15):8597–614.
35. Yin Y, Wunderink RG. MERS, SARS and other coronaviruses as causes of pneumonia. Respirology. 2018;23(2):130–7.
36. Yoshimoto FK. The proteins of severe acute respiratory syndrome Coronavirus-2 (SARS CoV-2 or n-COV19), the cause of COVID-19. Protein J. 2020;39(3):198–216.
37. Katsnelson A. What do we know about the novel coronavirus's 29 proteins? C&EN. 2020;98(15):19–21.

38. Jin Z, Du X, Xu Y, Deng Y, Liu M, Zhao Y, et al. Structure of M(pro) from SARS-CoV-2 and discovery of its inhibitors. Nature. 2020;582(7811):289–93.
39. Rathnayake AD, Zheng J, Kim Y, Perera KD, Mackin S, Meyerholz DK, et al. 3C-like protease inhibitors block coronavirus replication in vitro and improve survival in MERS-CoV-infected mice. Sci Transl Med. 2020;12(557):eabc5332.
40. Wishart DS, Feunang YD, Guo AC, Lo EJ, Marcu A, Grant JR, et al. DrugBank 5.0: a major update to the DrugBank database for 2018. Nucleic Acids Res. 2018;46(D1):D1074–D82.
41. Gaulton A, Hersey A, Nowotka M, Bento AP, Chambers J, Mendez D, et al. The ChEMBL database in 2017. Nucleic Acids Res. 2017;45(D1):D945–D54.
42. Forli S, Huey R, Pique ME, Sanner MF, Goodsell DS, Olson AJ. Computational protein-ligand docking and virtual drug screening with the AutoDock suite. Nat Protoc. 2016;11(5):905–19.
43. Kitchen DB, Decornez H, Furr JR, Bajorath J. Docking and scoring in virtual screening for drug discovery: methods and applications. Nat Rev Drug Discov. 2004;3(11):935–49.
44. Weng G, Gao J, Wang Z, Wang E, Hu X, Yao X, et al. Comprehensive evaluation of fourteen docking programs on protein-peptide complexes. J Chem Theor Comput. 2020;16(6):3959–69.
45. Pettersen EF, Goddard TD, Huang CC, Couch GS, Greenblatt DM, Meng EC, et al. UCSF Chimera--a visualization system for exploratory research and analysis. J Comp Chem. 2004;25(13):1605–12.
46. Laskowski RA, Swindells MB. LigPlot+: multiple ligand-protein interaction diagrams for drug discovery. J Chem Inf Mod. 2011;51(10):2778–86.
47. Zoete V, Cuendet MA, Grosdidier A, Michielin O. SwissParam: a fast force field generation tool for small organic molecules. J Comp Chem. 2011;32(11):2359–68.
48. Kohnke B, Kutzner C, Grubmuller H. A GPU-accelerated fast multipole method for GROMACS: performance and accuracy. J Chem Theor Comput. 2020;16(11):6938–49.
49. Baker NA, Sept D, Holst MJ, McCammon JA. The adaptive multilevel finite element solution of the Poisson-Boltzmann equation on massively parallel computers. IBM J Res Devel. 2001;45(3.4):427–38.
50. Piplani S, Singh P, Petrovsky N, Winkler DA. Computational screening of repurposed drugs and natural products against SARS-Cov-2 main protease as potential COVID-19 therapies. Front Mol Biosci. 2021;9:781039.
51. Piplani S, Singh P, Winkler DA, Petrovsky N. Computationally repurposed drugs and natural products against RNA dependent RNA polymerase as potential COVID-19 therapies. arXiv preprint arXiv:201114241. 2020;
52. Piplani S, Singh P, Winkler DA, Petrovsky N. Computationally repurposed drugs and natural products against RNA dependent RNA polymerase as potential COVID-19 therapies. Mol Biomed. 2021;2:28.
53. Issa NT, Stathias V, Schurer S, Dakshanamurthy S. Machine and deep learning approaches for cancer drug repurposing. Semin Cancer Biol. 2021;68:132–42.
54. Urbina F, Puhl AC, Ekins S. Recent advances in drug repurposing using machine learning. Curr Opin Chem Biol. 2021;65:74–84.
55. Kc GB, Bocci G, Verma S, Hassan MM, Holmes J, Yang JJ, et al. A machine learning platform to estimate anti-SARS-CoV-2 activities. Nat Mach Intell. 2021;3(6):527–35.
56. Mohapatra S, Nath P, Chatterjee M, Das N, Kalita D, Roy P, et al. Repurposing therapeutics for COVID-19: rapid prediction of commercially available drugs through machine learning and docking. PLoS One. 2020;15(11):e0241543.
57. Zhou Y, Wang F, Tang J, Nussinov R, Cheng F. Artificial intelligence in COVID-19 drug repurposing. Lancet Digit Health. 2020;2(12):e667–e76.

# Chapter 24
# In Silico Drug Repositioning for COVID-19: Progress and Challenges

**Suresh Kumar**

## Introduction

The process of discovering new uses for previously approved, discontinued, delayed, or drugs under investigation is referred to as drug repurposing. It is also referred to as repositioning, drug reprofiling, indication expansion, or indication shift [1]. Although drug reuse is not a new concept, it has gained popularity over the past few decades. More than a third of the authorized pharmaceutical products have been reconstituted, resulting in a 25% increase in overall annual revenue for the pharmaceutical operation [2].

According to CMR International's recent Pharmaceutical Research and Development Handbook, more than 55 drugs were phased out during Phase III clinical development between 2008 and 2010 [3]. Although some drugs have failed in preclinical and early human studies, they are safe. This aspect of drug safety is very attractive for drug repositioning. In general, approved drugs are more likely to be safe in new indications and patient populations. The growing body of drug knowledge will shorten the development cycle and reduce the risk of development costs and costs associated with new molecular entities [4].

While drug repurpose is possible at any stage, it is most promising for drugs that are already approved [5]. Currently, advanced computer technology is being utilized to forecast novel drug targets or drug reuse. In comparison to high-throughput screening, which requires the assessment of hundreds of compounds, computer technology is rapid and affordable and may be used as a preliminary filtering approach. They are also beneficial for high-priority therapies that require more investigation and testing. The rationale for drug recycling is that numerous diseases

---

S. Kumar (✉)
Faculty of Health and Life Sciences, Management and Science University, University Drive, Shah Alam, Selangor, Malaysia
e-mail: sureshkumar@msu.edu.my



S. Adibi et al. (eds.), *Frontiers of COVID-19*,
https://doi.org/10.1007/978-3-031-08045-6_24

may use the same metabolic processes [6]. Drug repurposing has significant regulatory and scientific consequences, notably in situations like the COVID-19. This chapter addresses drug repurposing techniques and methodologies.

## Drug Repurposing

Traditional de novo drug discovery is an expensive and risky approach. Computational techniques for drug repurposing can significantly speed up the traditional drug discovery process (Fig. 24.1). Developing drugs traditionally is costly and time-consuming. It takes an average of 14 years and costs more than U.S. $2 billion to bring a drug to market. Approximately 90% of drugs fail throughout the drug development process owing to safety concerns or a lack of efficacy. The computational drug repurposing technique, which combines and analyses huge data sets on tens of thousands of drugs and diseases automatically, has the potential to significantly speed the traditional drug development process. As the COVID-19 epidemic expanded, two more impediments emerged: the speed with which therapeutic approval could be obtained and the urgency with which clinical requirements could be met. Appropriate regulatory measures should take the risk–benefit ratio into account. Drugs must be developed and authorized quickly to halt the spread of diseases [7]. Even if the proposed drug shows early efficacy in animal and clinical studies, it will take at least 2 years to reach the market. Because the manufacturer will conduct safety studies before the start of the clinical trial, and the clinical study can be delayed for up to 2 years [8–10].

While rapid development and decision-making can result in a more rapid release of drugs, complete safety, and effectiveness data are compromised. Although drug development takes an average of 12 to 15 years, it can be completed in as little as 12 to 18 months if the process is accelerated. To accelerate the completion of phase III clinical trials, shorter, fewer, or no phase III trials are required [11]. As a result, drug approval will require less information than usual in the event of a pandemic. This is possible when the period of low incidence coincides with the pandemic's

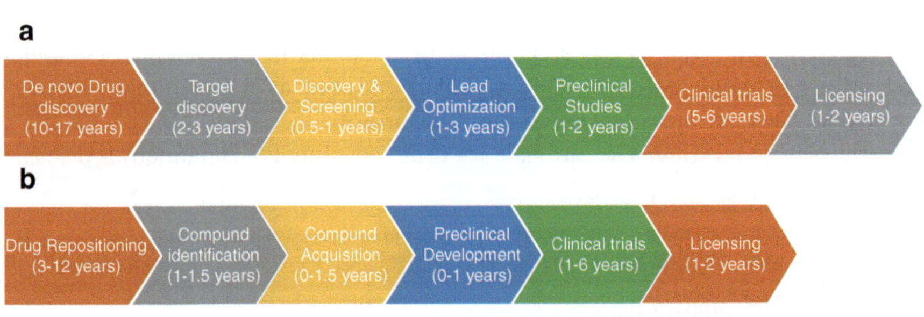


**Fig. 24.1** A comparison of traditional de novo drug discovery versus drug repositioning. (**a**) De novo drug discovery. (**b**) Drug repositioning

recruitment phase [12, 13]. Although COVID-19 lacks a broad legal framework because it is based on disease incidence, a small number of reusable drugs have been approved, owing in part to the evaluation of COVID-19's benefit–risk profile and biomarker evidence [14]. Drugs that have been repurposed for COVID-19 have been approved for an emergency, conditional marketing, or early access to drugs with limited clinical data [15].

Although postmarketing studies are commonly used to expand Phase II studies, approval decisions are typically based on data from Phase III clinical trials [16–20]. It is generally recognized that the safety information provided for all pharmaceutical drugs at the time of approval is insufficient. The goal of efficacy-focused clinical development is to improve efficacy. As a result, the postauthorization risk management plan is data-driven to address any safety concerns that occur following authorization. These problems are exacerbated by the need for rapid development and approval. As a result, this is strongly advised, although, in some circumstances, authorities will need to undertake a complete postapproval examination and report to the Food and Drug Administration (FDA) regularly [21].

## In Silico Drug Repurposing Methods

According to the Pharmaceutical Research and Manufacturers of America (PhRMA), only one out of every 5000–10,000 compounds discovered in drug research is likely to be commercialized [22]. The information age has transformed the process of drug development, providing massive amounts of data that have assisted in our knowledge of the molecular pathways behind human disease. While significant advances have been achieved in the postgenomic era, researchers continue to encounter problems in finding, collecting, and analyzing all relevant data on any human disease effectively and completely. This problem necessitates the efficient use of bioinformatics and computational methods. The primary obstacles include the following: (i) collecting relevant information from terabytes of data from various sources. (ii) data mining and knowledge management techniques are combined using coherent and manual search methods. (iii) effective data analysis to generate clinically relevant test hypotheses [23–25].

The complete sequencing of the human genome at the turn of the twentieth century reshaped the landscape of drug development. Currently, a large amount of data, such as the genome, transcriptome, proteome, metabolome, and pharmacological data, is dispersed among many databases that are publicly available through the Internet [26]. In addition, with the creation of complex protein and signaling pathway databases, the number of these databases has increased, and these databases collectively reflect the current understanding of disease mechanisms [27–30]. Likewise, the number of publications in scientific journals has increased along with the enormous amount of data. Due to these diverse resources, the development of bioinformatics and computational methods for collecting, analyzing, and interpreting data is essential [31]. This strategy has also led to the development of new

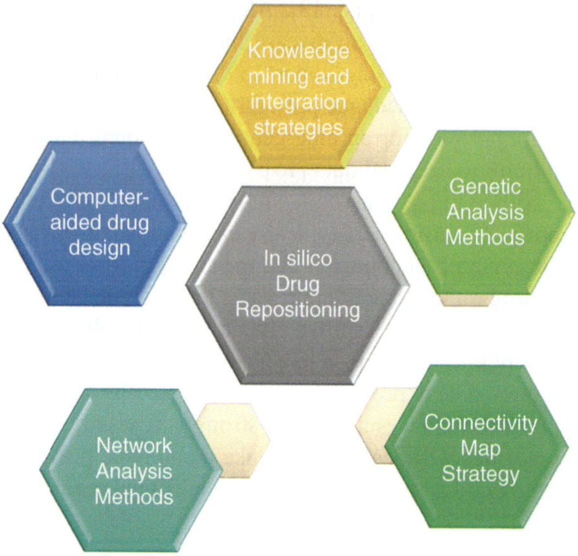


**Fig. 24.2** The computational approaches for drug repositioning:knowledge mining and integration strategies, genetic analysis methods, connectivity map strategy, network analysis methods and computer-aided drug design

theories linking disease with experimental or commercial drugs in conjunction with predictive algorithms [32–34]. These computational approaches to drug repositioning can be divided into the five strategies: knowledge mining and integration strategies, genetic analysis methods, connectivity map strategy, network analysis methods, and computer-aided drug design (Fig. 24.2).

## *Knowledge Mining and Integration Strategies*

Drug development is often divided into five stages: preclinical and discovery, safety evaluation, clinical research, FDA review, and FDA postmarketing surveillance. This is a lengthy and costly process with a high rate of failure. On the other side, drug repositioning is a four-stage process: The FDA is responsible for the identification, acquisition, development, and postmarket safety monitoring of drugs [35]. Recent research has produced a large amount of experimental data on COVID-19. To discover new and hidden knowledge, a computer evaluation of the use of data science techniques must be carried out. To fully understand the biology and mechanism of SARS-CoV-2 and its process, the data must be fully comprehended.

There has been a wealth of solutions because of the challenge computer biologists confront in gathering and understanding the most relevant data from many sources for the goal of hypothesis creation. At a high level, the main differences between these approaches relate to identifying and evaluating key sources. Consequently, the establishment of an opportunity to reposition a drug requires both a major computer effort and a biological evaluation of the feasibility of action for the new drug suggestion. A computer strategy for new drug suggestions in its systemic form is typically an automated approach. This oversees the evaluation of proposed diseases as well as the design of experimental study concepts to test with the assistance of biologists or disease experts [36].

To incorporate knowledgeable disease-related data, a target-based information technology method can be combined with high-throughput data mining strategies. The challenge is not only determining which data to extract or which methodologies to employ but also which high-quality rich-content databases to use for hypothesis creation [37]. A critical component of any new approach for disease indicators is the final prioritization or classification of the different types of data necessary to conduct a thorough evaluation of the evidence for each disease assumption. In addition, one disease hypothesis is compared to another via an absolute score system. The efficacy data from Phase II/III clinical trials are the most significant evidence for combining a biological target and a new indication for premarket drug candidates. Ongoing trial with no published data from clinical trials suggests preclinical data with slightly lower evidence [38]. The third level of evidence for target participation in a novel indication would be genetic evidence from functional polymorphic or associated human disease research, as well as mouse knockout data. Finally, evidence gathered from a variety of bibliographic databases can be used to generate new hypotheses for indications that can then be included in the disease classification system using advanced text mining techniques [39–42].

## *Genetic Analysis Methods*

Using genetic studies to identify "druggable" targets is one method to improve the chances of successful drug repositioning. The advent of large-scale genetic research, mostly in the form of genome-wide association studies (GWAS), has significantly expanded our understanding of the genetic basis of a variety of diseases and enabled researchers to use this information to develop therapeutic targets. Many GWAS conducted in recent years represents a large number of potential new drug retargeting libraries. Disease–gene associations are identified by combining functional genomic data with advanced computational approaches. Genetic analysis is an effective strategy for coming up with new therapeutic indication hypotheses. This information is especially useful when it is backed up by other sources of information, such as clinical expression analysis or preclinical research [43–45]. The approach can provide several high-end repositioning hypotheses depending on the nature and source of genomic data. Because of the success of this technology, many sequencing, expression, and phenotype genetic analytical methodologies have been developed [46, 47]. One of the limitations of the GWAS study is that some of the top genes identified may not be druggable. Second, relying exclusively on the impact of the most significant SNPs may lead to the omission of physiologically important target genes. Third, focusing upon only candidate genes may result in the omission of multi-target drugs, which may be more effective in some cases than single-target drugs. Fourth, due to the complexity of the human genome, there is no one-size-fits-all approach to accurate annotation.

## *Connectivity Map Strategy*

The Connectivity Map concept may be the most unique strategy for discovering new indications in the process of drug repositioning. This is a computational method that uses microarray-based transcription profile data to generate new ideas for disease indications and is easy to apply to other "omics" platforms [48]. This technique can theoretically link small molecule drugs to their mode of action as well as novel diseases by using their corresponding gene expression. The stronger the relationship between the disease signature and the inverse drug profile, the more likely the drug is to reverse the disease genotype/phenotype [49].

Connectivity mapping is a method for assembling reference transcriptional profiles obtained from microarrays by assessing the differential expression of a cell line treated with a series of drugs in comparison to untreated controls. The differential expressions' rank order for each compound is then generated. Disease signatures can be derived from a variety of sources, including disease microarrays and previously published data. By ranking all connection levels in descending order and setting the relevance threshold, the drug with the greatest score is chosen [50, 51]. As a result, the ideal treatment will have an exact inverse signature of the disease state, restoring the normal phenotype. This technique has the advantage of being platform-independent for compound reference profiles and disease signature sources. Because it is a computational approach, it has the potential to quickly identify many probable direct and inverse correlations between a wide range of disease conditions. The Connectivity Map method is based on the Kolmogorov-Smirnov statistic and employs Gene Set Enrichment Analysis, a nonparametric, rank-based pattern-matching tool. The expression profiles of the compound reference genes are also nonparametrically represented, but each gene is rank ordered depending on its degree of differential expression relative to untreated controls [52]. This method has a limitation in terms of experimental replicates, which can be challenging given that most small compounds have only one copy per cell line per experiment. Another potential limitation is the occurrence of batch processing effects.

## *Network Analysis Methods*

Network analysis tools greatly simplify the investigation of the complexity of biological systems and the diversity of different types of data defining a disease state. These techniques can be used to mathematically and graphically represent the various protein interactions that occur in higher species. In general, these strategies focus on concepts that are overrepresented in the pattern of the nodes and edges of a biological network [53, 54]. This approach could be extended to network hubs that appear to be key proteins in protein interactions. These hubs can be useful as important intervention sites in a specific disease condition, making them potential drug targets [55]. The current state of knowledge about molecular interaction networks is incomplete, and the associated configuration profiles are also very noisy, which are the limitations. Interactomes, on the other hand, only provide static snapshots of biological systems, whereas it contains dynamic systems. There is a paucity of information on precise interaction kinetics, and there is no obvious link between the molecular origin and the organism's reaction.

Transcriptome data in the gene regulatory network may capture the dynamic features of cells and give an in-depth knowledge of drug action mechanisms. A network analysis approach for differential expression data has been developed to identify genes from specific disease linkage and associated regions. Most gene prioritization methods necessitate prior knowledge of disease processes to identify potential drug targets. Differential gene expression studies show that gene expression patterns change systemically as diseases develop. Consequently, diverse gene expression patterns might be used as input to prioritize prospective therapeutic targets. However, this technique has certain drawbacks, such as the difficulty in defining robust gene features owing to noise in the expression of some genes. Furthermore, drug targets and genes controlled by targets may not always have significant expression changes [56].

Compounds and metabolites are depicted as nodes in the metabolic network. Excessive chemical concentrations (mass flow) produced by specific enzymes can result in disease. These enzymes may be therapeutic targets for this disease due to their ability to manipulate the concentration of disease-causing compounds via drug manipulation. Flux balance analysis is an example of an approach for identifying pharmacological targets.

The protein–protein interaction network (PPIN) is a form of a molecular interaction network that displays the interaction between a known drug target and other proteins, as well as proteins that interact indirectly with the target. Due to the difficulty of scanning the entire PPIN subnetwork space, advanced mathematical techniques will be required to detect out-of-tune subnetworks effectively. While PPIN's drug repositioning strategy has been extremely successful, it does have certain limitations. PPINs include links to undefined potential functionalities derived from several experimental sources. Additionally, the required data is noisy and incomplete, resulting in a bias in the generated network.

The network-based method is an effective way to link the molecular and phenotypic levels to determine drug targets. Determining the interaction between the drug and the target protein is an important step in drug discovery. Drug discovery and design are mainly based on the interaction between the drug and the target. Many drugs are nonspecific and respond to other targets in addition to the main target. In this case, a drug interaction is used to clarify the relationship between two drugs based on their similarity. The association with drug diseases includes various association modes, such as drug indications and drug side effects. In the disease–disease interaction, it has been proposed that two drugs with similar molecular pathophysiology can be interchanged. When effective drug repositioning is required, each network approach has limitations that can be overcome by combining data from several sources, such as molecular interaction networks and gene expression profiles.

## *Computer-Aided Drug Design*

Drug design may be divided into two categories: structural drug design and ligand-based drug design. A structural drug design is predicated on knowledge of the three-dimensional structure of the protein target as determined by X-ray crystallography or nuclear magnetic resonance spectroscopy. To carry out the structural drug design paradigm, an atomic-resolution three-dimensional protein structure of the receptor is required. A well-resolved crystal structure is preferred, with a resolution of at least 2.5 is often regarded as sufficient. If the target's three-dimensional structure is unknown, a protein model can be built by homology modeling to the nearest target-related protein having a known and accessible three-dimensional structure. Molecular docking can anticipate the intermolecular framework formed by a protein and a small molecule or another protein, as well as the binding modes that inhibit the protein. The virtual screening (VS) method compares the target protein to databases that contain millions of drug-like or lead-like compounds with well-defined three-dimensional structures [57]. To conduct the computational screening, the ligands' binding affinities are compared using a docking method. Ligand-based drug design is a method for finding compounds that bind to a protein target without knowledge of the three-dimensional receptor. The quantitative structure–activity relationship (QSAR) and pharmacophore modeling techniques are essential in ligand-oriented drug discovery because they provide statistical models for finding and optimizing leads [58]. However, using molecular docking for drug repositioning has several drawbacks. Docking applications are severely limited by the requirement for known chemical ligands and three-dimensional (3D) structures of protein targets because the structures of many physiologically significant proteins are still unknown. Furthermore, the molecular docking method is computationally intensive, which could lead to longer processing times. Furthermore, molecular docking studies have a high rate of false positives due to structural flaws in some proteins and inadequate modeling of atomic and molecular interactions. Machine learning approaches appear to be less expensive than docking simulations, since they can test more potential candidates for subsequent experimental screening.

# In Silico Drug Repurposing for COVID-19

Previously approved FDA drugs for other diseases were repositioned for COVID-19 treatment using various computational methods. Network-based algorithms, expression-based algorithms, and docking simulations were used to identify the drug that was predicted for drug repurposing in COVID-19 therapies. However, the accuracy of the predictions can be determined by comparing the reported computer studies' final candidate drug lists to the drugs currently undergoing clinical trials on clinicaltrials.gov (https://clinicaltrials.gov/). Numerous computational studies predicted and repurposed drugs for COVID-19 treatment, include chloroquine, hydroxychloroquine, remdesivir, lopinavir–ritonavir, ivermectin, favipiravir, oseltamivir, ribavirin, corticosteroids, and tocilizumab. This section will examine the clinical success of computationally predicted repurposed drugs [6]. This section contains comprehensive information on the drugs that have been largely repurposed and are currently being used to control SARS-CoV-2 infections as determined through computational methods. It is attempted to compile and review research on selected drugs using data from the WHO COVID guidelines, clinicaltrials.org, and a variety of other sources (at the time of writing this manuscript, September 2021).

## *Chloroquine*

Chloroquine has been repurposed as a COVID-19 drug due to its potent antiviral activity. Chloroquine is used to make chloroquine, a malarial drug that was traditionally found in the bark of Peruvian Kinchon trees. According to in-vitro research, chloroquine is a powerful bioactive agent against RNA viruses. Chloroquine has been found to have potential therapeutic effects against the coronavirus of SARS-CoV-1. The extensive antiviral activity against COVID-19 evaluated for chloroquine. While these results are preliminary, they are widely welcomed by the media, and some well-known personalities, including certain health regulatory authorities, have encouraged the use of chloroquine and hydroxychloroquine to treat COVID-19 [59]. However, little is known about the effect of chloroquine and hydroxychloroquine on the frequency and severity of adverse drug reactions (ADRs). Significant clinical studies have demonstrated that hydroxychloroquine and chloroquine are unlikely to be effective in treating or preventing COVID-19, prompting the U.S. Food and Drug Administration (FDA) to revoke the drug's emergency use authorization on June 15, 2020 [60]. According to the current meta-analysis of randomized studies, the use of chloroquine in COVID-19 patients has no benefit [61].

## *Hydroxychloroquine*

Hydroxychloroquine (a chloroquine derivative) is an antimalarial drug with anti-inflammatory characteristics. It has been used successfully as a safe anti-inflammatory medicine in auto-immune diseases, and preliminary research suggests that it may decrease pro-inflammatory cytokine expression in COVID-19. However, whether it is effective in eliminating the SARS-CoV-2 virus in ICU patients with overactive immune systems, particularly when the lungs are severely inflamed, has yet to be scientifically demonstrated [62, 63]. The available clinical evidence appears to be insufficient to prove the efficacy of HCQ in severely ill COVID-19 patients [61]. However, hydroxychloroquine, like chloroquine, has been demonstrated to be unsuccessful in the treatment or prevention of COVID-19, forcing the U.S. Food and Drug Administration (FDA) to revoke the drug's emergency use authorization on June 15, 2020. The recent solidarity trial, the UK's recovery trial, and a Cochrane review of other evidence on hydroxychloroquine conclusively showed that hydroxychloroquine did not reduce deaths among hospitalized COVID-19 patients.

## *Lopinavir–Ritonavir*

In vitro and animal studies have shown that lopinavir is effective against MERS-CoV. Additionally, lopinavir inhibits SARS-CoV by inhibiting a critical reproductive protease that appears to be highly conserved in SARS-CoV-2. In several countries, lopinavir–ritonavir therapy is recommended as first- or second-line treatment for COVID-19. Although several observational studies have demonstrated that lopinavir–ritonavir is associated with decreased viral shedding and fever in patients with COVID-19. Recent research on COVID-19, however, has found that regular lopinavir–ritonavir supplementation provides no benefit [64]. The lopinavir/ritonavir did not show efficacy in two large randomized controlled trials in hospitalized patients with COVID-19. The COVID-19 treatment guidelines panel recommends against the use of lopinavir/ritonavir for the treatment of COVID-19 in hospitalized patients [65].

## *Remdesivir*

Remdesivir is a novel and effective intravenous antiviral medication. It is effective against COVID-19 as well as other beta-coronaviruses in the same family. The laboratory investigation has shown that human cells can be protected from becoming infected with COVID-19. Furthermore, the findings suggest that in vitro remediation is highly successful in eradicating COVID-19 infection. Remdesivir was approved for emergency use in over 50 countries during the COVID-19 pandemic. The FDA has approved Remdesivir for the treatment of COVID-19 infection in adults and hospitalized children (over the age of 12 and weighing less than 45 kg). In adult COVID 19 patients, remdesivir, on the other hand, was not associated with statistically significant therapeutic benefits. Additional international research is necessary to establish the drug's efficacy and safety in COVID-19 patients [66]. An interesting study revealed that RDV's parent nucleotide, GS-441524, is more effective and less hazardous than its prodrug form and has been proven to be efficacious in vivo veterinary settings. As a result, future research into the parent nucleotide's usage against COVID-19 should proceed at a quicker speed.

### *Favipiravir*

Favipiravir is a novel RNA-dependent RNA polymerase (RdRp) inhibitor that is successful in the treatment of Ebola. Favipiravir is considered as a feasible treatment for COVID-19 due to its efficacy against a variety of viral diseases. Some research has demonstrated that favipiravir can accelerate virological clearance and clinical improvement, but most investigations are hampered by potential confounding factors (e.g., concurrent use of immunomodulators and other therapies). The study found no improvement in terms of mortality. A systematic review found that when given during the first seven days of hospitalization, there is a possibility of clinical improvement, but no statistically significant decrease in mortality for any of the groups studied, including hospitalized patients and those with mild or moderate symptoms. Other well-designed studies on dosage and duration of treatment, are essential to draw clear conclusions [67]. Any approval for the use of favipiravir, on the other hand, will require more clinical research, followed by approval for public use by the country's competent regulatory body [68].

### *Oseltamivir*

Oseltamivir inhibits the neuraminidase enzyme, which is expressed on the viral surface against the influenza virus and is also effective for various avian influenza virus strains. The enzyme promotes the release of virus from infected cells and facilitates viral movement within the respiratory tract. In the presence of neuraminidase inhibitors, virions stay attached to the membrane of infected cells and are also entrapped in respiratory secretions [69]. Clinical trials are also being conducted using oseltamivir in combination with various chloroquine and favipiravir regimens. A study showed that the drug exhibited no positive result on COVID-19. Additional clinical trials and larger, randomized controlled trials are required to demonstrate Oseltamivir's efficacy in patients with COVID-19 [70].

### *Ribavirin*

Ribavirin is an antiviral drug that prevents viruses from replicating and spreading [71]. Ribavirin has been approved for COVID-19 therapy in combination with interferon alfa or lopinavir–ritonavir. Ribavirin is effective against the Middle East respiratory syndrome corona virus (MERS-CoV) in vitro and in vivo, and case reports demonstrate that ribavirin paired with interferon alfa resulted in virologic clearance and survival. Clinical trial evidence demonstrating ribavirin's efficacy in treating COVID-19 is still insufficient [72].

## *Ivermectin*

Ivermectin is a medication used to treat parasite infestations and it was repositioned for COVID-19 treatment. Throughout the COVID-19 epidemic, misinformation suggesting that ivermectin helps treat and prevent COVID-19 has been extensively propagated. These claims are unsupported by reliable scientific evidence. Multiple major health organizations, including the Food and Drug Administration, the United States Centres for Disease Control, the European Medicines Agency, and the World Health Organization, have declared that ivermectin is not authorized or approved to treat COVID-19 [73].

## *Corticosteroid*

Corticosteroids are anti-inflammatory drugs that suppress the immune system. Dexamethasone is a glucocorticoid drug used in the treatment of rheumatoid arthritis, a range of skin diseases, severe allergies, asthma, and chronic obstructive pulmonary disease. According to WHO guidelines, corticosteroids should be used only in patients with severe or critical COVID-19 infection and not in individuals with nonsevere COVID-19 infection (absence of criteria for severe or critical infection). Dexamethasone was authorized by the European Medicines Agency (EMA) in September 2020 for use in adults and adolescents (12 years of age and a weight of at least 40 kg) who need supplemental oxygen therapy. Prolonged corticosteroid treatment may lead to the development of the so-called long COVID syndrome, which is characterized by tiredness and psychological problems and may be exacerbated by steroid-related adverse medication responses such as myopathy, neuromuscular weakness, and mental symptoms. Thus, corticosteroids seem to be a double-edged sword in the battle against COVID-19 and should be used with caution, considering the risk–benefit ratio, as a short-course treatment drug in a limited group of patients with COVID-19 who have been documented to benefit from survival. The safety and efficacy of corticosteroids in combination with antiviral medication for the treatment of COVID-19 have not been extensively studied in clinical trials [74].

## *Tocilizumab*

Tocilizumab (TCZ) is a recombinant humanized anti-interleukin-6 receptor monoclonal antibody used to treat systemic juvenile idiopathic arthritis (SJIA), polyarticular juvenile idiopathic arthritis (pJIA), and rheumatoid arthritis. In June 2021, the FDA issued tocilizumab an emergency use authorization for the treatment of COVID-19 in hospitalized patients aged two years and older who need supplementary oxygen, noninvasive or invasive mechanical ventilation. The COVID-19 Treatment Guidelines panel recommends tocilizumab in combination with dexamethasone in certain hospitalized patients who are having rapid respiratory decompensation due to COVID-19 [75]. The European Medicines Agency (EMA) is now assessing tocilizumab for the treatment of hospitalized individuals with severe COVID-19 who are already undergoing corticosteroid therapy and need additional oxygen or mechanical ventilation as of August 2021.

## Opportunities and Challenges

The traditional approach to pharmaceutical drug development is costly, time-consuming, and prone to failure. Repositioning, on the other hand, is a low-risk strategy that saves time and money. Experiments like cell-based assays, protein-based assays, animal models, and clinical trials provide a direct, evidence-based, and accurate understanding of the drug–disease connection. As a result of the availability of experimental data, computational techniques for drug repositioning have gained popularity in recent years, and they are frequently merged with them to provide accurate results. While there are many excellent computer models for drug repositioning, creating a reliable model is a difficult and time-consuming process. One of the major challenges is that theoretical calculation techniques are difficult to put into practice due to the difficulty of mapping such theoretical approaches to replicate biological activity, as well as other barriers such as missing, distorted, or erroneous data. For example, creating an accurate gene expression profile may be difficult due to a variety of factors, such as changes in experimental conditions throughout multiple trials, resulting in data mismatches in gene expression features and hence data bias. Furthermore, when these genes are employed as pharmacological targets, significant changes in gene expression may not occur consistently, resulting in incorrect findings. Furthermore, chemical structure and molecular information techniques are challenging to find probable drug–target interactions due to a lack of high-resolution structural data on drug targets. Another issue with computational drug repositioning models is the lack of a reliable gold standard data set for assessing their efficacy. Furthermore, the model's recommended potential repositioning drugs cannot be evaluated without clinical validation of safety criteria and proof of their effectiveness against anticipated diseases.

Clinical trials are typically preceded by preclinical investigations, both in vitro and in vivo. In the event of drug repurposing, preclinical research on the impact of a drug on disease should be prioritized. However, it requires a thorough knowledge of the disease process, which in the case of COVID-19 may be difficult. In contrast to clinical trials, preclinical research may rapidly assess whether a certain pharmacological approach is likely to be worth pursuing. Preclinical studies, by definition, offer an inadequate picture of disease biology and may produce inconsistent findings, and the knowledge they can provide regarding drug safety and efficacy is severely restricted. Randomized controlled trials are the gold standard for gathering evidence on drug efficacy in clinical trials because they allocate possible confounders to treated and untreated patients at random. The clinical proof is needed to demonstrate a drug's effectiveness and safety, even if preclinical research indicates biological plausibility. During a pandemic, conducting methodologically sound research may be difficult since the rapid spread of low-quality findings may have severe implications. Several considerations highlight the necessity of interpreting current clinical data with great care.

As a result, effective drug repositioning necessitates a combination of computer prediction and in-vitro validation or retrospective clinical history analysis. The comprehensive methodology, which includes a combination of computational and experimental methodologies, enables a comprehensive assessment of all repositioning possibilities. Effectiveness and timeliness of repositioned drugs are greatly improved using a multimodal approach to pharmacological reconstitution [76]. Certain legal concerns may make it difficult to patent a novel therapeutic application and/or enforce patent rights, reducing the incentives for drug repurposing. Certain national regulations make obtaining a patent for a second or subsequent medical use more challenging, although repurposed medicinal uses are protected in most of the major pharmaceutical markets. While patents can be awarded for off-patent drugs, enforcement may be an issue if the new indication makes use of currently available strengths and dose formulas.

Combining and integrating all the approaches will open up a plethora of new possibilities for drug development, most notably through the construction and access to massive databases of drug and disease omics data. Researchers now have access to the most up-to-date, reliable tools and data to investigate unknown mechanisms of action/pathways based on the target protein and/or biomarkers associated with disease progression. Thanks to advancements in techniques such as genomics, proteomics, transcriptomics, and metabolomics, numerous datasets and tools and pathway analysis are publicly available [77]. Several algorithms have been developed to improve the speed and convenience of the recalculation methods. Pharmaceutical repositioning is similarly fraught with difficulties. Repositioning an existing drug by adding a new therapeutic indication is a difficult and complex task because it involves numerous factors, like technology, commercial strategy, patents, investment, and market demand. Selection of an appropriate medicinal product sector, clinical trial issues such as outdated or inadequate clinical or preclinical data on the original pharmaceutical or drug product are few prominent challenges.

## Conclusion

There are currently no drugs available that are effective in treating COVID-19 patients. While research continues, some countries are experimenting with various combinations to treat their patients. While computing can aid in repurposing, data from in vitro drug screening, in vivo research, including animal models, ongoing clinical trials, electronic health records, literature mining, or expert knowledge must be used to evaluate computational drug repurposing methods. Numerous candidate drugs continue to exhibit experimental flaws, necessitating comprehensive validation of candidate therapeutics to establish a baseline for technique accuracy. Because this is impractical, it has become even more critical to combine projections with expert knowledge. Researchers and scientists should avoid duplicating studies and organize studies so that the outcomes can be compared. It is also necessary to conduct a critical analysis of existing data to determine the efficacy and safety of a drug for possible repurposing. As a result, additional clinical trials and large randomized control studies are required through international collaboration to improve the treatment options and safety of COVID-19 patients.

## References

1. Saini M, Parihar N, Soni SL, Sharma V. Drug repurposing: an overview. Asian J Pharm Res Dev. 2020;8(4):194–212.
2. Talevi A, Bellera CL. Challenges and opportunities with drug repurposing: finding strategies to find alternative uses of therapeutics. Expert Opin Drug Discovery. 2020;15(4):397–401.
3. Poduri R. Pharmaceutical industry, academia, regulatory authorities and end user collaboration in successful drug discovery and development. In: Drug Discovery and Development: From Targets and Molecules to Medicines. Singapore: Springer; 2021. p. 465–71.
4. Sonaye HV, Sheikh RY, Doifode CA. Drug repurposing: iron in the fire for older drugs. Biomed Pharmacother. 2021;1(141):111638.
5. Shyr ZA, Gorshkov K, Chen CZ, Zheng W. Drug discovery strategies for SARS-CoV-2. J Pharmacol Exp Ther. 2020;375(1):127–38.
6. Galindez G, Matschinske J, Rose TD, Sadegh S, Salgado-Albarrán M, Späth J, Baumbach J, Pauling JK. Lessons from the COVID-19 pandemic for advancing computational drug repurposing strategies. Nat Comput Sci. 2021;1(1):33–41.
7. Garrison LP Jr, Towse A, Bresnahan BW. Assessing a structured, quantitative health outcomes approach to drug risk-benefit analysis. Health Aff. 2007;26(3):684–95.
8. Ross JS, Mulvey GK, Hines EM, Nissen SE, Krumholz HM. Trial publication after registration in ClinicalTrials. Gov: a cross-sectional analysis. PLoS Med. 2009;6(9):e1000144.
9. Paul SM, Mytelka DS, Dunwiddie CT, Persinger CC, Munos BH, Lindborg SR, Schacht AL. How to improve R&D productivity: the pharmaceutical industry's grand challenge. Nat Rev Drug Discov. 2010;9(3):203–14.
10. Sultana J, Crisafulli S, Gabbay F, Lynn E, Shakir S, Trifirò G. Challenges for drug repurposing in the COVID-19 pandemic era. Front Pharmacol. 2020;6(11):1657.
11. Chong CR, Sullivan DJ. New uses for old drugs. Nature. 2007;448(7154):645–6.
12. Eichler HG, Pignatti F, Flamion B, Leufkens H, Breckenridge A. Balancing early market access to new drugs with the need for benefit/risk data: a mounting dilemma. Nat Rev Drug Discov. 2008;7(10):818–26.
13. Eichler HG, Oye K, Baird LG, Abadie E, Brown J, Drum CL, Ferguson J, Garner S, Honig P, Hukkelhoven M, Lim JC. Adaptive licensing: taking the next step in the evolution of drug approval. Clinical Pharmacology & Therapeutics. 2012;91(3):426–37.
14. Eichler HG, Bloechl-Daum B, Brasseur D, Breckenridge A, Leufkens H, Raine J, Salmonson T, Schneider CK, Rasi G. The risks of risk aversion in drug regulation. Nat Rev Drug Discov. 2013;12:907–16.
15. Sarkar C, Mondal M, Torequl Islam M, Martorell M, Docea AO, Maroyi A, Sharifi-Rad J, Calina D. Potential therapeutic options for COVID-19: current status, challenges, and future perspectives. Front Pharmacol. 2020;15(11):1428.

16. Baumfeld Andre E, Reynolds R, Caubel P, Azoulay L, Dreyer NA. Trial designs using real-world data: the changing landscape of the regulatory approval process. Pharmacoepidemiol Drug Saf. 2020;29(10):1201–12.
17. Schneeweiss S, Gagne JJ, Glynn RJ, Ruhl M, Rassen JA. Assessing the comparative effectiveness of newly marketed medications: methodological challenges and implications for drug development. Clin Pharmacol Therapeut. 2011;90(6):777–90.
18. Sharma MR, Schilsky RL. Role of randomized phase III trials in an era of effective targeted therapies. Nat Rev Clin Oncol. 2012;9(4):208.
19. Raphael MJ, Gyawali B, Booth CM. Real-world evidence and regulatory drug approval. Nat Rev Clin Oncol. 2020;17(5):271–2.
20. Swift B, Jain L, White C, Chandrasekaran V, Bhandari A, Hughes DA, Jadhav PR. Innovation at the intersection of clinical trials and real-world data science to advance patient care. Clin Transl Sci. 2018;11(5):450–60.
21. Angus DC. Optimizing the trade-off between learning and doing in a pandemic. JAMA. 2020;323(19):1895–6.
22. Prasad S, McOsker C, Foley M. Filling the drug discovery abyss. Drug Discovery. 2016;17:25.
23. Leelananda SP, Lindert S. Computational methods in drug discovery. Beilstein J Org Chem. 2016;12(1):2694–718.
24. Ou-Yang SS, Lu JY, Kong XQ, Liang ZJ, Luo C, Jiang H. Computational drug discovery. Acta Pharmacol Sin. 2012 Sep;33(9):1131–40.
25. Kumar N, Hendriks BS, Janes KA, de Graaf D, Lauffenburger DA. Applying computational modeling to drug discovery and development. Drug Discov Today. 2006;11(17–18):806–11.
26. Kumar S. Online resource and tools for the development of drugs against novel coronavirus. In: Silico Modeling of Drugs Against Coronaviruses. Methods in Pharmacology and Toxicology. New York, NY: Humana; 2021. https://doi.org/10.1007/7653_2020_53.
27. Kumar S. Protein–Protein Interaction Network for the Identification of New Targets Against Novel Coronavirus. In: Silico Modeling of Drugs Against Coronaviruses. Methods in Pharmacology and Toxicology. New York, NY: Humana; 2021. https://doi.org/10.1007/7653_2020_62.
28. Kumar S. COVID-19: A drug repurposing and biomarker identification by using comprehensive gene-disease associations through protein-protein interaction network analysis. Preprints. 2020:2020030440. https://doi.org/10.20944/preprints202003.0440.v1.
29. Nana KS, Karuppanan K, Kumar S. Identification of common key genes and pathways between Covid-19 and lung cancer by using protein-protein interaction network analysis. bioRxiv. 2021; https://doi.org/10.1101/2021.02.16.431364
30. Kumar S, Mathavan S, Jin WJ, Azman NA, Subramanaiam D, Zainalabidin NA, Lingadaran D, Sattar ZB, Manickam DL, Anbananthan PS, Taqiyuddin JA. COVID-19 Vaccine Candidates by Identification of B and T Cell Multi-Epitopes Against SARS-CoV-2. Preprints 2020. https://doi.org/10.20944/preprints202008.0092.v1.
31. Mathavan S, Kumar S. Evaluation of the Effect of D614G, N501Y and S477N Mutation in SARS-CoV-2 through Computational Approach. Preprints 2020. https://doi.org/10.20944/preprints202012.0710.v1.
32. Kumar S, Ramanujam M. Computational prediction of novel broad-spectrum drug targets against vibrio cholerae by integrated genomics and proteomics approach. Malaysian J Med Health Sci. 2020;16(2):99–104.
33. Kumar S. In Silico Identification of Novel Tuberculosis Drug Targets in Mycobacterium tuberculosisP450 Enzymes by Interaction Study with Azole Drugs. Preprints 2020.
34. Kumar S. Computational identification and binding analysis of orphan human cytochrome P450 4X1 enzyme with substrates. BMC Res Notes. 2015;8(1):1.
35. Karaman B, Sippl W. Computational drug repurposing: current trends. Curr Med Chem. 2019;26(28):5389–409.

36. Oprea TI, Nielsen SK, Ursu O, Yang JJ, Taboureau O, Mathias SL, Kouskoumvekaki I, Sklar LA, Bologa CG. Associating drugs, targets and clinical outcomes into an integrated network affords a new platform for computer-aided drug repurposing. Mol inform. 2011;30(2–3):100–11.
37. Xue H, Li J, Xie H, Wang Y. Review of drug repositioning approaches and resources. Int J Biol Sci. 2018;14(10):1232.
38. Mazzarella R, Webb C. Computational and bioinformatic strategies for drug repositioning. Drug Repositioning. 2012;9:91.
39. Deftereos SN, Andronis C, Friedla EJ, Persidis A, Persidis A. Drug repurposing and adverse event prediction using high-throughput literature analysis. Wiley Interdiscip Rev Syst Biol Med. 2011;3(3):323–34.
40. Rebholz-Schuhmann D, Oellrich A, Hoehndorf R. Text-mining solutions for biomedical research: enabling integrative biology. Nat Rev Genet. 2012;13(12):829–39.
41. Andronis C, Sharma A, Virvilis V, Deftereos S, Persidis A. Literature mining, ontologies and information visualization for drug repurposing. Brief Bioinform. 2011;12(4):357–68.
42. Loging W, Rodriguez-Esteban R, Hill J, Freeman T, Miglietta J. Cheminformatic/bioinformatic analysis of large corporate databases: application to drug repurposing. Drug Discov Today Ther Strateg. 2011;8(3–4):109–16.
43. Nabirotchkin S, Peluffo AE, Rinaudo P, Yu J, Hajj R, Cohen D. Next-generation drug repurposing using human genetics and network biology. Curr Opin Pharmacol. 2020;51:78–92.
44. Vilar S, Hripcsak G. The role of drug profiles as similarity metrics: applications to repurposing, adverse effects detection and drug–drug interactions. Brief Bioinform. 2017;18(4):670–81.
45. Grenier L, Hu P. Computational drug repurposing for inflammatory bowel disease using genetic information. Comput Struct Biotechnol J. 2019;17:127–35.
46. Hamid JS, Hu P, Roslin NM, Ling V, Greenwood CM, Beyene J. Data integration in genetics and genomics: methods and challenges. Hum Genomics Proteomics. 2009;2009:869093.
47. Hasin Y, Seldin M, Lusis A. Multi-omics approaches to disease. Genome Biol. 2017;18(1):1–5.
48. Michnick SW. The connectivity map. Nat Chem Biol. 2006;2(12):663–4.
49. Reka AK, Kuick R, Kurapati H, Standiford TJ, Omenn GS, Keshamouni VG. Identifying inhibitors of epithelial-mesenchymal transition by connectivity map–based systems approach. J Thorac Oncol. 2011;6(11):1784–92.
50. De Bastiani MA, Pfaffenseller B, Klamt F. Master regulators connectivity map: a transcription factors-centered approach to drug repositioning. Front Pharmacol. 2018;9:697.
51. Koehler AN. Microarrays in chemical biology. Wiley Encyclopedia Chem Biol. 2007;14:1.
52. Lamb J, Crawford ED, Peck D, Modell JW, Blat IC, Wrobel MJ, Lerner J, Brunet JP, Subramanian A, Ross KN, Reich M. The Connectivity Map: using gene-expression signatures to connect small molecules, genes, and disease. Science. 2006;313(5795):1929–35.
53. Eckhardt M, Hultquist JF, Kaake RM, Hüttenhain R, Krogan NJ. A systems approach to infectious disease. Nat Rev Genet. 2020;21(6):339–54.
54. Ideker T, Galitski T, Hood L. A new approach to decoding life: systems biology. Annu Rev Genomics Hum Genet. 2001;2(1):343–72.
55. Cheng F, Desai RJ, Handy DE, Wang R, Schneeweiss S, Barabási AL, Loscalzo J. Network-based approach to prediction and population-based validation of in silico drug repurposing. Nat Commun. 2018;9(1):1–2.
56. Sadegh S, Matschinske J, Blumenthal DB, Galindez G, Kacprowski T, List M, Nasirigerdeh R, Oubounyt M, Pichlmair A, Rose TD, Salgado-Albarrán M. Exploring the SARS-CoV-2 virus-host-drug interactome for drug repurposing. Nat Commun. 2020;11(1):1–9.
57. Surabhi S, Singh BK. Computer aided drug design: an overview. J Drug Deliv Ther. 2018;8(5):504–9.
58. Abdolmaleki A, Ghasemi B, J, Ghasemi F. Computer aided drug design for multi-target drug design: SAR/QSAR, molecular docking and pharmacophore methods. Curr Drug Targets. 2017;18(5):556–75.
59. Cortegiani A, Ingoglia G, Ippolito M, Giarratano A, Einav S. A systematic review on the efficacy and safety of chloroquine for the treatment of COVID-19. J Crit Care. 2020;57:279–83.

60. Manivannan E, Karthikeyan C, Moorthy NS, Chaturvedi SC. The rise and fall of chloroquine/hydroxychloroquine as compassionate therapy of COVID-19. Front Pharmacol. 2021;12:1057.
61. Axfors C, Schmitt AM, Janiaud P, van't Hooft J, Abd-Elsalam S, Abdo EF, Abella BS, Akram J, Amaravadi RK, Angus DC, Arabi YM. Mortality outcomes with hydroxychloroquine and chloroquine in COVID-19 from an international collaborative meta-analysis of randomized trials. Nat Commun. 2021;12(1):1–3.
62. Gasmi A, Peana M, Noor S, Lysiuk R, Menzel A, Benahmed AG, Bjørklund G. Chloroquine and hydroxychloroquine in the treatment of COVID-19: the never-ending story. Appl Microbiol Biotechnol. 2021;30:1–1.
63. Chen Y, Li MX, Lu GD, Shen HM, Zhou J. Hydroxychloroquine/chloroquine as therapeutics for COVID-19: truth under the mystery. Int J Biol Sci. 2021;17(6):1538.
64. Patel TK, Patel PB, Barvaliya M, Saurabh MK, Bhalla HL, Khosla PP. Efficacy and safety of lopinavir-ritonavir in COVID-19: a systematic review of randomized controlled trials. J Infect Public Health. 2021;14:740–8.
65. Young B, Tan TT, Leo YS. The place for remdesivir in COVID-19 treatment. Lancet Infect Dis. 2021;21(1):20.
66. Horby PW, Mafham M, Bell JL, Linsell L, Staplin N, Emberson J, Palfreeman A, Raw J, Elmahi E, Prudon B, Green C. Lopinavir–ritonavir in patients admitted to hospital with COVID-19 (RECOVERY): a randomised, controlled, open-label, platform trial. Lancet. 2020;396(10259):1345–52.
67. Dabbous HM, Abd-Elsalam S, El-Sayed MH, Sherief AF, Ebeid FF, Abd El Ghafar MS, Soliman S, Elbahnasawy M, Badawi R, Tageldin MA. Efficacy of favipiravir in COVID-19 treatment: a multi-center randomized study. Arch Virol. 2021;166(3):949–54.
68. Butler CC, van der Velden AW, Bongard E, Saville BR, Holmes J, Coenen S, Cook J, Francis NA, Lewis RJ, Godycki-Cwirko M, Llor C. Oseltamivir plus usual care versus usual care for influenza-like illness in primary care: an open-label, pragmatic, randomised controlled trial. Lancet. 2020;395(10217):42–52.
69. Hassanipour S, Arab-Zozani M, Amani B, Heidarzad F, Fathalipour M, Martinez-de-Hoyo R. The efficacy and safety of favipiravir in treatment of COVID-19: a systematic review and meta-analysis of clinical trials. Sci Rep. 2021;11(1):1.
70. Rosa SG, Santos WC. Clinical trials on drug repositioning for COVID-19 treatment. Rev Panam Salud Publica. 2020;8(44):e40.
71. Thomas E, Ghany MG, Liang TJ. The application and mechanism of action of ribavirin in therapy of hepatitis C. Antivir Chem Chemother. 2012;23(1):1–2.
72. Chen N, Zhou M, Dong X, Qu J, Gong F, Han Y, Qiu Y, Wang J, Liu Y, Wei Y, Yu T. Epidemiological and clinical characteristics of 99 cases of 2019 novel coronavirus pneumonia in Wuhan, China: a descriptive study. Lancet. 2020;395(10223):507–13.
73. Ali MJ, Hanif M, Haider MA, Ahmed MU, Sundas FN, Hirani A, Khan IA, Anis K, Karim AH. Treatment options for COVID-19: a review. Front Med. 2020;31(7):480.
74. Singh AK, Majumdar S, Singh R, Misra A. Role of corticosteroid in the management of COVID-19: a systemic review and a Clinician's perspective. Diabetes Metab Syndr Clin Res Rev. 2020;14(5):971–8.
75. Salama C, Han J, Yau L, Reiss WG, Kramer B, Neidhart JD, Criner GJ, Kaplan-Lewis E, Baden R, Pandit L, Cameron ML. Tocilizumab in patients hospitalized with Covid-19 pneumonia. N Engl J Med. 2021;384(1):20–30.
76. Hurle MR, Yang L, Xie Q, Rajpal DK, Sanseau P, Agarwal P. Computational drug repositioning: from data to therapeutics. Clin Pharmacol Ther. 2013;93(4):335–41.
77. Jin G, Wong ST. Toward better drug repositioning: prioritizing and integrating existing methods into efficient pipelines. Drug Discov Today. 2014;19(5):637–44.

# Chapter 25
# Computationally Repurposed Natural Products Targeting SARS-CoV-2 Attachment and Entry Mechanisms

**Mark Tristan J. Quimque, Kin Israel R. Notarte, Von Novi O. de Leon, Joe Anthony H. Manzano, John Emmanuel R. Muñoz, Delfin Yñigo H. Pilapil IV, Justin Allen K. Lim, and Allan Patrick G. Macabeo**

## Abbreviations

| | |
|---|---|
| ACE2 | Angiotensin-converting enzyme 2 |
| ADME | Absorption, distribution, metabolism, and excretion |
| BE | Binding energy |
| COVID-19 | Coronavirus disease 2019 |
| CT | Cytoplasmic tail |
| CTD | C-terminal domain |

M. T. J. Quimque
Laboratory of Organic Reactivity, Discovery and Synthesis, Research Center of Natural and Applied Sciences, University of Santo Tomas, Manila, Philippines

Department of Chemistry, College of Science and Mathematics, Mindanao State University—Iligan Institute of Technology, Iligan, Philippines
e-mail: marktristan.quimque@g.msuiit.edu.ph

K. I. R. Notarte
Faculty of Medicine and Surgery, University of Santo Tomas, Manila, Philippines
e-mail: krnotarte@ust.edu.ph

V. N. O. de Leon · J. A. H. Manzano · J. E. R. Muñoz · D. Y. H. Pilapil IV
Laboratory of Organic Reactivity, Discovery and Synthesis, Research Center of Natural and Applied Sciences, University of Santo Tomas, Manila, Philippines

Department of Biological Sciences, College of Science, University of Santo Tomas, Manila, Philippines
e-mail: vonnovi.deleon.sci@ust.edu.ph; joeanthony.manzano.sci@ust.edu.ph; johnemmanuel.munoz.sci@ust.edu.ph; delfinynigo.pilapil.sci@ust.edu.ph

J. A. K. Lim · A. P. G. Macabeo (✉)
Laboratory of Organic Reactivity, Discovery and Synthesis, Research Center of Natural and Applied Sciences, University of Santo Tomas, Manila, Philippines
e-mail: agmacabeo@ust.edu.ph


S. Adibi et al. (eds.), *Frontiers of COVID-19*,
https://doi.org/10.1007/978-3-031-08045-6_25

| | |
|---|---|
| ER | Endoplasmic reticulum |
| FP | Fusion peptide |
| GRP78 | Glucose-regulated protein 78/78-kDa glucose-regulated protein |
| hACE2 | Human angiotensin-converting enzyme 2 |
| HR1 | Heptad repeat 1 |
| HR2 | Heptad repeat 2 |
| LRo5 | Lipinski's Rule of Five |
| MDS | Molecular dynamics simulations |
| NRP1 | Neuropilin-1 |
| NTD | N-terminal domain |
| RBD | Receptor-binding domain |
| RBM | Receptor-binding motif |
| RMSD | Root-mean-square deviation |
| RMSF | Root-mean-square fluctuation |
| $S_1$ | Subunit 1 |
| $S_2$ | Subunit 2 |
| SARS-CoV-2 | Severe acute respiratory syndrome coronavirus 2 |
| SBD | Substrate-binding domain |
| TM | Transmembrane domain |
| TMPRSS2 | Transmembrane protein serine protease 2 |

## Introduction

The global effort on genomic sequencing led to the identification of structural proteins and enzymes that are crucial for SARS-CoV-2 inoculation and replication [1]. SARS-CoV-2 infection begins as the spikes interact with angiotensin-converting enzyme 2 (ACE2) receptor-enriched host cells. Viral fusion with the host cell is then triggered with the activation of transmembrane protease serine type 2 (TMPRSS2) [2]. Following endocytosis, the virus utilizes the host cellular machinery for its replication, assembly, and release of new virions [3]. Consequently, these pathologic mechanisms result to an overwhelming inflammatory response leading to multiple organ failure. In the absence of timely interventions, there could be worse prognosis and death becomes inevitable [4].

Although there are hundreds of clinical trials and preclinical studies designed to find cure for COVID-19, there are limited number of FDA-approved therapeutics for this widely spreading disease [1]. Most of these therapeutics are repurposed drugs, including hydroxychloroquine, remdesivir, and lopinavir [5]. There is also a delay in the global roll-out of vaccines due to increasing vaccine hesitancy [6]. Another impediment to wide-scale vaccine development is its delicate manufacturing, storage system, and safety [1, 6].

In addition, there have been reports of new variants which are more infectious and virulent than the Wuhan strain [7]. These novel variants are known to decrease efficacy of vaccines and therapeutic antiviral regimens [8, 9]. With the rise of infections, great efforts have been dedicated to discovering effective therapeutic and prophylactic agents against COVID-19 [1]. Computational methodologies have played an integral role in the discovery of new antiviral agents with the aim to accelerate and economize the process of drug design and development. Apart from the use of molecular docking and molecular dynamics simulations in screening drug candidates, the said computational tools have aided the mechanistic understanding of the potential drug's interaction with specific viral targets [10–12].

Natural products and herbal medicines have been used for the prevention of viral infections over the years. They have shown a wide array of biological activities against pathogenic viruses such as influenza virus, hepatitis C virus, Herpes simplex virus, flavivirus, and human immunodeficiency virus [13–17]. These medicinal products also exhibited favorable efficacy and tolerable toxicity [1]. In the face of a global health crisis, exploring prophylactics and therapeutic regimens from natural products is a promising and practical strategy to contain COVID-19 [18].

In this chapter, we explored the potential of alkaloids, fatty acids and sterols, peptides, polyphenols, and terpenoids which showed in silico activity against SARS-CoV-2 target proteins obtained through virtual screening. Herein, we present the potential druggability of the aforementioned natural products that target structural spike protein particularly the receptor domains for angiotensin-converting enzyme 2 (ACE2), glucose-regulated protein 78 (GRP78), and neuropilin-1 (NRP-1) and host cell transmembrane protease serine type 2 (TMPRSS2) which facilitate host cell recognition, viral attachment, and fusion.

## Structural Features of SARS-CoV-2 Spike Protein

The SARS-CoV-2 spike is a transmembrane homotrimeric glycoprotein that protrudes from the viral envelope crowning the virion surface. For coronaviruses, the ectodomain spike share the same structural organization composed of two functional subunits: the *N*-terminal $S_1$ subunit which is responsible for host cell receptor recognition and binding and the C-terminal $S_2$ subunit which is responsible for fusion of the viral and cellular membranes. Wrapp and coworkers determined the trimeric structure of SARS-CoV-2 spike using high-resolution cryogenic electron microscopy and reported the structural features of the prefusion conformation of SARS-CoV-2 spike [19]. Each protomer of the spike trimer is composed of 1260 amino acids. The $S_1$ subunit is composed of four sub-domains: an *N*-terminal domain (NTD), a receptor-binding domain (RBD, or the C-terminal domain, CTD), and two subdomains (SD1 and SD2). The transmembrane S2 subunit is composed of 588 amino acids and contains an *N*-terminal hydrophobic fusion peptide (FP), two heptad repeats (HR1 and HR2), a transmembrane domain (TM), and a cytoplasmic tail (CT) (Fig. 25.1) [19–21].

The highly glycosylated spike is a class I fusion protein and exists in a metastable prefusion conformation. Upon interaction of the virus with the host cell, triggered by the binding of the $S_1$ subunit to a host cell receptor, the spike protein

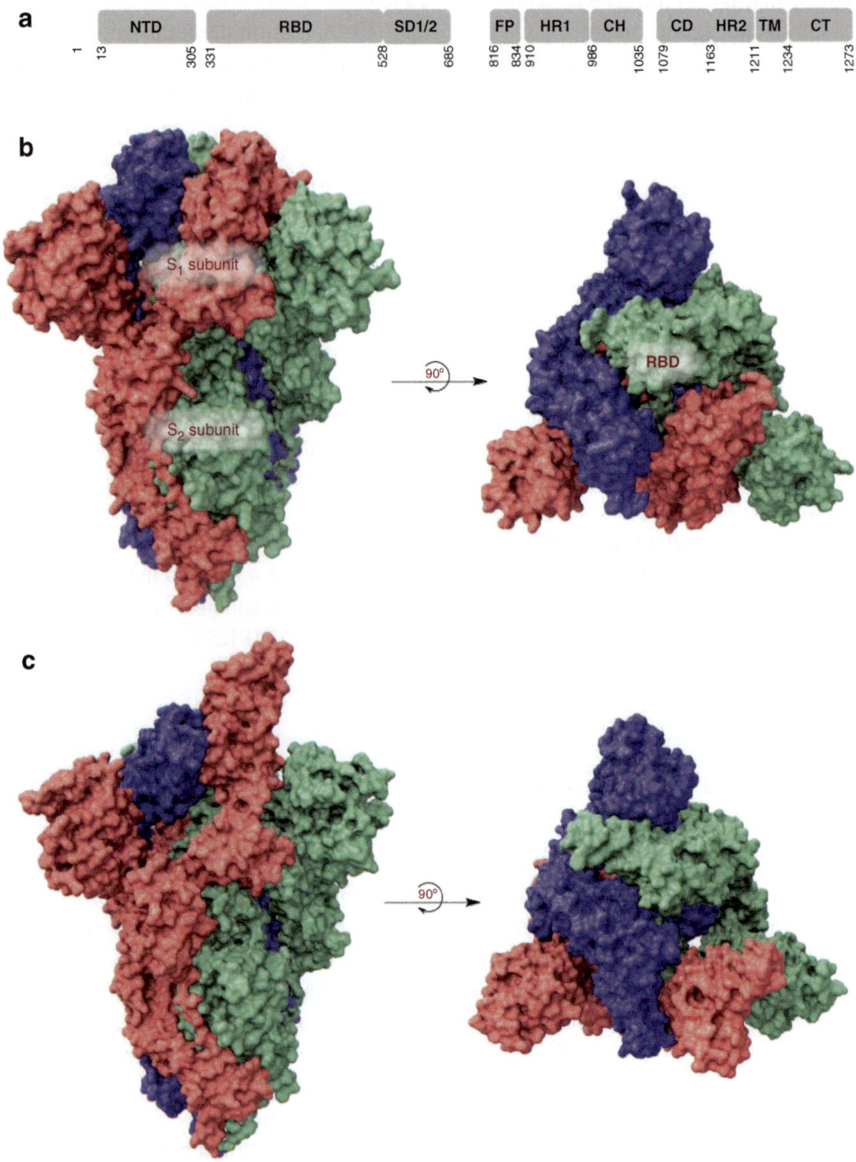


**Fig. 25.1** (**a**) Schematic representation of the overall topology of the SARS-CoV-2 spike monomer. (**b**) Molecular surface representation of the "down" state of SARS-CoV-2 spike (PDB 6VXX). (**c**) Molecular surface representation of the partially "up" state of SARS-CoV-2 spike (PDB 6VYB)

undergoes considerable structural rearrangement to allow for fusion of the virus with host cell membrane. This process of receptor binding prompts the $S_2$ subunit to transition from a metastable prefusion state to a more stable postfusion state which is essential for fusion [22]. Moreover, the RBD at the $S_1$ subunit could adopt to two conformational states— "down" and "up" (Fig. 25.1). The latter conformation is a result of hinging the RBD upward to transiently expose it during host cell receptor engagement corresponding to a receptor-accessible state [22–24].

As previously mentioned, the RBD is a critical part of the spike protein that is a target for development of inhibitors to viral attachment, neutralizing antibodies, and vaccines [25]. For coronaviruses, each viral species showcases distinct domains for the $S_1$ subunit, particularly the RBD, to recognize various host cell receptors. Two independent groups reported the structural features of the SARS-CoV-2 spike RBD via high-resolution X-ray crystallography [22, 26]. The RBD region of SARS-CoV-2 spike is composed of about 200 residues (amino acids 319–541) and share about 73–76% sequence similarity with SARS-CoV spike RBD [22, 27]. The portion of the RBD that makes direct contact to human ACE2 (hACE2) is called the receptor-binding motif (RBM). Lan and coworkers reported that the interface between the RBM and ACE2 is a network of hydrophilic interactions, where 13 hydrogen bonds from ten RBM residues (Asn487, Lys417, Gln493, Tyr505, Tyr449, Thr500, Asn501, Gly446, Tyr489, and Gly502) and two salt bridges from one RBM residue (Lys417) were shown to interact against the amino acid residues of ACE2 [22]. The SARS-CoV-2 RBM was found to have more residue contacts with ACE2, a larger binding interface, and a higher binding affinity to ACE2 compared with SARS-CoV RBM which can be attributed to the higher infectivity and virulence of the SARS-CoV-2 [22, 26, 28, 29]. Several computational simulations corroborated with this observation, showing a more stable complex and increased affinity between SARS-CoV-2 RBD and hACE2 versus between SARS-CoV and hACE2 [30–34].

Although the primary entry of the virus to the host cell is through ACE2, the SARS-CoV-2 spike RBD may interact with the master chaperone protein, Glucose Regulating Protein 78 (GRP78). In a computational study by Ibrahim et al., it is demonstrated that the cell-surface receptor GRP78 may mediate viral entry through binding with the spike RBD, particularly via residues 480–488 [35]. Under reasonable conditions, GRP78 is bound to the lumen of the endoplasmic reticulum (ER). However, under cellular stress, overexpression of GRP78 is initiated where this phenomenon leads to GRP78's dislodgement from the ER and its translocation to the host cell surface where it becomes susceptible to viral recognition by spike [35, 36].

Another secondary receptor for the viral spike or as coreceptor with ACE2 is a multifunctional transmembrane heptameric protein neuropilin-1 (NRP-1). NRP-1 was identified from the study of Cantuti-Castelvetri et al. as a host factor relevant for SARS-CoV-2 infection. NRP-1 is abundantly found in the respiratory and olfactory epithelium, particularly in endothelial and epithelial cells [37]. The SARS-CoV-2 spike features a cleavage site that proteolytically activated by host cell protease furin. Such cleavage site is located in the subunit junction between $S_1$ and $S_2$, which is absent in SARS-CoV spike. NRP-1 reinforces the infectivity of SARS-CoV-2 by binding to the spike $S_1$ fragments upon proteolytic furin cleavage and allow penetration of the virus to the host cell [37–39].

To date, experimental and computational studies regarding the entry of SARS-CoV-2 is primarily focused on ACE2 with potential assistance of TMPRSS2. However, evidence from researches do not discount the possibility that other membrane receptors such as GRP78 and NRP-1 may likewise serve as secondary host factors and facilitate viral entry under specified conditions. The exploration of targeting the various regions of SARS-CoV-2 spike responsible for binding to these host receptor proteins by small-molecule inhibitors is a promising direction to discover therapeutic and prophylactic potentials focused on viral entry.

## Inhibitors of SARS-CoV-2 Receptor Binding Domain (RBD) for Angiotensin-Converting Enzyme 2 (ACE2)

### *Alkaloids*

Alkaloids are a widely distributed class of nitrogen-containing natural products and have been extensively studied for their medical use [40–42]. A variety of biological activities are associated with alkaloids and their biosynthetic precursors, including antiviral activity particularly against human coronaviruses [43, 44] has been explored.

The alkaloids bicuculine (**1**) and withasomnine (**2**) (Fig. 25.2) showed high binding affinities to the SARS-CoV-2 receptor binding domain for ACE2 receptor with binding energies (BE) of −9.9 and −8.0 kcal/mol using AutoDock algorithm, respectively. Alkaloid **1** interacted via hydrogen bonding, $\pi$–$\pi$ and hydrophobic interactions with either one or more of the following residues of the receptor binding domain of SARS-CoV-2 spike protein: Tyr7020, Leu6820, Met6818, Leu6819, Ala7024, Arg6817, Val7021, and Asp7018 [45, 46].

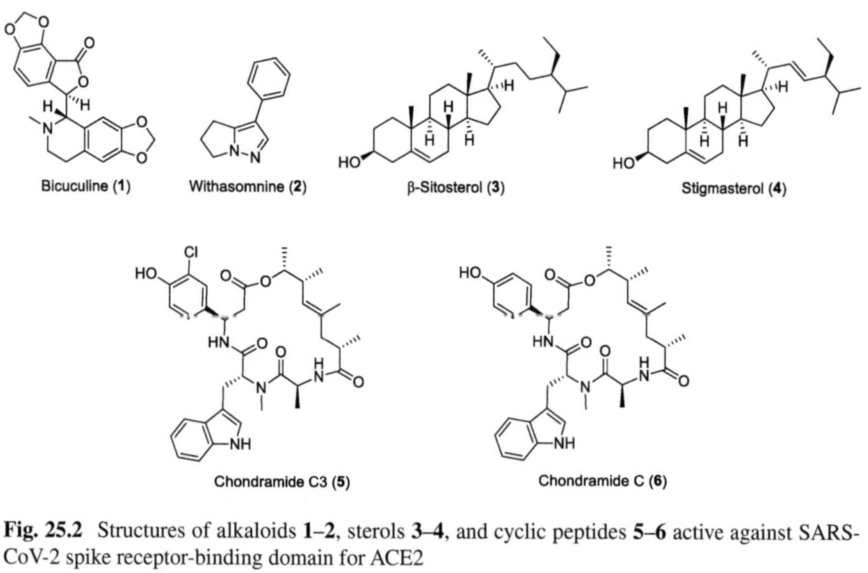


**Fig. 25.2** Structures of alkaloids **1–2**, sterols **3–4**, and cyclic peptides **5–6** active against SARS-CoV-2 spike receptor-binding domain for ACE2

## *Sterols*

Sterols are a subgroup of generally nonpolar steroids containing a 3-hydroxyl group in the A-ring of the cyclopentanoperhydrophenanthrene nucleus. Plant sterols, in particular, showcase a myriad of biological activities. Among them is their ability to block cholesterol absorption sites in the human intestine thereby controlling cholesterol levels. However, a small number of sterols, including their synthetic derivatives, have been shown to exhibit potent antiviral properties [47, 48].

$\beta$-sitosterol (**3**, BE = −8.1 kcal/mol) and stigmasterol (**4**, BE = −7.7 kcal/mol) (Fig. 25.2) docked onto the binding site of SARS-CoV-2 S-protein using AutoDock. Both compounds also showed in silico inhibitory effects against the host ACE2 receptor binding domain with binding energy of −10.9 kcal/mol for sterol **3** and −9.8 kcal/mol for sterol **4** [49].

## *Peptides*

Naturally occurring peptides form an interesting group of pharmaceutical compounds with structural resemblance between small molecules and proteins, but have distinct biochemical and pharmaceutical properties [50]. The cyclodepsipeptides chondramides exhibit biological properties such as antimicrobial, immunosuppressive, and antitumor activities [51, 52].

Among the myxobacterial chondramides molecularly docked against ACE2 receptor in the study of Fernandez and coworkers, chondramide C3 (**5**) exhibited highest binding propensity with binding energy of −8.7 kcal/mol (Figs. 25.2 and 25.3). Cyclic peptide **5** formed hydrogen bonds with Glu406, Tyr449, Tyr453, Ser494, Tyr495, Gly496, and Tyr505. The docked complex was also stabilized via several interactions with Arg403 ($\pi$–cation), Lys417 ($\pi$–alkyl), Tyr453 ($\pi$–$\pi$ stacked), Tyr505 ($\pi$–alkyl), and Gly496 (C–H bond). Evaluation of ADME properties and toxicity profile analysis revealed **5** to be highly druggable with no predicted toxicity risks [53]. Interestingly, the propensity of chondramide C3 (**5**) remained constant when docked against spike protein variants K417N/T, A475V, I472V, L452R, V483A, F490L, S477N, and N439K, while decreased binding affinity was observed for N501Y and E484K which may be attributed to the absence of interaction between the ligand and Tyr501 and Lys484, respectively. Thus, chondramide C3 (**5**) was shown to confer lesser in silico inhibitory activity against the N501Y and E484K variants. However, another myxobacterial depsipepide, chondramide C (**6**) showed a stronger antagonistic potential particularly against N501Y (−9.1 kcal/mol) and E484K (−8.7 kcal/mol) SARS-CoV-2 variants. One of the major differences between the structures of depsipeptides **5** and **6** is the presence of an *ortho*-chloro substituent in the phenol moiety in **5** where the electronegative group is likely to associate with the hydroxyl group of the phenol ring via intramolecular H-bonding hindering **5**'s potential to form intermolecular interactions with the polar

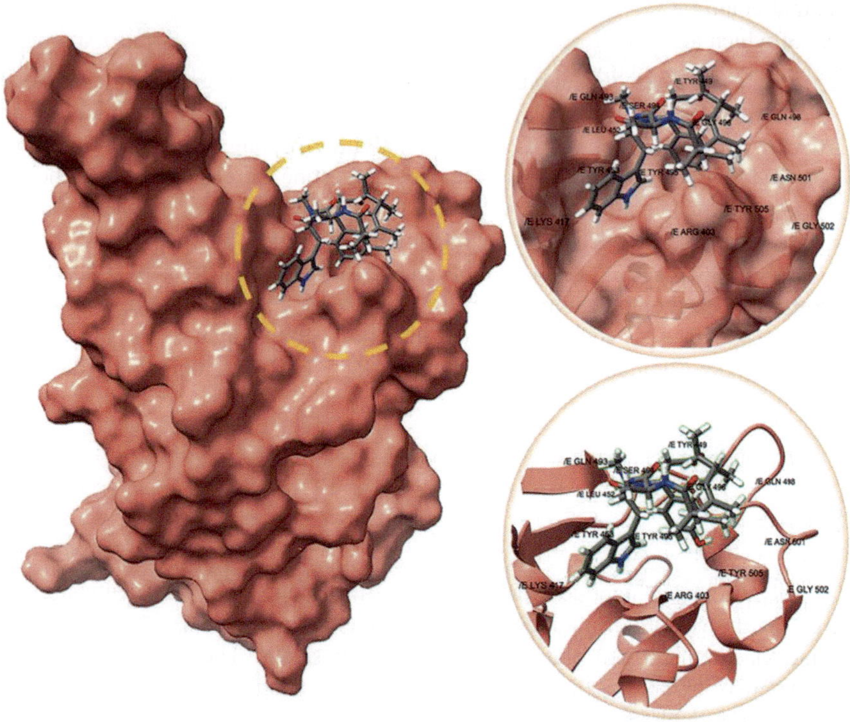

**Fig. 25.3** Putative binding site of SARS-CoV-2 spike RBD for ACE2 showing the docked pose of a cyclic peptide chondramide C3 (**5**)

residues present in the spike RBD variants. Aside from the single-substituted variants, depsipeptide **6** also showed similarly strong affinities against the South African (N501Y-E484K-K417N, BE = −9.3 kcal/mol) and the Brazilian (N501Y-E484K-K417T, BE = −8.4 kcal/mol) variants. Evaluation of ADME properties and toxicity profile analysis revealed these compounds as highly druggable with no predicted toxicity risks.

## *Polyphenols*

Polyphenols, a family of widely distributed natural products known for their profound antiviral activity, have been found to be potentially active at a molecular level against SARS-CoV-2 [54]. Polyphenols comprise the majority of screened natural compounds with in silico antagonistic effects on SARS-CoV-2 viral entry targeting its spike protein or the receptor binding domain of host ACE2 to the virus. Some curcuminoids, stilbenoids, flavonoids, and tannins were reported to exhibit this biological activity.

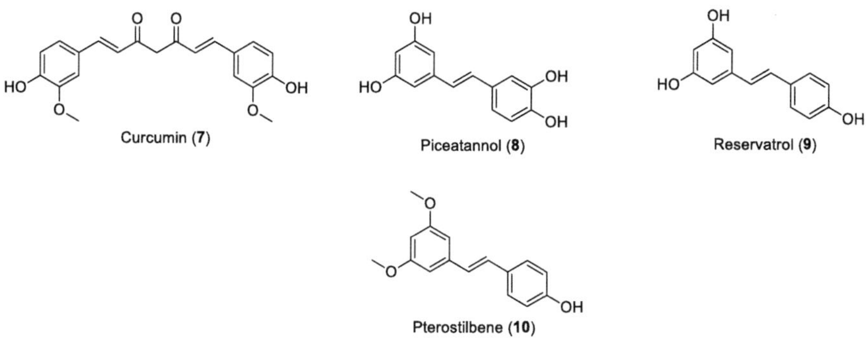


**Fig. 25.4** Structures of curcuminoid **7** and stilbenols **8–10** active against SARS-CoV-2 spike receptor-binding domain for ACE2

## Curcuminoid

Curcumin (**7**, Fig. 25.4) binds onto the active site of SARS-CoV-2 spike glycoprotein with binding energy of −9.3 kcal/mol using AutoDock Vina algorithm. Polyphenol **7** was reported to form four hydrogen bonds with the spike residues, namely, Gln744, Gln947, Ser985, and Gly981. This compound was also stabilized in the complex by a hydrophobic interaction with Phe741 [55].

## Stilbenols and Stilbenoid

Piceatannol (**8**), resveratrol (**9**), and pterostilbene (**10**) are stilbene derivatives reported to confer promising inhibitory activity against SARS-CoV-2 entry (Fig. 25.4). Polyphenols **8** and **9** demonstrated binding energies of −8.2 and −8.0 kcal/mol against the ACE2 receptor, respectively. Polyphenol **8** formed hydrogen bonds with Asn33, Phe390, Ser494, Gly496, and Lys353, and hydrophobic interactions with Asn33, His34, and Tyr505. Similarly, both Asn33 and Phe390 residues also interacted via hydrogen bonding with **9** which has shown stability in the receptor pocket of ACE2 to SARS-CoV-2 with RMSD of 1.78 Å and RMSF of 1.19 Å for 50 ns [56]. Meanwhile, compound **10** was molecularly docked onto the active site of viral spike protein and exhibited high binding affinity (BE = −8.9 kcal/mol). Polyphenol **10** was stabilized by hydrogen bonding with Gly496 and Ser494, and alkyl interaction with His34. Molecular dynamics experiments revealed stability of **10**–spike complex for 400 ns with RMSD of 1.96 Å and RMSF of 1.41 Å [57].

## Flavonoids

Twenty-seven flavonoidal compounds have been reported so far to confer in silico anti-SARS-CoV-2 activities by inhibiting viral entry by targeting either the host ACE2 receptor to SARS-CoV-2 or the spike protein of the virion itself (Figs. 25.5

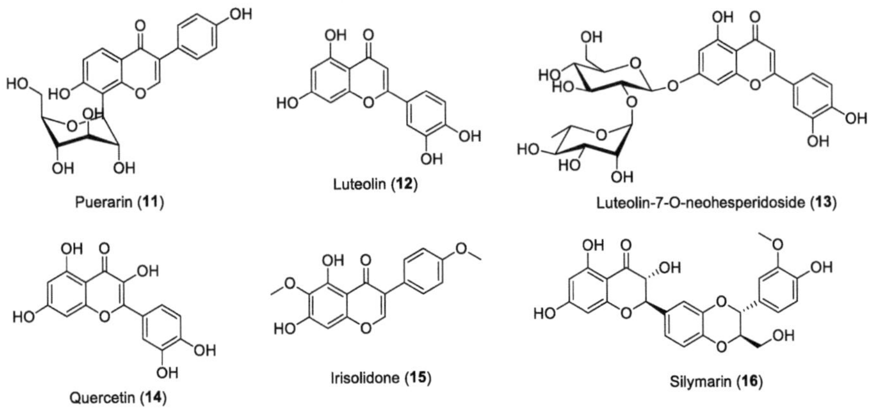


**Fig. 25.5** Structures of flavonoids **11–16** active against SARS-CoV-2 spike receptor-binding domain for ACE2

and 25.6). These flavonoids include puerarin (**11**), luteolin (**12**), luteolin 7-O-neohesperidoside (**13**), quercetin (**14**), irisolidone (**15**), silymarin (**16**), hesperidin (**17**), chrysin (**18**), kaempferol (**19**), delphinidin 3,5-diglucoside (**20**), scutellarein 7-glucoside (**21**), avicularin (**22**), procumbentin (**23**), catechin (**24**), epigallocatechin-3-gallate (**25**), theaflavin-3,3-digallate (**26**), isorhamnetin (**27**), morin (**28**), bergenin (**29**), and kobophenol A (**30**) [45, 49, 58–65]. Among these, anthocyanin delphinidin 3,5-diglucoside (**20**) conferred highest binding propensities onto the ACE2 receptor binding domain to SARS-CoV-2 with binding energy of −13.6 kcal/mol using Glide package of Schrodinger chemical simulation software. Notably, **20** also interacted via hydrogen bond with Tyr127 [64]. Kobophenol A (**30**), a tetrastilbene, also showed in silico potential with a binding energy of −11.2 kcal/mol. **30**–ACE2 receptor complex was revealed to be thermodynamically stable for 500 ns [59]. Flavonoligan silymarin (**16**) and flavonol isorhamnetin (**27**) passed Lipinski's rule of five (LRo5), which is used in drug discovery and development to computationally evaluate the oral bioavailability of a compound in line with its ADME and toxicity properties. A compound is classified to have good druggability when it satisfies at least three of the following parameters: (1) molecular weight of less than 500 Daltons (Da), (2) H-bond acceptors of less than or equal to 10, (3) H-bond donors of less than or equal to 5, and an octanol–water partition coefficient (log *P*) value of no more than 5 [66, 67]. On the other hand, anthocyanin delphinidin 3,5-diglucoside (**20**), flavone scutellarein 7-glucoside (**21**), flavonol avicularin (**22**), and flavanol epigallocatechin-3-gallate (**25**) showed poor druggability based on either LRo5 or absorption, distribution, metabolism, and excretion (ADME) properties, or both [62, 64, 65].

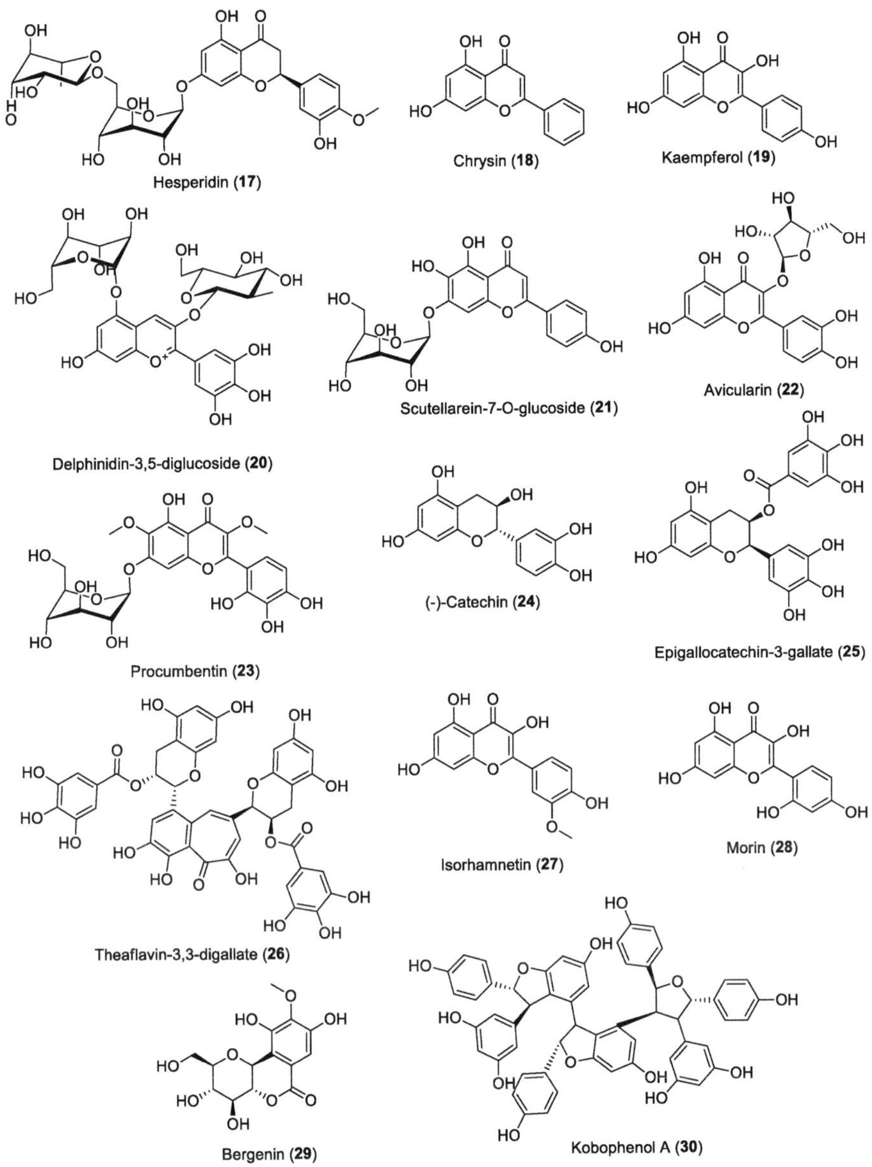


**Fig. 25.6** Structures of flavonoids **17–30** active against SARS-CoV-2 spike receptor-binding domain for ACE2

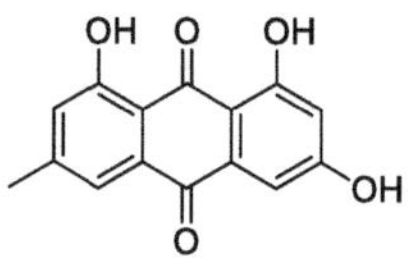

Emodin (**31**)

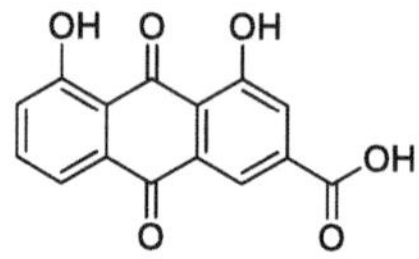

Rhein (**32**)

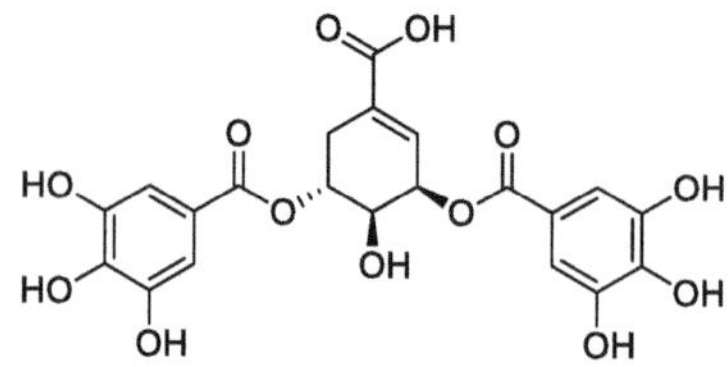

3,5-di-O-galloylshikimic acid (**33**)

**Fig. 25.7** Structures of anthraquinones **31–32** and tannin **33** active against SARS-CoV-2 spike receptor-binding domain for ACE2

### Anthraquinone

The anthraquinone emodin (**31**, Fig. 25.7) demonstrated high binding affinity against ACE2 receptor, with a binding energy of −9.8 kcal/mol, with Ala71, Asp67, and Lys74 as the interacting residues [58]. Similarly, molecular docking of rhein (**32**, Fig. 25.7) to ACE2 exhibited a good binding propensity of −9.1 kcal/mol. Anthraquinone **32** formed hydrogen bonds with Arg977, Arg977, and Thr980 [55].

### Tannin

3,5-Di-*O*-galloylshikimic acid (**33**, Fig. 25.7) was reported to demonstrate promising affinity (BE = −11.2 kcal/mol) against the ACE2 receptor to SARS-CoV-2 using the Glide package of Schrodinger chemical simulation software. While molecular dynamics simulations (MDS) revealed stable docked complex with several interacting ACE2 receptor residues such as His505, Arg273, His345, Tyr127, Glu406, and His345, tannin **33** failed to satisfy LRo5 [64].

## *Terpenoids*

Terpenoids, structurally characterized by a building block isoprene unit, represent the largest and most diverse class of natural products. They have a wide range of pharmaceutical applications which includes use as antimicrobial agents having exhibited activities against a number of viruses, bacteria, and fungi [68, 69]. In a molecular modeling study, several terpenoids were shown to display inhibitory activities against SARS-CoV-2 nonstructural proteins [70].

Terpenoids such as carvone (**34**), bicylogermacrene (**35**), andrographolide (**36**), glycyrrhizin (**37**), diosgenin (**38**), and withanolides (**39–45**) (Fig. 25.8), showed high binding affinities against ACE2 receptor with binding energies ranging from −8.5 to −11.0 kcal/mol [46, 55, 71–73]. Interestingly, terpenoids under the withanolide group, namely, withaferin A (**39**), withanolide A (**40**), withanolide B (**41**),

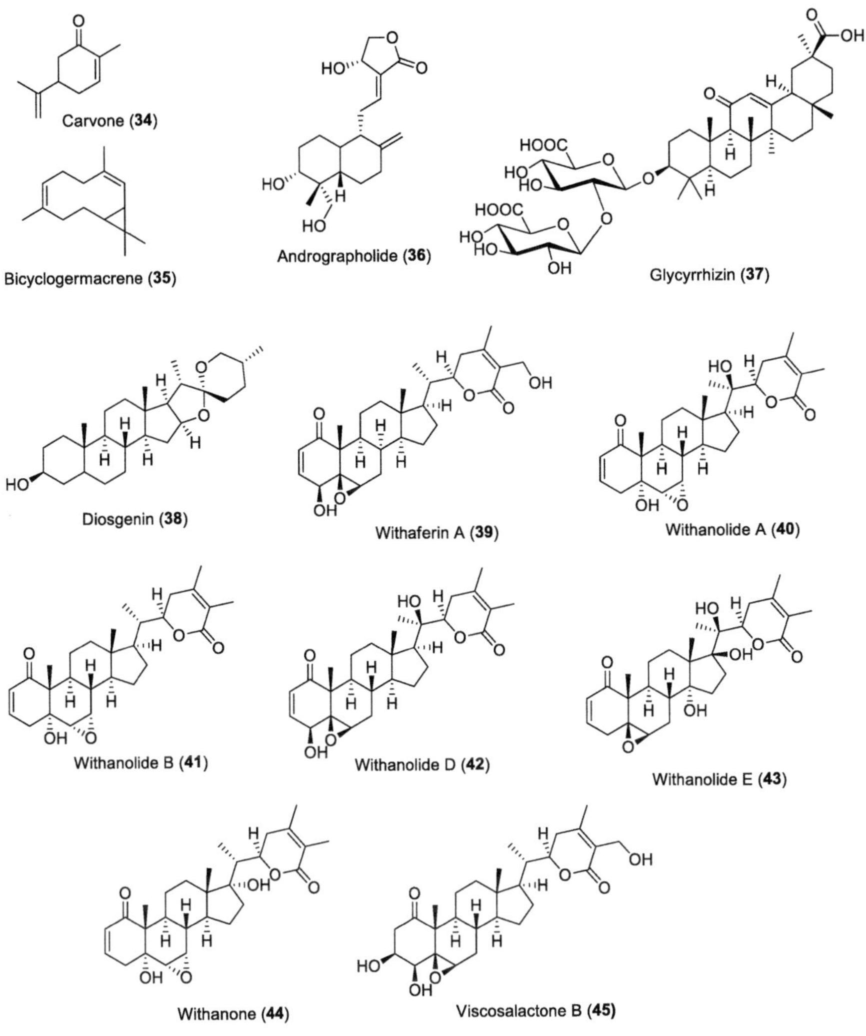


**Fig. 25.8** Structures of terpenoids **34–45** active against SARS-CoV-2 spike receptor-binding domain for ACE2

withanolide D (**42**), withanolide E (**43**), withanone (**44**), and viscosalactone B (**45**) exhibited binding energies better than −9.0 kcal/mol. Withanolide B (**41**) presented the best binding energy (BE = −11.0 kcal/mol) with Lys6844, Asn6841, Asp6928, Lys6968, Tyr6930, Gly6871, Gly6869, Asp6931, Leu6898, Cys6913, Met6929, Phe6947, Asp6897, Asn6899, Ser6872, and Pro6932 as the interacting residues [46]. Glycyrrhizin (**37**), a triterpenoid saponin, showed the second highest binding affinity with a binding energy of −10 kcal/mol. It interacted with the ACE2 receptor mostly via hydrogen bonding with Gln944, Tyr738, Gln984, and Thr980 [55].

## Organic Sulfides and Other Organosulfur Compounds

Many naturally occurring sulfur-containing compounds are showcase specific therapeutic and preventative effects on disease development and progression. Organosulfur compounds, such as those isolated from the garlic family, have been reported to have anti-inflammatory, bactericidal, antifungal, and antibiotic activities [74]. Interestingly, some of these compounds were found to combat the severity of dengue virus infection by inhibiting oxidative stress response which then hinders the production of inflammatory cytokines [75].

Allyl disulfide (**46**), allyl trisulfide (**47**), allyl (E)-1-propenyl disulfide (**48**), diallyl tetrasulfide (**49**), allyl methyl trisulfide (**50**), allyl (Z)-1-propenyl disulfide (**51**), 2-propenyl propyl trisulfide (**52**), methyl allyl disulfide (**53**), and 1,2-dithiole (**54**), are organic sulfides derived from garlic which demonstrated high binding affinities against ACE2 receptor-binding domain to SARS-CoV-2 ranging from −9.0 to −14.1 kcal/mol (Fig. 25.9) [73]. Compounds **49, 52, 53** exhibited binding energies better than −14.0 kcal/mol. For compound **49**, the interacting residues found were Gly205, Asp206, Lys562, and Ala396, while molecular dynamic simulations showed stability of the docked complex with an RMSD of 1.23 Å. Both organic sulfides **52** and **53** interacted with residues Trp566, Glu208, Val209, and Gln98 and were also thermodynamically stable (RMSD = 1.85 Å) inside the ACE2 receptor binding pocket. Additionally, 1,2-dithiole (**54**) presented a good binding of −7.89 kcal/mol, with an RMSD of 3.09 Å as per MDS.

## Phenolic Acids

Fulvic acid (**55**, Fig. 25.10) is effectively bound onto the active pocket of viral spike protein in silico with binding energy of −7.0 kcal/mol [76]. Chlorogenic acid (**56**, Fig. 25.10) on the other hand demonstrated antagonistic effects against ACE2 receptor with Gln42 and Asp38 as interacting residues [77].

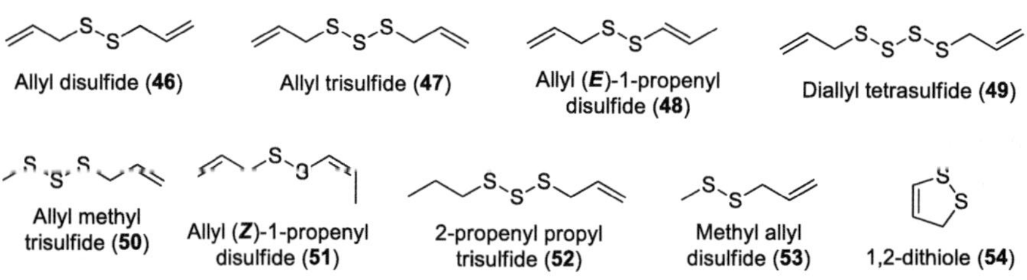


**Fig. 25.9** Structures of organosulfur compounds **46–54** active against SARS-CoV-2 spike receptor-binding domain for ACE2

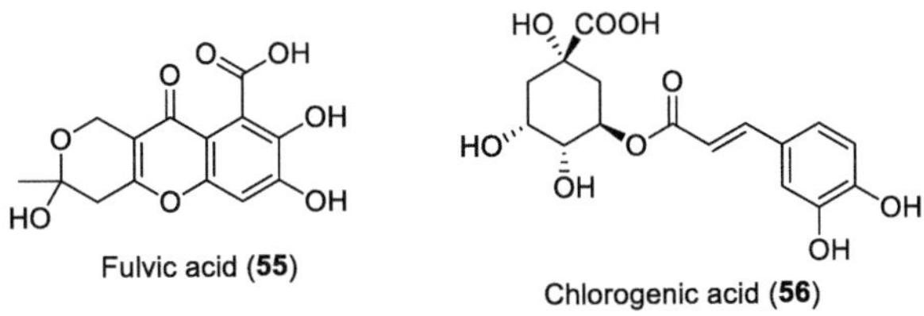


**Fig. 25.10** Structures of phenolic acids **55–56** active against SARS-CoV-2 spike receptor-binding domain for ACE2

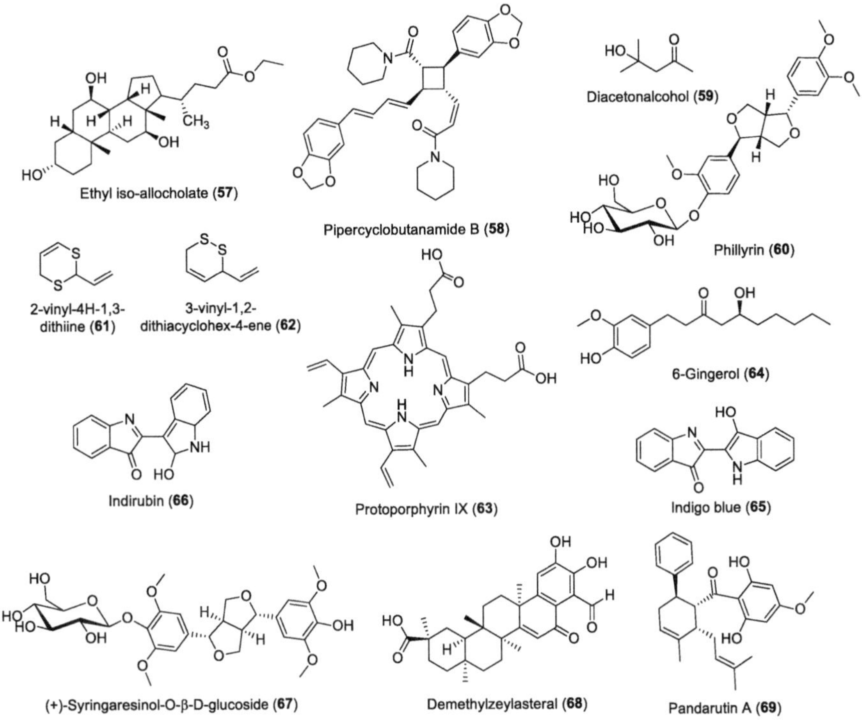


**Fig. 25.11** Structures of miscellaneous compounds **57–69** active against SARS-CoV-2 spike receptor-binding domain for ACE2

## *Miscellaneous Natural Products*

Molecular docking experiments on other natural product classes have been reported to confer inhibitory activity against ACE2 receptor (Fig. 25.11). These include ethyl iso-allocholate (**57**), pipercyclobutanamide B (**58**, alkamide), diacetonalcohol (**59**, beta-hydroxy ketone), phillyrin (**60**, lignan glucoside), dithiins 2-vinyl-4H-1,3-dithiine (**61**) and 3-vinyl-1,2-dithiacyclohex-4-ene (**62**), protoporphyrin IX (**63**), 6-gingerol (**64**, gingerol), indigo blue (**65**, indigoid), indirubin (**66**, indoline), (+)-syringaresinol-O-beta-D-glucoside (**67**, lignan), demethylzeylasteral (**68**, phenolic nor-triterpene), and panduratin A (**69**, phenylpropanoid) (Gu et al. 2020; [55, 71–73, 77–80]). Among these natural products, two dithiins **61** and **62**, scored highest binding affinities against ACE2 with binding energies of −11.8 and −10.6 kcal/mol, respectively. Diithin **61** showed interactions with Gln98, Val209, and Asn210 as well as an RMSD of 0.62 Å as per MDS. Diithin **62**, on the other hand, showed interactions with Trp566, Pro565, and Glu208 and stability inside the ACE2 receptor binding domain (RMSD = 1.19 Å).

## Inhibitors of SARS-CoV-2 Receptor Binding Domain for GRP78

### *Alkaloids*

A study conducted by Quimque and coworkers screened thirteen secondary metabolites using AutoDock Vina to determine their inhibitory activity against GRP78 binding region of spike. It was observed that among the secondary compounds, the quinazoline alkaloid quinadoline B (**70**) had the highest binding affinity with a molecular docking score of −10.5 kcal/mol (Figs. 25.12 and 25.13). Through

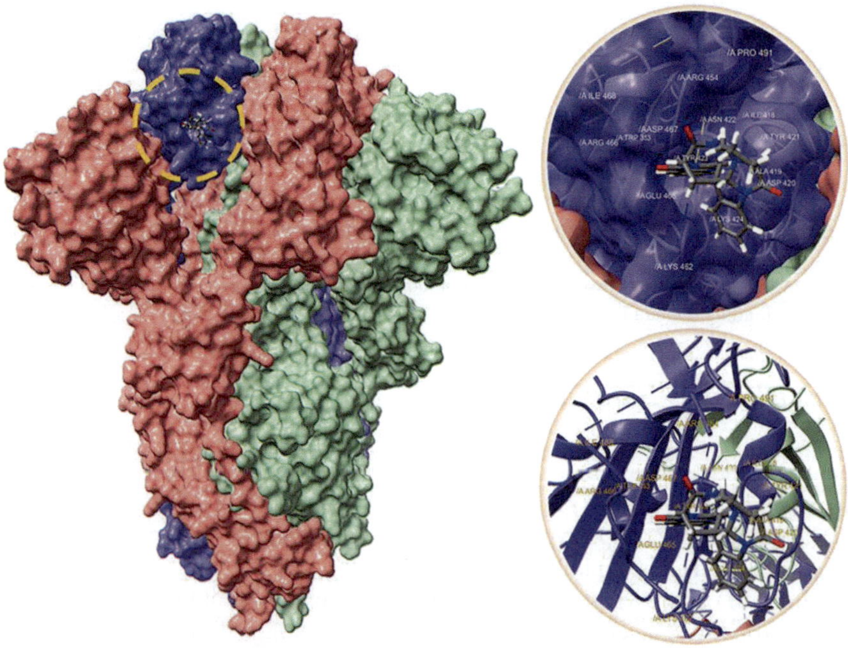

**Fig. 25.12** Putative binding site of SARS-CoV-2 spike binding receptor region for GRP78 showing the docked pose of alkaloid quinadoline B (**70**)

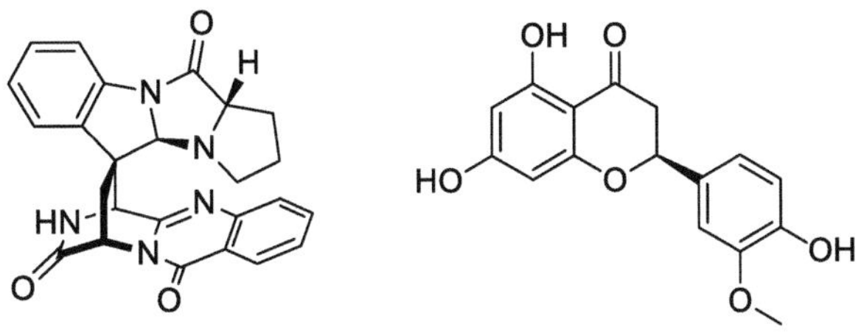


**Fig. 25.13** Structures of alkaloid **70** and polyphenol **71** active against SARS-CoV-2 spike receptor-binding region for GRP78

analyzing the compound–protein complex molecular interaction in the GRP78-binding region of the spike protein, it was determined that alkaloid **70** interacts with amino acid residues Phe430 ($\pi$–$\pi$ stacking), Asp441 ($\pi$–anion), Ala444 ($\pi$–alkyl stacking), and Cys454 ($\pi$–sulfur bonding). Molecular dynamics using the Amber 18 software revealed that the compound's average RMSD was 2.5 Å with acceptable fluctuations between 0 and 10 ns. Furthermore, the RMSF graph shows a high fluctuation with an average of 2.6 Å. Pharmacokinetic evaluation through ADME and toxicity profiling using the SwissADME and Osiris Property Explorer has demonstrated the compound's promising druggability despite its reported high irritant effect. Thus, quinadoline B (**70**) has shown great potential as a GRP78 inhibitor to induce anti-SARS-CoV-2 activity by blocking viral entry to the host cells [12].

## *Polyphenols*

Four polyphenolic compounds, namely, epigallocatechin gallate (**25**), isorhamnetin (**27**), homoeriodictyol (**71**, Fig. 25.13), and curcumin (**7**) were screened using AutoDock Vina against the ATPase domain of GRP78 and the GRP78-binding site of SARS-CoV-2 spike protein. These secondary metabolites are further classified as flavanol, flavonol, flavanone, and curcuminoid, respectively, with high affinity toward the GRP78's ATPase domain and especially regions III and IV of the spike protein that form several hydrogen bonds with the pocket residues of GRP78. Among the screened compounds, the natural ATP-competitive inhibitor epigallocatechin gallate (**25**) yielded the highest binding score of −10.5 kcal/mol through molecular docking against the ATP binding site of GRP78. Polyphenol **25** was found to interact with residues Gly228, Phe258, Gly364, Ser365, Ile368, and Asp224 by means of hydrogen bonding. Aside from its good binding affinity to host cell GRP78, **25** also had the best binding affinity toward the GRP78-binding region of spike with a docking score of −10.5 kcal/mol. Analysis of binding interactions revealed the compound and protein complex interacted with each other via hydrogen bonds with Glu427, Ser452, Ala454, Ser455, Gln458 and a hydrophobic interaction with residue Ile450. The binding of **25** induces improper functions of GRP78 as this compound attaches to SBD which results in its conformational changes.

Polyphenol **71** resulted with the second best binding score against the target protein with a docking score of −9.0 kcal/mol. Analysis of binding interactions of the complex revealed that **71** has hydrogen bonding interactions with residues Thr38, Thr39, Ile61, Glu201, Asp224, Phe258, Gly228, Glu249, and Asp249. In addition, **71** has the second highest recorded binding energy of −8.1 kcal/mol against the GRP78 spike binding site. The complex was also reported to have interactions with residues Glu427, Glu430, Ser448, and Gln485 through hydrogen bonding. The next top scoring compound is isorhamnetin (**27**) which had a binding score of −8.8 kcal/mol. The compound was able to interact with the ATPase domain of GRP78 through hydrogen bonding with Thr38, Thr39, Ile61, Glu201, Asp224, and Phe258 amino acid residues. Notably, this particular compound scored the lowest among the four compounds with a docking score of −7.2 kcal/mol against the spike binding region of GRP78. Polyphenol **27** has the same set of interacting residues with **71** also by means of H bond interactions. Lastly, curcumin (**7**) generated a binding energy of −8.2 kcal/mol. The residues Thr39, Ile61, Glu201, Asp224, Glu228, and Phe258 are observed to interact with compound **6** by means of hydrogen bonding. Curcumin scored the third highest binding affinity with the GRP78 spike binding site with a binding energy of −7.7 kcal/mol. Two residues Glu427 and Ile450 interacted with curcumin through hydrogen bonds while Ser425 and Thr441 had hydrophobic bonds with the aforementioned compound. Thus, all four compounds showed good inhibitory activity against the full-length GRP78 protein and spike-GRP78 interaction mitigating the viral entry to host cells [81].

## *Peptides*

Aside from screening polyphenols for GRP78 inhibitory activity, Allam and coworkers tested the GRP78 inhibitory activity of five peptides obtained from structurally annotated therapeutic peptides database (SATPdb), namely, satpdb12488 (**72**), satpdb14438 (**73**), satpdb28899 (**74**), satpdb18674 (**75**), and satpdb18446 (**76**) (Fig. 25.14). Using the ClusPro Server these peptides were found to bind to regions 1426–1459 of GRP78. Specifically, the satpdb18674 (**75**) peptide residues (Gln1, Ser, and Thr7) with the GRP78 residues Val429, Gln449, and Ser452. In the same target, the peptide **76** residues Val1, Tyr3, Asn4, and Thr10 interacted with GRP78 amino acid residues Val429, Thr434, Gln449, and Ser452. For peptide **72**, the amino acid residues Thr2, Met5, Asp16, and Asp19 interacted with the Val429, Thr434, Lys447, Phe451, and Ser452 amino acid residues of the GRP78. Thr9, Ser12, and Ile13 residues of peptide **73** reportedly interacted with the following GRP78 residues, namely, Val429, Thr434, and Thr458. Lastly, the residues of the peptide **74** which are Thr15, Serr16, Leu19, and Asp20 interacted with amino acid residues Val429 and Thr458 from the same region. Overall the five compounds were able to establish multiple hydrogen bonds with the residues of the GRP78 specifically located in the substrate-binding pocket. Among the five peptides, the authors stated

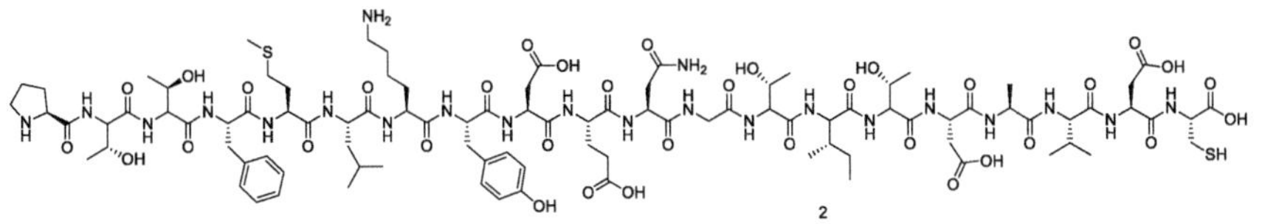

satpdb12488 (**71**)

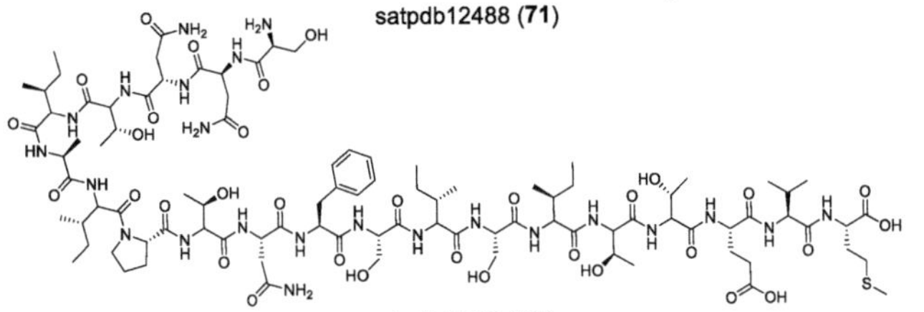

satpdb14438 (**73**)

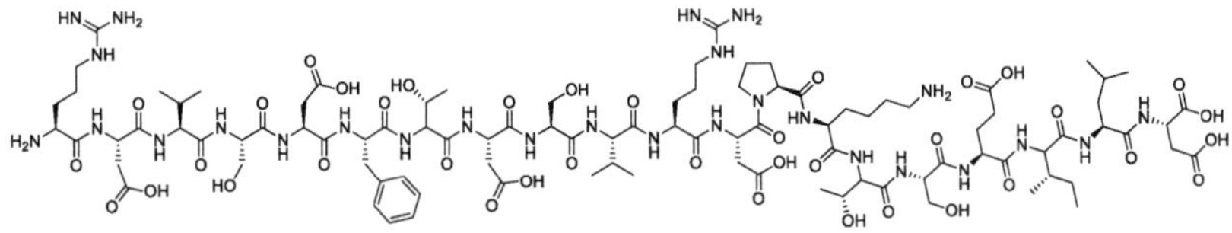

satpdb28899 (**74**)

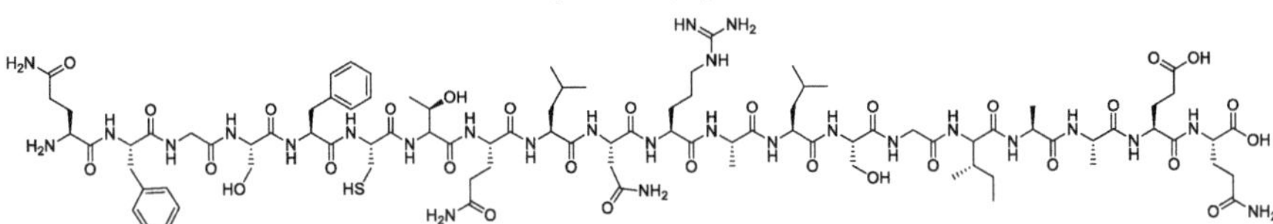

satpdb18674 (**75**)

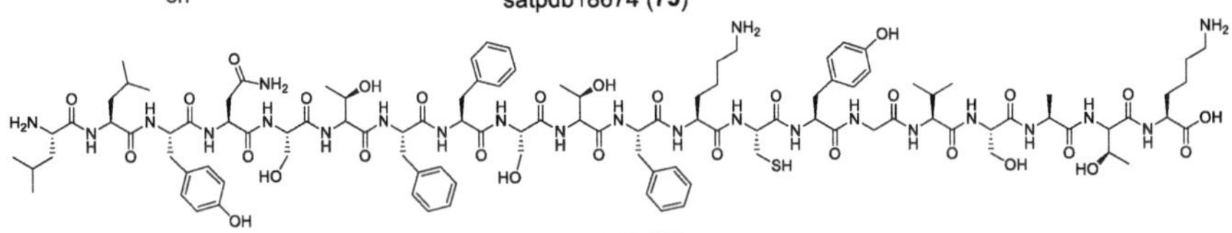

satpdb18446 (**76**)

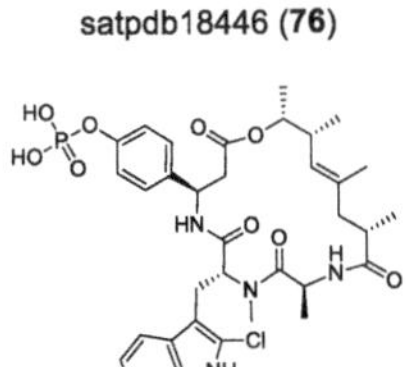

Chondramide C6 (**77**)

**Fig. 25.14** Structures of peptides **72–77** active against SARS-CoV-2 spike receptor-binding region for GRP78

that satpdb18674 as the best peptide to have SARS-CoV-2 antagonistic effects via the GRP78 due to its high affinity towards this protein [81].

Fernandez and coworkers screened different secondary metabolites obtained from myxobacteria to determine their potential SARS-CoV-2 inhibitory activity. Among those secondary metabolites, the chondramide C6 (**77**, Fig. 25.14) exhibited high binding affinity against GRP78 with a docking score of −8.8 kcal/mol. Postdock analysis revealed that cyclic peptide **77** was able to exhibit hydrogen bonding interactions with residues Asn506 and Gly495, π–sigma interaction with residue Leu474, π–alkyl interaction with residue Pro510, and π–anion interaction with residue Asp486 [53]. Overall, chondramide C6 (**77**) has shown good binding affinity to be potentially classified as a GRP78 inhibitor that would hinder SARS-CoV-2 viral entry.

### *Terpenoids*

The steroidal lactone withaferin A (**39**) exhibited the highest binding affinity against GRP78 with an AutoDock Tool docking score of −8.7 kcal/mol according to a study conducted by Sudeep and coworkers. Based on postdock analysis, **39** demonstrated noncovalent interactions with residues Ile426, Thr428, Thr434, and Phe451. Furthermore, terpenoid **39** was pharmacologically evaluated using SWISSADME and exhibited good druggability by adhering to Lipinski's Ro5 [82]. Thus, the terpenoid showed favorable binding affinities against GRP78 as a means in preventing SARS-CoV-2 viral entry.

## Inhibitors of SARS-CoV-2 Receptor Binding Domain for NRP-1 Binding Region

A study by Fernandez and coworkers demonstrated myxobacterial chondramides C1 (**78**), C2 (**79**), and E3 (**80**) as promising inhibitors of viral receptor binding domain for NRP-1 (Figs. 25.15 and 25.16). Compounds **78** and **79** passed LRo5 with no predicted toxicity risks. Reports on natural products as inhibitors of SARS-CoV-2 receptor for NRP-1 remain rudimentary [53].

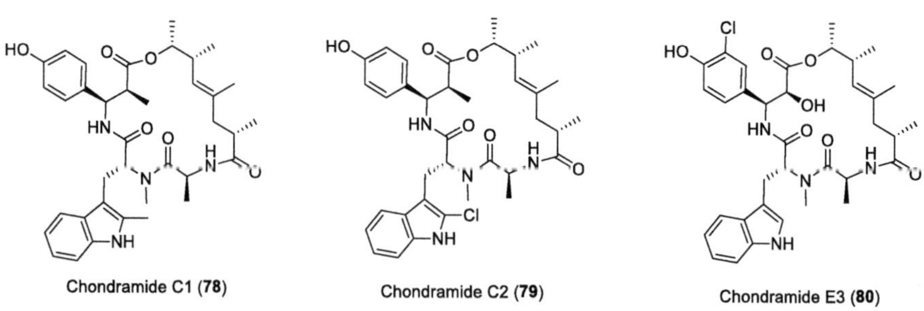


**Fig. 25.15** Structures of chondramides **78**–**80** active against SARS-CoV-2 spike receptor-binding region for NRP-1

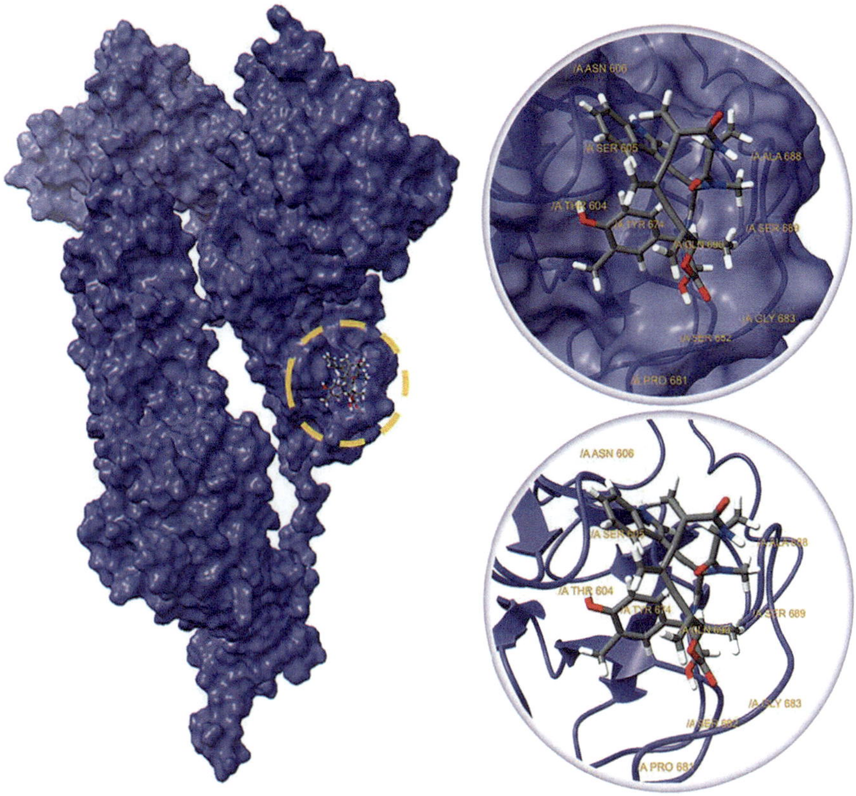


**Fig. 25.16** Putative binding site of SARS-CoV-2 spike (Chain A) binding receptor region for NRP-1 showing the docked pose of cyclic peptide chondramide E3 (**80**)

## Inhibitors of Host Cell TMPRSS2

### *Alkaloids*

Alkaloids of different subclasses exhibited favorable binding affinities with unique mechanisms mostly to the topological extracellular domain of TMPRSS2 according to AutoDock Vina scoring. The spirolepine alkaloid cryptospirolepine (**81**) bound Ser39, His40, and Ser151 of TMPRSS2 through conventional hydrogen bonding and Ile75, Tyr149, and Ser151 through hydrophobic interactions with an affinity of −9.9 kcal/mol (Figs. 25.17 and 25.18) [83]. Moreover, the cryptospirolepine–TMPRSS2 complex was thermodynamically stable with RMSD value of 1.99 Å and RMSF value of 0.66 Å throughout a 100-ns MDS performed using VMD Tk console scripts. Alkaloid **81** is non-AMES toxic, noncarcinogenic, has high gastrointestinal absorption potential with low acute toxicity, and also orally bioavailable as per

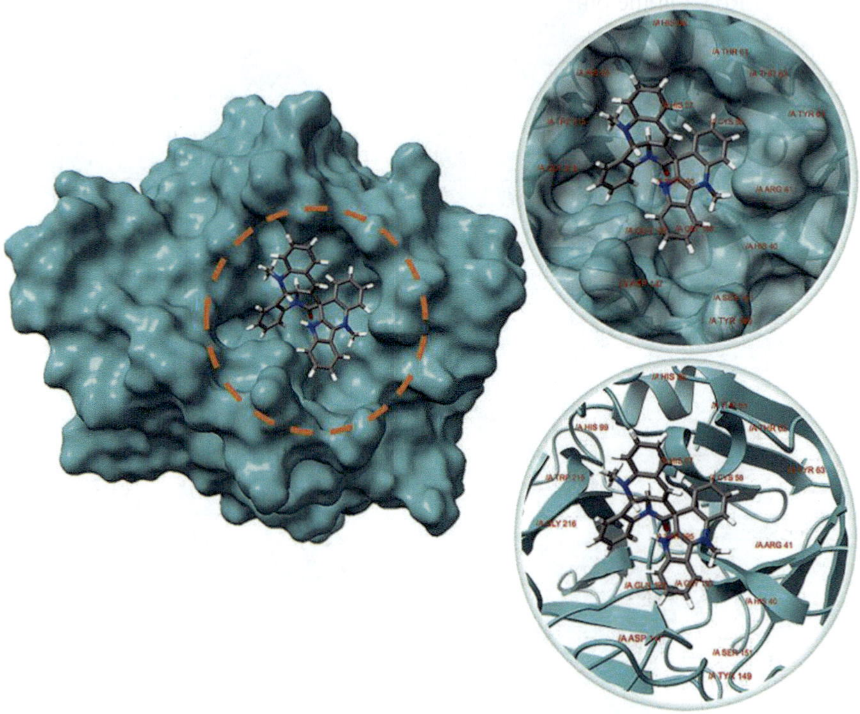

**Fig. 25.17** Putative binding site of host cell TRMPSS2 showing the docked pose of spirolepine alkaloid cryptospirolepine (**81**)

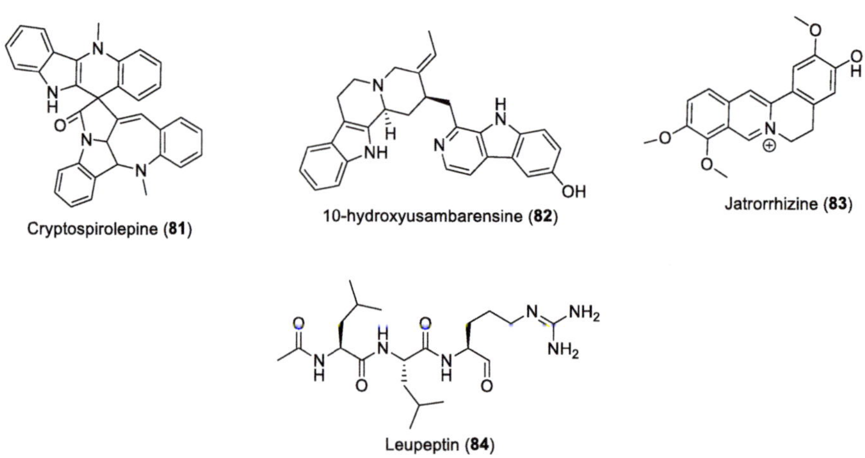


**Fig. 25.18** Structures of alkaloids **81**–**83** and peptide **84** active against host cell TMPRSS2

Lipinski's Ro5. On the other hand, the indole alkaloid, 10-hydroxyusambarensine (**82**, Fig. 25.18), docked with Asp189, Ala190, Ser195, and Ser214 of the protease through hydrogen bonding as well as with Arg41, His57, His96, Ala190, Cys191, Gln192, and Trp215 by hydrophobic interactions with a propensity of −10.4 kcal/mol [83]. This alkaloid is also non-AMES toxic, noncarcinogenic with low acute toxicity, and orally bioavailable based on Lipinski's Ro5. Another alkaloid, jatrorrhizine (**83**, Fig. 25.18), of the protoberberine type was bound to two of TMPRSS2 catalytic triad residues His296 and Ser441 through hydrogen bonding and van der Waals interaction, respectively, with an affinity of −7.5 kcal/mol [84]. Additional interactions that contributed to its affinity include hydrogen bonding with Gly439; $\pi$ interactions with Val275, Val280, Pro301, and Leu302; carbon–hydrogen bonding with Gln438; and van der Waals interactions with His279. As with all other reported top alkaloids against TMPRSS2, Alkaloid **83** has good oral bioavailability as per Lipinski's Ro5 with additional pharmacokinetic properties of high gastrointestinal absorption potential, and good blood–brain barrier penetrative property.

## *Peptides*

The tripeptide leupeptin (**84**, Fig. 25.18), formally known as N-acetyl-L-leucyl-L--leucyl-L-argininal, is the only reported natural peptide with virtual antagonistic effect against TMPRSS2. It conferred a binding affinity of −9.325 kcal/mol to TMPRSS2 determined through extra precision mode in induced fit docking. Leupeptin remarkably bound onto the TMPRSS2 catalytic triad His41, Asp180, and Ser186, noting that the homology model was based on hepsin serine protease. In addition, interactions with Ser 181, Gly209, Lys87, Gly184, Val125, and His24 of TMPRSS2 contributed to leupeptin's propensity. Notably, peptide **84** had thermodynamically similar RMSD value of less than 2 Å with known inhibitors camostat and nafamostat but the stability of bound TMPRSS2 with the peptide was more stable at 2.4 Å compared to the complexes formed by the known inhibitors [85].

## *Polyphenols*

Polyphenols appear as the most reported virtual inhibitors of TMPRSS2. Various polyphenolic subclasses of fungal, lichen, and plant origin comprise natural inhibitors of the serine protease. Flavones, chalcone, tannin, proanthocyanidins, anthraquinone, xanthone, and phenolic acids exhibit anti-TMPRSS2 properties.

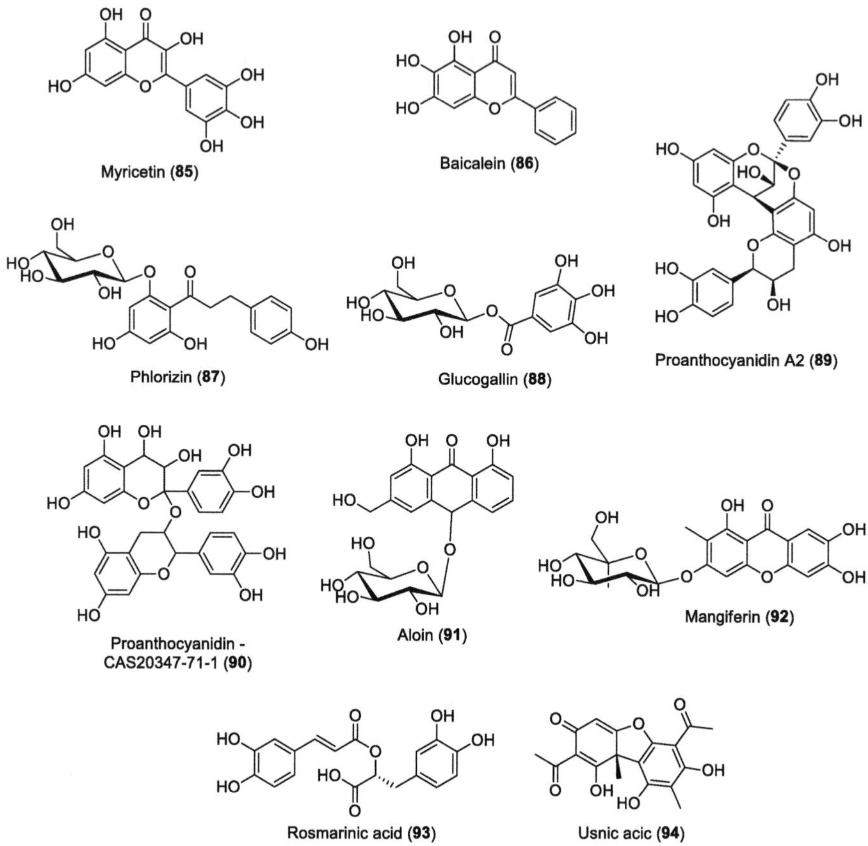


**Fig. 25.19** Structures of polyphenols **85–94** active against host cell TMPRSS2

## Flavonol and Flavone

Myricetin (**85**) and baicalein (**86**) bound His296 and Ser441 of the TMPRSS2 catalytic triad through hydrogen bonding and van der Waals interactions, respectively (Fig. 25.19) [84]. Myricetin (**85**), a hexahydroxyflavone, exhibited a higher binding affinity of −8.3 kcal/mol with good oral availability according to Lipinski's Ro5 than baicalein (**86**), a trihydroxyflavone, with an affinity of −7.7 kcal/mol as per AutoDock Vina scoring. Further interactions involved in the **85**–TMPRSS2 complex include hydrogen bonds with Glu389 and Ser460; $\pi$–anion interaction with Glu389; and van der Waals interactions with Asp 435, Ser 436, Gln 438, Ser441, Thr 459, Gly 462, Gly 464, Cys 465, and Gly 472. On the other hand, **86**-TMPRSS2 interactions also include hydrogen bonding with Ser460 and Ser436; $\pi$ interactions with Cys437, Cys465, and Trp461; and van der Waals interactions with Glu 389, Asp435, Gln438, Ser 441, Thr459, Gly462, Gly464, Gly472, and Val473.

### Chalcone

The dihydrochalcone glucoside, phlorizin (**87**, Fig. 25.19), bound His296 and Ser441 of the TMPRSS2 catalytic triad via π–cation interaction and hydrogen bonding, respectively [86]. This conferred an affinity of −7.7 kcal/mol through PyRx AutoDock Vina scoring function. Other interactions with the serine protease encompassed hydrogen bonding with Ser460 and Gly464; π–cation interaction with His296; π–alkyl interaction with Val280; π–sulfur bonding with Cys297; and van der Waals interactions with Cys281, Glu299, Leu302, Lys342,Ser436, Cys437, Gln438, Gly439, Asp440, Thr459, Trp461, Gly462, Ser463, and Cys465. Furthermore, the **87**–TMPRSS2 complex displayed stability of RMSD value 2 nm from 2.5 ns to 7.5 ns and RMSF value of less than 0.5 nm in a 10-ns GROMACS CHARMM36-march2019 force field TIP3P model molecular dynamics simulation. Chemically, this chalcone has good oral bioavailability, no AMES toxicity, no hepatotoxicity, and is non–skin sensitive.

### Hydrolysable Tannin

Glucogallin (**88**, Fig. 25.19) exhibited a binding affinity of −6.9 kcal/mol to TMPRSS2 as per PyRx AutoDock Vina scoring function, docking with catalytic triad residues His296 and Ser441 through van der Waals interaction and hydrogen bonding, respectively [86]. Tannin **88** also interacted with TMPRSS2 via hydrogen bonding with Val280, Gly439, and Gly462; π–sigma interaction with Gln438; and van der Waals interactions with His296, Ser436, Cys437, Asp440, Thr459, Ser460, Trp461, Ser463, and Cys464. Through a 10-ns GROMACS CHARMM36-march2019 force field TIP3P model molecular dynamics simulation, the **88**–TMPRSS2 complex was observed to be thermodynamically stable with an RMSD value of 0.1 nm at approximately 1.25 ns until the end of simulation and RMSF value of less than 0.5 nm. Pharmacologically, glucogallin (**88**) was found to have good oral bioavailability as per Lipinski's Ro5 and has no AMES toxicity, hepatotoxicity, and skin sensitivity properties.

### Proanthocyanidins

Proanthocyanidins A2 (**89**) and CAS20347–71-1 (**90**) exhibited binding affinities of −7.9 kcal/mol based on AutoDock Vina scoring and −5.5 kcal/mol according to Glide XP calculation, respectively (Fig. 25.19) [84, 87]. Proanthocyanidin **89** remarkably was bound to the catalytic triad residues His296 and Ser441 via hydrogen bonding. An amide–π interaction with Trp461 was also observed, accompanied by other interactions with Asp435, Cys437, Lys342, Gln438, Gly439, Thr459, Ser460, Ser463, Gly464, Gly472, and Val473.

#### Anthraquinone

The sole anthraquinone with reported potential anti-TMPRSS2 property is aloin (**91**, Fig. 25.19). This anthraquinone glycoside demonstrated a binding affinity of −6.5 kcal/mol to the serine protease based on a Glide XP calculation [87].

#### Xanthone

Mangiferin (**92**, Fig. 25.19) docked with TMPRSS2 through hydrogen bonding with Ala243 and Glu289; $\pi$–donor interactions with Phe357; $\pi$–$\pi$ alkyl interactions with Ile242 and Pro288; and van der Waals interactions with Lys191, Asn192, Cys244, Thr287, Trp290, and Pro363 [86]. Xanthone **92** had an affinity of −6.9 kcal/mol to TMPRSS2 based on PyRx AutoDock Vina scoring function; moreover, the complex was stable from 1 to 10 ns with an RMSD value of approximately 0.1 nm and RMSF value of less than 0.5 nm as demonstrated by a 10-ns GROMACS CHARMM36-march2019 force field TIP3P model molecular dynamics simulation. With regard to its pharmacological features, compound **92** is non-AMES toxic, nonhepatotoxic, and nonskin sensitive.

#### Phenolic Acids

Rosmarinic acid (**93**) and the dibenzofuran derivative usnic acid (**94**) demonstrated virtual anti-TMPRSS2 activities with affinities of −5.8 and −5.6 kcal/mol, respectively, based on Glide XP calculations [87]. Phenolic acid **93** is of plant origin while **94** can be found in lichens (Fig. 25.19).

### *Terpenoids*

Terpenoids of various degrees of isoprene units exhibited potential as inhibitors of TMPRSS2 (Fig. 25.20). The monoterpenoid iridoid glycoside, geniposide (**95**), exhibited a binding affinity of −14.69 kcal/mol as per MOE software and formed hydrogen bonds with TMPRSS2 residues Asn146, Arg147, Arg150, Lys449, and Asn450 [88]. Additionally, this monoterpenoid is non-toxic. On the other hand, the diterpenoid columbin (**96**) bound TMPRSS2 catalytic triad residues His296 and Ser441 through hydrogen bonding and van der Waals interaction, respectively [84]. These were accompanied by $\pi$ interactions with Ser 436, Cys 437, Ser 460, and Cys 465; and other interactions with Ser411, Gln438, Gly439, Thr459, Trp461, Gly462, and Gly464. This as a whole conferred an affinity of −8.2 kcal/mol according to AutoDock Vina scoring function. In addition, terpenoid **96** has good oral bioavailability based on Lipinski's Ro5. With regard to triterpenoids, the ianostanoid ganodermanontriol (**97**) and pentacyclic gedunin (**98**) both bound His296 and Ser441 of

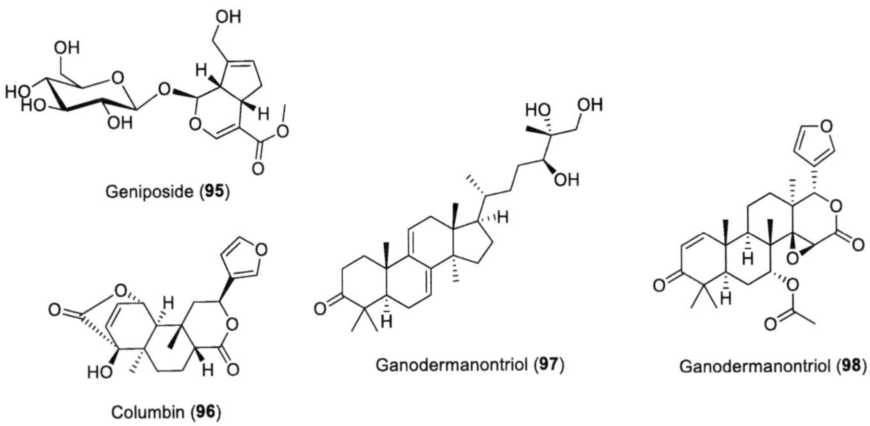


**Fig. 25.20** Structures of terpenoids **95–98** active against host cell TMPRSS2

the catalytic triad with terpenoid **97** specifically forming carbon–hydrogen bonding with His296 and conventional hydrogen bonding with Ser441 and terpenoid **98** forming noncovalent interactions with the residues [84, 89]. Additionally, **97** which has good oral bioavailability, exhibited hydrogen bonding with Gly462; carbon–hydrogen bonding with Trp461; and van der Waals interactions with Lys340, Thr341, Lys342, Glu389, Leu419, Cys437, Gln438, Ser460, and Cys465. On the other hand, **98** demonstrated additional noncovalent interactions with Cys297, Cys437, Ser460, Gly462, Gly464, and Cys465 of the serine protease.

# Prospects

Since the advent of the COVID-19 pandemic in the early 2020, various prophylactic and therapeutic regimens have been identified encompassing small molecules, neutralizing antibodies, and bioengineered products [18]. With the aid of computational chemistry and virtual screening, a comprehensive library of small molecules with favorable binding affinity with SARS-CoV-2 drug targets was established ([90]; Tahir ul [91]). However, the toxicity and efficacy of these drug leads need further testing in animal models and human subjects [18]. Natural products and herbal medicines have long been used in treating respiratory infections and may have been approved as drugs and over-the-counter nutraceuticals or food additives. In general, these natural products have shown satisfactory safety profiles with minimal toxicity risks making them ideal prophylactic or therapeutic drug candidates [1, 18]. With the aid of computational simulations, an array of natural products has been found highly potent in blocking SARS-CoV-2 spikes and membrane receptors of human coronavirus ([2, 12]; Tahir ul [91]). Furthermore, the stability of natural products and herbal medicines in human gastrointestinal tract is barely an issue. The gut microbiome, acidic gastric environment, and presence of digestive enzymes have less impact on the bioavailability of natural products and herbs compared to antibody and other prophylactic and therapeutic regimens. This advantage makes oral dosing rather than intravenous administration possible. Furthermore, the ease in production makes it possible for the mass deployment of herbal medicines to large population [1, 18]. With the emergence of new SARS-CoV-2 variants that are more transmissible and infectious, there is urgency to develop drug prototypes that are safe, efficacious, and stable as antiviral agents. Through computational-driven drug discovery, natural products such as alkaloids, sterols, peptides, polyphenols, and terpenoids were demonstrated to block host cell recognition, and viral attachment and fusion through binding with various receptor-binding regions of SARS-CoV-2 spike protein for ACE2, GRP78, and NRP-1 as well as host cell transmembrane TMPRSS2. Thus, to further probe the antiviral properties of these natural products, in vitro and in vivo assays have to be performed to understand the nature and behavior of these secondary compounds against the SARS-CoV-2 virus infecting a living biological model. Finally, the discovery of these drug leads could provide inspiration in the design and development of SARS-CoV-2 therapeutics.

## References

1. Antonio ADS, Wiedemann LSM, Veiga-Junior VF. Natural products' role against COVID-19. RSC Adv. 2020;10:23379–93. https://doi.org/10.1039/d0ra03774e.
2. Hoffmann M, Kleine-Weber H, Schroeder S, et al. SARS-CoV-2 cell entry depends on ACE2 and TMPRSS2 and is blocked by a clinically proven protease inhibitor. Cell. 2020;181:271–80. https://doi.org/10.1016/j.cell.2020.02.052.
3. Sadegh S, Matschinske J, Blumenthal DB, et al. Exploring the SARS-CoV-2 virus-host-drug interactome for drug repurposing. Nat Commun. 2020;11:1–9. https://doi.org/10.1038/s41467-020-17189-2.
4. Shamsi A, Mohammad T, Anwar S, et al. Potential drug targets of SARS-CoV-2: from genomics to therapeutics. Int J Biol Macromol. 2021;177:1–9. https://doi.org/10.1016/j.ijbiomac.2021.02.071.
5. Gil C, Ginex T, Maestro I, et al. COVID-19: drug targets and potential treatments. J Med Chem. 2020;63:12359–86. https://doi.org/10.1021/acs.jmedchem.0c00606.
6. Wouters OJ, Shadlen KC, Salcher-Konrad M, et al. Challenges in ensuring global access to COVID-19 vaccines: production, affordability, allocation, and deployment. Lancet. 2020;397:1023–34. https://doi.org/10.1016/S0140-6736(21)00306-8.
7. Karim SSA. New SARS-CoV-2 Variants — Clinical, Public Health, and Vaccine Implications. New Engl J Med. 2021;384:1866–8. https://doi.org/10.1056/NEJMc2100362.
8. Bian L, Gao F, Zhang J, et al. Effects of SARS-CoV-2 variants on vaccine efficacy and response strategies. Expert Rev Vaccines. 2021;20:365–73. https://doi.org/10.1080/14760584.2021.1903879.
9. Moore JP, Offit PA. SARS-CoV-2 vaccines and the growing threat of viral variants. J Am Med Assoc. 2021;325:821–2. https://doi.org/10.1001/jama.2021.1114.
10. Bharti R, Shukla SK. Molecules against COVID-19: an *in silico* approach for drug development. J Electron Sci Technol. 2021;19:1–8. https://doi.org/10.1016/j.jnlest.2021.100095.
11. Quimque MT, Notarte KI, Letada A, et al. Potential cancer- and Alzheimer's disease-targeting phosphodiesterase inhibitors from *Uvaria alba*: insights from *in vitro* and consensus virtual screening. ACS Omega. 2021;6:8403–17. https://doi.org/10.1021/acsomega.1c00137.

12. Quimque MTJ, Notarte KIR, Fernandez RAT, et al. Virtual screening-driven drug discovery of SARS-CoV-2 enzyme inhibitors targeting viral attachment, replication, post-translational modification and host immunity evasion infection mechanisms. J Biomol Struct Dyn. 2021;39:4316–33. https://doi.org/10.1080/07391102.2020.1776639.
13. Calland N, Sahuc M-E, Belouzard S, et al. Polyphenols inhibit hepatitis C virus entry by a new mechanism of action. J Virol. 2015;89:10053–63. https://doi.org/10.1128/JVI.01473-15.
14. Fioravanti R, Celestino I, Costi R, et al. Effects of polyphenol compounds on influenza a virus replication and definition of their mechanism of action. Bioorg Med Chem. 2012;20:5046–52. https://doi.org/10.1016/j.bmc.2012.05.062.
15. Hashimoto F, Kashiwada Y, Nonaka G, Nohara T. Evaluation of tea polyphenols as anti-HIV agents. Bioorg Med Chem Lett. 1996;6:695–700. https://doi.org/10.1016/0960-894X(96)00095-9.
16. Musarra-Pizzo M, Pennisi R, Ben-Amor I, et al. *In vitro* anti-HSV-1 activity of polyphenol-rich extracts and pure polyphenol compounds derived from pistachios kernels (*Pistacia vera* L.). Plants (Basel, Switzerland). 2020;9:1–11. https://doi.org/10.3390/plants9020267.
17. Vázquez-Calvo Á, Jiménez de Oya N, Martín-Acebes MA, et al. Antiviral properties of the natural polyphenols delphinidin and epigallocatechin gallate against the flaviviruses West Nile virus, zika virus, and dengue virus. Front Microbiol. 2017;8:1314. https://doi.org/10.3389/fmicb.2017.01314.
18. Huang J, Tao G, Liu J, et al. Current prevention of COVID-19: natural products and herbal medicine. Front Pharmacol. 2020;11:1–18. https://doi.org/10.3389/fphar.2020.588508.
19. Wrapp D, Wang N, Corbett KS, et al. Cryo-EM structure of the 2019-nCoV spike in the prefusion conformation. Science. 2020;367:1260–3. https://doi.org/10.1126/science.abb2507.
20. Duan L, Zheng Q, Zhang H, et al. The SARS-CoV-2 spike glycoprotein biosynthesis, structure, function, and antigenicity: implications for the Design of Spike-Based Vaccine Immunogens. Front Immunol. 2020;11:1–12. https://doi.org/10.3389/fimmu.2020.576622.
21. Walls AC, Park Y-J, Tortorici MA, et al. Structure, function, and antigenicity of the SARS-CoV-2 spike glycoprotein. Cell. 2020;181:281–292.e6. https://doi.org/10.1016/j.cell.2020.02.058.
22. Lan J, Ge J, Yu J, et al. Structure of the SARS-CoV-2 spike receptor-binding domain bound to the ACE2 receptor. Nature. 2020;581:215–20. https://doi.org/10.1038/s41586-020-2180-5.
23. Cai Y, Zhang J, Xiao T, et al. Distinct conformational states of SARS-CoV-2 spike protein. Science. 2020;369:1586–92. https://doi.org/10.1126/science.abd4251.
24. Henderson R, Edwards RJ, Mansouri K, et al. Controlling the SARS-CoV-2 spike glycoprotein conformation. Nat Struct Mol Biol. 2020;27:925–33. https://doi.org/10.1038/s41594-020-0479-4.
25. Tai W, He L, Zhang X, et al. Characterization of the receptor-binding domain (RBD) of 2019 novel coronavirus: implication for development of RBD protein as a viral attachment inhibitor and vaccine. Cell Mol Immunol. 2020;17:613–20. https://doi.org/10.1038/s41423-020-0400-4.
26. Shang J, Ye G, Shi K, et al. Structural basis of receptor recognition by SARS-CoV-2. Nature. 2020b;581:221–4. https://doi.org/10.1038/s41586-020-2179-y.
27. Song W, Gui M, Wang X, Xiang Y. Cryo-EM structure of the SARS coronavirus spike glycoprotein in complex with its host cell receptor ACE2. PLoS Pathog. 2018;14:e1007236. https://doi.org/10.1371/journal.ppat.1007236.
28. Shang J, Wan Y, Luo C, et al. Cell entry mechanisms of SARS-CoV-2. Proc Natl Acad Sci U S A. 2020a;117:11727–34. https://doi.org/10.1073/pnas.2003138117.
29. Sternberg A, Naujokat C. Structural features of coronavirus SARS-CoV-2 spike protein: targets for vaccination. Life Sci. 2020;257:118056. https://doi.org/10.1016/j.lfs.2020.118056.
30. Amin M, Sorour MK, Kasry A. Comparing the binding interactions in the receptor binding domains of SARS-CoV-2 and SARS-CoV. J Phys Chem Lett. 2020;11:4897–900. https://doi.org/10.1021/acs.jpclett.0c01064.
31. Brielle ES, Schneidman-Duhovny D, Linial M. The SARS-CoV-2 exerts a distinctive strategy for interacting with the ACE2 human receptor. Viruses. 2020;12:1–10. https://doi.org/10.3390/v12050497.

32. Chowdhury R, Boorla VS, Maranas CD. Computational biophysical characterization of the SARS-CoV-2 spike protein binding with the ACE2 receptor and implications for infectivity. Comput Struct Biotechnol J. 2020;18:2573–82. https://doi.org/10.1016/j.csbj.2020.09.019.
33. Spinello A, Saltalamacchia A, Magistrato A. Is the rigidity of SARS-CoV-2 spike receptor-binding motif the Hallmark for its enhanced infectivity? Insights from all-atom simulations. J Phys Chem Lett. 2020;11:4785–90. https://doi.org/10.1021/acs.jpclett.0c01148.
34. Wang Y, Liu M, Gao J. Enhanced receptor binding of SARS-CoV-2 through networks of hydrogen-bonding and hydrophobic interactions. Proc Natl Acad Sci U S A. 2020;117:13967–74. https://doi.org/10.1073/pnas.2008209117.
35. Ibrahim IM, Abdelmalek DH, Elshahat ME, Elfiky AA. COVID-19 spike-host cell receptor GRP78 binding site prediction. J Infect. 2020;80:554–62. https://doi.org/10.1016/j.jinf.2020.02.026.
36. Elfiky AA. SARS-CoV-2 spike-heat shock protein A5 (GRP78) recognition may be related to the immersed human coronaviruses. Front Pharmacol. 2020;11:1–3. https://doi.org/10.3389/fphar.2020.577467.
37. Cantuti-Castelvetri L, Ojha R, Pedro LD, et al. Neuropilin-1 facilitates SARS-CoV-2 cell entry and infectivity. Science. 2020;370:856–60. https://doi.org/10.1126/science.abd2985.
38. Daly JL, Simonetti B, Klein K, et al. Neuropilin-1 is a host factor for SARS-CoV-2 infection. Science. 2020;370:861–5. https://doi.org/10.1126/science.abd3072.
39. Kyrou I, Randeva HS, Spandidos DA, Karteris E. Not only ACE2—the quest for additional host cell mediators of SARS-CoV-2 infection: Neuropilin-1 (NRP1) as a novel SARS-CoV-2 host cell entry mediator implicated in COVID-19. Signal Transduct Target Ther. 2021;6:21. https://doi.org/10.1038/s41392-020-00460-9.
40. Macabeo APG, Krohn K, Gehle D, et al. Indole alkaloids from the leaves of Philippine *Alstonia scholaris*. Phytochemistry. 2005;66:1158–62. https://doi.org/10.1016/j.phytochem.2005.02.018.
41. Macabeo APG, Vidar WS, Chen X, et al. *Mycobacterium tuberculosis* and cholinesterase inhibitors from *Voacanga globosa*. Eur J Med Chem. 2011;46:3118–23. https://doi.org/10.1016/j.ejmech.2011.04.025.
42. Magpantay HD, Malaluan IN, Manzano JAH, et al. Antibacterial and COX-2 inhibitory Tetrahydrobisbenzylisoquinoline alkaloids from the Philippine medicinal plant *Phaeanthus ophthalmicus*. Plan Theory. 2021;10:1–16. https://doi.org/10.3390/plants10030462.
43. Fielding BC, da SMB FC, NSM I, de Sousa DP. Alkaloids: therapeutic potential against human coronaviruses. Molecules. 2020;25:1–16. https://doi.org/10.3390/molecules25235496.
44. Thawabteh A, Juma S, Bader M, et al. The biological activity of natural alkaloids against herbivores, cancerous cells and pathogens. Toxins. 2019;11:1–28. https://doi.org/10.3390/toxins11110656.
45. Gao L-Q, Xu J, Chen S-D. *In silico* screening of potential Chinese herbal medicine against COVID-19 by targeting SARS-CoV-2 3CLpro and angiotensin converting enzyme II using molecular docking. Chin J Integr Med. 2020;26:527–32. https://doi.org/10.1007/s11655-020-3476-x.
46. Srivastava A, Siddiqui S, Ahmad R, et al. Exploring Nature's bounty: identification of *Withania somnifera* as a promising source of therapeutic agents against COVID-19 by virtual screening and in silico evaluation. J Biomol Struct Dyn. 2020:1–51. https://doi.org/10.1080/07391102.2020.1835725.
47. Hisham Shady N, Youssif KA, Sayed AM, et al. Sterols and triterpenes: antiviral potential supported by *in-silico* analysis. Plan Theory. 2021;10:1–34. https://doi.org/10.3390/plants10010041.
48. Řezanka T, Siristova L, Sigler K. Sterols and triterpenoids with antiviral activity. Antiinfect Agents Med Chem. 2009;8:193–210. https://doi.org/10.2174/187152109788680207.
49. Yang L, Li Y-T, Miao J, et al. Network pharmacology studies on the effect of chai-Ling decoction in coronavirus disease 2019. Tradit Med Res. 2020a;5:145–59. https://doi.org/10.12032/TMR20200324170.

50. Lau JL, Dunn MK. Therapeutic peptides: historical perspectives, current development trends, and future directions. Bioorg Med Chem. 2018;26:2700–7. https://doi.org/10.1016/j.bmc.2017.06.052.
51. Joo SH. Cyclic peptides as therapeutic agents and biochemical tools. Biomol Ther (Seoul). 2012;20:19–26. https://doi.org/10.4062/biomolther.2012.20.1.019.
52. Sasse F, Kunze B, Gronewold TMA, Reichenbach H. The Chondramides: cytostatic agents from myxobacteria acting on the actin cytoskeleton. JNCI J Natl Cancer Inst. 1998;90:1559–63. https://doi.org/10.1093/jnci/90.20.1559.
53. Fernandez RAT, Quimque MTJ, Notarte KI, et al. Myxobacterial depsipeptide chondramides interrupt SARS-CoV-2 entry by targeting its broad, cell tropic spike protein. J Biomol Struct Dyn. 2021;1:1–20. https://doi.org/10.1080/07391102.2021.1969281.
54. de Leon VNO, Manzano JAH, Pilapil DYH, et al. Anti-HIV reverse transcriptase plant polyphenolic natural products with *in silico* inhibitory properties on seven non-structural proteins vital in SARS-Cov-2 pathogenesis. J Genet Eng Biotechnol. 2021a;19:104. https://doi.org/10.1186/s43141-021-00206-2.
55. Cheke RS, Narkhede RR, Shinde SD, et al. Natural product emerging as potential SARS spike glycoproteins-ACE2 inhibitors to combat COVID-19 attributed by *in-silico* investigations. Biointerface Res Appl Chem. 2021;11:10628–39. https://doi.org/10.33263/BRIAC113.1062810639.
56. Wahedi HM, Ahmad S, Abbasi SW. Stilbene-based natural compounds as promising drug candidates against COVID-19. J Biomol Struct Dyn. 2021;39:3225–34. https://doi.org/10.1080/07391102.2020.1762743.
57. Alazmi M, Motwalli O. Molecular basis for drug repurposing to study the Interface of the S protein in SARS-CoV-2 and human ACE2 through docking, characterization, and molecular dynamics for natural drug candidates. J Mol Model. 2020;26:1–10. https://doi.org/10.1007/s00894-020-04599-8.
58. Basu A, Sarkar A, Maulik U. Molecular docking study of potential Hytochemicals and their effects on the complex of SARS-COV-2 spike protein and human ACE2. Sci Rep. 2020;10:1–15. https://doi.org/10.1038/s41598-020-74715-4.
59. Gangadevi S, Badavath VN, Thakur A, et al. Kobophenol a inhibits binding of host ACE2 receptor with spike RBD domain of SARS-CoV-2, a Lead compound for blocking COVID-19. J Phys Chem Lett. 2021;12:1793–802. https://doi.org/10.1021/acs.jpclett.0c03119.
60. Gupta A, Ahmad R, Siddiqui S, et al. Flavonol morin targets host ACE2, IMP-α, PARP-1 and viral proteins of SARS-CoV-2, SARS-CoV and MERS-CoV critical for infection and survival: a computational analysis. J Biomol Struct Dyn. 2021;1:1–32. https://doi.org/10.1080/07391102.2021.1871863.
61. Jena AB, Kanungo N, Nayak V, et al. Catechin and curcumin interact with S protein of SARS-CoV2 and ACE2 of human cell membrane: insights from computational studies. Sci Rep. 2021;11:1–14. https://doi.org/10.1038/s41598-021-81462-7.
62. Mhatre S, Naik S, Patravale V. A molecular docking study of EGCG and theaflavin Digallate with the druggable targets of SARS-CoV-2. Comput Biol Med. 2021;129:1–10. https://doi.org/10.1016/j.compbiomed.2020.104137.
63. Sharbidre A, Dhage P, Duggal H, Meshram R. In silico investigation of *Tridax procumbens* phytoconstituents against SARS-CoV-2 infection. Biointerface Res Appl Chem. 2021;11:12120–48. https://doi.org/10.33263/BRIAC114.1212012148.
64. Sharma P, Shanavas A. Natural derivatives with dual binding potential against SARS-CoV-2 Main protease and human ACE2 possess low Oral bioavailability: a brief computational analysis. J Biomol Struct Dyn. 2020:1–12. https://doi.org/10.1080/07391102.2020.1794970.
65. Xu J, Gao L, Liang H, Dong CS. In silico screening of potential anti–COVID-19 bioactive natural constituents from food sources by molecular docking. Nutrition. 2021;82:1–7. https://doi.org/10.1016/j.nut.2020.111049.
66. Quimque MT, Notarte KI, Adviento XA, et al. Polyphenolic Natural Products Active In Silico against SARS-CoV-2 Spike Receptor Binding Domains and Non-Structural Proteins – A Review. Comb Chem High Throughput Screen. 2021;1:–40. https://doi.org/10.2174/1386207325666210917113207.

67. Lipinski CA, Lombardo F, Dominy BW, et al. Experimental and computational approaches to estimate solubility and permeability in drug discovery and development settings. Adv Drug Deliv Rev. 2001;46:3–26. https://doi.org/10.1016/s0169-409x(00)00129-0.
68. Cox-Georgian D, Ramadoss N, Dona C, Basu C. Therapeutic and medicinal uses of terpenes. Med Plants. 2019:333–59. https://doi.org/10.1007/978-3-030-31269-5_15.
69. Yang W, Chen X, Li Y, et al. Advances in pharmacological activities of terpenoids. Nat Prod Commun. 2020b;15:1–13. https://doi.org/10.1177/1934578X20903555.
70. Diniz LRL, Perez-Castillo Y, Elshabrawy HA, et al. Bioactive terpenes and their derivatives as potential SARS-CoV-2 proteases inhibitors from molecular modeling studies. Biomol Ther. 2021;11:1–19. https://doi.org/10.3390/biom11010074.
71. Asih SC, Irdiani R, Sahlan M, Nasikin M. Molecular docking study between 3 Thai medicinal plants compounds and Covid-19 therapeutic protein targets: SARS-CoV-2 Main protease, ACE-2, and PAK-1. Int J Appl Pharm. 2021;13:41–8. https://doi.org/10.22159/ijap.2021.v13s2.08
72. Mu C, Sheng Y, Wang Q, et al. Dataset of potential *Rhizoma polygonati* compound-druggable targets and partial pharmacokinetics for treatment of COVID-19. Data Brief. 2020;33:1–6. https://doi.org/10.1016/j.dib.2020.106475.
73. Thuy BTP, My TTA, Hai NTT, et al. Investigation into SARS-CoV-2 resistance of compounds in garlic essential oil. ACS Omega. 2020;5:8312–20. https://doi.org/10.1021/acsomega.0c00772.
74. Omar SH, Al-Wabel NA. Organosulfur compounds and possible mechanism of garlic in cancer. Saudi Pharm J. 2010;18:51–8. https://doi.org/10.1016/j.jsps.2009.12.007.
75. Hall A, Troupin A, Londono-Renteria B, Colpitts TM. Garlic organosulfur compounds reduce inflammation and oxidative stress during dengue virus infection. Viruses. 2017;9:1–10. https://doi.org/10.3390/v9070159.
76. Barros RO, Junior FLCC, Pereira WS, et al. Interaction of drug candidates with various SARS-CoV-2 receptors: an *in silico* study to combat COVID-19. J Proteome Res. 2020;19:4567–75. https://doi.org/10.1021/acs.jproteome.0c00327.
77. Yu J-W, Wang L, Bao L-D. Exploring the active compounds of traditional Mongolian medicine in intervention of novel coronavirus (COVID-19) based on molecular docking method. J Funct Foods. 2020;71:104016. https://doi.org/10.1016/j.jff.2020.104016.
78. Gutierrez-Villagomez JM, Campos-García T, Molina-Torres J, et al. Alkamides and piperamides as potential antivirals against the severe acute respiratory syndrome coronavirus 2 (SARS-CoV-2). J Phys Chem Lett. 2020;11:8008–16. https://doi.org/10.1021/acs.jpclett.0c01685.
79. Poochi SP, Easwaran M, Balasubramanian B, et al. Employing bioactive compounds derived from *Ipomoea obscura* (L.) to evaluate potential inhibitor for SARS-CoV-2 Main protease and ACE2 protein. Food Front. 2020;1:168–79. https://doi.org/10.1002/fft2.29.
80. Zhu Z-L, Qiu X-D, Wu S, et al. Blocking effect of Demethylzeylasteral on the interaction between human ACE2 protein and SARS-CoV-2 RBD protein discovered using SPR technology. Molecules. 2021;26:1–12. https://doi.org/10.3390/molecules26010057.
81. Allam L, Ghrifi F, Mohammed H, et al. Targeting the GRP78-Dependant SARS-CoV-2 cell entry by peptides and small molecules. Bioinform Biol Insights. 2020;14:1–11. https://doi.org/10.1177/1177932220965505.
82. Sudeep HV, Gouthamchandra K, Shyamprasad K. Molecular docking analysis of withaferin a from *Withania somnifera* with the glucose regulated protein 78 (GRP78) in comparison with the COVID-19 Main protease. Bioinformation. 2020;16:411–7. https://doi.org/10.6026/97320630016411.
83. Gyebi GA, Adegunloye AP, Ibrahim IM, et al. Prevention of SARS-CoV-2 cell entry: insight from *in silico* interaction of drug-like alkaloids with spike glycoprotein, human ACE2, and TMPRSS2. J Biomol Struct Dyn. 2020:1–25. https://doi.org/10.1080/07391102.2020.1835726
.
84. Pooja M, Reddy GJ, Hema K, et al. Unravelling high-affinity binding compounds towards transmembrane protease serine 2 enzyme in treating SARS-CoV-2 infection using molecular

modelling and docking studies. Eur J Pharmacol. 2021;890:1–12. https://doi.org/10.1016/j.ejphar.2020.173688.
85. Ramakrishnan J, Kandasamy S, Iruthayaraj A, et al. Strong binding of leupeptin with TMPRSS2 protease may be an alternative to Camostat and Nafamostat for SARS-CoV-2 repurposed drug: evaluation from molecular docking and molecular dynamics simulations. Appl Biochem Biotechnol. 2021;193:1909–23. https://doi.org/10.1007/s12010-020-03475-8.
86. Singh R, Gautam A, Chandel S, et al. Protease Inhibitory Effect of Natural Polyphenolic Compounds on SARS-CoV-2: An In Silico Study. Molecules. 2020;25:1–18. https://doi.org/10.3390/molecules25204604.
87. Coban M, Morrison J, Freeman W, et al. Attacking COVID-19 progression using multi-drug therapy for synergetic target engagement. Biomolecules. 2020;2:1–30. https://doi.org/10.26434/chemrxiv.12616151.
88. Rahman N, Basharat Z, Yousuf M, et al. Virtual screening of natural products against type II transmembrane serine protease (TMPRSS2), the priming agent of coronavirus 2 (SARS-CoV-2). Molecules. 2020;25:1–12. https://doi.org/10.3390/molecules25102271.
89. Vardhan S, Sahoo SK. Virtual screening by targeting proteolytic sites of Furin and TMPRSS2 to propose potential compounds obstructing the entry of SARS-CoV-2 virus into human host cells. J Tradit Complement Med. 2022;12(1):6–15. https://doi.org/10.1016/j.jtcme.2021.04.001.
90. Kupferschmidt K, Cohen J. Race to find COVID-19 treatments accelerates. Science. 2020;367:1412–3. https://doi.org/10.1126/science.367.6485.1412.
91. Qamar MTU, Alqahtani SM, Alamri MA, Chen L-L. Structural basis of SARS-CoV-2 3CLpro and anti-COVID-19 drug discovery from medicinal plants. J Pharm Anal. 2020;10:313–9. https://doi.org/10.1016/j.jpha.2020.03.009.

[illegible]

# Chapter 26
# Different Platforms, Immune Response Modulators and Challenges in SARS-CoV-2 Vaccination

**Amanda Izeli Portilho, Victor Araujo Correa, Emanuelle Baldo Gaspar, and Elizabeth De Gaspari**

## What Influences a Vaccine's Response?

The immune response differs according to the pathogen that triggers it and the host's inner characteristics. It is desired that the vaccine induces an immune response ideal for protection and when it comes to diseases transmitted from person to person, the diminution of the spread can improve the control of the disease [1–3].

Historically, the majority of vaccines induce a humoral immune response. The aluminum hydroxide, the main adjuvant used, also contributes to it [4]. Antibodies are very important for protection, acting in different mechanisms of protection, such as direct neutralization, opsonophagocytosis, and activation of the complement system. However, with the advances in the immunology field, it has become clear that the control of certain diseases can be improved by certain patterns of immune response, which can be modulated by vaccine formulation and administration [2]. For example, the yellow fever vaccine formulated with the 17D strain, currently in use in many countries, activates the innate immunity and elicits both neutralizing antibodies and CD4+/CD8+ lymphocytes [5]; the control of the Human papillomavirus (HPV) depends on T-cell mediated cytotoxicity, given the epithelial location of the infection [6]; the BCG (*Bacillus* Calmette–Guerin) vaccine, against tuberculosis (TB), elicits delayed tissue hypersensitivity (DTH), with CD4+ cells activating

A. I. Portilho · V. A. Correa · E. De Gaspari (✉)
Departamento de Imunologia, Instituto Adolfo Lutz, São Paulo, SP, Brazil

Programa de Pós-Graduação Interunidades em Biotecnologia, Instituto de Ciências Biomédicas, Universidade de São Paulo, São Paulo, SP, Brazil
e-mail: a.izeliportilho@usp.br; elizabeth.gaspari@ial.sp.gov.br

E. B. Gaspar
Embrapa Pecuária Sul, Bagé, RS, Brazil
e-mail: emanuelle.gaspar@embrapa.br


S. Adibi et al. (eds.), *Frontiers of COVID-19*,
https://doi.org/10.1007/978-3-031-08045-6_26

macrophages to kill the pathogen, whether if it is free or internalized by the host's cells [2].

Another issue is the systemic versus the mucosal immune response. It is known that many pathogens enter the body through the mucosa. Developing an immune response in such sites should contribute to control the disease since the initial contact. It can be successfully achieved by mucosal vaccination (e.g., intranasal or oral routes), which can induce both systemic and mucosal responses [7, 8]. However, only a few licensed vaccines are administered by mucosal routes, especially when compared with those administered by injections [9]. It can be explained by the challenges of the antigen to overcome mucosal barriers (pH, mucous, enzymes, microbiome, etc.), which explains the importance of suitable formulations to improve mucosal vaccines [10].

## SARS-CoV-2 Vaccines: Development Scenario, Platforms Used, and Their Particularities

The COVID-19 pandemic changed the vaccine development scenario. The pandemic's impact on health and economics ensured an incredible demand for efficient therapies against the disease [11]. Although several drugs were/are being tested, preventive measures to avoid transmission seems to be the key to control the disease, so the search for vaccines was stimulated across the world, resulting in more than 194 vaccines in preclinical trials and 121 in clinical trials around the world as of September 2021 [12, 13].

As never seen before, vaccines were available 1 year after their development had started. By the time this review was written (September 2021), there were 24 vaccines described in the WHO Evaluation Process datasheet, and 23 vaccines were approved and in use around the world, using several platforms, as further described in Table 26.1 [15–17]. This was made possible not only due to the scientific advances, which improved the understanding of the pathogen, allowing us to recognize vaccine targets and carry out tests in record time, and publishing the results obtained, but also to the partnerships between research institutes/universities and industry and changes in the regulation process [18].

Before COVID-19, it would be expected 15 years for new vaccines to be developed, with years to conclude each step, which would comprise preclinical and toxicology studies; phase 1, 2 and 3 trials; revision by regulatory agencies and, finally, production and distribution. In the case of COVID-19, we carried out these steps in months: preclinical researches were supported by known platforms and SARS-CoV/MERS-CoV studies; phases 1 and 2 of clinical trials were overlapped; the vaccine production started during phase 3, aiming to accelerate the process so that the final product would be available within 10–15 months [19]. Because immunization was needed to control the pandemic, the WHO suggested that vaccines demonstrating at least 50% of efficacy would be appropriate for use. The efficacy proved

**Table 26.1** SARS-CoV-2 approved vaccines and platforms used

| Platform | Vaccine | Developer/manufacturer | No. of countries approved |
|---|---|---|---|
| Recombinant-subunit | ZF2001/RBD-Dimer | Anhui Zhifei Longcon | 2 |
| | CIGB-66/Abdala | BioCubaFarma | 3 |
| | Soberana 02 | BioCubaFarma | 1 |
| | MVC-COV1901 | MedGen | 1 |
| | Covavax | Novavax | 5 |
| | COVIran Barekat | Shifa Pharmed Industrial | 1 |
| | EpiVacCorona | Vector Center of Virology | 2 |
| Whole-inactivated virus | Covaxin | Bharat Biotech | 9 |
| | KoviVac | Chumakov Center | 1 |
| | KCONVAC | Minhai Biotechnology | 1 |
| | QazCovid-in/QazVac | Research Institute for Biological Safety Problems | 2 |
| | BBIBP-CorV/Covilo | Sinopharm (Beijing) | 64 |
| | BBIBP-CorV | Sinopharm (Wuhan) | 2 |
| | CoronaVac | Sinovac | 40 |
| Recombinant-vector | Covishield | AstraZeneca | 177 |
| | Vaxzevria | AstraZeneca | 122 |
| | Ad5-nCoV/Convidecia | CanSino Biologicals | 9 |
| | Sputnik V | Gamaleya Institute | 71 |
| | Sputnik Light | Gamaleya Institute | 15 |
| | Ad26.COV 2-S | Janssen | 66 |
| mRNA | mRNA-1273 | Moderna | 72 |
| | Comirnaty | Pfizer/BioNTech | 100 |
| DNA | ZyCoV-D | Zydus Cadila | 1 |

(Table developed with data from [14] and [15])

by clinical trials, however, does not agree with the effectiveness, which is elucidated only on phase 4 trials, because it considers field characteristics that are not represented in randomized trials—herd immunity, differences provided by socioeconomic status or geographical location, and immunogenicity disparity according to age groups (especially the youngest and the elderly), among others [20, 21].

Age was especially challenging in SARS-CoV-2 vaccine trials: since the elderly are the ones more affected by the severity of the disease, it would be important to include this population in trials. However, the acceptance of the elderly to participate in clinical trials has been historically low and, in the pandemic scenario, we should consider the likelihood of higher-risk groups to adopt prophylactic actions that diminish their exposure, providing data that should be cautiously analyzed [20, 21]. Furthermore, phase 4 is also important to assess rare adverse effects, and it is important to keep them under control [22–24].

To efficiently respond to the pandemic, a large-scale production of vaccines would be needed. Adapting existing platforms would help to address this need [25]. Indeed, different platforms were tested to develop vaccines against COVID-19: among the licensed ones, there are whole, inactivated pathogen; protein subunit; viral vector (which used adenovirus) and mRNA vaccines [17, 18]. The vaccines in response to COVID-19 showed how classic platforms, using the inactivated microorganism or its subunits, are still effective. However, it also proved that new technologies, as vector-based and nucleic acid vaccines, can be successful. Efforts to establish different platforms and to refine the existing ones were necessary. Here, we briefly describe the platforms employed to develop SARS-CoV-2 vaccines.

## Vaccine Platforms

### *Whole-Pathogen Vaccine*

The traditional whole-pathogen vaccine is divided into two types, live-attenuated (live pathogen with reduced virulence) and inactivated (thermally or chemically inactivated pathogen). This strategy has been used by many vaccines [26, 27].

Live attenuated vaccines are usually very effective and a single dose is often enough to induce long-lasting immunity, once the vaccine induces a mild infection that seems like a real infection, leading to a strong immune response with immunological memory. The disadvantage of this vaccine is the risk for the organism to recover its virulence and cause disease. For that reason, not everyone can receive live attenuated vaccines, as people with a compromised, damaged, or weakened immune system. Besides, it needs a cold chain to stay potent [26, 27].

The inactivated vaccines were first applied to pathogens such as typhoid fever, plague, and cholera bacilli at the end of nineteenth century [28]. This kind of vaccine is made from killed virulent microorganisms; for this reason, it is safer than attenuated vaccines. It presents good immunogenicity, but lesser if compared with attenuated vaccines. It needs a large amount of killed pathogen for the immune system to recognize the antigens and often require multiple doses to induce an immune memory [18, 29]. To overcome this issue, adjuvants and virosomes are added to improve the protective immune response [30]. Currently, vaccines like BBIBP-CorV, CoronaVac and Covaxin use this method.

Covaxin is a vaccine of two-dose regimen, recommended to be taken 28 days apart. In a phase III study that enrolled 25,800 participants, the vaccine demonstrated 81% of efficacy [31]. An analysis indicates that the vaccine induced antibodies that can neutralize the UK variant and other heterologous strains [32, 33].

A phase 1/2 study demonstrated that the BBIBP-CorV is tolerable and immunogenic in healthy people, with a rapid humoral immune response against SARS-CoV-2 that can be detected 4 days after the first dose and reaches 100% of seroconversion in all participants on day 42. Immunization schedules with vaccination on days 0 and 21, and days 0 and 28, demonstrated to elicit great neutralizing antibody titers [34].

CoronaVac demonstrated to be safe and immunogenic. In healthy adults aged from 18 to 59 years, with an immunization regimen of two doses, on days 0 and 28, the seroconversion was seen in 97% of the group that received a 3 μg dose and 100% in the group that received the 6 μg dose [35]. One study demonstrated that efficacy of CoronaVac is not reduced in older adults, since it was immunogenic in adults of 60 years and older [36].

## *Adenovirus-Vectored Vaccine*

Adenovirus is an attractive vehicle to transfer foreign genes in genetic therapy, and it is also a promising vector for the vaccine-vectored platform because it is safe, easy to manipulate and able to stimulate a robust cellular and/or humoral immune response in clinical trials [37, 38].

A large number of adenoviruses from human and nonhuman primates, which have a low seroprevalence in humans, have been vectorized and tested as vaccine vehicle in animal models and humans. However, the prevalence of preexisting immunity to adenoviral vector is considered as a serious problem in its use; moreover, the vector can infect a diverse mammalian cells by the binding of adenoviral fiber protein to the host cell surface, and the adenoviral epitopes can induce an immunodominance over the interested gene epitope, hindering the induction of gene-specific immunity [39]. There are many licensed and on clinical trial vaccines using adenovirus as vectors, such as ChAdOx1 nCoV-19 (AZD1222), Sputnik V (Gam-COVID-Vac), Ad26.COV2.S, and Ad5nCov.

The ChAdOx1 nCoV-19 consists of the replicon-deficient chimpanzee adenovirus vector ChAOx1, containing the SARS-CoV-2 Spike protein gene. This vaccine was demonstrated to be safe and effective across three continents (Brazil, South America; UK, Europe; and South Africa, Africa), showing a vaccine efficacy of 70–74% after two doses, on days 0 and day 28. After one standard dose, it presented protection of 60–61% against symptomatic disease, with no safety concern [40].

Sputnik V is a heterologous recombinant adenovirus approach. It uses the human adenovirus (Ad) 26 and Ad 5 to express the Spike protein from SARS-Cov-2. The use of different adenoviruses in each dose (one in day 0 and other on day 21) intends to overcome any preexisting Ad immunity in population [41]. In a phase III analysis, the vaccine showed safety and an efficacy of 91–96% in a large cohort, also showing a neutralizing activity against SARS-CoV-2 variants [42, 43].

Ad26.COV2.S vaccine comprises a recombinant, replication-incompetent human Ad 26 encoding Spike protein, administered in a single dose, which demonstrated to be safe and induced an excellent humoral and cellular immune response with antibody neutralizing activity [44]. Efficacy against moderate to severe–critical COVID-19 was 67% at least 14 days after immunization and 66% after 28 days of administration, whereas efficacy against severe disease was 77% after 14 days of immunization and 85% after 28 days [45].

## *Protein Subunit Vaccine*

Protein subunit vaccine utilizes the recombinant protein technology, which is efficient; not expensive; safe, once it is non-replicating and lacks the infectious component; and widely available. It allows for the cost-effective production of recombinant proteins in diverse organisms, such as microbial, yeast, insect, and mammalian cells. Each organism has its benefits and handicaps; this way, the choice of what kind of cell to be used to express the protein is an important factor that has to be considered [46].

There are many vaccines being developed using this methodology, such as NVX-CoV2373/Covavax and EpiVacCorona [17]. NVX-CoV2373 is a recombinant SARS-CoV-2 nanoparticle vaccine, composed of the full-length SARS-CoV-2 Spike protein and Matrix-M1 adjuvant. The vaccine is administered by a two-dose schedule, at day 0 and day 21. It has been demonstrated to be safe and elicited cellular immunity, inducing an CD4+ response biased to a T helper 1 response [47]. In a phase III clinical trial, it was showed that the vaccine was 89.3% effective against the B.1.1.7 UK variant and 49.4% against the B.1.351 variant [48].

## *Nucleic Acid Vaccine*

The nucleic acid vaccine has become a famous platform because it combines the positive attributes of live attenuated and subunit vaccines; this way, it has the potential to be safe, once it does not involve the live organism and effective, by mimicking the live infection, expressing the antigen in situ after immunization, and the immune response will be directed toward the antigen of interest [49].

The nucleic acid vaccine is composed of DNA or RNA sequences encoding the antigen, delivered by a virus-like particle to enter the host cell, formulated with lipids or emulsion, or using electroporation [50]. Once plasmid DNA (pDNA) or messenger RNA (mRNA) is injected intramuscularly, the genetic sequence encoding the target antigen is processed through different pathways for each platform. For immunization with pDNA, the DNA has to overcome cytoplasmic and nuclear membranes to be transcribed into mRNA and move back to cytoplasm, where the translation is initiated. The secreted antigen will stimulate the cellular and humoral immune response. However, the integration of exogenous DNA into the host genome is a risk of using a DNA vaccine, which may cause severe mutagenesis and diseases [50, 51]. For the mRNA vaccine, the mRNA encoding the target antigen is delivered into the cells and will translate the interest protein in situ, then the host immune system will mount a robust immune response against the target antigen. Differently from the DNA vaccine, it does not integrate into the host genome, but the main issue would be the instability of mRNA. Both platforms presented poor immunogenicity in the past, but nowadays, mRNA technology leads to highly effective SARS-CoV-2 vaccines [51, 52].

Some licensed vaccines that use this platform are BNT162b2 and mRNA-1273. BNT16b2 is a nucleoside-modified mRNA formulated in a lipid nanoparticle, the mRNA encodes the spike protein from SARS-CoV-2 modified by 2 proline mutations to stabilize the protein in an antigenically preferred, prefusion conformation [53]. The vaccine schedule is 2 doses within 21 days apart. A study demonstrated that using this schedule the vaccine induces a strong antibody response in healthy adults aged 19–55 years in a nonrandomized, open-label phase I/II, with a significant increase in IgG after 21 days of first dose with a strong booster response after 7 days of second dose, inducing a neutralizing antibody activity. Moreover, BNT162b2 elicits a robust expansion of CD4+ and CD8+ cells to SARS-CoV-2 in vaccinated individuals [54]. In a phase II/III study, the vaccine shows efficacy of 95% in persons of 16 years or older [55]. The vaccine also demonstrated to neutralize mutant strains of SARS-CoV-2 [56].

The mRNA-1273 developed by Moderna consists of mRNA encoding the Spike protein stabilized in the prefusion conformation, formulated into a lipid nanoparticle. Two doses of vaccine intramuscularly with 28 days apart is recommended. It was noticed that after the last dose the vaccine induced a strong CD4+ response involving Th1 pattern, inducing neutralizing antibodies in individuals of 18 years and older [57, 58]. Besides that, in a phase III study the vaccine showed an efficacy of 95.5% [59].

## Immune Response Modulators

### *Immunization Routes*

It is known that the immunization route helps modulate the immune response. The intramuscular route is the route used for the current licensed SARS-CoV-2 vaccines, but there are other vaccines that use other routes ongoing clinical trials [13, 17]. Concerning mucosal pathogens, a local immune response would be interesting, since it helps to control the disease at the site of infection [8]. Parenteral routes can generate a robust systemic humoral response after the injection of low antigenic doses, but they are poor inducers of mucosal immunity [60].

Mucosal vaccination can elicit both local and systemic immune responses, mimicking the natural course of the disease. The presence of innate immunity and adaptive responders, as secretory IgA (sIgA) and cytotoxic T cells, protects the site of infection, in a way that the pathogen cannot disseminate throughout the body. The mucosal protection can also control the transmission of the disease, reducing carriage rates, which improves the vaccine's impact [7, 8]. Thus, the administration (via intranasal or oral route) is not invasive, so it might increase the uptake of vaccination, besides reducing the risks and costs of working with perforating material. This kind of administration is a good fit for the pandemic scenario, where there is an urge to vaccinate the maximum of individuals and achieve the control of the disease [61].

Despite all these benefits, only a few oral and intranasal vaccines are licensed, because their development faces several challenges. It needs higher antigenic doses to ensure a mucosal and systemic response, given that the regional immune system is more tolerogenic than the sterile sites, such as the muscle. The antigen has to overcome the mucosa barriers: pH differences, presence of enzymes and mucus, and competition with the microbiome [7]. Including adjuvants in mucosa-aimed formulations might be the key to overcome these limitations. The ideal adjuvant should be capable of protecting the antigen in the hostile mucosa environment while improving its immunogenicity and delivering it to the site where the immune response should happen [25].

## *Adjuvants and Delivery Systems*

Vaccines adjuvants are synthetic or natural materials that enhance the immune response. It allows the use of lower antigenic concentration and fewer vaccine doses. Adjuvants also increase the stability of the formulation, making it less susceptible to degradation during storage or administration. Adjuvants are a heterogeneous group of compounds, which can be classified as delivery systems or immunostimulatory molecules according to their mechanism of action [12].

Aluminum salts are the main adjuvants we know, which were started to be used during the 1930s. The mechanism of alum adjuvanticity is related to the activation of the NLRP3 inflammasome, the release of proinflammatory cytokines, and monocyte recruitment to the site of injection, which moves to lymph nodes, differentiating in dendritic cells (DCs) that prime CD4+ cells. The cytokine environment, with the presence of IL1β, leads the response to a Th2 pattern, which supports antibody production by lymphocytes B. The ideal immune response against SARS-CoV-2 is being studied and lacks elucidation, but authors agree that a synergetic response, which mobilizes different arms of the immune response (innate, humoral, and cellular), should be the way to effectively control the disease [12, 62]. If it is proven to be right, the ideal vaccine for COVID-19 can rely on the use of different adjuvants, since the alum mechanism might not be the better suit [18].

Immunostimulatory adjuvants improve immunogenicity by stimulating the immune system. Pathogen-associated molecular patterns (PAMPs) can stimulate the innate immunity and are promising adjuvants. Also, they might confer cross-reactivity with different microorganisms expressing the similar structures and are easy to obtain [63]. Lipopolysaccharide (LPS), from Gram-negative bacteria, and monophosphoryl lipid A (MPL), from *Salmonella minnesota*, are Toll-like receptor (TLR)-4 ligands; flagellin is a TLR-5 ligand and CpG oligonucleotides are TLR-9 ligands, providing activation of innate mechanisms, which stimulates cytokine release and activates antigen-presenting cells [63, 64]. Cholera toxin subunit B (CTb), from *Vibrio cholerae*, and heat-labile enterotoxin subunit B (HTb), from *Escherichia coli*, are recognized by the GM1 receptor, present on B cells, both of them improving sIgA production at the mucosa and systemic IgG [65]. Outer membrane vesicles (OMVs) of Gram-negative bacteria, like *Neisseria meningitidis*, present several PAMPs that activate the immune system. It was used as an adjuvant for a SARS-CoV-2 vaccine platform tested in mice and induced both humoral and cellular responses [66, 67].

The combination of aluminum salts along with PAMPs led to adjuvant systems, like AS04, which comprises aluminum salts with MPL, improving the recognition by TLR-4, enhancing both humoral and cellular response [68]. There are a lot of SARS-CoV-2 vaccines in clinical trial that use at least one immunostimulatory adjuvant, for example, the trimeric S-protein vaccine SCB-2019, that comprises a native-like trimeric subunit Spike protein adjuvanted by CpG plus alum, currently on phase II/III (NCT04672395); the FINLAY-FR2 anti-SARS-CoV-2 vaccine, which is composed by the RBD antigen chemically conjugated to tetanus toxoid, which is on phase III, among others [17].

The use of cytokines and chemokines as adjuvants not only activates the immune system but also orchestrates it toward the desired type of response. For example, IL-12 signaling enhances B cell growth; CCL28 and CCL27 help to achieve mucosal and epidermis immunity; CCL2, CCL3, and CCL4 act on the linkage between the innate and adaptative immunity, improving immune response maturation. They can be used alone or complexed with other adjuvants [64, 69].

MF29 and AS03 are human-approved adjuvants, composed of emulsions that use naturally occurring phospholipids, and proved to induce humoral and cell-mediated immunity in clinical trials, including in SARS-CoV and MERS-CoV vaccine candidates and in influenza vaccine candidates [70].

Delivery systems are especially of interest in mucosa vaccination, since it comprises the encapsulation or inclusion of the antigen in a particulate system that protects it from degradation, so that it can be presented to antigen-presenting cells (APCs). These adjuvants can be nanoparticles, liposomes, microspheres, polymers or even specific cell ligands, like M cell ligands [71].

Polymers are often used in nanoparticle vaccines, encapsulating the antigen and providing its slow liberation. By definition, nanoparticles are situated between 1 and 100 nm, which is a good fit for uptake by DCs [64]. Liposomes, composed of phospholipids bilayers surrounding an aqueous antigenic suspension, are another example of nanotechnology applied to vaccines. Besides the protection, delivery to specific site and slow liberation of the antigen, it is possible to manipulate the liposome's size, charge, shape and composition, so that it addresses the specific target [72]. Microcarriers, which reach the μm scale, may not be well sized for DCs uptake, but can be suitable for M cells, in mucosa vaccination [64]. The nucleic acid vaccines (DNA or mRNA) are supported by delivery systems, which allow the entrance into the host cells, thus protecting the nucleic acid, especially mRNA, which is less stable [73]. The lipid nanoparticles (e.g., ionic lipids, lipid-linked polyethylene glycol, phospholipids and cholesterols) converge with mRNA vaccines: studies verified activation of CD4+ and CD8+ cells by this combination [12]. Currently, there are two mRNA vaccines against COVID-19 in use, developed by Moderna and Pfizer-BioNTech. Both of them use delivery systems: the SN-102 nanoparticle (Moderna) and ALC-0315 (Pfizer-BioNTech), which protects the mRNA from degradation and allows it to enter the vaccine's cells. It is expected that studies about delivery systems will be continued, improving the stability of vaccines during transport and storage, making them more suitable for a pandemic scenario [19, 73, 74].

It should be stated that not all adjuvants are adequate for all immunization routes and that, despite their qualities, the use of adjuvants may increase the cost of vaccines and limit its manufacturing. Such a point deserves attention, especially during a pandemic, where economy is struggling and high vaccine coverage could be improved by manufacturing vaccines in each country. In that way, finding suitable adjuvants for low-income countries (e.g., adjuvants based on microorganisms that are a product of other vaccines, like outer membrane vesicles from gram-negative pathogens or LPS from acellular *Pertussis* vaccine) can improve vaccine development and manufacturing [63, 64].

The urge to develop SARS-CoV-2 vaccines makes it more logical to use approved adjuvants [12]. However, we should keep looking for adjuvant options that suit different needs and manufacturing realities.

## *The Use of Mucosa Vaccines for SARS-CoV-2*

The mucosa airway is related to SARS-CoV-2 infection and COVID-19 progress. The pathogen entrance occurs through the nasopharynx and moves to the lungs. The mucosa immune system associated with the nasopharynx is named nasopharynx-associated lymphoid tissue (NALT) [62]. The cells in the nasal airway express both the angiotensin-converting enzyme (ACE-2) and the cellular serine protease TMPRSS2, which SARS-CoV-2 uses to bind and infect cells. However, recent studies highlight the gut symptoms in COVID-19, probably due the expression of ACE-2 and TMPRSS2 in this niche, and the presence of replicating virus in the oral cavity, which could indicate a deeper compromising of mucosa tissues in COVID-19, thus restating the importance of studying mucosa immunity against it [75–77].

It is proposed that the initial NALT response to SARS-CoV-2 would help to control the infection. After its entrance into the nose, natural antibodies and lectins, components of the innate immune response, could recognize glycoside structures of the virus. Infected cells and DCs would release type I IFNs, leading to antiviral response, and innate cells, activated by PAMPs and damage-associated molecular patterns (DAMPs), would support the adaptive immunity, presenting antigens, so that specific T and B lymphocytes could differentiate. Finally, the pathogen would be eliminated in the upper respiratory system. On the other hand, an ineffective mucosa response would allow the virus to reach the lower respiratory system; also, the high viral load would lead to the release of pro-inflammatory cytokines, the recruitment of neutrophils to the lung, and the tissue injury by the uncoordinated immune response [62]. Studies regarding viral infections suggest that the presence of T lymphocytes on the airway is more effective than activating central T cells to control the pathogen and provide immunologic memory [12]. Regarding SARS-CoV-2, IgA seems to display an important role in neutralizing the virus [78]. If the compromising of other mucosa tissues is proved to be an issue, mucosal delivery of vaccines could also stimulate other niches: because of expression of certain cellular receptors, the administration of antigenic preparations in one mucosa site may elicit the immune response in a different one—for example, intranasal administration may induce immune response in the respiratory, gastrointestinal and genital tracts, expanding the protection throughout the body [25].

The manufacturing and administration of vaccines can be just as challenging as its development, especially for low- and middle-income countries. When it comes to administration by injection, it requires trained people and disposable material. Another issue is the cold chain to transport and the immunogen [18]. As described above, mucosa vaccines and novel adjuvants could help overcome these issues, supporting more effective immunization.

Some studies report interesting results from intranasal immunization against SARS-CoV-2 in animal models. Prime-booster immunization with intramuscular/intranasal doses of RBD protein adjuvanted by outer membrane vesicles of *Neisseria meningitidis* elicited high-avidity, neutralizing antibodies in mice [66]. When intramuscular and intranasal delivery of an Adenovirus vectored vaccine expressing S protein were compared, the latter conferred protection against upper and lower respiratory system infection, inducing IgA, neutralizing antibodies, and CD8+ cells in the lung of mice. In hamsters, the same vaccine induced higher antibodies levels and less inflammation, minimizing lung pathology [79, 80]. Putting these descriptions together, it seems that mucosa vaccines would be more adequate to prevent COVID-19 [25]. At the time of writing (September 2021), there were 3 oral, 7 intranasal, 2 intramuscular/intranasal, and 1 subcutaneous/oral vaccines against SARS-CoV-2 in clinical trials [13].

In the past years, mucosa immunization has been discussed and studied. It presents several benefits, but those are accompanied by some challenges. The parenteral immunization, however, allowed to start vaccination and has been helping control the COVID-19 pandemic, showing how effective vaccines, regardless of its administration site or platform used, are important.

## Potentially Modified Response to Vaccination

The response to vaccination can be impaired in some situations. Here, we briefly describe how specific populations would respond to SARS-CoV-2 vaccines and the concern about the new variants causing COVID-19.

## Disease-Modifying Therapies and Immunocompromised Patients

Patients using immunomodulatory or immunosuppressive medication might have their response to vaccination affected [81]. SARS-CoV-2 vaccines in these populations are expected to be safe and present some variability on efficacy, but are not completely elucidated, so the decision to vaccinate these patients has to balance the need for protection and the risk of adverse events. Solutions like the temporary withdrawal of the immunotherapy to ensure a better response to the vaccine can be studied, but knowing the risks related to it—an increase of disease's severity and loss of response to the drugs [82].

It is early to recognize the SARS-CoV-2 vaccine's effects on immunocompromised patients and previous data about other vaccines is often variable: some studies show impairment of the humoral response and reduced neutralizing antibodies, while others present adequate response if booster doses were administrated. When it comes to cellular response, there are even fewer studies focused on it [81–83]. However, a phase 4 trial described overall decreased, but acceptable IgG and neutralizing antibody seroconversion after two doses of inactivated-SARS-CoV-2 vaccine in autoimmune rheumatic disease patients; also, there was no moderate or severe adverse effects reported [84]. Interestingly, a study described that B cells depleted patients developed T cell response to the BNT162b2 mRNA vaccine, which was effective to prevent COVID-19 [85].

Such data support the vaccination of immunocompromised patients. However, the platform used has an important role in this question. Live-attenuated and inactivated vaccines are related to greater risks, and studies often point to a variable immune response to this type of vaccines, while nonviral vaccines are safer and data do not indicate overall decreased immune response [82, 86]. The importance of using diverse platforms in vaccine development and employing adequate adjuvants to increase the immunogenicity of subunit vaccines, which are usually safer, is restated, so patients on immunotherapy can continue their treatments and be protected from COVID-19 [87].

## Childhood

When compared to adults and the elderly, childen rarely develop severe COVID-19 and progress to death [88]. This aspect, along with the ethical issues to address clinical trials for kids, led to the initial focus of approving vaccines for adult use [20].

An important concern is that SARS-CoV-2 infection could lead to multisystem inflammatory syndrome in children (MIS-C), which presents elevated severity [89]. Even though this is rarer, seeing children sick by preventable diseases calls for attention [90]. The impact of social isolation and interruption of education should also be a driving force to immunizing kids [91].

Other important issues are the part that children play in the transmission of the virus and the achievement of herd immunity. Some studies pointed that children are less likely to transmit SARS-CoV-2; however, it might be underestimated by the asymptomatic infections, minor frequency of pediatric testing and rapid closure of schools [91, 92]. With the rise of more transmissible variants, the transmission by the younger is likely to become an issue [90]. To achieve herd immunity, the majority of the population, including children, should be vaccinated [93].

## Pregnancy

The COVID-19 implications on pregnancy have been revised. Increased risks of admission to intensive-care units, iatrogenic preterm birth and caesarean delivery, besides strong suggestions of vertical transmission, were described [94, 95]. The influence of COVID-19, especially leading to poor delivery that compromises both mother and newborn, sustains the claim to vaccinate pregnant women, along with the benefit of protecting both mother and fetus [96, 97].

The immune response mechanisms change during pregnancy, which is needed for the fetus development. It is known that antigen-presenting cells and B cells undergo variations, which is likely to impair humoral response as well. However, there is a lack of studies in the literature that directly compare groups of pregnant and nonpregnant women [98]. Despite these changes on the immune system, there is no evidence suggesting that pregnancy would lead to a different response to mRNA vaccines concerning their safety [99]. However, pregnant women had been excluded from clinical trials, making it complicated to indicate the current vaccines for this population [93]. So far, obstetricians have to weigh the characteristics of each woman, according to her underlying conditions and exposure risk, thus following data from vaccinated pregnant women [99].

Another important issue related to vaccination in pregnant women is passive immunity, which can protect the newborn [98]. The data obtained from natural infection suggests a reduced passive-immunization through the placenta, which could lead to the newborn being at risk of infection [100]. However, antibody transference following the mother's immunization should be studied to understand it in the vaccine context [101].

## *SARS-CoV-2 Variants*

New strains of SARS-CoV-2 have emerged. The so-called variants of concern (VOC) present mutations that allow them to spread more easily and/or to be more virulent, thus aggravating the pandemic. The B.1.1.7; the B.1.351; the P.1; and the B.1.617.2 strains, which respectively emerged in the UK, South Africa, Brazil, and India, are examples of it [102, 103]. Such variants present mutations in the Spike protein, especially on the RBD, which rendered attention to the vaccine efficacy, given that most vaccines are using the spike protein as antigen [104].

The current SARS-CoV-2 vaccines present an overall decreased efficiency against the new variants. It should be stated that a lot of studies were based on neutralization assays, which rely on the humoral response [105].

The cellular response should also be assessed, along with in vivo studies, following the infection by SARS-CoV-2 variants in vaccinated subjects [106]. In a study conducted in South Africa, which accompanied 1010 vaccine recipients of ChAdOx1 nCoV-19, the neutralization activity presented an overall decrease, peptide studies pointed that one mutation of B.1.351 was located in a T cell response region, and, of the 42 volunteers who had mild or moderate COVID-19 during the study, 39 were infected with the B.1.351 strain, showing a decreased efficacy [107]. On the other hand, a study based on vaccine status and COVID-19 reports in England tested the ChAdOx1 nCoV-19 and BNT162b2 vaccines against the B.1.617.2 strain and showed a minor difference on effectiveness when two doses were administrated, reinforcing the importance of booster doses [102].

Cases of prolonged infections and higher-risk populations should be watched closely, because they contribute to the emergence of new variants [105]. The emergence of new variants can affect the achievement of herd immunity, thus compromising the control of the pandemic. Improving the current vaccination campaigns, keeping the genetic surveillance of SARS-CoV-2 and adapting vaccine platforms to provide vaccines against new variants, will be needed to respond to the evolving SARS-CoV-2 [103, 106].

## *Booster Doses and Heterologous Prime-Booster Schemes*

The prime-boost strategy can be performed using the same vaccine formulation and different administration routes, or the same route and different formulations [108, 109]. Currently, some countries have started administering booster doses of SARS-CoV-2 vaccines, which might fall into the prime-booster strategy with heterologous vaccine formulations [110]. Even though there is a lack of reports about boosting one of the current SARS-CoV-2 vaccines with another, the strategy of using different formulations was successful with other pathogens, like the human immunodeficiency virus (HIV), hepatitis C virus (HCV) and rabies virus [109, 111, 112].

The reason why heterologous prime-boost regimen provides better results is not completely elucidated, however, it was suggested that it confers a synergistically stronger response, since different formulations can trigger different immune mechanisms, therefore, this strategy can potentially confer a broad response, activating both humoral and cellular immunity [108, 109].

Recently, we reported results from prime-booster immunization with intramuscular/intranasal doses of RBD protein adjuvanted by OMVs of *Neisseria meningitidis*, which elicited high-avidity, neutralizing antibodies in mice. Using heterologous immunization routes might also confer benefits, especially to activate a mucosa immune response [66].

As we know, many countries still face difficulties as the lack of vaccines. Hence, it is important to use preestablished protocols, discussed in the literature, to guide intervention plans and improve SARS-CoV-2 vaccine coverage.

## Conclusion

Since the beginning of the COVID-19 pandemic, the world has searched for adequate therapies. Despite the advances in the treatment field, preventive measures had proven to be the key to control the disease, as seen before. However, the development of vaccines was only possible due to exhaustive work in different areas: basic biology to understand the host–pathogen interaction, biotechnology, immunology, among others. The success of vaccination will be supported by public communication and the control of SARS-CoV-2 will probably demand a surveillance system. Now, the different niches of society should work together not only to address effective SARS-CoV-2 vaccines but also to be prepared against other emerging pathogens and to improve in-use vaccines. Another important point is to balance the concern about booster doses and refined vaccines in high-income settings with the need to immunize millions of people in the developing world.

## References


1. Coughtrie AL, Jefferies JM, Cleary DW, Doncaster CP, Faust SN, Kraaijeveld AR, et al. Microbial epidemiology and carriage studies for the evaluation of vaccines. J Med Microbiol. 2019;68(10):1408–18. https://doi.org/10.1099/jmm.0.001046.
2. Sell S. How vaccines work: immune effector mechanisms and designer vaccines. Expert Rev Vaccines. 2019;18(10):993–1015. https://doi.org/10.1080/14760584.2019.1674144.
3. Stern PL. Key steps in vaccine development. Ann Allergy Asthma Immunol. 2020;125(1):17–27. https://doi.org/10.1016/j.anai.2020.01.025.
4. Shah RR, Hassett KJ, Brito LA. Overview of vaccine adjuvants: introduction, history, and current status. Methods Mol Biol. 2017;1494:1–13. https://doi.org/10.1007/978-1-4939-6445-1_1.
5. Beck AS, Barrett ADT. Current status and future prospects of yellow fever vaccines. Expert Rev Vaccines. 2015;14(11):1479–92. https://doi.org/10.1586/14760584.2015.1083430.
6. Mekonnen ZA, Grubor-Bauk B, Masavuli MG, Shrestha AC, Ranasinghe C, Bull RA, et al. Toward DNA-based T-cell mediated vaccines to target HIV-1 and hepatitis C virus: approaches to elicit localized immunity for protection. Front Cell Infect Microbiol. 2019;9:91. https://doi.org/10.3389/fcimb.2019.00091.
7. Li M, Wang Y, Sun Y, Cui H, Zhu SJ, Qiu HJ. Mucosal vaccines: strategies and challenges. Immunol Lett. 2020;217:116–25. https://doi.org/10.1016/j.imlet.2019.10.013.
8. Zheng Z, Diaz-Arévalo D, Guan H, Zeng M. Noninvasive vaccination against infectious diseases. Hum Vaccin Immunother. 2018;14(7):1717–33. https://doi.org/10.1080/21645515.2018.1461296.
9. Savelkoul HFJ, Ferro VA, Strioga MM, Schijns VEJC. Choice and design of adjuvants for parenteral and mucosal vaccines. Vaccine. 2015;3(1):148–71. https://doi.org/10.3390/vaccines3010148.
10. Wang YB, Wang LP, Li P. Perspectives on novel vaccine development. Pol J Vet Sci. 2018;21(3):643–9. https://doi.org/10.24425/124302.
11. Ali I, Alharbi OML. COVID-19: disease, management, treatment and social impact. Sci Total Environ. 2020;728:138861. https://doi.org/10.1016/j.scitotenv.2020.138861.
12. Chung JY, Thone MN, Kwon YJ. COVID-19 vaccines: the status and perspectives in delivery points of view. Adv Drug Deliv Rev. 2021;170:1–25. https://doi.org/10.1016/j.addr.2020.12.011.
13. World Health Organization. COVID-19 vaccine tracker and landscape. 2021a. Updated in September 24, 2021. https://www.who.int/publications/m/item/draft-landscape-of-covid-19-candidate-vaccines. Accessed 26 Sept 2021.
14. World Health Organization. COVID-19 vaccine coverage. 2021d. Updated July 6, 2021. https://www.who.int/docs/default-source/coronaviruse/act-accelerator/1-covid-19-vaccine-coverage.pdf?sfvrsn=b4b17450_5. Accessed 26 Sept 2021.
15. COVID-19 Vaccine Tracker. Approved vaccines. 2021. https://covid19.trackvaccines.org/vaccines/approved/. Accessed 26 Sept 2021.
16. World Health Organization. WHO Coronavirus (COVID-19) Dashboard. 2021b. https://covid19.who.int/. Accessed 26 Sept 2021.
17. World Health Organization. Status of COVID-19 Vaccines within WHO EUL/PQ evaluation process. 2021c. Updated in August 19, 2021. https://extranet.who.int/pqweb/sites/default/files/documents/Status_COVID_VAX_19August2021.pdf. Accessed 26 Sept 2021.
18. Wang J, Peng Y, Xu H, Cui Z, Williams RO. The COVID-19 vaccine race: challenges and opportunities in vaccine formulation. AAPS PharmSciTech. 2020a;21(6):225. https://doi.org/10.1208/s12249-020-01744-7.
19. Krammer F. SARS-CoV-2 vaccines in development. Nature. 2020;586(7830):516–27. https://doi.org/10.1038/s41586-020-2798-3.
20. Hodgson SH, Mansatta K, Mallett G, Harris V, Emary KRW, Pollard AJ. What defines an efficacious COVID-19 vaccine? A review of the challenges assessing the clinical efficacy of vac-

cines against SARS-CoV-2. Lancet Infect Dis. 2021;21(2):e26–35. https://doi.org/10.1016/S1473-3099(20)30773-8.
21. Trzewikoswki de Lima G, De Gaspari E. Study of the immune response in the elderly: is it necessary to develop a vaccine against *Neisseria meningitidis* for the aged? J Aging Res. 2019;2019:9287121. https://doi.org/10.1155/2019/9287121.
22. Forni G, Mantovani A, Forni G, Mantovani A, Moretta L, Rappuoli R, et al. COVID-19 vaccines: where we stand and challenges ahead. Cell Death Differ. 2021;28(2):626–39. https://doi.org/10.1038/s41418-020-00720-9.
23. Petousis-Harris H. Assessing the safety of COVID-19 vaccines: a primer. Drug Saf. 2020;43(12):1205–10. https://doi.org/10.1007/s40264-020-01002-6.
24. Verger P, Dubé E. Restoring confidence in vaccines in the COVID-19 era. Expert Rev Vaccines. 2020;19(11):991–3. https://doi.org/10.1080/14760584.2020.1825945.
25. Mudgal R, Nehul S, Tomar S. Prospects for mucosal vaccine: shutting the door on SARS-CoV-2. Hum Vaccine Immunother. 2020;16(12):2921–31. https://doi.org/10.1080/21645515.2020.1805992.
26. Mark TW, Saunders ME. Vaccines and clinical immunization. In The immune response: basic and clinic principles; 2006. p. 695–749. https://doi.org/10.1016/B978-012088451-3.50025-9.
27. Yadav DK, Yadav N, Khurana SMP. Vaccines: present status and applications. In Animal biotechnology: models in discovery and translation. New York: Academic Press; 2014. p. 491–508. https://doi.org/10.1016/B978-0-12-416002-6.00026-2.
28. Plotkin S. History of vaccination. PNAS. 2014;111(34):12283–7. https://doi.org/10.1073/pnas.1400472111.
29. Green MD, Al-Humadi NH. Preclinical toxicology of vaccines. In A comprehensive guide to toxicology in nonclinical drug development. 2nd ed; 2017. p. 709–35. https://doi.org/10.1016/B978-0-12-803620-4.00027-X.
30. Zepp F. Principles of vaccine design—lessons from nature. Vaccine. 2010;28(Suppl 3):C14–24. https://doi.org/10.1016/j.vaccine.2010.07.020.
31. Thiagarajan K. What do we know about India's Covaxin vaccine? BMJ. 2021;373:n997. https://doi.org/10.1136/bmj.n997.
32. Sapkal GN, Yadav PD, Ella R, Deshpande GR, Sahay RR, Gupta N, et al. Neutralization of UK-variant VUI-202012/01 with COVAXIN vaccinated human serum. bioRxiv. 2021a;2021:426986. https://doi.org/10.1101/2021.01.26.426986.
33. Sapkal GN, Yadav PD, Ella R, Deshpande GR, Sahay RR, Gupta N, et al. Inactivated COVID-19 vaccine BBV152/COVAXIN effectively neutralizes recently emerged B 1.1.7 variant of SARS-CoV-2. J Travel Med. 2021b;28:taab051. https://doi.org/10.1093/jtm/taab051.
34. Xia S, Zhang Y, Wang Y, Wang H, Yang Y, Gao GF, et al. Safety and immunogenicity of an inactivated SARS-CoV-2 vaccine, BBIBP-CorV: a randomised, double-blind, placebo-controlled, phase 1/2 trial. Lancet. 2021;21(1):39–51. https://doi.org/10.1016/S1473-3099(20)30831-8.
35. Zhang Y, Zeng G, Pan H, Li C, Hu Y, Chu K, et al. Safety, tolerability, and immunogenicity of an inactivated SARS-CoV-2 vaccine in healthy adults aged 18–59 years: a randomised, double-blind, placebo-controlled, phase 1/2 clinical trial. Lancet Infect Dis. 2021;21(2):181–92. https://doi.org/10.1016/S1473-3099(20)30843-4.
36. Wu Z, Hu Y, Xu M, Chen Z, Yang W, Jiang Z, et al. Safety, tolerability, and immunogenicity of an inactivated SARS-CoV-2 vaccine (CoronaVac) in healthy adults aged 60 years and older: a randomised, double-blind, placebo-controlled, phase 1/2 clinical trial. Lancet Infect Dis. 2021;21(6):803–12. https://doi.org/10.1016/S1473-3099(20)30987-7.
37. Coughlan L. Factors which contribute to the immunogenicity of non-replicating adenoviral vectored vaccines. Front Immunol. 2019;11:909. https://doi.org/10.3389/fimmu.2020.00909.
38. Tatsis N, Ertl HCJ. Adenoviruses as vaccine vectors. Mol Ther. 2004;10(4):626–9. https://doi.org/10.1016/j.ymthe.2004.07.013.

39. Singh S, Kumar R, Agrawal B. Adenoviral vector-based vaccines and gene therapies: current status and future prospects. London: IntechOpen; 2018. https://doi.org/10.5772/intechopen.79697.
40. Voysey M, Clemens SAC, Madhi SA, Weckx L, Folegatti PM, Aley PK, et al. Safety and efficacy of the ChAdOx1 nCoV-19 vaccine (AZD1222) against SARS-CoV-2: an interim analysis of four randomised controlled trials in Brazil, South Africa, and the UK. Lancet. 2021;397(10269):99–111. https://doi.org/10.1016/S0140-6736(20)32661-1.
41. Jones I, Roy P. Sputnik V COVID-19 vaccine candidate appears safe and effective. Lancet. 2021;397(10275):642–3. https://doi.org/10.1016/S0140-6736(21)00191-4.
42. Ikegame S, Siddiquey M, Hung CT, Haas G, Brambilla L, Oguntuyo K, et al. Neutralizing activity of Sputnik V vaccine sera against SARS-CoV-2 variants. Nat Commun. 2021;12(1):400230. https://doi.org/10.21203/rs.3.rs-400230/v1.
43. Logunov DY, Dolzhikova IV, Shcheblyakov DV, Tukhvatulin AI, Zubkova OV, Dzharullaeva AS, et al. Safety and efficacy of an rAd26 and rAd5 vector-based heterologous prime-boost COVID-19 vaccine: an interim analysis of a randomised controlled phase 3 trial in Russia. Lancet. 2021;397(10275):671–81. https://doi.org/10.1016/S0140-6736(21)00234-8.
44. Stephenson KE, Le Gars M, Sadoff J, de Groot AM, Heerwegh D, Truyers C, et al. Immunogenicity of the Ad26.COV2.S vaccine for COVID-19. JAMA. 2021;325(15):1535–44. https://doi.org/10.1001/jama.2021.3645.
45. Sadoff J, Gray G, Vandebosch A, Cárdenas V, Shukarev G, Grinsztejn B, et al. Safety and efficacy of single-dose Ad26.COV2.S vaccine against Covid-19. N Engl J Med. 2021;384:2187–201. https://doi.org/10.1056/NEJMoa2101544.
46. Pollet J, Chen WH, Strych U. Recombinant protein vaccines, a proven approach against coronavirus pandemics. Adv Drug Deliv Rev. 2021;170:71–82. https://doi.org/10.1016/j.addr.2021.01.001.
47. Keech C, Albert G, Cho I, Robertson A, Reed P, Neal S, et al. Phase 1–2 trial of a SARS-CoV-2 recombinant spike protein nanoparticle vaccine. N Engl J Med. 2020;383:2320–32. https://doi.org/10.1056/NEJMoa2026920.
48. Yang ZP, Yang M, Lai CL. COVID-19 vaccines: a review of the safety and efficacy of current clinical trials. Pharmaceuticals. 2021;14(5):406. https://doi.org/10.3390/ph14050406.
49. Deering RP, Kommareddy S, Ulmer JB, Brito LA, Geall AJ. Nucleic acid vaccines: prospects for non-viral delivery of mRNA vaccines. Expert Opin Drug Deliv. 2014;11(6):885–99. https://doi.org/10.1517/17425247.2014.901308.
50. Kumar A, Meldgaard TS, Bertholet S. Novel platforms for the development of a universal influenza vaccine. Front Immunol. 2018;9:600. https://doi.org/10.3389/fimmu.2018.00600.
51. Zhang C, Maruggi G, Shan H, Li J. Advances in mRNA vaccines for infectious diseases. Front Immunol. 2019;10:594. https://doi.org/10.3389/fimmu.2019.00594.
52. Bettini E, Locci M. SARS-CoV-2 mRNA vaccines: immunological mechanism and beyond. Vaccines (Basel). 2021;9(2):147. https://doi.org/10.3390/vaccines9020147.
53. Lamb YN. BNT162b2 mRNA COVID-19 vaccine: first approval. Drugs. 2021;81(4):495–501. https://doi.org/10.1007/s40265-021-01480-7.
54. Sahin U, Muik A, Vogler I, Derhovanessian E, Kranz LM, Vormehr M, et al. BNT162b2 induces SARS-CoV-2-neutralising antibodies and T cells in humans. medRxiv. 2020;2020:20245175. https://doi.org/10.1101/2020.12.09.20245175.
55. Polack FP, Thomas SJ, Kitchin N, Absalon J, Gurtman A, Lockhart S, et al. Safety and efficacy of the BNT162b2 mRNA Covid-19 vaccine. N Engl J Med. 2020;383(27):2603–15. https://doi.org/10.1056/NEJMoa2034577.
56. Xie X, Zou J, Fontes-Garfias CR, Xia H, Swanson KA, Cutler M, et al. Neutralization of N501Y mutant SARS-CoV-2 by BNT162b2 vaccine-elicited sera. bioRxiv. 2021;2021:425740. https://doi.org/10.1101/2021.01.07.425740.
57. Anderson EJ, Rouphael NG, Widge AT, Jackson LA, Roberts PC, Makhene M, et al. Safety and immunogenicity of SARS-CoV-2 mRNA-1273 vaccine in older adults. N Engl J Med. 2020;383(25):2427–38. https://doi.org/10.1056/NEJMoa2028436.

58. Baden LR, El Sahly HM, Essink B, Kotloff K, Frey S, Novak R, et al. Efficacy and safety of the mRNA-1273 SARS-CoV-2 vaccine. N Engl J Med. 2020;384(5):403–16. https://doi.org/10.1056/NEJMoa2035389.
59. Moderna. Moderna's COVID-19 vaccine candidate meets its primary efficacy endpoint in the first InterimAnalysis of the phase 3 COVE Study. 2020. https://investors.modernatx.com/node/10316/pdf. Accessed 6 May 2021.
60. Zimmermann P, Curtis N. Factors that influence the immune response to vaccination. Clin Microbiol Rev. 2019;32(2):e00084–18. https://doi.org/10.1128/CMR.00084-18.
61. Rauch S, Jasny E, Schmidt KE, Petsch B. New vaccine technologies to combat outbreak situations. Front Immunol. 2018;9:1963. https://doi.org/10.3389/fimmu.2018.01963.
62. Gallo O, Locatello LG, Mazzoni A, Novelli L, Annunziato F. The central role of the nasal microenvironment in the transmission, modulation, and clinical progression of SARS-CoV-2 infection. Mucosal Immunol. 2021;14(2):305–16. https://doi.org/10.1038/s41385-020-00359-2.
63. Miyaji EN, Carvalho E, Oliveira MLS, Raw I, Ho PL. Trends in adjuvant development for vaccines: DAMPs and PAMPs as potential new adjuvants. Braz J Med Biol Res. 2011;44(6):500–13. https://doi.org/10.1590/S0100-879X2011007500064.
64. Hellfritzsch M, Scherlie R. Mucosal vaccination via the respiratory tract. Pharmaceutics. 2019;11(8):1–24. https://doi.org/10.3390/pharmaceutics11080375.
65. Lycke N, Lebrero-Fernández C. ADP-ribosylating enterotoxins as vaccine adjuvants. Curr Opin Pharmacol. 2018;41:42–51. https://doi.org/10.1016/j.coph.2018.03.015.
66. Gaspar EB, De Gaspari E. Avidity assay to test functionality of anti-SARS-Cov-2 antibodies. Vaccine. 2021;39(10):1473–5. https://doi.org/10.1016/j.vaccine.2021.02.003.
67. Gaspar EB, Prudencio CR, De Gaspari E. Experimental studies using OMV in a new platform of SARS-CoV-2 vaccines. Hum Vaccin Immunother. 2021;17(9):2965–8. https://doi.org/10.1080/21645515.2021.1920272.
68. Del Giudice G, Rappuoli R, Didierlaurent AM. Correlates of adjuvanticity: a review on adjuvants in licensed vaccines. Semin Immunol. 2018;39:14–21. https://doi.org/10.1016/j.smim.2018.05.001.
69. Mohan T, Zhu W, Wang Y, Wang B-Z. Applications of chemokines as adjuvant for vaccine immunotherapy. Immunobiology. 2018;223(6–7):477–85. https://doi.org/10.1016/j.imbio.2017.12.001.
70. Liang Z, Zhu H, Wang X, Jing B, Li Z, Xia X, et al. Adjuvants for coronavirus vaccines. Front Immunol. 2020;11:2896. https://doi.org/10.3389/fimmu.2020.589833.
71. Kaurav M, Madan J, Sudheesh MS, Pandey RS. Combined adjuvant-delivery system for new generation vaccine antigens: alliance has its own advantage. Artif Cells Nanomed Biotechnol. 2018;46(sup3):S818–31. https://doi.org/10.1080/21691401.2018.1513941.
72. Karch CP, Burkhard P. Vaccine technologies: from whole organisms to rationally designed protein assemblies. Biochem Pharmacol. 2016;120:1–14. https://doi.org/10.1016/j.bcp.2016.05.001.
73. Wang F, Kream RM, Stefano GB. An evidence based perspective on mRNA-SARS-Cov-2 vaccine development. Med Sci Monit. 2020b;26:1–8. https://doi.org/10.12659/MSM.924700.
74. Buschmann MD, Carrasco MJ, Alishetty S, Paige M, Alameh MG, Weissman D. Nanomaterial delivery systems for mRNA vaccines. Vaccines (Basel). 2021;9(1):65. https://doi.org/10.3390/vaccines9010065.
75. D'Amico F, Baumgart DC, Danese S, Peyrin-Biroulet L. Diarrhea during COVID-19 infection: pathogenesis, epidemiology, prevention, and management. Clin Gastroenterol Hepatol. 2020;18(8):1663–72. https://doi.org/10.1016/j.cgh.2020.04.001.
76. Huang N, Pérez P, Kato T, Mikami Y, Okuda K, Gilmore RC, et al. SARS-CoV-2 infection of the oral cavity and saliva. Nat Med. 2021;27(5):892–903. https://doi.org/10.1038/s41591-021-01296-8.

77. Marian AJ. Current state of vaccine development and targeted therapies for COVID-19: impact of basic science discoveries. Cardiovasc Pathol. 2021;50:107278. https://doi.org/10.1016/j.carpath.2020.107278.
78. Sterlin D, Mathian A, Miyara M, Mohr A, Anna F, Claër L, et al. IgA dominates the early neutralizing antibody response to SARS-CoV-2. Sci Transl Med. 2021;13(577):eabd2223. https://doi.org/10.1126/scitranslmed.abd2223.
79. Bricker TL, Darling TL, Hassan A. A single intranasal or intramuscular immunization with chimpanzee adenovirus vectored SARS-CoV-2 vaccine protects against pneumonia in hamsters. bioRxiv. 2020;2020:408823. https://doi.org/10.1101/2020.12.02.408823.
80. Hassan AO, Kafai NM, Dmitriev IP, Fox JM, Smith BK, Harvey IB, et al. A single-dose intranasal ChAd vaccine protects upper and lower respiratory tracts against SARS-CoV-2. Cell. 2020;183(1):169–84. https://doi.org/10.1016/j.cell.2020.08.026.
81. Sonani B, Aslam F, Goyal A, Patel J, Bansal P. COVID-19 vaccination in immunocompromised patients. Clin Rheumatol. 2021;40(2):797–8. https://doi.org/10.1007/s10067-020-05547-w.
82. Gresham LM, Marzario B, Dutz J, Kirchhof MG. An evidence-based guide to SARS-CoV-2 vaccination of patients on immunotherapies in dermatology. J Am Acad Dermatol. 2021;84(6):1652–66. https://doi.org/10.1016/j.jaad.2021.01.047.
83. Ciotti JR, Valtcheva MV, Cross AH. Effects of MS disease-modifying therapies on responses to vaccinations: a review. Mult Scler Relat Disord. 2020;45:102439. https://doi.org/10.1016/j.msard.2020.102439.
84. Medeiros-Ribeiro AC, Aikawa NE, Saad CGS, Yuki EFN, Pedrosa T, Fusco SRG, et al. Immunogenicity and safety of the CoronaVac inactivated vaccine in patients with autoimmune rheumatic diseases: a phase 4 trial. Nat Med. 2021;27(10):1744–51. https://doi.org/10.1038/s41591-021-01469-5.
85. Simon D, Tascilar K, Schmidt K, Manger B, Weckwerth L, Sokolova M, et al. Brief report: Humoral and cellular immune responses to SARS-CoV-2 infection and vaccination in B cell depleted autoimmune patients. Arthritis Rheumatol. 2021;74(1):33–7. https://doi.org/10.1002/art.41914.
86. Ortega Rodríguez NR, Audícana Berasategui MT, de la Hoz CB, Valero SA. The century of mRNA vaccines: COVID-19 vaccines and allergy. J Investig Allergol Clin Immunol. 2021;31(1):89–91. https://doi.org/10.18176/jiaci.0665.
87. Baker D, Roberts CAK, Pryce G, Kang AS, Marta M, Reyes S, et al. COVID-19 vaccine-readiness for anti-CD20-depleting therapy in autoimmune diseases. Clin Exp Immunol. 2020;202(2):149–61. https://doi.org/10.1111/cei.13495.
88. Ludvigsson JF. Systematic review of COVID-19 in children shows milder cases and a better prognosis than adults. Acta Paediatr. 2020;109(6):1088–95. https://doi.org/10.1111/apa.15270.
89. Simpson JM, Newburger JW. Multisystem inflammatory syndrome in children in association with COVID-19. Circulation. 2020;142(5):437–40. https://doi.org/10.1161/CIRCULATIONAHA.120.048726.
90. Callaway E. COVID vaccines and kids: five questions as trials begin. Nature. 2021;592:670–1. https://doi.org/10.1038/d41586-021-01061-4.
91. Kamidani S, Rostad CA, Anderson EJ. COVID-19 vaccine development: a pediatric perspective. Curr Opin Pediatr. 2021;33(1):144–51. https://doi.org/10.1097/MOP.0000000000000978.
92. Lee B, Raszka WV Jr. COVID-19 transmission and children: the child is not to blame. Pediatrics. 2020;146(2):e2020004879. https://doi.org/10.1542/peds.2020-004879.
93. Blasi F, Gramegna A, Sotgiu G, Saderi L, Voza A, Alibert S, et al. SARS-CoV-2 vaccines: a critical perspective through efficacy data and barriers to herd immunity. Respir Med. 2021;180:106355. https://doi.org/10.1016/j.rmed.2021.106355.
94. Alzamora MC, Paredes T, Caceres D, Webb CM, Valdez LM, La Rosa M. Severe COVID-19 during pregnancy and possible vertical transmission. Am J Perinatol. 2020;37(8):861–5. https://doi.org/10.1055/s-0040-1710050.

95. Khalil A, Kalafat E, Benlioglu C, O'Brien P, Morris E, Draycott T, et al. SARS-CoV-2 infection in pregnancy: a systematic review and meta-analysis of clinical features and pregnancy outcomes. EClinicalMedicine. 2020;25:100446. https://doi.org/10.1016/j.eclinm.2020.100446.
96. Maykin MM, Heuser C, Feltovich H, Society for Maternal-Fetal Medicine Health Policy Advocacy Committee. Pregnant people deserve the protection offered by SARS-CoV-2 vaccines. Vaccine. 2021;39(2):171–2. https://doi.org/10.1016/j.vaccine.2020.12.007.
97. Whitehead CL, Walker SP. Consider pregnancy in COVID-19 therapeutic drug and vaccine trials. Lancet. 2020;395(10237):23–9. https://doi.org/10.1016/S0140-6736(20)31029-1.
98. Loubet P, Anselem O, Launay O. Immunization during pregnancy. Expert Rev Vaccines. 2018;17(5):383–93. https://doi.org/10.1080/14760584.2018.1471988.
99. Rasmussen SA, Kelley CF, Horton JP, Jamieson DJ. Coronavirus disease 2019 (COVID-19) vaccines and pregnancy: what obstetricians need to know. Obstet Gynecol. 2021;137(3):408–14. https://doi.org/10.1097/AOG.0000000000004290.
100. Edlow AG, Li JZ, Collier ARY, Atyeo C, James KE, Boatin AA, et al. Assessment of maternal and neonatal SARS-CoV-2 viral load, transplacental antibody transfer, and placental pathology in pregnancies during the COVID-19 pandemic. JAMA Netw Open. 2020;3(12):e2030455. https://doi.org/10.1001/jamanetworkopen.2020.30455.
101. Moore KM, Suthar MS. Comprehensive analysis of COVID-19 during pregnancy. Biochem Biophys Res Commun. 2021;538:180–6. https://doi.org/10.1016/j.bbrc.2020.12.064.
102. Bernal JL, Andrews N, Gower C, Gallagher E, Simmons R, Thelwall S, et al. Effectiveness of COVID-19 vaccines against the B.1.617.2 variant. medRxiv. 2021;385(7):585–94. https://doi.org/10.1101/2021.05.22.21257658.
103. Bian L, Gao F, Zhang J, He Q, Mao Q, Xu M, et al. Effects of SARS-CoV-2 variants on vaccine efficacy and response strategies. Expert Rev Vaccines. 2021;20(4):365–73. https://doi.org/10.1080/14760584.2021.1903879.
104. Boehm E, Kronig I, Neher RA, Eckerle I, Vetter P, Kaiser L, et al. Novel SARS-CoV-2 variants: the pandemics within the pandemic. Clin Microbiol Infect. 2021;27(8):1109–17. https://doi.org/10.1016/j.cmi.2021.05.022.
105. Gupta RK. Will SARS-CoV-2 variants of concern affect the promise of vaccines? Nat Rev Immunol. 2021;21(6):340–1. https://doi.org/10.1038/s41577-021-00556-5.
106. Altmann DM, Boyton RJ, Beale R. Immunity to SARS-CoV-2 variants of concern. Science. 2021;371(6534):1103–4. https://doi.org/10.1126/science.abg7404.
107. Madhi SA, Baillie V, Cutland CL, Voysey M, Koen AL, Fairlie L, et al. Efficacy of the ChAdOx1 nCoV-19 Covid-19 vaccine against the B.1.351 variant. N Engl J Med. 2021;384(20):1885–98. https://doi.org/10.1056/NEJMoa2102214.
108. Kardani K, Bolhassani A, Shahbazi S. Prime-boost vaccine strategy against viral infections: mechanisms and benefits. Vaccine. 2016;34:413–23. https://doi.org/10.1016/j.vaccine.2015.11.062.
109. Lu S. Heterologous prime-boost vaccination. Curr Opin Immunol. 2009;21:346–51. https://doi.org/10.1016/j.coi.2009.05.016.
110. Burki T. Booster shots for COVID-19-the debate continues. Lancet. 2021;21:1359–60. https://doi.org/10.1016/S1473-3099(21)00574-0.
111. Dory D, Fischer T, Béven V, Cariolet R, Rziha HJ, Jestin A. Prime-boost immunization using DNA vaccine and recombinant Orf virus protects pigs against Pseudorabies virus (Herpes suid 1). Vaccine. 2006;24:6256–63. https://doi.org/10.1016/j.vaccine.2006.05.078.
112. Rollier C, Verschoor E, Paranhos-Baccala G, Drexhage JAR, Verstrespen BE, Berland JL, et al. Modulation of vaccine-induced immune responses to hepatitis C virus in rhesus macaques by altering priming before adenovirus boosting. J Infect Dis. 2005;192:920–9. https://doi.org/10.1086/432517.

# Chapter 27
# SARS-CoV-2 Vaccine Against Virus: Mission Accomplished!?

**Clara Luzia Magnus and Barbara Schmidt**

## Abbreviations

| | |
|---|---|
| ACE-2 | Angiotensin-converting enzyme 2 |
| COVID-19 | Coronavirus disease-19 |
| nsps | Nonstructural proteins |
| SARS-CoV-2 | Severe acute respiratory syndrome coronavirus-2 |
| VOC | Variant of concern |
| VOI | Variant of interest |

## A Virus with Potential

In autumn 2019, the SARS-CoV-2 pandemic started with a viral strain, whose closest relatives circulate in bats and pangolins [1, 2]. The sequence of Wuhan-Hu-1 obtained by next generation sequencing was quickly deposited in GenBank (accession no. MN908947) and became publicly available on January 12, 2020 [3]. This reference genome served as a blueprint for all currently available vaccines against

C. L. Magnus
Institute of Medical Microbiology and Hygiene, University of Regensburg, Regensburg, Germany

B. Schmidt (✉)
Institute of Medical Microbiology and Hygiene, University of Regensburg, Regensburg, Germany

Institute of Clinical Microbiology and Hygiene, Clinical Virology and Infection Immunology, University Medical Center, Regensburg, Germany
e-mail: barbara.schmidt@ukr.de


S. Adibi et al. (eds.), *Frontiers of COVID-19*,
https://doi.org/10.1007/978-3-031-08045-6_27

COVID-19, namely the inactivated SARS-CoV-2 vaccine of Sinovac [4]; the mRNA vaccines BNT162b2 of Pfizer/BioNTech [5] and mRNA-1273 of Moderna [6]; and the vector-based vaccines. Among the latter are the ChAdOx1-based AZD1222 of AstraZeneca [7], the Adenovirus type 5 (Ad5)-recombinant vaccine of CanSino Biologics [8], the Ad5/Ad26-based Gam-COVID-Vac of the Gamaleya Research Institute of Epidemiology and Microbiology [9], the *Ad26*.COV2.S vaccine of Janssen-Cilag/Johnson & Johnson [10], and the first protein-based vaccine of Novavax [11]. Further candidates are still to come.

Coronaviruses are large single-stranded RNA viruses with a positive sense genome coding for spike, envelope, membrane, and nucleocapsid structural proteins as well as 16 nonstructural proteins (nsps). These nsps include an RNA-dependent RNA polymerase (nsp12) and, as a special feature for an RNA virus, an exonuclease (nsp14) [12]. Its proofreading activity has been held responsible for the relatively low mutation rate among the RNA viruses, which lulled scientists into false security that SARS-CoV-2 may remain a relatively stable virus. Yet, starting from a common ancestor, SARS-CoV-2 has developed into different clades and accumulated diversity through extensive transmission (Fig. 27.1), which may reflect not only random mutation but also targeted adaptation to the human host [13]. The virus uses the angiotensin-converting enzyme 2 of many species as receptor for entry [14, 15]. Occasionally, the virus has been transmitted to carnivores such as cats, dogs, tigers, and lions; SARS-CoV-2 can also be transmitted experimentally to other species, for example, Syrian hamsters, ferrets, and nonhuman primates, showing the zoonotic potential of the virus [16–18].

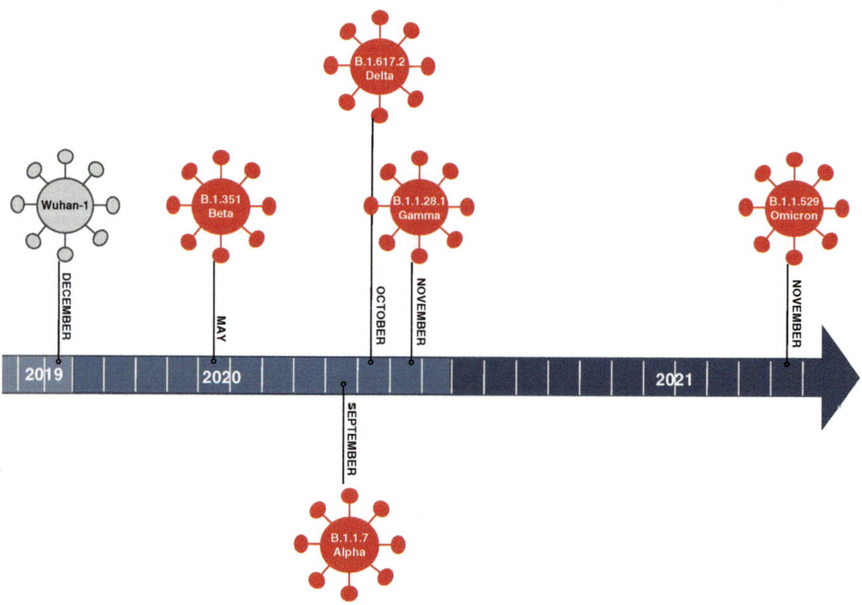


**Fig. 27.1** Timeline of SARS-CoV-2 variants of concern (VOC) since first appearance in late 2019. Placement in the timeline refers to tracking information provided by the WHO (https://www.who.int/en/activities/tracking-SARS-CoV-2-variants/)

## Mutations in the Viral Spike Protein and Beyond

Since January 2020, the virus has started mutating to increase its transmissibility and infectiousness. One of the first mutations to appear was the exchange of aspartate to glycine at position 614 (D614G) of the SARS-CoV-2 spike protein [19]. This variant quickly dominated the European pandemic, suggesting either a founder effect, initiated and supported by multiple superspreading events, or an increased infectivity of the viral particle (Fig. 27.2). The latter has turned out to be true by showing that D614G disrupts an interprotomeric contact, which shifts the spike protein to a more efficient receptor-binding open conformation [20]. In addition, vesicular stomatitis virus-based pseudoparticles carrying 614G instead of 614D were found to be significantly more infectious, as SARS-CoV-2 spike proteins with 614G were packed more densely into the viral envelope [21]. The higher amount of functional spike trimer into the viral envelope enabled a more efficient entry of the virus into ACE2-expressing target cells [21].

Unexpectedly, the virus crossed the species barrier from human to mink in April 2020. In connection with the fur industry in the Netherlands and Denmark, some minks were infected with a new SARS-CoV-2 variant called "cluster 5" (Fig. 27.2), causing respiratory infections and increased mortality in these animals [22–24]. This virus had acquired multiple mutations in the receptor-binding motif of the spike protein (Y453F), in the N-terminal domain (deletions at positions 69/70), near the S1/S2 cleavage site (I692V) and near or in the transmembrane domain (S1147L and M1229I), most likely representing an adaptation to the mink angiotensin-converting

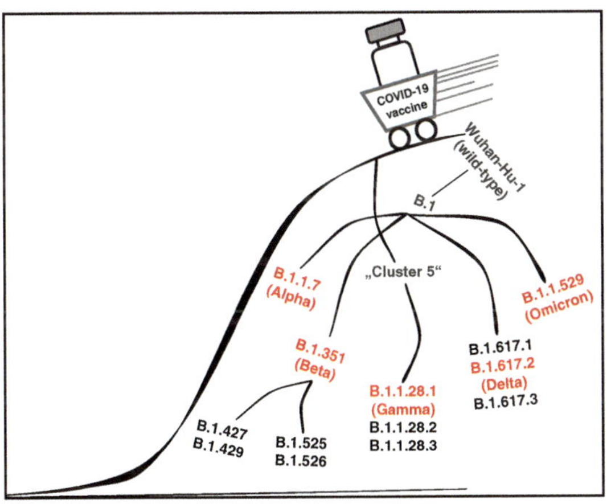


**Fig. 27.2** Cartoon showing the race of the COVID-19 vaccine based on the original Wuhan-Hu-1 strain against the evolution of SARS-CoV-2 spike variants of concern (VOC) from 2019 to 2021. Virus phylogeny is based on a rectangular tree generated with Nextstrain/ncov (https://nextstrain.org/ncov/global?c=emerging_lineage) and data from GISAID (https://www.gisaid.org/)

enzyme 2 (ACE-2) receptor [25, 26]. Residue Y453F also mediates enhanced binding of the viral spike protein to the human ACE-2 receptor [27]. Spillover infections from minks to farm residents and further close contacts confirmed frequent mink-to-human transmission with secondary human cases [28]. Culling and burying millions of mink was intended to eradicate this cluster, but whether this approach was successful is still unclear. Subsequently, the bodies were exhumed and incinerated to prevent the virus from resurfacing and potentially triggering vaccine failure.

In the summer and autumn of 2020, SARS-CoV-2 variants with deletions in the spike protein at positions 69 and 70 emerged in several immunocompromised patients with B-cell deficiencies in malignant diseases [29–31]. Reduced immunological competence of the hosts supported prolonged virus replication and evolution, which began to undermine the effectiveness of convalescent plasma therapy.

From October to December 2020, a SARS-CoV-2 variant of interest (VOI) turned into a variant of concern (VOC), when it quickly took over the southeast and southwest of UK [32–34]. This variant belonged to strain B.1.1.7 and was renamed VOC Alpha by the WHO. It combined deletions in the spike protein with mutations in the receptor-binding domain, in particular key mutation N501Y, which was shown to enhance binding to ACE-2 [35] and increase infectivity by 50–70% as evident from contact tracing [36]. Although initial studies could not readily detect an increased pathogenicity of the virus, large observational cohort studies ultimately found a higher risk for admission to intensive care units and an increased mortality compared to patients with non-B.1.1.7 SARS-CoV-2 infections [37–41].

The next variant to surface was B.1.351, now renamed VOC Beta, which quickly became the dominant virus in South Africa [42]. The virus is characterized by key mutations K417N, E484K and N501Y within the receptor-binding domain. Mutation E484K in the context of N501Y is responsible for a reduced neutralizing activity of monoclonal antibodies and sera from convalescent patients [43]. This variant was the first to be shown to undermine the response to the vaccine, while VOC Alpha is still targeted by current vaccines [44–46].

A similar list of mutations in the receptor-binding domain was detected in a SARS-CoV-2 variant emerging in Brazil [47]. This variant belonging to lineage B.1.1.28.1 (identical to P.1) and now renamed VOC Gamma, shows a similar profile of immune escape compared to VOC Beta, but also an augmented infectivity due to increased ACE-2 binding [47]. These combined characteristics appear to have contributed to the second deadly wave in Manaus, despite the high seroprevalence from the first wave [48].

A fourth SARS-CoV-2 variant, which has surged in India [49] and many other countries of the world [50, 51], is lineage B.1.617.2, now renamed VOC Delta. In the meantime, sublines of the Delta variant have been detected. No phenotypic differences are observed so far, but this may change with further mutations. Mutation P681R facilitates cleavage of the spike protein and enhances pathogenicity of the Delta variant [52]. In addition, VOC Delta demonstrates higher replication efficiency [53] and higher infectious viral loads in vaccinated and unvaccinated people [54].

The most recent VOC to appear was Omicron, identified from the respiratory specimen of an immunocompromised subject in South Africa in November 2021 [55, 56]. This SARS-CoV-2 variant has quickly displaced the other virus variants worldwide, mainly because it is a true immune escape variant that carried, among others, mutations K417N, E484A and Q493R [57–59]. Fortunately, Omicron sub-lineage BA.1 showed attenuated replication and pathogenicity due to its inefficient use of transmembrane serine protease 2 (TMPRSS2) [60, 61]. These viral properties resulted in reduced lung infiltration in a rodent models of respiratory disease [62].

Large phylogenetic analyses indicate that the diversity of SARS-CoV-2 increases with replication, as the development of viral quasispecies was limited only in countries with effective quarantine measures such as Asia and Oceania [63]. Notably, SARS-CoV-2 does not only mutate in the spike protein but throughout the viral genome. Mutations in the viral polymerase, but also in the exonuclease [64] may be particularly detrimental because they have the potential to enhance virus replication and to sabotage viral proofreading, which would allow for even more efficient mutational escape. As long as viral replication is not effectively slowed down, new VOI and—most likely VOC—will emerge.

Very early on, SARS-CoV-2 began to optimize itself—and is still doing so. To date, E484K/Q, N501Y, L452R and P681R mutations have evolved independently in different SARS-CoV-2 VOCs (Table 27.1). Of note, position E484 is mutated in all currently circulating VOCs, demonstrating the importance of this amino acid within the viral spike protein. This remarkably convergent evolution demonstrates the evolutionary capacity of the virus to escape selection pressure and to adapt specifically. The aforementioned mutations provide better transmissibility, higher infection rates and/or immune evasion. With the exception of one variant that contained a larger deletion in an open reading frame [65], the infectivity of SARS-CoV-2 increased with evolution.

**Table 27.1** Mutations within the spike protein of the five SARS-CoV-2 variants of concern (VOC)

| VOC (Pango lineage) | Alpha | Beta | Gamma | Delta | Omicron |
|---|---|---|---|---|---|
| S-protein mutation | B.1.1.7 | B.1.351 | B.1.1.28.1/P.1 | B.1.617.2 | B.1.1. 529 |
| L18F | | (x) | x | | |
| T19I/R | | | | x (R) | (x) (I) |
| T20N | | | x | | |
| L24S | | | | | (x) |
| Δ25/Δ27 | | | | | (x) |
| P26S | | | x | | |
| A67V | | | | | (x) |
| Δ69/Δ70 | x | | | | (x) |
| D80A | | x | | | |
| T95I | | | | | (x) |
| D138Y | | | x | | |

(continued)

**Table 27.1** (continued)

| VOC (Pango lineage) | Alpha | Beta | Gamma | Delta | Omicron |
|---|---|---|---|---|---|
| G142D | | | | x | x |
| Δ143/Δ145 | | | | | (x) |
| Δ144/Δ145 | x | | | | |
| E156G | | | | x | |
| Δ157/Δ158 | | | | x | |
| R190S | | | x | | |
| N211I | | | | | (x) |
| Δ212 | | | | | (x) |
| V213G | | | | | (x) |
| 214EP (insertion) | | | | | (x) |
| D215G | | | | | |
| Δ241–Δ243 | | x | | | |
| *G339D* | | | | | x |
| *S371F/L* | | | | | x (F/L) |
| *S373P* | | | | | x |
| *S375F* | | | | | x |
| *S376A* | | | | | (x) |
| *P384L* | | x | | | |
| *D405N* | | | | | (x) |
| *D408S* | | | | | (x) |
| *K417N/T* | | x (N) | x (T) | x (N) | x (N) |
| *N440K* | | | | | x |
| *G446S* | | | | | x |
| *L452R* | | | | x | |
| *S477N* | | | | | x |
| *T478K* | | | | x | x |
| *E484K/Q/A* | (x) (K) | x (K) | x (K) | x (Q) | x (A) |
| *Q493R* | | | | | x |
| *S494P* | (x) | | | | |
| *G496S* | | | | | (x) |
| *G498R* | | | | | x |
| *N501Y* | x | x | x | | x |
| *Y505H* | | | | | x |
| *E516Q* | | (x) | | | |
| T547K | | | | | (x) |
| A570D | x | | | | |
| Q613H | | | | | |
| D614G | x | x | x | x | x |
| H655Y | | | x | | x |
| N679K | | | | | x |
| P681H/R | x (H) | | x (H) | x (R) | x (H) |
| I692V | | | | | |
| A701V | | x | | | |

**Table 27.1** (continued)

| VOC (Pango lineage) | Alpha | Beta | Gamma | Delta | Omicron |
|---|---|---|---|---|---|
| T716I | x | | | | |
| N764K | | | | | x |
| D769Y | | | | | x |
| N856K | | | | | (x) |
| D950N | | | | x | |
| Q954H | | | | | x |
| S982A | x | | | | |
| N969K | | | | | x |
| L981F | | | | | (x) |
| T1027I | | | x | | |
| D1118H | x | | | | |
| V1176F | | | x | | |

The table lists the mutations that have been described for each virus strain with reference to the Stanford University Coronavirus Antiviral & Resistance Database (https://covdb.stanford.edu/, last updated on 4/20/2022). Brackets indicate that either the position or the amino acid at this position is not present in all isolates of this lineage. Mutations within the receptor-binding domain of SARS-CoV-2 (amino acid residues 333–527) [66] are marked in italics. B.1.1.529 comprises Omicron sublineages BA.1 and BA.2. Evolutionary convergence within SARS-CoV-2 lineages can be recognised by the presence of identical mutations in different viral strains

## The Pressure is on

In the current situation, the virus gets under increasing pressure. Patients suffering from severe courses of COVID-19 receive convalescent plasma or recently licensed monoclonal antibodies. Modeling of this scenario predicted that resistance to single and double monoclonal combinations can develop quickly under positive selection. In fact, monoclonal antibodies targeting different epitopes of the viral spike protein have selected resistant virus variants in vitro, which was not observed using an antibody cocktail [67]. The immune pressure from vaccination as well as from natural infections is also rising. On the other hand, humoral immune responses against SARS-CoV-2 do not seem to be long-lasting, so that this situation still provides sufficient opportunities for virus replication. That this assumption has already become reality is shown by the fact that VOC Omicron has escaped most monoclonal antibodies.

What should we do? First, laboratories should initiate a worldwide surveillance of mutant viruses to get a real glimpse on viral evolution. This should include monitoring of SARS-CoV-2 infections in animals to cover cross-species transmission, which may be an important source for reinfection. Second, academics and industries should start producing and testing of SARS-CoV-2 vaccines against immune escape variants. Preliminary data show that a variant vaccine of Moderna boosters the immunity against the original as well a mutant strains [68]. However, we do not yet know in how far vaccine-induced humoral and cellular immune responses will be cross-reactive against modified spike trimers. In addition, we should work on vaccines inducing mucosal immunity more effectively than current vaccines do. Third, governments and industries should evaluate all possibilities to upscale vaccine production. We do not need a snowball of vaccines; we need an avalanche.

**Acknowledgements** The authors thank the Bavarian Ministry of Science and Art for financial support through the pandemic responsiveness fund. The authors have no affiliations or financial involvement with any organization or entity with a financial interest in or financial conflict with the subject matter or materials discussed in the chapter.

## References

1. Lu R, Zhao X, Li J, Niu P, Yang B, Wu H, Wang W, Song H, Huang B, Zhu N, Bi Y, Ma X, Zhan F, Wang L, Hu T, Zhou H, Hu Z, Zhou W, Zhao L, Chen J, Meng Y, Wang J, Lin Y, Yuan J, Xie Z, Ma J, Liu WJ, Wang D, Xu W, Holmes EC, Gao GF, Wu G, Chen W, Shi W, Tan W. Genomic characterisation and epidemiology of 2019 novel coronavirus: implications for virus origins and receptor binding. Lancet. 2020;395(10224):565–74. https://doi.org/10.1016/S0140-6736(20)30251-8.
2. Zhang T, Wu Q, Zhang Z. Probable pangolin origin of SARS-CoV-2 associated with the COVID-19 outbreak. Curr Biol. 2020;30(7):1346–51. https://doi.org/10.1016/j.cub.2020.03.022.
3. Wu F, Zhao S, Yu B, Chen YM, Wang W, Song ZG, Hu Y, Tao ZW, Tian JH, Pei YY, Yuan ML, Zhang YL, Dai FH, Liu Y, Wang QM, Zheng JJ, Xu L, Holmes EC, Zhang YZ. A new coronavirus associated with human respiratory disease in China. Nature. 2020;579(7798):265–9. https://doi.org/10.1038/s41586-020-2008-3.
4. Zhang Y, Zeng G, Pan H, Li C, Hu Y, Chu K, Han W, Chen Z, Tang R, Yin W, Chen X, Hu Y, Liu X, Jiang C, Li J, Yang M, Song Y, Wang X, Gao Q, Zhu F. Safety, tolerability, and immunogenicity of an inactivated SARS-CoV-2 vaccine in healthy adults aged 18–59 years: a randomised, double-blind, placebo-controlled, phase 1/2 clinical trial. Lancet Infect Dis. 2020;21(2):181–92. https://doi.org/10.1016/S1473-3099(20)30843-4.
5. Polack FP, Thomas SJ, Kitchin N, Absalon J, Gurtman A, Lockhart S, Perez JL, Perez Marc G, Moreira ED, Zerbini C, Bailey R, Swanson KA, Roychoudhury S, Koury K, Li P, Kalina WV, Cooper D, Frenck RW Jr, Hammitt LL, Tureci O, Nell H, Schaefer A, Unal S, Tresnan DB, Mather S, Dormitzer PR, Sahin U, Jansen KU, Gruber WC, Group CCT. Safety and efficacy of the BNT162b2 mRNA Covid-19 vaccine. N Engl J Med. 2020;383(27):2603–15. https://doi.org/10.1056/NEJMoa2034577.
6. Baden LR, El Sahly HM, Essink B, Kotloff K, Frey S, Novak R, Diemert D, Spector SA, Rouphael N, Creech CB, McGettigan J, Kehtan S, Segall N, Solis J, Brosz A, Fierro C, Schwartz H, Neuzil K, Corey L, Gilbert P, Janes H, Follmann D, Marovich M, Mascola J, Polakowski L, Ledgerwood J, Graham BS, Bennett H, Pajon R, Knightly C, Leav B, Deng W, Zhou H, Han S, Ivarsson M, Miller J, Zaks T, Group CS. Efficacy and safety of the mRNA-1273 SARS-CoV-2 vaccine. N Engl J Med. 2020;384(5):403–16. https://doi.org/10.1056/NEJMoa2035389.
7. Voysey M, Clemens SAC, Madhi SA, Weckx LY, Folegatti PM, Aley PK, Angus B, Baillie VL, Barnabas SL, Bhorat QE, Bibi S, Briner C, Cicconi P, Collins AM, Colin-Jones R, Cutland CL, Darton TC, Dheda K, Duncan CJA, Emary KRW, Ewer KJ, Fairlie L, Faust SN, Feng S, Ferreira DM, Finn A, Goodman AL, Green CM, Green CA, Heath PT, Hill C, Hill H, Hirsch I, Hodgson SHC, Izu A, Jackson S, Jenkin D, Joe CCD, Kerridge S, Koen A, Kwatra G, Lazarus R, Lawrie AM, Lelliott A, Libri V, Lillie PJ, Mallory R, Mendes AVA, Milan EP, Minassian

AM, McGregor A, Morrison H, Mujadidi YF, Nana A, O'Reilly PJ, Padayachee SD, Pittella A, Plested E, Pollock KM, Ramasamy MN, Rhead S, Schwarzbold AV, Singh N, Smith A, Song R, Snape MD, Sprinz E, Sutherland RK, Tarrant R, Thomson EC, Torok ME, Toshner M, Turner DPJ, Vekemans J, Villafana TL, Watson MEE, Williams CJ, Douglas AD, Hill AVS, Lambe T, Gilbert SC, Pollard AJ, Oxford CVTG. Safety and efficacy of the ChAdOx1 nCoV-19 vaccine (AZD1222) against SARS-CoV-2: an interim analysis of four randomised controlled trials in Brazil, South Africa, and the UK. Lancet. 2021;397(10269):99–111. https://doi.org/10.1016/S0140-6736(20)32661-1.
8. Zhu FC, Li YH, Guan XH, Hou LH, Wang WJ, Li JX, Wu SP, Wang BS, Wang Z, Wang L, Jia SY, Jiang HD, Wang L, Jiang T, Hu Y, Gou JB, Xu SB, Xu JJ, Wang XW, Wang W, Chen W. Safety, tolerability, and immunogenicity of a recombinant adenovirus type-5 vectored COVID-19 vaccine: a dose-escalation, open-label, non-randomised, first-in-human trial. Lancet. 2020;395(10240):1845–54. https://doi.org/10.1016/S0140-6736(20)31208-3.
9. Logunov DY, Dolzhikova IV, Zubkova OV, Tukhvatulin AI, Shcheblyakov DV, Dzharullaeva AS, Grousova DM, Erokhova AS, Kovyrshina AV, Botikov AG, Izhaeva FM, Popova O, Ozharovskaya TA, Esmagambetov IB, Favorskaya IA, Zrelkin DI, Voronina DV, Shcherbinin DN, Semikhin AS, Simakova YV, Tokarskaya EA, Lubenets NL, Egorova DA, Shmarov MM, Nikitenko NA, Morozova LF, Smolyarchuk EA, Kryukov EV, Babira VF, Borisevich SV, Naroditsky BS, Gintsburg AL. Safety and immunogenicity of an rAd26 and rAd5 vector-based heterologous prime-boost COVID-19 vaccine in two formulations: two open, non-randomised phase 1/2 studies from Russia. Lancet. 2020;396(10255):887–97. https://doi.org/10.1016/S0140-6736(20)31866-3.
10. Sadoff J, Gray G, Vandebosch A, Cardenas V, Shukarev G, Grinsztejn B, Goepfert PA, Truyers C, Fennema H, Spiessens B, Offergeld K, Scheper G, Taylor KL, Robb ML, Treanor J, Barouch DH, Stoddard J, Ryser MF, Marovich MA, Neuzil KM, Corey L, Cauwenberghs N, Tanner T, Hardt K, Ruiz-Guinazu J, Le Gars M, Schuitemaker H, Van Hoof J, Struyf F, Douoguih M, Group ES. Safety and efficacy of single-dose Ad26.COV2.S vaccine against Covid-19. N Engl J Med. 2021;384(23):2187–201. https://doi.org/10.1056/NEJMoa2101544.
11. Heath PT, Galiza EP, Baxter DN, Boffito M, Browne D, Burns F, Chadwick DR, Clark R, Cosgrove C, Galloway J, Goodman AL, Heer A, Higham A, Iyengar S, Jamal A, Jeanes C, Kalra PA, Kyriakidou C, McAuley DF, Meyrick A, Minassian AM, Minton J, Moore P, Munsoor I, Nicholls H, Osanlou O, Packham J, Pretswell CH, San Francisco Ramos A, Saralaya D, Sheridan RP, Smith R, Soiza RL, Swift PA, Thomson EC, Turner J, Viljoen ME, Albert G, Cho I, Dubovsky F, Glenn G, Rivers J, Robertson A, Smith K, Toback S, nCo VSG. Safety and efficacy of NVX-CoV2373 Covid-19 vaccine. N Engl J Med. 2021;385(13):1172–83. https://doi.org/10.1056/NEJMoa2107659.
12. Kim D, Lee JY, Yang JS, Kim JW, Kim VN, Chang H. The architecture of SARS-CoV-2 transcriptome. Cell. 2020;181(4):914–21. https://doi.org/10.1016/j.cell.2020.04.011.
13. Alm E, Broberg EK, Connor T, Hodcroft EB, Komissarov AB, Maurer-Stroh S, Melidou A, Neher RA, O'Toole A, Pereyaslov D, Laboratories WHOERs, Group GE, Laboratories WHOERs, Group* GE. Geographical and temporal distribution of SARS-CoV-2 clades in the WHO European region, January to June 2020. Euro Surveill. 2020;25(32):2001410. https://doi.org/10.2807/1560-7917.ES.2020.25.32.2001410.
14. Letko M, Marzi A, Munster V. Functional assessment of cell entry and receptor usage for SARS-CoV-2 and other lineage B betacoronaviruses. Nat Microbiol. 2020;5(4):562–9. https://doi.org/10.1038/s41564-020-0688-y.
15. Hoffmann M, Kleine-Weber H, Schroeder S, Kruger N, Herrler T, Erichsen S, Schiergens TS, Herrler G, Wu NH, Nitsche A, Muller MA, Drosten C, Pohlmann S. SARS-CoV-2 cell entry depends on ACE2 and TMPRSS2 and is blocked by a clinically proven protease inhibitor. Cell. 2020;181(2):271–80. https://doi.org/10.1016/j.cell.2020.02.052.
16. Jo WK, de Oliveira-Filho EF, Rasche A, Greenwood AD, Osterrieder K, Drexler JF. Potential zoonotic sources of SARS-CoV-2 infections. Transbound Emerg Dis. 2020;68(4):1824–34. https://doi.org/10.1111/tbed.13872.

17. Abdel-Moneim AS, Abdelwhab EM. Evidence for SARS-CoV-2 infection of animal hosts. Pathogens. 2020;9(7):529. https://doi.org/10.3390/pathogens9070529.
18. Schlottau K, Rissmann M, Graaf A, Schon J, Sehl J, Wylezich C, Hoper D, Mettenleiter TC, Balkema-Buschmann A, Harder T, Grund C, Hoffmann D, Breithaupt A, Beer M. SARS-CoV-2 in fruit bats, ferrets, pigs, and chickens: an experimental transmission study. Lancet Microbe. 2020;1(5):e218–25. https://doi.org/10.1016/S2666-5247(20)30089-6.
19. Korber B, Fischer WM, Gnanakaran S, Yoon H, Theiler J, Abfalterer W, Hengartner N, Giorgi EE, Bhattacharya T, Foley B, Hastie KM, Parker MD, Partridge DG, Evans CM, Freeman TM, de Silva TI, Sheffield C-GG, McDanal C, Perez LG, Tang H, Moon-Walker A, Whelan SP, LaBranche CC, Saphire EO, Montefiori DC. Tracking changes in SARS-CoV-2 spike: evidence that D614G increases infectivity of the COVID-19 virus. Cell. 2020;182(4):812–27. https://doi.org/10.1016/j.cell.2020.06.043.
20. Yurkovetskiy L, Wang X, Pascal KE, Tomkins-Tinch C, Nyalile TP, Wang Y, Baum A, Diehl WE, Dauphin A, Carbone C, Veinotte K, Egri SB, Schaffner SF, Lemieux JE, Munro JB, Rafique A, Barve A, Sabeti PC, Kyratsous CA, Dudkina NV, Shen K, Luban J. Structural and functional analysis of the D614G SARS-CoV-2 spike protein variant. Cell. 2020;183(3):739–51. https://doi.org/10.1016/j.cell.2020.09.032.
21. Zhang L, Jackson CB, Mou H, Ojha A, Peng H, Quinlan BD, Rangarajan ES, Pan A, Vanderheiden A, Suthar MS, Li W, Izard T, Rader C, Farzan M, Choe H. SARS-CoV-2 spike-protein D614G mutation increases virion spike density and infectivity. Nat Commun. 2020;11(1):6013. https://doi.org/10.1038/s41467-020-19808-4.
22. Oreshkova N, Molenaar RJ, Vreman S, Harders F, Oude Munnink BB, Hakze-van der Honing RW, Gerhards N, Tolsma P, Bouwstra R, Sikkema RS, Tacken MG, de Rooij MM, Weesendorp E, Engelsma MY, Bruschke CJ, Smit LA, Koopmans M, van der Poel WH, Stegeman A. SARS-CoV-2 infection in farmed minks, the Netherlands, April and May 2020. Euro Surveill. 2020;25(23):2001005. https://doi.org/10.2807/1560-7917.ES.2020.25.23.2001005.
23. Molenaar RJ, Vreman S, Hakze-van der Honing RW, Zwart R, de Rond J, Weesendorp E, Smit LAM, Koopmans M, Bouwstra R, Stegeman A, van der Poel WHM. Clinical and pathological findings in SARS-CoV-2 disease outbreaks in farmed mink (Neovison vison). Vet Pathol. 2020;57(5):653–7. https://doi.org/10.1177/0300985820943535.
24. Hammer AS, Quaade ML, Rasmussen TB, Fonager J, Rasmussen M, Mundbjerg K, Lohse L, Strandbygaard B, Jorgensen CS, Alfaro-Nunez A, Rosenstierne MW, Boklund A, Halasa T, Fomsgaard A, Belsham GJ, Botner A. SARS-CoV-2 transmission between mink (Neovison vison) and humans. Denmark Emerg Infect Dis. 2021;27(2):547–51. https://doi.org/10.3201/eid2702.203794.
25. Laussaunière R, Fonager J, Rasmussen M, Frische A, Polacek Strandh C, Rasmussen TB, Botner A, Fomsgaard A. SARS-CoV-2 spike mutations arising in Danish mink and their spread to humans. 2021. https://files.ssi.dk/Mink-cluster-5-short-report_AF02-1.pdf.
26. Tan CCS, Lam SD, Richard D, Owen C, Berchtold D, Orengo C, Nair MS, Kuchipudi SV, Kapur V, van Dorp L, Balloux F. Transmission of SARS-CoV-2 from humans to animals and potential host adaptation. bioRxiv. 2022;2022:384743. https://doi.org/10.1101/2020.11.16.384743.
27. Bayarri-Olmos R, Rosbjerg A, Johnsen LB, Helgstrand C, Bak-Thomsen T, Garred P, Skjoedt MO. The SARS-CoV-2 Y453F mink variant displays a pronounced increase in ACE-2 affinity but does not challenge antibody neutralization. J Biol Chem. 2021;296:100536. https://doi.org/10.1016/j.jbc.2021.100536.
28. Oude Munnink BB, Sikkema RS, Nieuwenhuijse DF, Molenaar RJ, Munger E, Molenkamp R, van der Spek A, Tolsma P, Rietveld A, Brouwer M, Bouwmeester-Vincken N, Harders F, Hakze-van der Honing R, Wegdam-Blans MCA, Bouwstra RJ, GeurtsvanKessel C, van der Eijk AA, Velkers FC, Smit LAM, Stegeman A, van der Poel WHM, Koopmans MPG. Transmission of SARS-CoV-2 on mink farms between humans and mink and back to humans. Science. 2021;371(6525):172–7. https://doi.org/10.1126/science.abe5901.
29. Choi B, Choudhary MC, Regan J, Sparks JA, Padera RF, Qiu X, Solomon IH, Kuo HH, Boucau J, Bowman K, Adhikari UD, Winkler ML, Mueller AA, Hsu TY, Desjardins M, Baden

LR, Chan BT, Walker BD, Lichterfeld M, Brigl M, Kwon DS, Kanjilal S, Richardson ET, Jonsson AH, Alter G, Barczak AK, Hanage WP, Yu XG, Gaiha GD, Seaman MS, Cernadas M, Li JZ. Persistence and evolution of SARS-CoV-2 in an immunocompromised host. N Engl J Med. 2020;383(23):2291–3. https://doi.org/10.1056/NEJMc2031364.

30. Avanzato VA, Matson MJ, Seifert SN, Pryce R, Williamson BN, Anzick SL, Barbian K, Judson SD, Fischer ER, Martens C, Bowden TA, de Wit E, Riedo FX, Munster VJ. Case study: prolonged infectious SARS-CoV-2 shedding from an asymptomatic immunocompromised individual with cancer. Cell. 2020;183(7):1901–12. https://doi.org/10.1016/j.cell.2020.10.049.
31. Kemp SA, Collier DA, Datir RP, Ferreira I, Gayed S, Jahun A, Hosmillo M, Rees-Spear C, Mlcochova P, Lumb IU, Roberts DJ, Chandra A, Temperton N, Collaboration C-NBC, Consortium C-GU, Sharrocks K, Blane E, Modis Y, Leigh KE, JAG B, van Gils MJ, KGC S, Bradley JR, Smith C, Doffinger R, Ceron-Gutierrez L, Barcenas-Morales G, Pollock DD, Goldstein RA, Smielewska A, Skittrall JP, Gouliouris T, Goodfellow IG, Gkrania-Klotsas E, CJR I, LE MC, Gupta RK. SARS-CoV-2 evolution during treatment of chronic infection. Nature. 2021;592(7853):277–82. https://doi.org/10.1038/s41586-021-03291-y.
32. https://www.gov.uk/government/publications/investigation-of-novel-sars-cov-2-variant-variant-of-concern-20201201.
33. Leung K, Shum MH, Leung GM, Lam TT, Wu JT. Early transmissibility assessment of the N501Y mutant strains of SARS-CoV-2 in the United Kingdom, October to November 2020. Euro Surveill. 2021;26(1):2002106. https://doi.org/10.2807/1560-7917.ES.2020.26.1.2002106.
34. Davies NG, Abbott S, Barnard RC, Jarvis CI, Kucharski AJ, Munday JD, CAB P, Russell TW, Tully DC, Washburne AD, Wenseleers T, Gimma A, Waites W, KLM W, van Zandvoort K, Silverman JD, Group CC-W, Consortium C-GU, Diaz-Ordaz K, Keogh R, Eggo RM, Funk S, Jit M, Atkins KE, Edmunds WJ. Estimated transmissibility and impact of SARS-CoV-2 lineage B.1.1.7 in England. Science. 2021;372(6538):abg3055. https://doi.org/10.1126/science.abg3055.
35. Laffeber C, de Koning K, Kanaar R, Lebbink JHG. Experimental evidence for enhanced receptor binding by rapidly spreading SARS-CoV-2 variants. J Mol Biol. 2021;433(15):167058. https://doi.org/10.1016/j.jmb.2021.167058.
36. Volz E, Mishra S, Chand M, Barrett JC, Johnson R, Geidelberg L, Hinsley WR, Laydon DJ, Dabrera G, O'Toole A, Amato R, Ragonnet-Cronin M, Harrison I, Jackson B, Ariani CV, Boyd O, Loman NJ, McCrone JT, Goncalves S, Jorgensen D, Myers R, Hill V, Jackson DK, Gaythorpe K, Groves N, Sillitoe J, Kwiatkowski DP, Consortium C-GU, Flaxman S, Ratmann O, Bhatt S, Hopkins S, Gandy A, Rambaut A, Ferguson NM. Assessing transmissibility of SARS-CoV-2 lineage B.1.1.7 in England. Nature. 2021;593(7858):266–9. https://doi.org/10.1038/s41586-021-03470-x.
37. Davies NG, Jarvis CI, Group CC-W, Edmunds WJ, Jewell NP, Diaz-Ordaz K, Keogh RH. Increased mortality in community-tested cases of SARS-CoV-2 lineage B.1.1.7. Nature. 2021;593(7858):270–4. https://doi.org/10.1038/s41586-021-03426-1.
38. Nyberg T, Twohig KA, Harris RJ, Seaman SR, Flannagan J, Allen H, Charlett A, De Angelis D, Dabrera G, Presanis AM. Risk of hospital admission for patients with SARS-CoV-2 variant B.1.1.7: cohort analysis. BMJ. 2021;373:n1412. https://doi.org/10.1136/bmj.n1412.
39. Challen R, Brooks-Pollock E, Read JM, Dyson L, Tsaneva-Atanasova K, Danon L. Risk of mortality in patients infected with SARS-CoV-2 variant of concern 202012/1: matched cohort study. BMJ. 2021;372:n579. https://doi.org/10.1136/bmj.n579.
40. Grint DJ, Wing K, Williamson E, McDonald HI, Bhaskaran K, Evans D, Evans SJ, Walker AJ, Hickman G, Nightingale E, Schultze A, Rentsch CT, Bates C, Cockburn J, Curtis HJ, Morton CE, Bacon S, Davy S, Wong AY, Mehrkar A, Tomlinson L, Douglas IJ, Mathur R, Blomquist P, MacKenna B, Ingelsby P, Croker R, Parry J, Hester F, Harper S, DeVito NJ, Hulme W, Tazare J, Goldacre B, Smeeth L, Eggo RM. Case fatality risk of the SARS-CoV-2 variant of concern B.1.1.7 in England, 16 November to 5 February. Euro Surveill. 2021;26(11):2100256. https://doi.org/10.2807/1560-7917.ES.2021.26.11.2100256.

41. Patone M, Thomas K, Hatch R, Tan PS, Coupland C, Liao W, Mouncey P, Harrison D, Rowan K, Horby P, Watkinson P, Hippisley-Cox J. Mortality and critical care unit admission associated with the SARS-CoV-2 lineage B.1.1.7 in England: an observational cohort study. Lancet Infect Dis. 2021;21(11):1518–28. https://doi.org/10.1016/S1473-3099(21)00318-2.
42. Tegally H, Wilkinson E, Giovanetti M, Iranzadeh A, Fonseca V, Giandhari J, Doolabh D, Pillay S, San EJ, Msomi N, Mlisana K, von Gottberg A, Walaza S, Allam M, Ismail A, Mohale T, Glass AJ, Engelbrecht S, Van Zyl G, Preiser W, Petruccione F, Sigal A, Hardie D, Marais G, Hsiao NY, Korsman S, Davies MA, Tyers L, Mudau I, York D, Maslo C, Goedhals D, Abrahams S, Laguda-Akingba O, Alisoltani-Dehkordi A, Godzik A, Wibmer CK, Sewell BT, Lourenco J, Alcantara LCJ, Kosakovsky Pond SL, Weaver S, Martin D, Lessells RJ, Bhiman JN, Williamson C, de Oliveira T. Detection of a SARS-CoV-2 variant of concern in South Africa. Nature. 2021;592(7854):438–43. https://doi.org/10.1038/s41586-021-03402-9.
43. Li Q, Nie J, Wu J, Zhang L, Ding R, Wang H, Zhang Y, Li T, Liu S, Zhang M, Zhao C, Liu H, Nie L, Qin H, Wang M, Lu Q, Li X, Liu J, Liang H, Shi Y, Shen Y, Xie L, Zhang L, Qu X, Xu W, Huang W, Wang Y. SARS-CoV-2 501Y.V2 variants lack higher infectivity but do have immune escape. Cell. 2021;184(9):2362–71. https://doi.org/10.1016/j.cell.2021.02.042.
44. Collier DA, De Marco A, Ferreira I, Meng B, Datir RP, Walls AC, Kemp SA, Bassi J, Pinto D, Silacci-Fregni C, Bianchi S, Tortorici MA, Bowen J, Culap K, Jaconi S, Cameroni E, Snell G, Pizzuto MS, Pellanda AF, Garzoni C, Riva A, Collaboration C-NBC-, Consortium C-GU, Elmer A, Kingston N, Graves B, LE MC, KGC S, Bradley JR, Temperton N, Ceron-Gutierrez L, Barcenas-Morales G, Harvey W, Virgin HW, Lanzavecchia A, Piccoli L, Doffinger R, Wills M, Veesler D, Corti D, Gupta RK. Sensitivity of SARS-CoV-2 B.1.1.7 to mRNA vaccine-elicited antibodies. Nature. 2021;593(7857):136–41. https://doi.org/10.1038/s41586-021-03412-7.
45. Muik A, Wallisch AK, Sanger B, Swanson KA, Muhl J, Chen W, Cai H, Maurus D, Sarkar R, Tureci O, Dormitzer PR, Sahin U. Neutralization of SARS-CoV-2 lineage B.1.1.7 pseudovirus by BNT162b2 vaccine-elicited human sera. Science. 2021;371(6534):1152–3. https://doi.org/10.1126/science.abg6105.
46. Wang P, Nair MS, Liu L, Iketani S, Luo Y, Guo Y, Wang M, Yu J, Zhang B, Kwong PD, Graham BS, Mascola JR, Chang JY, Yin MT, Sobieszczyk M, Kyratsous CA, Shapiro L, Sheng Z, Huang Y, Ho DD. Antibody resistance of SARS-CoV-2 variants B.1.351 and B.1.1.7. Nature. 2021;593(7857):130–5. https://doi.org/10.1038/s41586-021-03398-2.
47. Faria NR, Mellan TA, Whittaker C, Claro IM, Candido DDS, Mishra S, Crispim MAE, Sales FCS, Hawryluk I, McCrone JT, Hulswit RJG, Franco LAM, Ramundo MS, de Jesus JG, Andrade PS, Coletti TM, Ferreira GM, Silva CAM, Manuli ER, Pereira RHM, Peixoto PS, Kraemer MUG, Gaburo N Jr, Camilo CDC, Hoeltgebaum H, Souza WM, Rocha EC, de Souza LM, de Pinho MC, Araujo LJT, Malta FSV, de Lima AB, Silva JDP, Zauli DAG, Ferreira ACS, Schnekenberg RP, Laydon DJ, Walker PGT, Schluter HM, Dos Santos ALP, Vidal MS, Del Caro VS, Filho RMF, Dos Santos HM, Aguiar RS, Proenca-Modena JL, Nelson B, Hay JA, Monod M, Miscouridou X, Coupland H, Sonabend R, Vollmer M, Gandy A, Prete CA Jr, Nascimento VH, Suchard MA, Bowden TA, Pond SLK, Wu CH, Ratmann O, Ferguson NM, Dye C, Loman NJ, Lemey P, Rambaut A, Fraiji NA, Carvalho M, Pybus OG, Flaxman S, Bhatt S, Sabino EC. Genomics and epidemiology of the P.1 SARS-CoV-2 lineage in Manaus, Brazil. Science. 2021;372(6544):815–21. https://doi.org/10.1126/science.abh2644.
48. Sabino EC, Buss LF, Carvalho MPS, Prete CA Jr, Crispim MAE, Fraiji NA, Pereira RHM, Parag KV, da Silva PP, Kraemer MUG, Oikawa MK, Salomon T, Cucunuba ZM, Castro MC, de Souza Santos AA, Nascimento VH, Pereira HS, Ferguson NM, Pybus OG, Kucharski A, Busch MP, Dye C, Faria NR. Resurgence of COVID-19 in Manaus, Brazil, despite high seroprevalence. Lancet. 2021;397(10273):452–5. https://doi.org/10.1016/S0140-6736(21)00183-5.
49. Choudhary OP, Priyanka SI, Rodriguez-Morales AJ. Second wave of COVID-19 in India: dissection of the causes and lessons learnt. Travel Med Infect Dis. 2021;43:102126. https://doi.org/10.1016/j.tmaid.2021.102126.
50. Sheikh A, McMenamin J, Taylor B, Robertson C, Public Health S, the EIIC. SARS-CoV-2 Delta VOC in Scotland: demographics, risk of hospital admission, and vaccine effectiveness. Lancet. 2021;397(10293):2461–2. https://doi.org/10.1016/S0140-6736(21)01358-1.

51. Campbell F, Archer B, Laurenson-Schafer H, Jinnai Y, Konings F, Batra N, Pavlin B, Vandemaele K, Van Kerkhove MD, Jombart T, Morgan O, le Polain de Waroux O. Increased transmissibility and global spread of SARS-CoV-2 variants of concern as at June 2021. Euro Surveill. 2021;26(24):2100509. https://doi.org/10.2807/1560-7917.ES.2021.26.24.2100509.
52. Saito A, Irie T, Suzuki R, Maemura T, Nasser H, Uriu K, Kosugi Y, Shirakawa K, Sadamasu K, Kimura I, Ito J, Wu J, Iwatsuki-Horimoto K, Ito M, Yamayoshi S, Loeber S, Tsuda M, Wang L, Ozono S, Butlertanaka EP, Tanaka YL, Shimizu R, Shimizu K, Yoshimatsu K, Kawabata R, Sakaguchi T, Tokunaga K, Yoshida I, Asakura H, Nagashima M, Kazuma Y, Nomura R, Horisawa Y, Yoshimura K, Takaori-Kondo A, Imai M, Genotype to Phenotype Japan C, Tanaka S, Nakagawa S, Ikeda T, Fukuhara T, Kawaoka Y, Sato K. Enhanced fusogenicity and pathogenicity of SARS-CoV-2 Delta P681R mutation. Nature. 2022;602(7896):300–6. https://doi.org/10.1038/s41586-021-04266-9.
53. Mlcochova P, Kemp SA, Dhar MS, Papa G, Meng B, Ferreira I, Datir R, Collier DA, Albecka A, Singh S, Pandey R, Brown J, Zhou J, Goonawardane N, Mishra S, Whittaker C, Mellan T, Marwal R, Datta M, Sengupta S, Ponnusamy K, Radhakrishnan VS, Abdullahi A, Charles O, Chattopadhyay P, Devi P, Caputo D, Peacock T, Wattal C, Goel N, Satwik A, Vaishya R, Agarwal M, Indian S-C-GC, Genotype to Phenotype Japan C, Collaboration C-NBC, Mavousian A, Lee JH, Bassi J, Silacci-Fegni C, Saliba C, Pinto D, Irie T, Yoshida I, Hamilton WL, Sato K, Bhatt S, Flaxman S, James LC, Corti D, Piccoli L, Barclay WS, Rakshit P, Agrawal A, Gupta RK. SARS-CoV-2 B.1.617.2 Delta variant replication and immune evasion. Nature. 2021;599(7883):114–9. https://doi.org/10.1038/s41586-021-03944-y.
54. Luo CH, Morris CP, Sachithanandham J, Amadi A, Gaston D, Li M, Swanson NJ, Schwartz M, Klein EY, Pekosz A, Mostafa HH. Infection with the SARS-CoV-2 Delta variant is associated with higher infectious virus loads compared to the alpha variant in both unvaccinated and vaccinated individuals. medRxiv. 2021;2021:21262077. https://doi.org/10.1101/2021.08.15.21262077.
55. Viana R, Moyo S, Amoako DG, Tegally H, Scheepers C, Althaus CL, Anyaneji UJ, Bester PA, Boni MF, Chand M, Choga WT, Colquhoun R, Davids M, Deforche K, Doolabh D, du Plessis L, Engelbrecht S, Everatt J, Giandhari J, Giovanetti M, Hardie D, Hill V, Hsiao NY, Iranzadeh A, Ismail A, Joseph C, Joseph R, Koopile L, Kosakovsky Pond SL, Kraemer MUG, Kuate-Lere L, Laguda-Akingba O, Lesetedi-Mafoko O, Lessells RJ, Lockman S, Lucaci AG, Maharaj A, Mahlangu B, Maponga T, Mahlakwane K, Makatini Z, Marais G, Maruapula D, Masupu K, Matshaba M, Mayaphi S, Mbhele N, Mbulawa MB, Mendes A, Mlisana K, Mnguni A, Mohale T, Moir M, Moruisi K, Mosepele M, Motsatsi G, Motswaledi MS, Mphoyakgosi T, Msomi N, Mwangi PN, Naidoo Y, Ntuli N, Nyaga M, Olubayo L, Pillay S, Radibe B, Ramphal Y, Ramphal U, San JE, Scott L, Shapiro R, Singh L, Smith-Lawrence P, Stevens W, Strydom A, Subramoney K, Tebeila N, Tshiabuila D, Tsui J, van Wyk S, Weaver S, Wibmer CK, Wilkinson E, Wolter N, Zarebski AE, Zuze B, Goedhals D, Preiser W, Treurnicht F, Venter M, Williamson C, Pybus OG, Bhiman J, Glass A, Martin DP, Rambaut A, Gaseitsiwe S, von Gottberg A, de Oliveira T. Rapid epidemic expansion of the SARS-CoV-2 omicron variant in southern Africa. Nature. 2022;603(7902):679–86. https://doi.org/10.1038/s41586-022-04411-y.
56. Karim SSA, Karim QA. Omicron SARS-CoV-2 variant: a new chapter in the COVID-19 pandemic. Lancet. 2021;398(10317):2126–8. https://doi.org/10.1016/S0140-6736(21)02758-6.
57. Cao Y, Wang J, Jian F, Xiao T, Song W, Yisimayi A, Huang W, Li Q, Wang P, An R, Wang J, Wang Y, Niu X, Yang S, Liang H, Sun H, Li T, Yu Y, Cui Q, Liu S, Yang X, Du S, Zhang Z, Hao X, Shao F, Jin R, Wang X, Xiao J, Wang Y, Xie XS. Omicron escapes the majority of existing SARS-CoV-2 neutralizing antibodies. Nature. 2022;602(7898):657–63. https://doi.org/10.1038/s41586-021-04385-3.
58. Liu L, Iketani S, Guo Y, Chan JF, Wang M, Liu L, Luo Y, Chu H, Huang Y, Nair MS, Yu J, Chik KK, Yuen TT, Yoon C, To KK, Chen H, Yin MT, Sobieszczyk ME, Huang Y, Wang HH, Sheng Z, Yuen KY, Ho DD. Striking antibody evasion manifested by the omicron variant of SARS-CoV-2. Nature. 2022;602(7898):676–81. https://doi.org/10.1038/s41586-021-04388-0.

59. Dejnirattisai W, Shaw RH, Supasa P, Liu C, Stuart AS, Pollard AJ, Liu X, Lambe T, Crook D, Stuart DI, Mongkolsapaya J, Nguyen-Van-Tam JS, Snape MD, Screaton GR, Com COVsg. Reduced neutralisation of SARS-CoV-2 omicron B.1.1.529 variant by post-immunisation serum. Lancet. 2022;399(10321):234–6. https://doi.org/10.1016/S0140-6736(21)02844-0.
60. Suzuki R, Yamasoba D, Kimura I, Wang L, Kishimoto M, Ito J, Morioka Y, Nao N, Nasser H, Uriu K, Kosugi Y, Tsuda M, Orba Y, Sasaki M, Shimizu R, Kawabata R, Yoshimatsu K, Asakura H, Nagashima M, Sadamasu K, Yoshimura K, Genotype to Phenotype Japan C, Sawa H, Ikeda T, Irie T, Matsuno K, Tanaka S, Fukuhara T, Sato K. Attenuated fusogenicity and pathogenicity of SARS-CoV-2 omicron variant. Nature. 2022;603(7902):700–5. https://doi.org/10.1038/s41586-022-04462-1.
61. Shuai H, Chan JF, Hu B, Chai Y, Yuen TT, Yin F, Huang X, Yoon C, Hu JC, Liu H, Shi J, Liu Y, Zhu T, Zhang J, Hou Y, Wang Y, Lu L, Cai JP, Zhang AJ, Zhou J, Yuan S, Brindley MA, Zhang BZ, Huang JD, To KK, Yuen KY, Chu H. Attenuated replication and pathogenicity of SARS-CoV-2 B.1.1.529 omicron. Nature. 2022;603(7902):693–9. https://doi.org/10.1038/s41586-022-04442-5.
62. Halfmann PJ, Iida S, Iwatsuki-Horimoto K, Maemura T, Kiso M, Scheaffer SM, Darling TL, Joshi A, Loeber S, Singh G, Foster SL, Ying B, Case JB, Chong Z, Whitener B, Moliva J, Floyd K, Ujie M, Nakajima N, Ito M, Wright R, Uraki R, Warang P, Gagne M, Li R, Sakai-Tagawa Y, Liu Y, Larson D, Osorio JE, Hernandez-Ortiz JP, Henry AR, Ciuoderis K, Florek KR, Patel M, Odle A, Wong LR, Bateman AC, Wang Z, Edara VV, Chong Z, Franks J, Jeevan T, Fabrizio T, DeBeauchamp J, Kercher L, Seiler P, Gonzalez-Reiche AS, Sordillo EM, Chang LA, van Bakel H, Simon V, Consortium Mount Sinai Pathogen Surveillance study g, Douek DC, Sullivan NJ, Thackray LB, Ueki H, Yamayoshi S, Imai M, Perlman S, Webby RJ, Seder RA, Suthar MS, Garcia-Sastre A, Schotsaert M, Suzuki T, ACM B, Diamond MS, Kawaoka Y. SARS-CoV-2 omicron virus causes attenuated disease in mice and hamsters. Nature. 2022;603(7902):687–92. https://doi.org/10.1038/s41586-022-04441-6.
63. van Dorp L, Acman M, Richard D, Shaw LP, Ford CE, Ormond L, Owen CJ, Pang J, Tan CCS, Boshier FAT, Ortiz AT, Balloux F. Emergence of genomic diversity and recurrent mutations in SARS-CoV-2. Infect Genet Evol. 2020;83:104351. https://doi.org/10.1016/j.meegid.2020.104351.
64. Pachetti M, Marini B, Benedetti F, Giudici F, Mauro E, Storici P, Masciovecchio C, Angeletti S, Ciccozzi M, Gallo RC, Zella D, Ippodrino R. Emerging SARS-CoV-2 mutation hot spots include a novel RNA-dependent-RNA polymerase variant. J Transl Med. 2020;18(1):179. https://doi.org/10.1186/s12967-020-02344-6.
65. Young BE, Fong SW, Chan YH, Mak TM, Ang LW, Anderson DE, Lee CY, Amrun SN, Lee B, Goh YS, Su YCF, Wei WE, Kalimuddin S, Chai LYA, Pada S, Tan SY, Sun L, Parthasarathy P, Chen YYC, Barkham T, Lin RTP, Maurer-Stroh S, Leo YS, Wang LF, Renia L, Lee VJ, Smith GJD, Lye DC, Ng LFP. Effects of a major deletion in the SARS-CoV-2 genome on the severity of infection and the inflammatory response: an observational cohort study. Lancet. 2020;396(10251):603–11. https://doi.org/10.1016/S0140-6736(20)31757-8.
66. Lan J, Ge J, Yu J, Shan S, Zhou H, Fan S, Zhang Q, Shi X, Wang Q, Zhang L, Wang X. Structure of the SARS-CoV-2 spike receptor-binding domain bound to the ACE2 receptor. Nature. 2020;581(7807):215–20. https://doi.org/10.1038/s41586-020-2180-5.
67. Baum A, Fulton BO, Wloga E, Copin R, Pascal KE, Russo V, Giordano S, Lanza K, Negron N, Ni M, Wei Y, Atwal GS, Murphy AJ, Stahl N, Yancopoulos GD, Kyratsous CA. Antibody cocktail to SARS-CoV-2 spike protein prevents rapid mutational escape seen with individual antibodies. Science. 2020;369(6506):1014–8. https://doi.org/10.1126/science.abd0831.
68. Wu K, Choi A, Koch M, Ma L, Hill A, Nunna N, Huang W, Oestreicher J, Colpitts T, Bennett H, Legault H, Paila Y, Nestorova B, Ding B, Pajon R, Miller JM, Leav B, Carfi A, McPhee R, Edwards DK. Preliminary analysis of safety and immunogenicity of a SARS-CoV-2 variant vaccine booster. medRxiv. 2021;2021:21256716. https://doi.org/10.1101/2021.05.05.21256716.

# Chapter 28
# COVID-19 Vaccines Authorized by Stringent Regulatory Authorities and Vaccine Candidates Expecting Approval in 2021

**Melvin Sanicas, T. Anh Wartel, and Merlin Sanicas**

## Introduction

The COVID-19 pandemic has had sweeping effects that disrupted every part of society worldwide necessitating the development of vaccines against this novel virus, SARS-CoV-2. Different approaches are currently used to develop COVID-19 vaccines from traditional live-attenuated, inactivated, subunit vaccines, to more novel technologies such as DNA or mRNA vaccines. Of the over 300 vaccine candidates, approximately 100 are in clinical trials while 18 have been authorized for use. In this chapter, we discuss the different technologies used in vaccine development and the COVID-19 vaccines developed for each modality. We then describe in detail the different vaccines that have been approved by any national regulatory authority and the publicly available data for these vaccines. Here we have included vaccines that have received emergency use approval (EUA) or full approval from stringent regulatory authorities (SRA) or World Health Organization (WHO) Emergency Use Listing (EUL). We also discuss how the vaccines have been developed in less than a year. We have also identified the knowledge gaps that need to be filled to understand the important questions like durability of protection, the need for a booster, long-term safety and efficacy against emerging SARS-CoV-2 variants.

M. Sanicas
Clinical - Vaccines, Clover Biopharmaceuticals, Zürich, Switzerland

Grupo de Genética de Micobacterias, Dpto. Microbiología, Medicina Preventiva y Salud Pública, Universidad de Zaragoza, Zaragoza, Spain

T. A. Wartel (✉)
International Vaccine Institute, Seoul, Republic of Korea
e-mail: anh.wartel@ivi.int

M. Sanicas
Centre de Recherche en Cancérologie de Marseille, Aix-Marseille Université, Marseille, France


S. Adibi et al. (eds.), *Frontiers of COVID-19*,
https://doi.org/10.1007/978-3-031-08045-6_28

## Vaccine Development and Production Timeline

Prior to the COVID-19 pandemic and the unprecedented achievement that is the speed of producing the COVID-19 vaccines, the development and production process of a vaccine is long and arduous. The phases of a vaccine production process can be divided roughly into the following phases: the pre-clinical phase, the clinical phase and the licensing and post-market surveillance [1–4] these phases often span more than a decade for each vaccine being produced (Fig. 28.1), especially if it was the first for a specific disease or vaccine type. To understand this process, we will discuss each of the phases.

1. *Pre-clinical phase*. This is the initial phase of any vaccine development process and can be subdivided into the following:

   (a) *Exploratory phase*: This phase includes gathering data such as disease burden, the infectious organism's life cycle and the pathologic mechanism of the disease. This is then followed by identifying candidate antigens to target. These antigens can be surface molecules or regulatory molecules that are conserved within the species that can be related to the pathogen's mechanism of entry or a critical component of its life cycle. These target antigens may include entire pathogens that have been attenuated or inactivated; molecules such as recombinant proteins or polysaccharides. For recombinant proteins or polysaccharide antigens, specific formulation and optimization steps may be necessary to enhance the immunogenicity through the addition of adjuvants. Immunogenicity, defined as a vaccine candidate's ability to induce the immune response is tested using in vitro methods at this stage. The phase ends with several iterations of the vaccine candidate that will then undergo the following stage.

   (b) *Animal model*: A set of animal models are chosen based on its similarity to the disease condition in humans, oftentimes mice and non-human primates. This step will provide the vaccine candidates' immunogenicity in vivo, its initial safety and toxicology profile, initial dosing and method of delivery, its ability to protect and reduce disease burden on the animal models using challenge studies.

   (c) *Submission for an investigational new drug (IND) to the National Regulatory Authorities (NRA)*: This application includes the manufacturing process of the vaccine candidates that are planned to move forward with clinical testing, the formulation of the vaccine, and the results of the in vitro and the in vivo animal models. This application also includes the proposed clinical study and how it will validate the efficacy and safety of the vaccine candidates.

2. *Clinical trials*. After the NRA approves the application, the vaccine candidates will now undergo the proposed clinical trial design. The gold standard study design being a randomized double-blind placebo-controlled study [6]. This can be subdivided into the following.

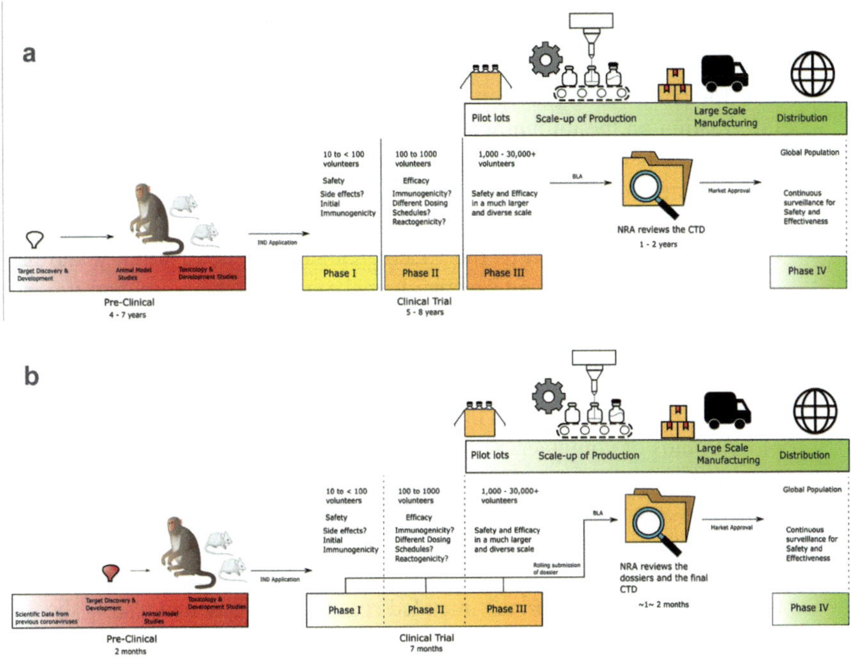


**Fig. 28.1** Vaccine Development and Production Timeline difference between previously produced vaccines and the COVID-19 Vaccines. (**a**) Previous vaccines followed a development and production timeline that lasts around 15 years in total. The pre-clinical phase lasting around 4-7 years begins with discovery and development of candidate targets followed by the animal models. The traditional clinical trial phase follows a sequential progression from phase I to III, spanning around 5-8 years where each phase has to close, the data be analyzed, meet the clinical objectives and be approved prior to progressing into the next phase. Once all 3 phases are finished it is then followed by the preparation of the CTD to be submitted for a BLA. Scale up of production occurs alongside the application and once approved, global distribution and post-marketing surveillance begins. (**b**) In contrast to the canonical vaccines, the development and production timeline of the SARS-CoV-2 vaccines was modified in response to the ongoing pandemic. Thanks to a global coordinated effort to identify the best target antigen and the already existing scientific data on previous coronaviruses, the pre-clinical phase only lasted 2 months and entered the clinical phase shortly after. The COVID-19 vaccines' clinical trial had the current phase running in parallel with the next phase if interim data analysis showed promising results which shortened the overall clinical trial duration. Instead of one final document submitted at the end of the 3 clinical trials in the traditional sense, COVID-19 vaccines had a rolling submission to the NRA which also decreased the time for approval. Manufacturing scale-up and production was occurring simultaneous to the Phase III trials which allowed for immediate global distribution once approved and followed by post-marketing surveillance

(a) *Phase I clinical trial*: This phase includes ten to less than a hundred healthy volunteers, usually in adults and lasts several months. The primary objective is to prove that the vaccine candidates are safe and no serious adverse events are related to the vaccine. Common side effects are noted such as local and systemic adverse reactions. The immunogenicity is also measured.

(b) *Phase II clinical trial*: This phase includes hundreds to a thousand volunteers and could last up to a few years. They may also begin to include groups that are at higher risk of acquiring the disease to represent the target population for protection. The primary emphasis of this phase is to have more information on the immunogenicity such as the optimal dose strength, how many doses is necessary, the interval between the doses and comparing different routes of administration. This phase also consists of validating the assays necessary to measure the immunogenicity. Safety data is continuously monitored as well as the vaccine candidate's compatibility and harmony with already existing vaccines to make sure that there is no interference with the immune response of each. The manufacturing and the formulation processes are also finalized at this point in preparation for the production of the pilot lots.

(c) *Phase III clinical trial*: This final phase of the clinical trial enrols up to tens of thousands of volunteers in different geographic locations and ethnicity to have a more global representation of the clinical database and may last a few years. Vaccine efficacy, defined as the estimated reduction in the chance to develop the disease in the vaccinated group in comparison to the placebo group [7] is also established at this point. This also includes the upscaling of the production process to the intended commercial scale and testing the first three sets produced called the pilot lots. This is to validate and document the consistency of the production process and the quality of the vaccines produced (i.e. lot-to-lot consistency).

3. *Licensing and post-market surveillance.*

(a) *License application*: If the clinical trial succeeds, the vaccine developers and sponsors can now submit for a Biologics License Application (BLA) to regulatory authority. They submit a common technical document (CTD) that compiles information from all the previous stages: the pre-clinical data, the clinical trial data, and the quality of the manufacturing process. The regulatory authority will then assess the information provided and will decide whether to approve the vaccine or not. This process takes up to 2 years.

(b) *Stringent regulatory authority*: A stringent regulatory authority or SRA is a regulatory authority which is: a member of the International Council for Harmonisation of Technical Requirements for Pharmaceuticals for Human Use (ICH), being the European Commission, the U.S. Food and Drug Administration and the Ministry of Health, Labour and Welfare of Japan also represented by the Pharmaceuticals and Medical Devices Agency (as before 23 October 2015); or an ICH observer, being the European Free Trade Association, as represented by Swissmedic, and Health Canada (as before 23 October 2015); or a regulatory authority associated with an ICH member through a legally binding, mutual recognition agreement [8].

(c) *Phase IV clinical trial*: Once approved, the vaccine may then begin its large-scale production and distribution to the countries where the marketing authorization is obtained. A phase IV trial, or the post-marketing surveillance, is also started to assess the effectiveness of the vaccine in the general population (i.e. real world setting) and also continuously monitor for serious adverse events or possible long-term side effects or rare events that cannot be detected within the well-controlled setting of clinical trials.

## How Were COVID-19 Vaccines Developed in Less Than a Year

Development for most of the vaccines we currently have took several years to several decades. Here is a summary of the different vaccine-preventable diseases, the year when the pathogens were discovered and the year when the respective vaccines became available (Table 28.1).

The COVID-19 vaccines were developed in less than a year. Several factors contributed to the unprecedented speed of development:

**Table 28.1** Pathogens, year of discovery, year of vaccine availability, duration in years from discovery to vaccine availability [9]

| Pathogen | Discovery | Vaccine availability | Discovery to vaccine (years) |
|---|---|---|---|
| *Mycobacterium tuberculosis* | 1882 | 1921 | 39 |
| *Haemophilus influenzae* B | 1892 | 1985 | 93 |
| Malaria parasite | 1897 | 2015 (not yet widely used) | 118 |
| Yellow fever | 1900 | 1935 | 35 |
| *Bordetella pertussis* | 1906 | 1926 | 20 |
| Polio | 1908 | 1953 (inactivated), 1956 (oral) | 45 (inactivated), 48 (oral) |
| Herpes (HSV-1) | 1919 | No vaccine | 100 + |
| Influenza | 1933 | 1945 | 12 |
| Dengue virus | 1943 | 2015 | 72 |
| Mumps | 1945 | 1948 (inactivated), 1967 (attenuated) | 3 (inactivated), 22 (attenuated) |
| Measles | 1954 | 1963 | 9 |
| Hepatitis B | 1965 | 1981 | 16 |
| Ebola virus | 1976 | 2019 | 43 |
| Hepatitis A | 1973 | 1995 | 22 |
| Human papillomavirus (HPV) | 1974 | 2006 | 32 |
| Human immunodeficiency virus (HIV) | 1983 | No vaccine | 38 + |
| SARS coronavirus/ SARS-CoV | 2002 | No vaccine (virus disappeared!) | XX |
| MERS coronavirus | 2012 | No vaccine | 9 + |
| SARS-CoV-2 (COVID-19) | 2019 | 2020 | 0.875 |

## *Vaccine Trials Were Done in Parallel Instead of Sequential*

When doing clinical studies, typically Phase 1 is completed, results are gathered, a manuscript is prepared for submission to a peer-reviewed journal, while funding for Phase 2 is secured. Then Phase 2 is performed, results are gathered, a manuscript is prepared for submission to a peer-reviewed journal, while funding for Phase 3 is secured similarly. Many COVID-19 vaccine studies combined Phase 1 and Phase 2 or Phase 2 and Phase 3. If the vaccine appears to be safe without any safety signals, more participants were added. Developing vaccines in a pandemic requires a fast start and several steps executed in parallel before confirming a successful outcome of another step [10].

## *Rolling Submission of Regulatory Dossier*

In a non-pandemic situation, submission for review to National or stringent regulatory agencies only happen once Phase 1, 2, and 3 studies are completed, and regulatory dossiers are prepared detailing the product's efficacy, safety and quality. Only then can a formal application for marketing authorization to National or stringent regulatory agencies (NRA/SRA) be submitted and reviewed by the agency's internal or external statisticians, medical and clinical reviewers, regulatory scientists and external advisory board of scientific and medical experts. For COVID-19 vaccines, data from clinical trials were submitted on a rolling basis. Developers were sending the data to the regulators as they become available and the regulators were reviewing the data as they were submitted [11]. The guidance for emergency use approval (EUA) for COVID-19 vaccine by the U.S. Food and Drugs Administration (FDA) allowed developers to submit regulatory dossier with a median duration of 2 months for clinical data [12].

## *Scientific Data from Other Coronaviruses*

SARS-CoV-2 is not the first coronavirus. Scientists have been studying coronaviruses for over half a century now starting from the non-pandemic human coronaviruses including types 229E, NL63, OC43 and HKU1. All of these coronaviruses usually cause mild to moderate upper respiratory tract illnesses, like the common cold. For years, researchers had been studying related coronaviruses, which cause SARS (severe acute respiratory syndrome) and MERS (Middle East respiratory syndrome) and knowledge has been gained from the initial development of vaccines for SARS and MERS so the discovery phase was omitted and some processes were adopted to help accelerate the timeline [5]. Vaccine developers had existing data on the structure, genome and life cycle of coronaviruses [9].

## *Global Collaboration and Data Sharing*

Chinese researchers quickly sequenced the virus and shared their data with other scientists early in January 2020. Once the genomic sequence became available to the global scientific community, vaccine developers started creating SARS-CoV-2 vaccine candidates. Many labs working on other pathogens stopped their research to focus on COVID-19.

## *Funding for COVID-19 Vaccine Research*

Vaccine development is expensive—the cost of developing a vaccine—from research and discovery to product registration—is estimated to be between U.S. $200 million and U.S. $500 million per vaccine. However, for the COVID-19 pandemic, the USA, European Union, UK and several other developed countries together with philanthropic organizations and funding agencies like the Bill & Melinda Gates Foundation, Wellcome Trust and CEPI pledged billions of dollars to fund vaccine research. Even celebrities like Dolly Parton donated $1 M to coronavirus vaccine research. The U.S. government's Operation Warp Speed invested over 18 billion USD to support the development of 7 vaccine candidates [13]. In a non-pandemic situation, developers need to apply for funding to start new studies or continue existing ones. Even in private companies doing vaccine development, projects may be postponed or completely stopped because of competing priorities or lack of funding.

## *Coalition for Epidemic Preparedness Innovations (CEPI)*

CEPI is an innovative global partnership between public, private, philanthropic and civil society organizations launched in 2017 in Davos, Switzerland at the World Economic Forum. CEPI aims to develop vaccines to stop future epidemics. CEPI has invested in 12 COVID-19 vaccine candidates, including mRNA vaccine from Moderna, a protein-based coronavirus vaccine developed by Novavax, and the ChAdOx1 viral vector vaccine developed by Oxford University and AstraZeneca [14].

## *Advancements in Science and Technology*

The vaccine platforms that enabled the first COVID-19 vaccines to reach the finish line used the mRNA technology (i.e. Pfizer/Biotech vaccine, Moderna vaccine). These are the first mRNA vaccines licensed but scientists have been studying this technology since the 1990s. Another mRNA vaccine in Phase 3 clinical trials is being developed by CureVac, the world's first company to successfully harness mRNA for medical purposes. The company was founded in 2000 and CureVac has started mRNA vaccine research since then [15]. The basic research on DNA vaccines began at least 25 years ago, and RNA vaccines have benefited from 10–15 years of strong research [16]. The viral vector vaccines (i.e. Oxford Astra Zeneca and Janssen vaccine) also benefited from having existing vaccines already licensed and used (i.e. Ebola vaccine).

## *COVID-19 Community Transmission in Many Countries*

Apart from Taiwan and New Zealand, COVID-19 community transmission still happens. Countries like the USA, UK, Russia, Mexico, France, India, Indonesia, Portugal and Italy record over 10,000 new cases per day. When doing efficacy trials for vaccines, one group is given the vaccine candidate, the other group gets a placebo or an existing vaccine. Then they are monitored for months until the clinical trial reaches a pre-specified number of COVID-19 cases. Then the data will be analyzed to calculate vaccine efficacy by looking at how many of the infected individuals were vaccinated and unvaccinated. Because there is widespread transmission, the different trials reached the required number of cases faster [9].

## Different Types of Vaccines for COVID-19

Vaccine developers working on a coronavirus vaccine are using different vaccine types, with their respective advantages and disadvantages (Table 28.2 and Fig. 28.2).

Many conventional vaccines use whole viruses to trigger an immune response. There are two main approaches. *Live-attenuated vaccines*, such as the measles–mumps–rubella (MMR) vaccine, contain attenuated (weakened) forms of the disease-causing pathogen that can still replicate without causing illness. This attenuated organism acts as an antigen and stimulates the body to create a robust antibody response but may risk causing disease in people with weak or compromised immune systems. There are no approved live-attenuated vaccines for COVID but there are candidate vaccines, developed by Mehmet Ali Aydinlar University and Acibadem Labmed Health Services A.S., Meissa Vaccines, Indian Immunologicals LTD and Griffith University, and Codagenix/Serum Institute of India [19].

*Inactivated vaccines*, including most influenza vaccines and the inactivated polio vaccine, contain a version of an organism that has been killed or inactivated using chemicals, heat or radiation. This killed form acts as an antigen and stimulates the body to create an antibody response. Inactivated virus vaccines can be given to people with compromised immune systems. Both types use well-established technology and pathways for regulatory approval however, both require special laboratory facilities to grow the virus or bacterium safely before it can be inactivated or weakened [17, 20].

**Table 28.2** Different vaccine approaches—their advantages and disadvantage [17, 18]

| | Live attenuated | Inactivated | Protein subunit | Vector-based | mRNA |
|---|---|---|---|---|---|
| + | Single dose can provide long lasting and effective immunity<br>No adjuvants needed<br>May have cross protection<br>Well-established technology<br>Relatively simple to manufacture | Safer—No risk of recovering virulence and causing disease<br>Suitable for people with compromised immune systems<br>Well-established technology<br>Relatively simple to manufacture | Safer<br>Applicable to populations who are immuno-compromised/ immunosenescent long-term immunity<br>Well-established technology | Innate immune response stimulation, T and B cell response induction<br>Versatility based on vector used<br>Well-established technology | Not infectious, no live components, no risk of triggering disease<br>No risk for genome integration<br>Relatively easy to manufacture |
| – | May recover virulence and cause disease<br>Horizontal spread of vaccine strain possible<br>Relatively temperature sensitive<br>Transient immunosuppression | Short-lived immunity without adjuvants<br>Booster shots may be required | Low immunogenicity<br>Needs multiple dosing for long-term protection<br>Adjuvants and booster shots may be required<br>Relatively complex to manufacture<br>Identifying the best antigen takes time | Possibility of anti-vector immunity or pre-existing anti-vector immunity<br>Relatively complex to manufacture | Instability concern<br>Require ultra-cold storage<br>Booster shots may be required |

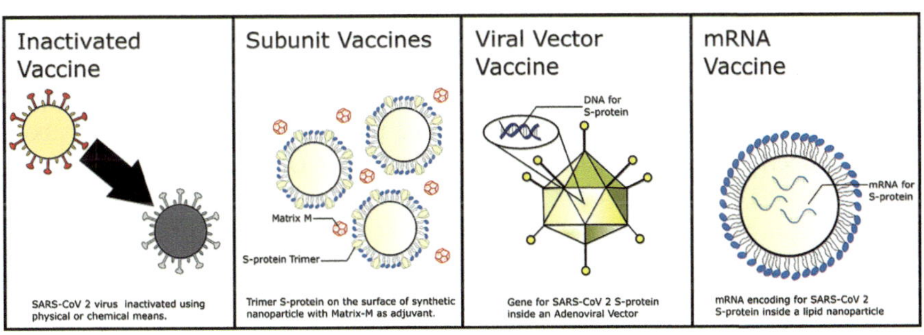


**Fig. 28.2** COVID-19 vaccine types available as of June 2021

## *CoronaVac (SinoVac Biotech)*

CoronaVac is an inactivated COVID-19 vaccine developed and manufactured by Beijing-based SinoVac Biotech. CoronaVac's main advantages is that it can be stored in a standard refrigerator at 2–8 °C. A randomised, double-blind, placebo-controlled phase I/II study was conducted on healthy adults aged 18–59 years old in

Suining County of Jiangsu province, China [21] and 60 and over in Renqiu, Hebei, China [22]. The trials found immunogenicity in most subjects and that the vaccine was generally safe and well tolerated, with few adverse effects. At the time of writing, no phase III trial data have been published in a peer reviewed journal but interim data from late-stage trials in Turkey, Indonesia and Brazil showed that the vaccine efficacy was 91.25% [23], 65.3% [24], and 50.4% [25] respectively. Final Phase III results from Turkey announced in March 2021 showed an efficacy of 83.5% [26]. A real-world study of millions of Chileans who received the vaccine found it 67% effective against symptoms, reduced hospitalizations by 85%, intensive care visits by 89%, and deaths by 80% [27]. Similar real-world data from Indonesia that followed 128,290 health workers in Jakarta showed 94% of vaccinated healthcare professionals were protected against symptomatic infection, 98% of them were protected from death and 96% from hospitalization as soon as 7 days after the second dose [28].

### *BBIBP-CorV (Sinopharm)*

BBIBP-CorV, an inactivated vaccine co-developed by SinoPharm and Beijing Bio-Institute of Biological Products (BBIBP), is the first Chinese COVID-19 vaccine given emergency use listing (EUL) by the World Health Organization (WHO) on May 7, 2021, 5 months after China's National Medical Products Administration authorized it on December 31, 2020 [29]. BBIBP-CorV contains SARS-CoV-2 that has undergone treatment with a chemical called beta-propiolactone which binds to SARS-CoV-2's genetic material and stops it from replicating and causing disease. The vaccine also contains the adjuvant aluminium hydroxide. WHO's Strategic Advisory Group of Experts on Immunization (SAGE) recommends the vaccine for people 18 years old and above with an interval of 3–4 weeks between the two doses. The WHO estimates overall vaccine efficacy to be around 78% while noting that data on adults over the age of 60 years are lacking [30]. Published data to support BBIBP-CorV vaccine are lacking. Data from a phase I/II trial that involved about 600 volunteers was published in The Lancet Infectious Diseases [31].

### *Covaxin (Bharat Biotech)*

Covaxin (also known as BBV152) is an inactivated COVID-19 vaccine formulated with a toll-like receptor 7/8 agonist molecule (IMDG) adsorbed to alum (Algel) developed by Hyderabad-based Indian biotechnology company Bharat Biotech in collaboration with the Indian Council of Medical Research. Phase I trial results showed that the vaccine was well-tolerated and enhanced immune responses [32].

In Phase I, BBV152 induced high neutralizing antibody responses that remained elevated in all participants at 3 months after the second vaccination. In Phase II, BBV152 showed better reactogenicity and safety outcomes, and enhanced humoral and cell-mediated immune responses compared with the phase I trial as doses in Phase II were given at 4 weeks interval as opposed to 2 weeks in Phase I [33]. Bharat Biotech reported via a press release that efficacy is 78%, in its interim analysis of its phase III trial [34].

*Subunit vaccines* do not contain the organism itself but use fragments of protein from the pathogen as antigens to trigger an immune response. Doing so minimizes the risk of side effects but also means a weaker immune response as compared to vaccines using the whole pathogen. Because of this, subunit vaccine often requires adjuvants [35] to improve the immune response. An example of an existing subunit vaccine is the hepatitis B vaccine [17, 18]. There are over 60 protein subunit vaccines against SARS-CoV-2 under development, including RBD-trimer of S protein, S1, recombinant S proteins, N, M proteins and others.

## *NVX-CoV2373 (Novavax)*

NVX-CoV2373 is a protein-based vaccine candidate engineered from the genetic sequence of the first strain of SARS-CoV-2 and created using Novavax's recombinant nanoparticle technology using the Sf9 insect cell baculovirus system to generate antigen derived from the coronavirus spike (S) protein and is adjuvanted with the company's saponin-based Matrix-M™ to enhance the immune response. It was generally well-tolerated and elicited robust antibody response in Phase I/II clinical testing [36]. NVX-CoV2373 is being evaluated in two pivotal Phase III trials: a trial in the UK included more than 15,000 people aged 18–84 years old which showed 100% protection against severe disease, efficacy of 96.4% against the original virus strain, 86.3% against the B.1.1.7/501Y.V1 variant and 89.7% overall; and the PREVENT-19 trial in the USA and Mexico that began in December 2020 [37]. In a Phase II study, NVX-CoV2373 vaccine was efficacious in preventing COVID-19, with higher vaccine efficacy observed among HIV-negative participants. Most infections in this trial conducted in South Africa were caused by the B.1.351 variant [38].

*Viral vector vaccines* use either a harmless virus or plasmids, different from the one the vaccine is targeting, to giving cells genetic instructions to produce antigens [39]. Genes of a pathogen are inserted into the genome of the vector which infects host cells and then travels to the nucleus to express the genes of the pathogen. Viral vector vaccines can mimic natural viral infection and trigger a strong immune response. Vectored vaccines can be replicating (viral vector is produced and able to infect new cells, which then create more viral antigen) or non-replicating (vaccine antigen is produced but the viral vector cannot be reproduced) [40].

## ChAdOx1/AZD1222 (Oxford University/Astra-Zeneca)

The ChAdOx1, also known as AZD1222, was developed at Oxford University and its technology consists of a replication-deficient chimpanzee adenoviral vector ChAdOx1, containing the SARS-CoV-2 structural surface glycoprotein antigen (spike protein) gene. The original pooled efficacy analysis of four randomized controlled studies in Brazil, South Africa, and UK in study participants who received two standards doses or a low dose followed by a standard dose showed vaccine efficacy of 62.1% (95% CI 41.0–75.7; 27 [0.6%] of 4440 in the ChAdOx1 group vs. 71 [1.6%] of 4455 in the control group) and vaccine efficacy of 90.0% (95% CI 67.4–97.0; 3 [0.2%] of 1367 in the ChAdOx1 group vs. 30 [2.2%] of 1374 in the control group), respectively. Overall vaccine efficacy on average was 70.4% (95% CI 54.8–80.6; 30 [0.5%] of 5807 in the ChAdOx1 group vs. 101 [1.7%] of 5829 in the control group) against confirmed symptomatic COVID-19. The timing of priming and booster dose could not be given within 4 weeks as initially planned due to manufacturing process, thus varied between studies, and ranged from 6 to 12 weeks after the first dose [41]. Emerging real world effectiveness data has started emerging to confirm or not the findings in well-controlled setting such as the phase III randomized controlled trial. Thus, with ChAdOx1 vaccine, effects were observed from 2 to 3 weeks after vaccination, reaching an effectiveness of 60% (41–73%) from 4 to 5 weeks, increasing to 73% (27–90%) from 5 weeks onwards [42].

## Sputnik V (Gamaleya Institute)

The Sputnik V COVID-19 vaccine (rAd26 and rAd5 vector-based COVID-19 vaccine Gam-COVID-19, both vectors carrying the gene for the full-length SARS-CoV-2 glycoprotein S) is developed at Gamaleya Institute administered in two-dose regimen, 21 days apart. The phase III efficacy study conducted in 21,977 adults randomly assigned to the vaccine group ($n$ = 16, 501) and the placebo group ($n$ = 5476) showed an overall efficacy of 91.6% (95% CI 85.6–95.2) against COVID-19 from day 21 after the first dose, the day of receiving the second dose. Vaccine efficacy was consistently equal or greater than 90% by age groups (i.e. 18–30 years, 31–40 years, 41–50 years; 51–60 years; >60 years). Furthermore, protection against moderate or severe COVID-19 was 100% (95% CI 94.4–100.0%) [43].

## Ad26.COV2.S (Johnson & Johnson)

Ad26.COV2.S vaccine manufactured by Johnson & Johnson is a recombinant, replication-incompetent human adenovirus type 26 vector encoding full-length spike protein in a prefusion-stabilized conformation. Per protocol analysis after single dose showed a protection level of 66.9% (116 cases in the vaccine group vs. 348 in the placebo group; adjusted 95% CI 59.0–73.4) against moderate to severe–critical COVID-19 cases and 66.1% (66 cases in the vaccine group vs. 193 in the placebo group; adjusted 95% CI 55.0–74.8) with onset at least 14 days and 28 days after injection, respectively. Vaccine efficacy against the severe COVID-19 cases was higher, 76.7% (adjusted 95% CI 54.6–89.1) and 85.4% (adjusted 95% CI 54.2–96.9) with onset at least 14 days and 28 days after injection, respectively [44].

All the three COVID-19 viral vectored vaccines have to be stored in refrigerator temperature between 2 and 8 °C.

*Nucleic acid vaccines* use genetic material—either RNA or DNA—to provide cells with the instructions to make the antigen. mRNA vaccines contain messenger RNA (mRNA), a single-stranded RNA molecule that complements DNA and created when DNA is transcribed by RNA polymerase to create pre-mRNA [45] Once the genetic material enters human cells, it uses our cells' machinery to make the antigen that will trigger an immune response. Because the antigen is produced inside our cells and in large amounts, the immune response is expected to be strong. The existing RNA vaccines need to be kept at ultra-cold temperatures which may prove challenging for countries in low- and middle-income countries [17, 18]. The concept of mRNA vaccines was first developed in the early 1990s [46].

## *Comirnaty mRNA Vaccine (Pfizer, BioNTech, Fosun)*

Comirnaty or Tozinameran or BNT162b2 is an mRNA vaccine developed by the German biotech company BioNTech in cooperation with the U.S. pharmaceutical company Pfizer and the Chinese pharmaceutical company Fosun. Comirnaty received emergency use authorization from the U.S. Food and Drug Administration in December 2020 for use in individuals 16 years of age and older, making it the first COVID-19 m-RNA vaccine authorized in the USA. The vaccine, given by intramuscular injection, is composed of nucleoside-modified mRNA (modRNA) encoding a mutated form of the full-length spike protein of SARS-CoV-2 encapsulated in lipid nanoparticles. The ongoing Phase III clinical trial, scheduled to run from 2020 to 2022, assesses the safety, efficacy, tolerability and immunogenicity of 2 doses of BNT162b2 separated by 21 days in three age groups: 12–15 years, 16–55 years or above 55 years. The trial involved over 44,000 participants half given the vaccine and half given placebo. Vaccine efficacy was calculated from over 36,000 participants (including people over 75 years of age. The study showed a 95% reduction in the number of symptomatic COVID-19 cases in the people who received the vaccine (8 cases out of 18,198 developed COVID-19 symptoms) compared with people who received a dummy injection (162 cases out of 18,325 developed COVID-19 symptoms) [47]. Since 31st December 2020, Comminate has been the first COVID-19 vaccine to receive emergency use validation from the World Health Organization [18].

## *SpikeVax (mRNA-1273) (Moderna, National Institutes of Health)*

mRNA-1273 COVID-19 vaccine is a lipid nanoparticle-encapsulated, nucleoside-modified mRNA vaccine encoding the stabilized prefusion spike glycoprotein of SARS-CoV-2 developed by Moderna Therapeutics and the U.S. National institutes of Health. On December 18, 2020, the Food and Drug Administration issued an Emergency Use Authorization (EUA) for the Moderna COVID-19 vaccine [48]. Moderna's vaccine remains stable at −20 °C, the temperature of a household freezer, for up to 6 months. It can remain refrigerated at 4 °C for up to 30 days [49]. By contrast, Pfizer's mRNA COVID-19 vaccine needs to be stored long-term below −60 °C, though unopened vials can be stored at freezer temperatures for up to 2 weeks [50]. Phase 3 clinical trials of the vaccine, with 30,420 volunteers, showed 94.1% efficacy at preventing COVID-19 as well as complete protection against severe forms of the disease. Symptomatic Covid-19 illness was confirmed in 185 participants in the placebo group (56.5 per 1000 person-years; 95% confidence interval [CI] 48.7–65.3) and in 11 participants in the mRNA-1273 group (3.3 per 1000 person-years; 95% CI 1.7–6.0); vaccine efficacy was 94.1% (95% CI 89.3–96.8%; $P < 0.001$) [51]. WHO's SAGE recommends the use of the Moderna mRNA-1273 vaccine at a schedule of two doses (100 μg, 0.5 mL each) 28 days apart. If necessary, the interval between the doses may be extended to 42 days [52].

## *Zy-CoV-D COVID-19 DNA vaccine (Zydus Cadila)*

ZyCov-D, also India's first needle-free COVID-19 vaccine, uses plasmids to deliver the vaccine between two layers of the skin. It is administered with a disposable needle-free injector, which uses a narrow stream of the fluid to penetrate the skin and deliver the vaccine to the proper tissue. Once the plasmids enter the nuclei of cells, they are converted into mRNA, which travels to the cytoplasm and is translated into the spike protein itself. According to an interim study that has yet to be published in a scientific journal, ZyCoV-D has been found to be 67% protective against symptomatic COVID-19. The efficacy figure of 67% came from trials involving more than 28,000 participants, which saw 21 symptomatic cases of COVID-19 in the vaccinated group and 60 among people who received a placebo. The Phase 3 clinical trial in India was conducted at the peak of the second wave of the pandemic in India with the SARS-CoV-2 variants circulating. Several other DNA vaccines against COVID-19 are in clinical trials globally [53].

## Current Knowledge Gaps

Per U.S. FDA guidance, the vaccines that have been authorized for emergency use have included a median follow-up duration of at least 2 month-clinical data after the primary series following U.S. FDA guideline [54]. It is thus essential to continue generating safety and efficacy data even though the COVID-19 vaccines are being used under EUA to address the waning immunity and the enhanced disease that has been of concern at the beginning of SARS-CoV-2 pandemic and remains of concern [55]. Furthermore, other gaps such as the need for a booster dose, heterologous prime-boost regimen (related to interchangeability question which is often time raised for programmatic supply issue), applicable to the COVID-19 pandemic and the need to also vaccinate the paediatric population have been raised [5]. Additional complementary studies in paediatric population have been conducted leading to the authorization of the COVID-19 vaccines in adolescents with Pfizer/BioNtech m-RNA vaccine [56]. Heterologous prime-boost interim safety data under com-COV protocol (a topic of high interest in light of the anticipated vaccine shortages that may slow down the vaccine roll-out), found that following prime-boost permutations of ChAdOx and Pfizer/BioNtech there was an increase of systemic reactogenicity after the boost dose in heterologous vaccine schedules in comparison to homologous vaccine schedules requiring an increased paracetamol use from the study participants [57].

As with any other vaccines, pregnant women should be considered in clinical trials and can also benefit from vaccination [58] since they may be at potential risk of severe COVID-19 and adverse pregnancy outcomes [59]. Vaccine trial with m-RNA has been conducted—m-RNA vaccine was shown to be immunogenic in pregnant women, and vaccine-elicited antibodies were transported to infant cord blood and breast milk. Pregnant and nonpregnant women who were vaccinated developed cross-reactive antibody responses and T-cell responses against SARS-CoV-2 variants of concern [60]. More studies in lactating and pregnant women should be performed with other COVID-19 vaccine platforms.

The side effects of SARS-CoV-2 vaccines are nearly always mild and transient. Fatigue and headache after vaccination are often troubling but these side effects merely reflect that the vaccine is doing its job of stimulating production of interferons [61]. With the data coming from the continuous post-marketing surveillance, certain treatable adverse events have been detected. This includes the risk of myocarditis in 1–25/1 million doses of mRNA vaccines [62]. Another is the heparin-induced thrombocytopenia (HIT) detected in patients receiving the AstraZeneca vaccine although the risks are debatable considering its risk of 1/100,000 is within the range of specific thrombotic events in the general population, 0.22–1.57/100,000 per year [63]. It should be emphasized still that the benefits provided by the vaccines as protection against morbidity and mortality to COVID-19 far outweighs these extremely rare side effects.

No well-established correlate of protection is known (yet) for SARS-CoV-2, but Khoury et al. [64] analyzed the relationship between in vitro neutralization levels and the observed protection from severe acute respiratory syndrome coronavirus 2 (SARS-CoV-2) infection using data from seven current vaccines and from convalescent cohorts and showed that neutralization level is highly predictive of immune protection [64].

While the world starts getting back to certain normalcy with the vaccines roll-out deployment worldwide, hope has been undermined with the emergence of variants of concern that may affect the impact of vaccination which is also another question being addressed either in vitro or in vivo by vaccine manufacturers [65].

**Acknowledgements** MS, AW and MS would like to thank all physicians, scientists and healthcare workers around the world who are dealing with this pandemic; we express their deepest condolences to all colleagues who have fallen while fighting COVID-19. We would like to credit Servier (https://smart.servier.com/) and DBCLS (https://togotv.dbcls.jp/en/pics.html) for the mouse and Rhesus monkey figures used in Fig. 28.1.

**Disclosure Statement** MS is an employee of Clover Biopharmaceuticals, but did not receive any financial support for writing this chapter. AW is an employee of the International Vaccine Institute and did not receive any financial support for writing this chapter. MS declares no conflict of interest and did not receive any financial aid for writing this chapter.

## References

1. Institute of Medicine (US) Committee on the Children's Vaccine Initiative: Planning Alternative Strategies, Mitchell VS, Philipose NM, Sanford JP. The children's vaccine initiative: achieving the vision. Washington, DC: National Academies Press; 1993.
2. The Complex Journey of a Vaccine. 2021. https://www.ifpma.org/wp-content/uploads/2019/07/IFPMA-ComplexJourney-2019_FINAL.pdf. Accessed 24 Jun 2021.
3. Vaccine Development, Testing, and Regulation. 2021. https://www.historyofvaccines.org/content/articles/vaccine-development-testing-and-regulation. Accessed 24 Jun 2021.
4. Vaccine Development-101. 2021. https://www.fda.gov/vaccines-blood-biologics/development-approval-process-cber/vaccine-development-101. Accessed 24 Jun 2021.
5. Krammer F. SARS-CoV-2 vaccines in development. Nature. 2020;586(7830):516–27. https://doi.org/10.1038/s41586-020-2798-3.
6. Misra S. Randomized double blind placebo control studies, the "Gold Standard" in intervention based studies. Indian J Sex Transm Dis AIDS. 2012;33(2):131–4. https://doi.org/10.4103/0253-7184.102130.
7. Weinberg GA, Szilagyi PG. Vaccine epidemiology: efficacy, effectiveness, and the translational research roadmap. J Infect Dis. 2010;201(11):1607–10. https://doi.org/10.1086/652404.
8. List of Stringent Regulatory Authorities. 2021. https://www.who.int/initiatives/who-listed-authority-reg-authorities/SRAs. Accessed 24 Jun 2021.
9. Sanicas M, The Diarist.PH. Vaccine development—from 10 years to 10 months—how did that happen? 2021. https://www.thediarist.ph/vaccine-development-from-10-years-to-10-months-how-did-that-happen/. Accessed 24 Jun 2021.
10. Lurie N, Saville M, Hatchett R, Halton J. Developing Covid-19 vaccines at pandemic speed. N Engl J Med. 2020;382(21):1969–73. https://doi.org/10.1056/NEJMp2005630.
11. Banerjea A. What is rolling review? Europe starts real-time review of another Covid vaccine. 2020. https://www.livemint.com/news/world/what-is-rolling-review-europe-starts-real-time-review-of-another-covid-vaccine-11601978882290.html. Accessed 24 Jun 2021.

12. Emergency Use Authorization for Vaccines to Prevent COVID-19. 2021. https://www.fda.gov/regulatory-information/search-fda-guidance-documents/emergency-use-authorization-vaccines-prevent-covid-19. Accessed 24 Jun 2021.
13. Lancet Commission on COVID-19 Vaccines and Therapeutics Task Force Members. Operation warp speed: implications for global vaccine security. Lancet Glob Health. 2021;9(7):e1017–21. https://doi.org/10.1016/S2214-109X(21)00140-6.
14. CEPI. Our portfolio—coalition for epidemic preparedness innovations. 2021. https://cepi.net/research_dev/our-portfolio/. Accessed 24 Jun 2021.
15. Historie Rework—CureVac. 2021. https://www.curevac.com/en/about-us/historie-rework/. Accessed 24 Jun 2021.
16. Dolgin E. Unlocking the potential of vaccines built on messenger RNA. Nature. 2019;574(7778):S10–2. https://doi.org/10.1038/d41586-019-03072-8.
17. Sanicas M, Sanicas M, Diop D, Montomoli E. A review of COVID-19 vaccines in development: 6 months into the pandemic. Pan Afr Med J. 2020;5(37):124. https://doi.org/10.11604/pamj.2020.37.124.24973.
18. WHO. WHO issues its first emergency use validation for a COVID-19 vaccine and emphasizes need for equitable global access. 2021b. https://www.who.int/news/item/31-12-2020-who-issues-its-first-emergency-use-validation-for-a-covid-19-vaccine-and-emphasizes-need-for-equitable-global-access. Accessed 24 Jun 2021.
19. Zhao J, Zhao S, Ou J, Zhang J, Lan W, Guan W, Wu X, Yan Y, Zhao W, Wu J, Chodosh J, Zhang Q. COVID-19: coronavirus vaccine development updates. Front Immunol. 2020;23(11):602256. https://doi.org/10.3389/fimmu.2020.602256.
20. WHO. The different types of COVID-19 vaccines. 2021a. https://www.who.int/news-room/feature-stories/detail/the-race-for-a-covid-19-vaccine-explained. Accessed 24 Jun 2021.
21. Zhang Y, Zeng G, Pan H, et al. Safety, tolerability, and immunogenicity of an inactivated SARS-CoV-2 vaccine in healthy adults aged 18–59 years: a randomised, double-blind, placebo-controlled, phase 1/2 clinical trial. Lancet Infect Dis. 2021;21:181–92. https://doi.org/10.1016/S1473-3099(20)30843-4.
22. Wu Z, Hu Y, Xu M, et al. Safety, tolerability, and immunogenicity of an inactivated SARS-CoV-2 vaccine (CoronaVac) in healthy adults aged 60 years and older: a randomised, double-blind, placebo-controlled, phase 1/2 clinical trial. Lancet Infect Dis. 2021;21:803–12. https://doi.org/10.1016/S1473-3099(20)30987-7.
23. Gumrukcu T, Kucukgocmen A. Turkey says China's Sinovac COVID vaccine 91.25% effective in late trials. 2020. https://www.reuters.com/article/health-coronavirus-turkey-china-int-idUSKBN28Y1R3. Accessed 24 Jun 2021.
24. Widianto S. Indonesia approves China's Sinovac vaccine as infections surge. 2021. https://www.reuters.com/article/us-health-coronavirus-indonesia-idUSKBN29G0RP. Accessed 24 Jun 2021.
25. Simões E. New Brazil data shows disappointing 50.4% efficacy for China's CoronaVac vaccine. 2021. https://www.reuters.com/article/us-health-coronavirus-brazil-coronavirus-idUSKBN29H2CE. Accessed 24 Jun 2021.
26. Reuters. Turkish study revises down Sinovac COVID-19 vaccine efficacy to 83.5%. 2021. https://www.reuters.com/article/health-coronavirus-turkey-sinovac-int-idUSKBN2AV18P. Accessed 24 Jun 2021.
27. Vergara E. Big Chile study finds Chinese vaccine slashes COVID deaths. 2021. https://abcnews.go.com/Health/wireStory/big-chile-study-finds-chinese-vaccine-slashes-covid-77120616. Accessed 24 Jun 2021.
28. Aditya A, O'Brien E, Lyu D, Che C, Sipahutar T, Permatasari S. China Sinovac shot seen highly effective in real world study. 2021. https://www.bloomberg.com/news/articles/2021-05-11/china-s-sinovac-shot-found-highly-effective-in-real-world-study. Accessed 24 Jun 2021.
29. China grants conditional approval for first COVID vaccine. 2021. http://english.nmpa.gov.cn/2020-12/31/c_579192.htm. Accessed 24 Jun 2021.
30. The Sinopharm COVID-19 vaccine: what you need to know. 2021. https://www.who.int/news-room/feature-stories/detail/the-sinopharm-covid-19-vaccine-what-you-need-to-know. Accessed 24 Jun 2021.

31. Xia S, Zhang Y, Wang Y, Wang H, Yang Y, Gao GF, Tan W, Wu G, Xu M, Lou Z, Huang W, Xu W, Huang B, Wang H, Wang W, Zhang W, Li N, Xie Z, Ding L, You W, Zhao Y, Yang X, Liu Y, Wang Q, Huang L, Yang Y, Xu G, Luo B, Wang W, Liu P, Guo W, Yang X. Safety and immunogenicity of an inactivated SARS-CoV-2 vaccine, BBIBP-CorV: a randomised, double-blind, placebo-controlled, phase 1/2 trial. Lancet Infect Dis. 2021;21(1):39–51. https://doi.org/10.1016/S1473-3099(20)30831-8.
32. Ella R, Reddy S, Jogdand H, Sarangi V, Ganneru B, Prasad S, Das D, Raju D, Praturi U, Sapkal G, Yadav P, Reddy P, Verma S, Singh C, Redkar SV, Gillurkar CS, Kushwaha JS, Mohapatra S, Bhate A, Rai S, Panda S, Abraham P, Gupta N, Ella K, Bhargava B, Vadrevu KM. Safety and immunogenicity of an inactivated SARS-CoV-2 vaccine, BBV152: interim results from a double-blind, randomised, multicentre, phase 2 trial, and 3-month follow-up of a double-blind, randomised phase 1 trial. Lancet Infect Dis. 2021a;21(7):950–61. https://doi.org/10.1016/S1473-3099(21)00070-0.
33. Ella R, Vadrevu KM, Jogdand H, et al. Safety and immunogenicity of an inactivated SARS-CoV-2 vaccine, BBV152: a double-blind, randomised, phase 1 trial [published correction appears in Lancet Infect Dis. 2021 Apr;21(4):e81]. Lancet Infect Dis. 2021b;21(5):637–46. https://doi.org/10.1016/S1473-3099(20)30942-7.
34. Koshy J. Updated data from Covaxin phase 3 trial shows 78% efficacy. 2021. https://www.thehindu.com/sci-tech/health/updated-data-from-covaxin-phase-3-trial-shows-78-efficacy/article34376018.ece. Accessed 24 Jun 2021.
35. Rambe D, Giudice G, Rossi S, Sanicas M. Safety and mechanism of action of licensed vaccine adjuvants. Int Curr Pharm J. 2015;4(8):420–31. https://doi.org/10.3329/icpj.v4i8.24024.
36. Novavax. Novavax COVID-19 vaccine demonstrates 89.3% efficacy in UK phase 3 trial. 2021. https://ir.novavax.com/news-releases/news-release-details/novavax-covid-19-vaccine-demonstrates-893-efficacy-uk-phase-3. Accessed 24 Jun 2021.
37. Park A. Novavax reports its COVID-19 vaccine is 96% efficacious. 2021. https://time.com/5946225/novavax-covid-19-phase-3-results/. Accessed 24 Jun 2021.
38. Shinde V, Bhikha S, Hoosain Z, Archary M, Bhorat Q, Fairlie L, Lalloo U, Masilela MSL, Moodley D, Hanley S, Fouche L, Louw C, Tameris M, Singh N, Goga A, Dheda K, Grobbelaar C, Kruger G, Carrim-Ganey N, Baillie V, de Oliveira T, Lombard Koen A, Lombaard JJ, Mngqibisa R, Bhorat AE, Benadé G, Lalloo N, Pitsi A, Vollgraaff PL, Luabeya A, Esmail A, Petrick FG, Oommen-Jose A, Foulkes S, Ahmed K, Thombrayil A, Fries L, Cloney-Clark S, Zhu M, Bennett C, Albert G, Faust E, Plested JS, Robertson A, Neal S, Cho I, Glenn GM, Dubovsky F, Madhi SA, 2019nCoV-501 Study Group. Efficacy of NVX-CoV2373 Covid-19 vaccine against the B.1.351 variant. N Engl J Med. 2021;384(20):1899–909. https://doi.org/10.1056/NEJMoa2103055.
39. Vrba SM, Kirk NM, Brisse ME, Liang Y, Ly H. Development and applications of viral vectored vaccines to combat zoonotic and emerging public health threats. Vaccines (Basel). 2020;8(4):680. https://doi.org/10.3390/vaccines8040680.
40. van Riel D, de Wit E. Next-generation vaccine platforms for COVID-19. Nat Mater. 2020;19:810–2. https://doi.org/10.1038/s41563-020-0746-0.
41. Voysey M, Clemens SAC, Madhi SA, Weckx LY, Folegatti PM, Aley PK, Angus B, Baillie VL, Barnabas SL, Bhorat QE, Bibi S, Briner C, Cicconi P, Collins AM, Colin-Jones R, Cutland CL, Darton TC, Dheda K, Duncan CJA, Emary KRW, Ewer KJ, Fairlie L, Faust SN, Feng S, Ferreira DM, Finn A, Goodman AL, Green CM, Green CA, Heath PT, Hill C, Hill H, Hirsch I, Hodgson SHC, Izu A, Jackson S, Jenkin D, Joe CCD, Kerridge S, Koen A, Kwatra G, Lazarus R, Lawrie AM, Lelliott A, Libri V, Lillie PJ, Mallory R, Mendes AVA, Milan EP, Minassian AM, McGregor A, Morrison H, Mujadidi YF, Nana A, O'Reilly PJ, Padayachee SD, Pittella A, Plested E, Pollock KM, Ramasamy MN, Rhead S, Schwarzbold AV, Singh N, Smith A, Song R, Snape MD, Sprinz E, Sutherland RK, Tarrant R, Thomson EC, Török ME, Toshner M, Turner DPJ, Vekemans J, Villafana TL, Watson MEE, Williams CJ, Douglas AD, Hill AVS, Lambe T, Gilbert SC, Pollard AJ; Oxford COVID Vaccine Trial Group. Safety and efficacy of the ChAdOx1 nCoV-19 vaccine (AZD1222) against SARS-CoV-2: an interim

analysis of four randomised controlled trials in Brazil, South Africa, and the UK. Lancet. 2021;397(10269):99–111. https://doi.org/10.1016/S0140-6736(20)32661-1. Epub 2020 Dec 8. Erratum in: Lancet. 2021 Jan 9;397(10269):98. PMID: 33306989; PMCID: PMC7723445.
42. LopezBernal J, Andrews N, Gower C, Robertson C, Stowe J, Tessier E, et al. Effectiveness of the Pfizer-BioNTech and Oxford-AstraZeneca vaccines on covid-19 related symptoms, hospital admissions, and mortality in older adults in England: test negative case-control study. BMJ. 2021;373:n1088. https://doi.org/10.1136/bmj.n1088.
43. Logunov DY, Dolzhikova IV, Shcheblyakov DV, et al. Safety and efficacy of an rAd26 and rAd5 vector-based heterologous prime-boost COVID-19 vaccine: an interim analysis of a randomised controlled phase 3 trial in Russia [Erratum in: Lancet. 2021 Feb 20;397(10275):670]. Lancet. 2021;397(10275):671–81. https://doi.org/10.1016/S0140-6736(21)00234-8.
44. Sadoff J, et al. Safety and efficacy of single-dose Ad26.COV2.S vaccine against Covid-19. N Engl J Med. 2021;384(23):2187–201. https://doi.org/10.1056/NEJMoa2101544.
45. Lodish H, Berk A, Zipursky SL, et al. Molecular cell biology. Section 4.4, The three roles of RNA in protein synthesis. 4th ed. New York: W. H. Freeman; 2000.
46. Schlake T, Thess A, Fotin-Mleczek M & Karl-Josef Kallen KJ. Developing mRNA-vaccine technologies, RNA Biology, 2012;9(11):1319–30, https://doi.org/10.4161/rna.22269.
47. Comirnaty COVID-19 mRNA vaccine. 2021. https://www.ema.europa.eu/en/medicines/human/EPAR/comirnaty. Accessed 25 May 2021.
48. Oliver S, Gargano J, Marin M, et al. The advisory committee on immunization practices' interim recommendation for use of Moderna COVID-19 vaccine—United States, December 2020. MMWR Morb Mortal Wkly Rep. 2021;69:1653–6. https://doi.org/10.15585/mmwr.mm695152e1.
49. Moderna Inc. Moderna announces longer shelf life for its COVID-19 Vaccine candidate at refrigerated temperatures. 2021. https://investors.modernatx.com/news-releases/news-release-details/moderna-announces-longer-shelf-life-its-covid-19-vaccine. Accessed 28 May 2021.
50. Wider storage and transportation conditions for the Pfizer COVID-19 vaccine now approved. 2021. https://www.tga.gov.au/media-release/wider-storage-and-transportation-conditions-pfizer-covid-19-vaccine-now-approved. Accessed 24 Jun 2021.
51. Baden LR, El Sahly HM, Essink B, et al. Efficacy and safety of the mRNA-1273 SARS-CoV-2 vaccine. N Engl J Med. 2021;384(5):403–16. https://doi.org/10.1056/NEJMoa2035389.
52. The Moderna COVID-19 (mRNA-1273) vaccine: what you need to know. 2021. https://www.who.int/news-room/feature-stories/detail/the-moderna-covid-19-mrna-1273-vaccine-what-you-need-to-know. Accessed 24 Jun 2021.
53. Mallapaty S. India's DNA COVID vaccine is a world first—more are coming. [online]. Nature.com. 2021. https://www.nature.com/articles/d41586-021-02385-x. Accessed 15 Sept 2021.
54. Krause PR, Gruber MF. Emergency use Authorization of Covid vaccines—safety and efficacy follow-up considerations. N Engl J Med. 2020;383(19):e107. https://doi.org/10.1056/NEJMp2031373.
55. Zellweger RM, Wartel TA, Marks F, Song M, Kim JH. Vaccination against SARS-CoV-2 and disease enhancement—knowns and unknowns. Expert Rev Vaccines. 2020;19(8):691–8. https://doi.org/10.1080/14760584.2020.1800463.
56. Wallace M, Woodworth KR, Gargano JW, et al. The Advisory Committee on Immunization Practices' interim recommendation for use of Pfizer-BioNTech COVID-19 vaccine in adolescents aged 12–15 years—United States, May 2021. MMWR Morb Mortal Wkly Rep. 2021;70(20):749–52. https://doi.org/10.15585/mmwr.mm7020e1.
57. Shaw RH, Stuart A, Greenland M, Liu X, Van-Tam JSN, Snape MD; Com-COV Study Group. Heterologous prime-boost COVID-19 vaccination: initial reactogenicity data [Erratum in: Lancet. 2021 May 18]. Lancet. 2021;397(10289):2043–6. https://doi.org/10.1016/S0140-6736(21)01115-6.
58. Farrell R, Michie M, Pope R. Pregnant women in trials of Covid-19: a critical time to consider ethical frameworks of inclusion in clinical trials. Ethics Hum Res. 2020;42(4):17–23. https://doi.org/10.1002/eahr.500060.

59. Delahoy MJ, Whitaker M, O'Halloran A, et al. Characteristics and maternal and birth outcomes of hospitalized pregnant women with laboratory-confirmed COVID-19—COVID-NET, 13 states, March 1–August 22, 2020. MMWR Morb Mortal Wkly Rep. 2020;69(38):1347–54. https://doi.org/10.15585/mmwr.mm6938e1.
60. Collier AY, McMahan K, Yu J, et al. Immunogenicity of COVID-19 mRNA vaccines in pregnant and lactating women. JAMA. 2021;325(23):2370–80. https://doi.org/10.1001/jama.2021.7563.
61. Sprent J, King C. COVID-19 vaccine side effects: the positives about feeling bad. Sci Immunol. 2021;6(60):eabj9256. https://doi.org/10.1126/sciimmunol.abj9256.
62. Haelle T. Covid-19 vaccines and teens: what to know about myocarditis risk. 2021. https://elemental.medium.com/covid-19-vaccines-and-teens-what-to-know-about-myocarditis-risk-920d09648b13. Accessed 24 Jun 2021.
63. Cines DB, Bussel JB. SARS-CoV-2 vaccine-induced immune thrombotic thrombocytopenia. N Engl J Med. 2021;384:2254–6. https://doi.org/10.1056/NEJMe2106315.
64. Khoury DS, Cromer D, Reynaldi A, et al. Neutralizing antibody levels are highly predictive of immune protection from symptomatic SARS-CoV-2 infection. Nat Med. 2021;27(7):1205–11. https://doi.org/10.1038/s41591-021-01377-8.
65. Gupta RK. Will SARS-CoV-2 variants of concern affect the promise of vaccines? [Erratum in: Nat Rev Immunol. 2021 May 10]. Nat Rev Immunol. 2021;21(6):340–1. https://doi.org/10.1038/s41577-021-00556-5.

# Chapter 29
# The Global Evolution of Clinical Practice During a Pandemic

**Sulaiman Karim, Brittany K. Bankhead, and Brian A. Kendall**

## Regional Variations in the Evolution of COVID-19

While the coronavirus disease 2019 (COVID-19) outbreak disrupted medical care across the entire nation and globe, regional differences among health-care facilities and resources introduced heterogeneity into the experiences of different populations. Regional variations influenced clinical practice and ultimately influenced health outcomes.

The comparison of rural and urban populations highlights regional variations and the evolution of COVID-19. For example, traveling distance, limited qualified providers in an area, and reduced bed capacity relative to urban health institutions have historically challenged clinical practice in remote areas [1]. In addition, urban areas are often associated with close living quarters, such as co-housing and apartment living [2]. This style of living presented numerous opportunities for super spreader events during the pandemic. Furthermore, various living conditions characteristic of urban areas, such as higher population density and higher rates of household overcrowding, demonstrated positive associations with COVID-19 transmission and mortality rates [3]. Moreover, metropolitan health-care facilities were further

S. Karim
Texas Tech University Health Sciences Center School of Medicine, Lubbock, TX, USA
e-mail: Sulaiman.karim@ttuhsc.edu

B. K. Bankhead
Department of Surgery, Texas Tech University Health Sciences Center School of Medicine, Lubbock, TX, USA
e-mail: Brittany.K.Bankhead@ttuhsc.edu

B. A. Kendall (✉)
Division of Emergency Medicine, Texas Tech University Health Sciences Center School of Medicine, Lubbock, TX, USA
e-mail: brian.kendall@ttuhsc.edu


S. Adibi et al. (eds.), *Frontiers of COVID-19*,
https://doi.org/10.1007/978-3-031-08045-6_29

burdened by the influx of patients transferred from outside facilities unable to meet such acutely heightened demand for critical care. For example, the total number of critical care transfers reported by Northwest London Critical Care Network between March 17th and May 6th of 2020 was 238, more than double the 106 transfers reported during an equivalent 50-day period in 2019. Notably, 94% of the 2020 period transfers were related to ICU capacity, while none of the 2019 period transfers were attributable to this reason [4].

Other socioeconomic factors appear to have played a role in the pandemic's regional manifestations. Individuals living in high-income neighborhoods substantially increased their days spent at home compared to individuals in low-income neighborhoods, who were more likely to work outside the home [5]. These findings suggest that lower-income areas faced unique barriers to social distancing during the pandemic. Furthermore, inequities in the testing and diagnosis of COVID-19 highlighted regional disparities during COVID-19. During the first several months of 2020, lower testing rates were reported in neighborhoods with higher levels of social vulnerability [6]. Other population characteristics, such as advanced age, smoking history, obesity prevalence, and high unemployment rates, were associated with higher viral reproduction rates and increased critical COVID-19 cases and mortality [7].

Taken together, these findings illustrate how the unique features of a population within a given region further influenced the pandemic's varying evolution across different areas of the globe. As a result, macro and micro variability in patient populations and clinical guidelines forced clinicians to adapt their practice of critical care and management of patients infected with severe acute respiratory syndrome coronavirus 2 (SARS-CoV-2).

## Potential Advanced-Stage Pathology of Disease Processes

The implication of backlog on hospital system recovery during the pandemic leads to the potential for disease progression. In addition, the mass disruption of patient care induced by the pandemic will likely result in worsened health outcomes and heightened mortality for patients, primarily due to diagnosis and treatment deferment delays. Considering this, appropriate preparation for advanced-stage pathological conditions is vital for clinical practice.

The disruption of acute care during the pandemic resulted in avoidable harm for many patients. De Luca et al. showed that throughout the COVID-19 global health crisis, primary percutaneous coronary intervention (PCI) procedures—a treatment strategy for a life-threatening type of heart attack—decreased, time to treatment, ischemia duration, and mortalities rose [8]. Furthermore, cases of delayed treatment occurred in hospitals stressed by the pandemic. A frontline account of the pandemic, shared by the New England Journal of Medicine, reported that two patients died while waiting for their surgeries after their transthoracic aortic valvular replacements were postponed [9]. This case highlights how global health crises such as the

COVID-19 pandemic complicate the distinction between "elective" and "medically necessary" procedures.

Another area of medicine where providers should anticipate advanced-stage pathology is oncology since 1-year relative survival rates for those with various types of cancer decrease with an increasing stage at diagnosis [10]. For instance, a study from Italy found that after a 2-month interruption of mammographic screenings, the pathological findings of diagnosed breast cancers showed clinical progression, increasing stage III morphology [11]. Furthermore, due to diagnostic delays in the UK alone, approximately 3500 avoidable cancer deaths are estimated to occur for lung, breast, esophageal, and colorectal cancer within 5 years after diagnosis, totaling roughly 60,000 years of life lost [12]. These findings were especially concerning considering the multitude of treatable cancer types with modern medicine and preventable with the diagnostic techniques currently available.

The mass disruption in diagnosis, treatment, and routine patient management limited clinical practice and increased mortality. Clinical practice will require modifications to adjust for these worsened health outcomes and increases in mortality as some of the leading causes of worldwide mortality. Heart disease and cancer treatment are especially concerning.

## Managing Surgical Backlog

Modern health-care systems witnessed a dramatic reduction in surgical volumes throughout the COVID-19 pandemic, creating an enormous backlog of cases [13]. Estimates suggest that over 28 million elective operations were canceled across the globe during the first 3 months of the pandemic [14]. This mass disruption, directly and indirectly, impacted patients and providers across a broad range of medical specialties, and it also necessitates careful consideration by physicians in navigating the subsequent management and care of their patients. This backlog presents significant strain on entire health systems in the post-COVID era as already-exhausted facilities trying to recover from the pandemic will need to increase capacities even further than prepandemic times. Furthermore, even as services resume and restrictions lift, operations will be only fractionally as efficient as before [15]. The recovery from backlog has unique implications for patients under different forms of care.

Elective surgery cancellation has countless unanticipated ramifications on patient well-being. Previous research showed that patients awaiting total hip arthroplasties have a 50% chance of worse postoperative outcomes when surgery was delayed more than 6 months, suggesting that surgical delays worsen the patient's quality of life postoperatively [16]. In addition, research during the COVID-19 era revealed that elective orthopedic surgery cancellations resulted in significantly higher reported pain levels and, consequently, higher analgesic use [17].

In addition to impacting patients' mental and physical well-being, mandatory cancellations of nonemergent hospital procedures and the resultant surgery backlog have tremendous economic implications for health-care facilities. Progression of disease states—such as metastatic breast, colorectal, and lung cancer—is ultimately associated with higher costs of care [18]. Thus, the backlog is costly on the levels of both institutions as well as individuals. Reduced institutional income may ultimately lead to provider contract restructuring and pay cuts, as well as facility downsizing, both of which have the potential to compromise the quality of care delivered in clinical practice.

The coronavirus pandemic rerouted treatment trajectories so that many conventionally operative cases were pushed toward nonoperative and potentially more conservative treatment routes. Such shifts in treatment approach posed an increased risk of mortality and unruly health outcomes for individuals. However, shifting emphasis away from invasive procedures as the first-line treatment could mean that patients avoided unnecessary, risky interventions that posed more significant risks for infection and post-operative complications. Despite these findings, withholding invasive surgical procedures until alternative treatments have failed may lengthen case resolution and lead to adverse patient outcomes. For example, previous research demonstrated that patients who underwent initial surgery for mitral valve regurgitation had better long-term clinical outcomes, including reduced overall mortality than patients treated with a conservative management strategy [19]. These findings highlight how abstaining from initial surgical intervention may present harm to patients in the long run. Moreover, the delayed use of surgical intervention could also heighten the risk for more advanced pathological states that ultimately require more aggressive treatments than what would have been required initially.

The impact of the pandemic on surgical backlog has negatively impacted some specialties more than others. In ophthalmology, 2 years post-suspension of elective procedures, the backlog for cataracts surgery alone is predicted to involve 1.1–1.6 million cases [20]. Similarly, elective orthopedic surgeries are predicted to be behind by over a million cases by 2 years post-deferment, assuming prepandemic growth in volume [21]. Cardiac surgery volumes decreased from baseline by 54% following COVID-related restrictions [22]. Case backlog in cardiac surgery is perhaps most concerning, given that heart disease reigns as the leading cause of death worldwide [23]. Furthermore, predictions show that it could take up to 8 months to clear this case backlog; even so, that is stringent upon when hospitals can resume and how much they can increase capacity [22].

Changes to clinical practice to reduce the growing surgical backlog will require collaboration among industry leaders and providers. Though reportedly taking various measures to increase surgical throughput, less than 50% of health system leaders surveyed by McKinsey & Company in 2020 were employing strategies to maximize capacity. At the time of the survey, actions taken by the correspondents included extending hours of operation, hiring additional staff, optimizing room turnover times, and contacting patients in advance to limit cancellations. McKinsey & Company outlined several recommendations for health-care systems facing an overwhelming backlog, one of which was reducing unnecessary deferral of care. Other helpful strategies for managing backlog include the employment of data analytics to help prioritize and reschedule delayed or canceled surgeries [24]. Hospitals may consider transitioning to relying more heavily upon outpatient settings for surgical care [25].

## Ambulatory Care and the Outpatient Setting

The COVID-19 pandemic altered ambulatory care in various ways, impacting providers and patients across many outpatient settings, most notably primary care, psychiatry, and physical rehabilitation. These effects included decreased accessibility to care, delays in care, modified modes of care delivery, and reductions in revenue generation. Nevertheless, despite similar adverse implications of COVID-19 on the landscape of outpatient care, the different specialties experienced unique challenges.

The impact of COVID-19 on primary care had significant deleterious consequences for patients regarding preventative screening, routine follow-up care, and patient referrals to secondary and tertiary care providers. For instance, in the UK, estimates predicted tremendous increases in the number of avoidable deaths among cancer patients due to delays in diagnosis, with up to a 16.6% estimated increase in deaths due to lung cancer alone [12]. Furthermore, laboratory test orders from outpatient clinics declined during the pandemic, illustrating the harmful effects on routine follow-up care [26].

The clinical practice of psychiatric care was also vulnerable to change as mental health disorders imparted unique vulnerabilities to patients during the pandemic, such as simply having a comorbidity that heightened the risk for severe SARS-CoV-2 infection, behavioral issues impacting conformity to public health guidelines, and impaired coping mechanisms to deal with the psychological toll of lockdown [27]. The psychological harm inflicted by the pandemic also posed unique implications for psychiatric medicine. Reported symptoms of anxiety and depression rose significantly between April and June 2020 relative to the same period in 2019 [28, 29]. Unfortunately, these psychological impacts also heightened vulnerability to harmful coping mechanisms. For instance, 13.3% of people aged 18 or older in the USA reported having started or increased substance use to help cope with the negative emotions induced by the pandemic [30]. This pandemic-induced substance abuse may have exacerbated other health issues that patients had or may have worsened existing substance use disorders and thus is imperative to consider.

The restrictions and stay-at-home orders implemented in response to the pandemic disrupted the delivery of rehabilitative medicine. This restriction is particularly concerning considering that it was shown that initiating physical therapy earlier improves an individual's functional abilities [31]. Other previous studies indicated that physical therapy results in significant long-term improvement in patients with chronic pain [32]. Taken collectively, these findings suggest that the pandemic's impact on rehabilitative care likely negatively affected the functional capabilities and quality of life of many patients overall. Moreover, research showing that SARS-CoV-2 infection can manifest as skeletal muscle injury symptoms suggests potential increased demand for physical therapy in the pain management of COVID-19 patients [33].

## Employee Screening Protocols

Uncertainty about the SARS-CoV-2 virus and an already worn-down workforce on the pandemic frontlines raised concerns for intrahospital infections, especially susceptible were high-risk health-care workers. Coupled with frayed supply chains and dwindling personal protective equipment (PPE), hospitals were forced to adapt to an increased number of critically ill patients with a decreased number of available and healthy health-care workers due to SARS-CoV-2 infections. Given concerns for nosocomial viral transmission, employee screening protocols were implemented and updated as the COVID-19 pandemic unfolded. In early 2020, landmark research regarding symptomatic and asymptomatic transmission encouraged testing of asymptomatic health-care workers to curb the nosocomial spread, requiring a dramatic increase in testing capabilities [34–36]. Other means to slow transmission include institutional changes regarding employee screening protocols, contact tracing, and travel restrictions.

Early changes in clinical practice warranted the need for developing screening protocols and managing risk. However, the implementation of screening protocols, especially early in the pandemic, relied on the locoregional and international availability of resources [37]. Infrastructure considerations regarding testing capacity have been addressed from the private sector with increased testing kit development and distribution availability. In the USA, as SARS-CoV-2 spread rapidly and political pressure mounted against the government, a national emergency was declared on March 13, 2020 to divert $50 billion toward fighting the virus and improved telehealth access to several states [38]. In response to the USA declaring the COVID-19 pandemic a national emergency, the American Medical Association called the emergency declaration "necessary to help ensure that America's health system has sufficient resources" [38]. In the time lag between policy development and resource mobilization, adapted screening protocols like serological testing or radiographic imaging and risk management methods were used.

Some institutions recognized the limitations of real-time polymerase chain reaction (RT-PCR) testing as the sole tool for systemic screening protocols, which prompted these institutions to supplement screening protocols with serological testing. Serological screening helped prevent the need for repeat RT-PCR testing, reduced laboratory resource use, and mitigated potential exposures. This screening method detects antibodies created by the immune system in response to a specific antigen rather than detecting the virus itself, as with traditional RT-PCR tests [39]. Despite the limitations of serological screening, several major US government organizations, including the NIH and DHHS, established the Serological Sciences Network for COVID-19 (SeroNet) to develop serological tests and increase testing capacity via the Public Readiness and Emergency Preparedness Act [40]. In addition to serological testing, CT and X-ray imaging have been used as an alternative to RT-PCR testing, especially in the early days of the pandemic with limited testing capacity due to decentralized federal coordination [41].

In a study conducted by Quattrone et al. [39], baseline serial serological screening followed by second-line viral RT-PCR testing for positive or symptomatic cases was an effective method of screening health-care workers. The possible systemic serological screening protocol to test health-care workers is summarized in Fig. 29.1 [39].

Risk management has also been used to decrease transmission with the use of contact tracing and travel restrictions. Additionally, some hospitals recognized both the vulnerability and value of senior clinicians, thereby taking measures to distance them from direct exposure and manage risk. A JAMA publication outlines how older clinicians should be considered for roles with less exposure, like advisory, executive, or communication roles [42]. However, despite increased screening protocols and concern for older clinicians, some places, such as New York City, relied on older clinicians to address workforce shortages during surges [43]. With health informatics support, risk management through contact tracing has made considerable progress in outbreak management.

In a study conducted by Reeves et al. [44], electronic health record (EHR)-based tools were used for screening protocols, including scripted triaging, standard messaging, and real-time data analytics. In Taiwan, for instance, the application of health informatics support leveraged national health resources with its immigration and customs database to risk stratify travelers. As a result, low-risk flight passengers were able to pass to immigration clearance, while high-risk individuals were required to quarantine and report symptoms with mobile device applications. Because health-care workers were at increased risk of COVID-19 exposure, the WHO recommends contact tracing to prevent intrahospital infections [45, 46]. Furthermore, because of rigorous contact tracing and screening protocols of health-care workers, the interval and incubation period of COVID-19 infection in health-care workers was much shorter than the general population [45].

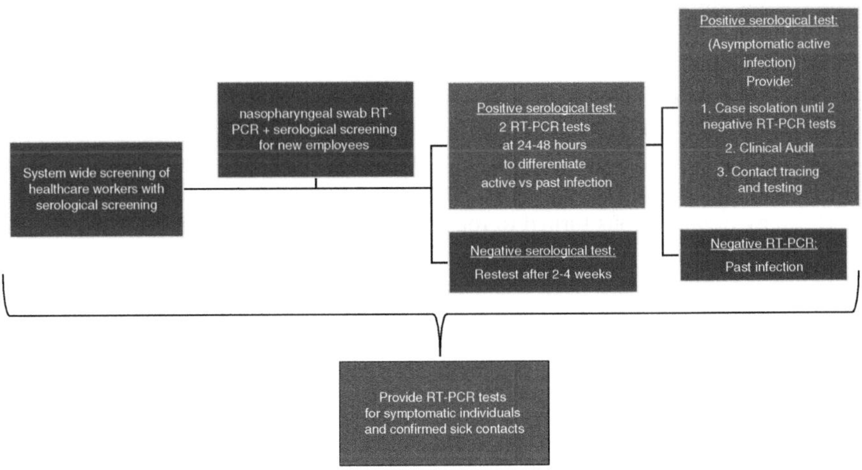


**Fig. 29.1** Systematic serological screening protocol of health-care workers [39]

## Personal Protective Equipment

The global supply of PPE drastically fell as China, the largest producer of masks and clinical gowns, experienced a surge of the first reported cases of COVID-19. Early in the pandemic, the World Health Organization director stated that "the chronic global shortage of personal protective equipment is now one of the most urgent threats to our collective ability to save lives" [47]. Cohen and van der Rodgers [48] argued that health is not a public good, and therefore, market prices are inappropriate mechanisms for rationing PPE. Health-care systems were forced to make creative changes and partnerships to keep their workers safe despite the global PPE shortage.

Early studies established the effectiveness of N95 masks and respirators in preventing bacterial and viral infections among hospital workers [49]. COVID-19 dramatically increased hospitalization rates and regionally overwhelmed health-care systems. Reduced supply of N95 masks, hospital gowns, and other PPE reduced the quality and quantity of care due to increased intrahospital viral transmission [48]. With a compromised health-care workforce, the health-care system was prone to destabilization as intrahospital infection rates increased. Global shortages of PPE worsened for many low-income countries as they rely on the same global supply chains, and more countries halt exports of PPE. UNICEF reported it only acquired 10% of its initial 240 million masks request for low-income countries [50, 51]. Increased access to PPE, especially for low-income countries, required an international commitment.

One notable case of PPE shortages came from the USA as the Defense Production Act was needed to mandate private production of PPE used by frontline health-care workers [48, 52]. The inability to stockpile PPE amid a pandemic coupled with budget cuts to the CDC and an implementation time lag after invoking the Defense Production Act in April 2020 resulted in creative changes across the country out of desperation. Studies have found multiple causes for the U.S. shortage of PPE, but many studies cite the lack of an immediate and robust response as a significant contributing factor [48, 52–54]. Additionally, the U.S. and China trade war made acquiring PPE from China more complicated as China's COVID-19 cases declined, and production resumed.

During the height of the PPE shortage, the CDC recommended reusing one-use masks and potentially even cloth masks, despite limited evidence of their efficacy [54]. Many organizations turned to reuse masks as a last resort; others sought creative solutions to the PPE shortage, as evident in the call for ideas published by Bauchner et al. [55] and Reid and Hurst [56]. Institutions like the University of Nebraska Medical Center began using UV light to disinfect N95 masks under the direction of Dr. John Lowe [57]. Additionally, recent research has used photothermal decontamination devices to safely decontaminate masks up to 3 cycles without compromising the masks' integrity [58]. Many institutions relied on homemade PPE alternatives as supplies became scarce. However, a study conducted by the University of Cambridge found cloth masks to be 50% effective compared to surgical masks at 80% [56, 59]. In July of 2020, the CDC announced there was consideration for releasing stockpiled N95 masks that had expired because of the dire PPE shortage [60]. By July of 2020, global supply chains stabilized, and China produced 110 million masks a day; however, high demand for PPE continued to exist as countries built their stockpiles in anticipation of subsequent viral surges [47].

## Bed Allocation

The ethical dilemma of bed allocation posed challenges amid hospitals overwhelmed by regional surges in COVID-19 cases. Given the rapidly changing nature of the SARS-CoV-2 virus, hospital administrators and clinicians required rapid adaptations to circumstances with a limited federal response. Federal guidelines varied widely based on local factors such as patient population, availability of resources, and politics. Countries with inadequate bed capacity were more prone to crisis level surges in COVID-19 cases with the inability to properly provide care to patients. Concerns for patient and employee safety amid both resource and personnel shortages prompted hospitals to find creative solutions to continue operations and prevent systemic collapse.

The Johns Hopkins Bloomberg School of Public Health found that all sub-Saharan Africa has roughly 2000 beds, excluding South Africa [61]. The scarcity of hospital beds starkly contrasts wealthier countries' capacity to care for their COVID-19 patients. However, Italy and the USA suffered massive bed shortages as COVID-19 surged early in 2020 and late 2020 for each country, respectively.

While China's reported cases of COVID-19 fell, Italy became the European epicenter for the pandemic. Craxì et al. [62] found some hospitals hardest hit by the surges admitted over 200 critical respiratory failures every day. Additionally, ethics committees from the Italian Society of Anesthesia, Analgesia, Resuscitation, and Intensive Care (SIAARTI) published guidelines amid scarce resource rationing. Italy's allocation strategy was modeled closely to their organ transplant guidelines optimizing maximum cost-benefit in years gained for the patient [62, 63]. Many Italian hospitals converted operating rooms, medical wards, and changing rooms into temporary negative pressure intensive care units [64]. Rapid policy and institutional changes developed in conjunction with ethical boards to allocate limited hospital beds properly.

Several surges riddled the USA throughout the COVID-19 pandemic. The interplay between civil liberties and public health has resulted in several efforts to reopen the economy with subsequent spikes in COVID-19 cases. First, surges in the USA consumed NYC as the largest and most densely populated city in the USA. By June 11, 2020, New York's death toll accounted for 7% of the world's death toll and 27% of American deaths [65]. Although New York was shocked by how ill-prepared it was to manage the pandemic, the US developed protocols, published in 2018, to manage bed and resource allocation during a public health emergency such as severe influenza [66]. By September 2020, nearly half of US hospitals reported to the Department of Health and Human Services reached critical capacity [67]. Finally, U.S. institutional changes in response to bed shortage led to development of surge capacity and increased focus on triage.

The development of surge capacity and triage protocols aided in lessening the disruption of bed shortages, especially in the USA. Early in the pandemic, care models were developed. One particularly well-received care model placed traditional ICU attendings in charge of physician lead teams to accommodate the dramatic increase in ICU beds [68]. Similarly, many institutions, such as the University of Washington School of Medicine, redirected research and teaching faculty into clinical practice to accommodate increased ICU care [69]. Schaye Verity et al. [70] cite tertiary and quaternary-care referral hospitals were critical for system expansion as smaller hospitals had fewer resources and were more easily overwhelmed.

## Reliance Upon Communication and Social Media for Clinical Updates

Our understanding of the SARS-CoV-2 virus was limited, despite the growing number of worldwide SARS-CoV-2 patients. Health agencies and health-care providers implemented institutional changes as data-sharing became more collective with an influx of research since the pandemic. However, due to the rapidly evolving nature of the COVID-19 pandemic, clinicians were forced to increasingly rely on social media for clinical updates as traditional dissemination strategies, like academic journals or conferences, could not keep up. With a heavier reliance on peer-to-peer communication, institutions found creative ways to adapt their pandemic response, such as reliance on mobile health platforms, videoconferences, and social media for clinical updates.

Relying on social media was not unique to the SARS-CoV-2 pandemic. A study conducted by Odlum and Yoon [71] drew a parallel when lawmakers questioned the CDC's ability to manage the Ebola health crisis following several confusing messages issued by the CDC. Instead, a quick and forceful public response is favored with mass dissemination media such as Twitter, much like Nigeria's response coordinated with the WHO. Odlum and Yoon [71] also cite how real-time Twitter data supports early detection of an infection outbreak. As a more significant percentage of the general population uses social media sites, we may better analyze regional health trends and improve global health outcomes with population-specific and literacy-appropriate health education messages. A study examining racial disparities and the SARS-CoV-2 virus found disseminating information on social media to be more effective than waiting for an academic publication [72].

As the pandemic unfolded within the USA, many communication media were used to supplement the federal response. The SARS-CoV-2, much like the Ebola epidemic, pressured health workers and agencies to increasingly rely on social media for clinical updates [73]. In late December 2019, CDC guidelines for health agencies and health-care providers remained focused on slowing transmission, but guidelines fell short anticipating impending disruptions to clinical practice [74]. Pharmacists' extemporaneous preparation of sanitizers using WHO guidelines following a sanitizer shortage is one example of changed clinical practice informed by timely advice from the WHO [75]. Moreover, local population and social factors influenced the CDC guidelines, and therefore, required strategic modification to best prepare hospitals for disease surges [70]. The pandemic response in NYC prompted new strategies for effectively disseminating clinical updates, such as delivering bidaily site-specific meetings, videoconferences, townhalls, business communication platforms, and traditional email [70].

Other health-care institutions such as the University Hospital of Geneva implemented a dedicated mobile health platform to disseminate clinical updates for their staff. Zamberg et al. [76] found medical staff use of mobile health platforms to significantly increase to more than double when viewing information about SARS-CoV-2. In the early stages, where contradictory information was published almost daily, and health professionals dealt with increasing patients and workload, traditional communication strategies like email or printed materials fell short as they were more difficult to sort, find, and update.

Increased reliance on social media for clinical updates was also likely tied to both the need for faster and more accessible data dissemination. Traditionally, disseminating public health knowledge is slow, ineffective, and leads to a gap in discovery and practice or policy development; thus, a "translation gap" often develops [77]. Among researchers, only 28% agreed their dissemination efforts were rated excellent or good, indicating traditional or passive dissemination methods such as academic journals or conferences are relatively ineffective [77]. Additionally, clinical safety infographics are associated with a higher preference and lower cognitive load according to the cognitive load theory and coding theory [78, 79]. The limitations of "echo chambers" and the inability to enforce accountability were also cited in the literature [72]. Despite the limitations of social media, a global effort to communicate scientific findings has challenged traditional dissemination strategies and encouraged unconventional ones.

## The Influx of Case Reports and Preliminary Data in Journals

The scientific community responded to the COVID-19 pandemic with a dramatic influx of case reports and preliminary data in journal publications. Increased publication of scientific data and case reports may be another silver lining in the pandemic. However, while the rapid dissemination of scientific work has greatly aided our understanding of the SARS-CoV-2 virus, concerns regarding the accuracy and the peer review process have been raised.

Submission of preprint publications has grown steadily for the past 5 years but has dramatically increased in the past 2 years with the pandemic's inception [80].

Open-access research has followed a similar growth trend as the scientific community aims to disseminate clinical updates and virus-related data. For example, a recent Lancet publication found that the number of publications, including preprints, exceeded publications during the Ebola and Zika virus, despite both epidemics also increasing open-access publications [81, 82].

In addition to increased preprint publications, the peer review process has also shortened for COVID-19 related articles. Horbach [83] found the average peer review time to be shortened by 49% for COVID-19 related articles and no acceleration in the peer review turnaround for non-COIVD-19 articles. Additionally, he found publishers made tremendous efforts to expand their pool of reviewers to assist in the rapid publication of new findings. The Medical Journal of Australia and the Royal Society Open Publishing were among many publishers to establish a fast-track peer review of COVID-19 manuscripts, preprint publications, and submissions to rapidly disseminate new findings [84, 85]. Publishers addressed the need to shorten the peer review time considerably, something traditionally considered a critical hurdle in publishing.

This unprecedented flood of research, both by preprints and journal publications, has undoubtedly changed the research landscape. The MIT Press [86] launched Rapid Reviews: COVID-19, in which they plan to use artificial intelligence (AI) to identify promising preprints and conduct expert peer reviews. In addition to AI, literature hubs like LitCovid increased accessibility to published work relating to COVID-19. The influx of research coupled with the increased publication rate has undoubtedly aided our ability to respond to the SARS-CoV-2 virus.

Publishers adapted to the increased demand for novel information about the SARS-CoV-2 virus with rapid review models and amassing a growing number of reviewers. However, as research evolves amid the influx of research, many in the scientific community were wary of preprints and scientific credibility. Traditionally, reviewers acted as filters to ensure only high-quality works get published, often taking months to a year to complete a peer review [87]. Quicker peer reviews introduce the possible tradeoff between speed and quality. Horbach [83] argues that false information in journal articles is more damaging because it appears "peer-reviewed" and is infrequently verified. The dramatic increase in preprints also contributed to public misinformation as research was presented without review. BioRxiv, one of the leading search engines for preprint papers, has addressed these concerns by adding a disclaimer that emphasizes that preprints do not undergo peer-review and should not be considered as conclusive or reported in media. Additionally, this has led scientists like Liam Brierley [81] to issue general guidelines to read preprint research.

## Novel Collaborations for Large-Scale Data

Large-scale data use has played an increasingly significant role in both science and technological development. Prospective meta-analysis (PMA), the Open Access (OA) initiative, and many other tools substantially aided data pooling and opened global collaboration opportunities. Collaboration for open data was particularly significant for lower-income or developing countries unable to access publicly funded research. However, large-scale data sharing was not immune to its challenges and limitations, but considerable progress came about during the COVID-19 pandemic.

Scientific progress has often relied on collaboration to advance our understanding and ability to solve novel problems. The need for large-scale data collaboration amid a pandemic becomes evident by the need to rapidly disseminate information, especially to inform policy and clinical practice. Chan et al. [88] recognized the need for collaborative large-scaled data sharing and open access as a means to increasing the stability and economic development of poorer nations. Additionally, the need for large-scale data collaboration has surfaced several deficiencies in open data sharing, particularly in Latin American countries. Curioso and Carrasco-Escobar [89] cite the existence of the Scientific Electronic Library Online (SciElo) that includes over 16 Latin American and Caribbean countries with over a million scientific articles from over 200 universities. However, they also emphasize the need for interoperable open data repositories, modeled after SciElo, to increase transparency, reproducibility of results, and aid in evidence-based policymaking. The push for collaborative open access to large-scale data has, however, raised legal and ethical concerns.

Chan et al. [88] cite that developing countries were often receptive to collaborative data sharing but face resistance from developed countries' academic institutions. Challenges to collaboration for large-scale data present cultural and systemic challenges, individual consent, and privacy [90]. Redundancy in possible overlapping publications was also a common challenge against large-scale data collaboration [91]. Nonetheless, resistance to collaboration has eased gradually over the years, accelerated by the COVID-19 pandemic.

Despite several challenges facing large-scale data collaboration, considerable progress has come to light during the COVID-19 pandemic. For instance, Gao et al. [92] recently published an extensive report detailing the collaboration of large-scale data in the USA, including the use of Research Electronic Data Capture (REDCap), consisting of 4421 active international nonprofit organizations by the CDC and NIH to support COVID-19 surveillance and research. One principle example of large-scale data collaborations comes from the John Hopkins University (JHU) COVID-19 dashboard. Gardner et al. [93] cite the JHU COVID-19 dashboard as the authoritative source of global COVID-19 epidemiological data, with over 1200 citations in the first 4 months of its publication.

Rios et al. [94] describe data sharing during the COVID-19 pandemic as "one of the pillars of scientific progress, cooperation between different countries and cultures is the fastest way to accumulate valuable knowledge and face challenges like the current pandemic." Likewise, the COVID-19 crisis impacted international collaboration and research practices by creating unprecedented information sharing and research demand.

## Conclusion

While the COVID-19 pandemic disrupted modern health-care systems, creative solutions emerged out of clinical necessity to address the rapidly evolving clinical landscape, resource shortages, and gaps in knowledge. The subsequent recovery process will undoubtedly highlight the pandemic's evolution across the globe and institutional changes in clinical practice. Mass disruptions in routine surgical volume led to massive surgical backlog resulting in treatment delays and the potential for disease progression. Coupled with frayed supply chains, uncertainty about the SARS-CoV-2 virus, and an already worn-down workforce forced health institutions to slow transmission with limited PPE or clinical guidelines. Global surges in COVID-19 cases posed ethical and logistical concerns for institutions, but the development of surge capacity and triage protocols aided in lessening the disruption of bed shortages. Despite the tragic toll of the COVID-19 pandemic, one silver lining may be the unprecedented data sharing and research evolution that informed clinical practice. Regardless of limited resources, information, or staff, the evolution of clinical practice in response to the COVID-19 pandemic is one of the beacons of modern scientific progress.

## References

1. Morgan JM, Calleja P. Emergency trauma care in rural and remote settings: challenges and patient outcomes. Int Emerg Nurs. 2020;51:100880. https://doi.org/10.1016/j.ienj.2020.100880.
2. Tummers L. Understanding co-housing from a planning perspective: why and how? Urban Res Pract. 2015;8(1):64–78. https://doi.org/10.1080/17535069.2015.1011427.
3. Lee W, Kim H, Choi HM, Heo S, Fong KC, Yang J, Bell ML. Urban environments and COVID-19 in three Eastern States of the United States. Sci Total Environ. 2021;779:146334. https://doi.org/10.1016/j.scitotenv.2021.146334.
4. Pett E, Leung HL, Taylor E, Chong MSF, Hla TTW, Sartori G, Wigmore T. Critical care transfers and COVID-19: managing capacity challenges through critical care networks. J Intensive Care Soc. 2020;23(2):203–9. https://doi.org/10.1177/1751143720980270.
5. Jay J, Bor J, Nsoesie EO, Lipson SK, Jones DK, Galea S, Raifman J. Neighbourhood income and physical distancing during the COVID-19 pandemic in the United States. Nat Hum Behav. 2020;4(12):1294–302. https://doi.org/10.1038/s41562-020-00998-2.
6. Bilal U, Barber S, Tabb L, Diez-Roux AV. Spatial inequities in COVID-19 testing, positivity, incidence and mortality in 3 US cities: a longitudinal ecological study. medRxiv. 2020;2020:20087833. https://doi.org/10.1101/2020.05.01.20087833.
7. Chaudhry R, Dranitsaris G, Mubashir T, Bartoszko J, Riazi S. A country level analysis measuring the impact of government actions, country preparedness and socioeconomic factors on COVID-19 mortality and related health outcomes. EClinicalMedicine. 2020;25:100464. https://doi.org/10.1016/j.eclinm.2020.100464.
8. De Luca G, Cercek M, Jensen LO, Vavlukis M, Calmac L, Johnson T, Verdoia M. Impact of COVID-19 pandemic and diabetes on mechanical reperfusion in patients with STEMI: insights from the ISACS STEMI COVID 19 registry. Cardiovasc Diabetol. 2020;19(1):215. https://doi.org/10.1186/s12933-020-01196-0.

9. Rosenbaum L. The untold toll—the pandemic's effects on patients without Covid-19. N Engl J Med. 2020;382(24):2368–71. https://doi.org/10.1056/NEJMms2009984.
10. McPhail S, Johnson S, Greenberg D, Peake M, Rous B. Stage at diagnosis and early mortality from cancer in England. Br J Cancer. 2015;112(Suppl 1):S108–15. https://doi.org/10.1038/bjc.2015.49.
11. Toss A, Isca C, Venturelli M, Nasso C, Ficarra G, Bellelli V, Tazzioli G. Two-month stop in mammographic screening significantly impacts on breast cancer stage at diagnosis and upfront treatment in the COVID era. ESMO Open. 2021;6(2):100055. https://doi.org/10.1016/j.esmoop.2021.100055.
12. Maringe C, Spicer J, Morris M, Purushotham A, Nolte E, Sullivan R, Aggarwal A. The impact of the COVID-19 pandemic on cancer deaths due to delays in diagnosis in England, UK: a national, population-based, modelling study. Lancet Oncol. 2020;21(8):1023–34. https://doi.org/10.1016/S1470-2045(20)30388-0.
13. Berlin, G, , Bueno D, Gibler K, Schulz J (2020). Cutting through the COVID-19 surgical backlog. McKinsey & Co, Atlanta
14. COVID Surg Collaborative. Elective surgery cancellations due to the COVID-19 pandemic: global predictive modelling to inform surgical recovery plans. BJS (Br J Surg). 2020;107(11):1440–9. https://doi.org/10.1002/bjs.11746.
15. Macdonald N, Clements C, Sobti A, Rossiter D, Unnithan A, Bosanquet N. Tackling the elective case backlog generated by Covid-19: the scale of the problem and solutions. J Public Health (Oxf). 2020;42(4):712–6. https://doi.org/10.1093/pubmed/fdaa155.
16. Garbuz DS, Xu M, Duncan CP, Masri BA, Sobolev B. Delays worsen quality of life outcome of primary total hip arthroplasty. Clin Orthop Relat Res. 2006;447:79–84.
17. Knebel C, Ertl M, Lenze U, Suren C, Dinkel A, Hirschmann MT, Pohlig F. COVID-19-related cancellation of elective orthopaedic surgery caused increased pain and psychosocial distress levels. Knee Surg Sports Traumatol Arthrosc. 2021;29:2379–85. https://doi.org/10.1007/s00167-021-06529-4.
18. Reyes C, Engel-Nitz NM, DaCosta Byfield S, Ravelo A, Ogale S, Bancroft T, Matasar M. Cost of disease progression in patients with metastatic breast, lung, and colorectal cancer. Oncologist. 2019;24(9):1209–18. https://doi.org/10.1634/theoncologist.2018-0018.
19. Kang DH, Heo R, Lee S, Baek S, Kim DH, Song JM, Lee JW. Initial surgery versus conservative management of symptomatic severe mitral regurgitation in the elderly. Heart. 2018;104(10):849–54. https://doi.org/10.1136/heartjnl-2017-311759.
20. Aggarwal S, Jain P, Jain A. COVID-19 and cataract surgery backlog in Medicare beneficiaries. J Cataract Refract Surg. 2020;46(11):1530–3. https://doi.org/10.1097/j.jcrs.0000000000000337.
21. Jain A, Jain P, Aggarwal S. SARS-CoV-2 impact on elective orthopaedic surgery: implications for post-pandemic recovery. J Bone Jt Surg Am. 2020a;102(13):e68. https://doi.org/10.2106/jbjs.20.00602.
22. Salenger R, Etchill EW, Ad N, Matthew T, Alejo D, Whitman G, Gammie JS. The surge after the surge: cardiac surgery post-COVID-19. Ann Thorac Surg. 2020;110(6):2020–5. https://doi.org/10.1016/j.athoracsur.2020.04.018.
23. Pan American Health Organization. WHO reveals leading causes of death and disability worldwide: 2000–2019. 2020. https://www.paho.org/en/news/9-12-2020-who-reveals-leading-causes-death-and-disability-worldwide-2000-2019.
24. Tank A. 4 strategies for addressing an elective surgery backlog. 2020. https://chghealthcare.com/blog/elective-surgery-backlog/.
25. Jain, A, , Dai TBK, Myers CG (2020b). Covid-19 created an elective surgery backlog: how can hospitals get back on track?. Harv Bus Rev 10: 346
26. Kruger EC, Banderker R, Erasmus RT, Zemlin AE. The impact of COVID-19 on routine patient care from a laboratory perspective. S Afr Med J. 2020;110(12):1201–5. https://doi.org/10.7196/SAMJ.2020.v110i12.15294.
27. Chevance A, Gourion D, Hoertel N, Llorca PM, Thomas P, Bocher R, Gaillard R. Ensuring mental health care during the SARS-CoV-2 epidemic in France: a narrative review. Encéphale. 2020;46(3s):S3–s13. https://doi.org/10.1016/j.encep.2020.03.001.

28. The Centers for Disease Control and Prevention. Early release of selected mental health estimates based on data from the January–June 2019 National Health Interview Survey. 2019. https://www.cdc.gov/nchs/data/nhis/earlyrelease/ERmentalhealth-508.pdf.
29. The Centers for Disease Control and Prevention. Indicators of anxiety or depression based on reported frequency of symptoms during last 7 days. 2020. https://www.cdc.gov/nchs/covid19/pulse/mental-health.htm.
30. Czeisler MÉ, Lane RI, Petrosky E, Wiley JF, Christensen A, Njai R, Rajaratnam SMW. Mental health, substance use, and suicidal ideation during the COVID-19 pandemic—United States, June 24–30, 2020. MMWR Morb Mortal Wkly Rep. 2020;69(32):1049–57. https://doi.org/10.15585/mmwr.mm6932a1.
31. Ojha HA, Wyrsta NJ, Davenport TE, Egan WE, Gellhorn AC. Timing of physical therapy initiation for nonsurgical management of musculoskeletal disorders and effects on patient outcomes: a systematic review. J Orthop Sports Phys Ther. 2016;46(2):56–70. https://doi.org/10.2519/jospt.2016.6138.
32. Şahin N, Karahan AY, Albayrak İ. Effectiveness of physical therapy and exercise on pain and functional status in patients with chronic low back pain: a randomized-controlled trial. Turk J Phys Med Rehabil. 2017;64(1):52–8. https://doi.org/10.5606/tftrd.2018.1238.
33. Mao L, Jin H, Wang M, Hu Y, Chen S, He Q, Hu B. Neurologic manifestations of hospitalized patients with coronavirus disease 2019 in Wuhan, China. JAMA Neurol. 2020;77(6):683–90. https://doi.org/10.1001/jamaneurol.2020.1127.
34. Bai Y, Yao L, Wei T, Tian F, Jin D-Y, Chen L, Wang M. Presumed asymptomatic carrier transmission of COVID-19. JAMA. 2020;323(14):1406–7. https://doi.org/10.1001/jama.2020.2565.
35. He X, Lau EHY, Wu P, Deng X, Wang J, Hao X, Leung GM. Temporal dynamics in viral shedding and transmissibility of COVID-19. Nat Med. 2020;26(5):672–5. https://doi.org/10.1038/s41591-020-0869-5.
36. Rivett L, Sridhar S, Sparkes D, Routledge M, Jones NK, Forrest S, Weekes MP. Screening of healthcare workers for SARS-CoV-2 highlights the role of asymptomatic carriage in COVID-19 transmission. Elife. 2020;9:58728. https://doi.org/10.7554/eLife.58728.
37. Fields BKK, Demirjian NL, Gholamrezanezhad A. Coronavirus disease 2019 (COVID-19) diagnostic technologies: a country-based retrospective analysis of screening and containment procedures during the first wave of the pandemic. Clin Imaging. 2020;67:219–25. https://doi.org/10.1016/j.clinimag.2020.08.014.
38. Tanne JH, Hayasaki E, Zastrow M, Pulla P, Smith P, Rada AG. Covid-19: how doctors and healthcare systems are tackling coronavirus worldwide. BMJ. 2020;368:m1090. https://doi.org/10.1136/bmj.m1090.
39. Quattrone F, Vabanesi M, Borghini A, De Vito G, Emdin M, Passino C. The value of hospital personnel serological screening in an integrated COVID-19 infection prevention and control strategy. Infect Control Hosp Epidemiol. 2021;42(3):373–4. https://doi.org/10.1017/ice.2020.242.
40. Chau CH, Strope JD, Figg WD. COVID-19 clinical diagnostics and testing technology. Pharmacotherapy. 2020;40(8):857–68. https://doi.org/10.1002/phar.2439.
41. Hersher R. 'It's like something's right in your grasp': hospitals struggle to test for virus. New York: New York University; 2020. p. 1–12.
42. Buerhaus PI, Auerbach DI, Staiger DO. Older clinicians and the surge in novel coronavirus disease 2019 (COVID-19). JAMA J Am Med Assoc. 2020;323(18):1777–8. https://doi.org/10.1001/jama.2020.4978.
43. Marsh BJ. In one day, 1000 NYC doctors and nurses enlist to battle coronavirus. New York Post. 2020;18:21–3.
44. Reeves JJ, Hollandsworth HM, Torriani FJ, Taplitz R, Abeles S, Tai-Seale M, Longhurst CA. Rapid response to COVID-19: health informatics support for outbreak management in an academic health system. J Am Med Inform Assoc. 2020;27(6):853–9. https://doi.org/10.1093/jamia/ocaa037.

45. Emecen AN, Basoglu Sensoy E, Sezgin E, Yildirim Ustuner B, Keskin S, Siyve N, Ergor G. Transmission dynamics and timing of key events for SARS-CoV-2 infection in healthcare workers. Infect Dis (Lond). 2021;53(7):531–7. https://doi.org/10.1080/23744235.2021.1900599.
46. Wells KJ, Dwyer AJ, Calhoun E, Valverde PA. Community health workers and non-clinical patient navigators: a critical COVID-19 pandemic workforce. Prev Med. 2021;146:106464. https://doi.org/10.1016/j.ypmed.2021.106464.
47. Burki T. Global shortage of personal protective equipment. Lancet Infect Dis. 2020;20(7):785–6. https://doi.org/10.1016/S1473-3099(20)30501-6.
48. Cohen J, van der Rodgers YM. Contributing factors to personal protective equipment shortages during the COVID-19 pandemic. Prev Med. 2020;141:106263. https://doi.org/10.1016/j.ypmed.2020.106263.
49. MacIntyre CR, Wang Q, Rahman B, Seale H, Ridda I, Gao Z, Dwyer DE. Efficacy of face masks and respirators in preventing upper respiratory tract bacterial colonization and co-infection in hospital healthcare workers. Prev Med. 2014;62:1–7. https://doi.org/10.1016/j.ypmed.2014.01.015.
50. Bradley J. In scramble for coronavirus supplies, rich countries push poor aside. The New York Times. 2020;9:9–10. https://www.nytimes.com/2020/04/09/world/coronavirus-equipment-rich-poor.html?smid=nytcore-ios-share
51. McMahon DE, Peters GA, Ivers LC, Freeman EE. Global resource shortages during COVID-19: bad news for low-income countries. PLoS Negl Trop Dis. 2020;14(7):e0008412. https://doi.org/10.1371/journal.pntd.0008412.
52. Devi S. US public health budget cuts in the face of COVID-19. Lancet Infect Dis. 2020;20(4):415. https://doi.org/10.1016/S1473-3099(20)30182-1.
53. Emanuel EJ, Persad G, Upshur R, Thome B, Parker M, Glickman A, Phillips JP. Fair allocation of scarce medical resources in the time of Covid-19. N Engl J Med. 2020;382(21):2049–55. https://doi.org/10.1056/NEJMsb2005114.
54. Hunter DJ. Engla, Journal—2010—New England Journal. N Engl J Med. 2020;31(1):1969–73.
55. Bauchner H, Fontanarosa PB, Livingston EH. Conserving supply of personal protective equipment—a call for ideas. JAMA. 2020;323(19):1911. https://doi.org/10.1001/jama.2020.4770.
56. Reid V, Hurst T. When desperation breeds creativity: how US hospitals are approaching a PPE shortage. Washington, DC: The Advisory Board Company; 2020. p. 1–4.
57. Lowe J. Nebraska medicine pioneering technique to re-use PPE. Omaha: UNMC; 2020. p. 1–3.
58. Muñoz M, Comtois-Bona M, Cortes D, Cimenci CE, Du Q, Thompson C, Alarcon EI. Integrated photothermal decontamination device for N95 respirators. Sci Rep. 2021;11(1):1822. https://doi.org/10.1038/s41598-020-80908-8.
59. Davies A, Thompson K-A, Giri K, Kafatos G, Walker J, Bennett A. Testing the efficacy of homemade masks: would they protect in an influenza pandemic? Disaster Med Public Health Prep. 2013;7(4):413–8. https://doi.org/10.1017/dmp.2013.43.
60. CDC. COVID-19 considerations for release of stockpiled N95s beyond the manufacturer-designated shelf life considerations to inform product release decisions. Washington, DC: CDC; 2020. p. 1–5.
61. Ma X, Vervoort D. COVID-19 and the critical shortage in critical care. Glob Health Now. 2020;58:1–5.
62. Craxì L, Vergano M, Savulescu J, Wilkinson D. Rationing in a pandemic: lessons from Italy. Asian Bioethics Rev. 2020;12(3):325–30. https://doi.org/10.1007/s41649-020-00127-1.
63. Cillo U, Burra P, Mazzaferro V, Belli L, Pinna AD, Spada M, on behalf of the, I. B. A multi-step, consensus-based approach to organ allocation in liver transplantation: toward a "blended principle model". Am J Transplant. 2015;15(10):2552–61. https://doi.org/10.1111/ajt.13408.
64. Carenzo L, Costantini E, Greco M, Barra FL, Rendiniello V, Mainetti M, Cecconi M. Hospital surge capacity in a tertiary emergency referral centre during the COVID-19 outbreak in Italy. Anaesthesia. 2020;75(7):928–34. https://doi.org/10.1111/anae.15072.

65. Ramachandran BS, Kusisto L, Honan K. How New York's coronavirus response made the pandemic worse. Wall Street J. 2020;11:3–5.
66. Daugherty Biddison EL, Faden R, Gwon HS, Mareiniss DP, Regenberg AC, Schoch-Spana M, Toner ES. Too many patients... a framework to guide statewide allocation of scarce mechanical ventilation during disasters. Chest. 2019;155(4):848–54. https://doi.org/10.1016/j.chest.2018.09.025.
67. Tsai TC, Jacobson BH, Jha AK. Effect of COVID-19 on critical ICU capacity in US acute care hospitals. medRxiv. 2020;2020:20248366. https://doi.org/10.1101/2020.12.16.20248366.
68. Kumaraiah D, Yip N, Ivascu N, Hill L. Innovative ICU physician care models: Covid-19 pandemic at New York–Presbyterian. NEJM Catal Innov Care Deliv. 2020;28:1–6. https://doi.org/10.1056/CAT.20.0158.
69. Murray CJL. Forecasting COVID-19 impact on hospital bed-days, ICU-days, ventilator-days and deaths by US state in the next 4 months. medRxiv. 2020;114:20043752. https://doi.org/10.1101/2020.03.27.20043752.
70. Schaye Verity E, Reich Jenna A, Bosworth Brian P, Stern David T, Volpicelli F, Shapiro Neil M, Bails Douglas B. Collaborating across private, public, community, and Federal Hospital Systems: lessons learned from the Covid-19 pandemic response in NYC. NEJM Catal. 2020;1(6):343. https://doi.org/10.1056/CAT.20.0343.
71. Odlum M, Yoon S. What can we learn about the Ebola outbreak from tweets? Am J Infect Control. 2015;43(6):563–71. https://doi.org/10.1016/j.ajic.2015.02.023.
72. Jain R, Kelly CA, Mehta S, Tolliver D, Stewart A, Perdomo J. A trainee-led social media advocacy campaign to address COVID-19 inequities. Pediatrics. 2021;147(3):8456. https://doi.org/10.1542/peds.2020-028456.
73. Fung IC-H, Duke CH, Finch KC, Snook KR, Tseng P-L, Hernandez AC, Tse ZTH. Ebola virus disease and social media: a systematic review. Am J Infect Control. 2016;44(12):1660–71. https://doi.org/10.1016/j.ajic.2016.05.011.
74. Patel A, Jernigan DB, nCo, V. C. D. C. R. T. Initial public health response and interim clinical guidance for the 2019 novel coronavirus outbreak—United States, December 31, 2019–February 4, 2020. MMWR Morb Mortal Wkly Rep. 2020;69(5):140–6. https://doi.org/10.15585/mmwr.mm6905e1.
75. Mallhi TH, Liaqat A, Abid A, Khan YH, Alotaibi NH, Alzarea AI, Khan TM. Multilevel engagements of pharmacists during the COVID-19 pandemic: the way forward. Front Public Health. 2020;8:561924. https://doi.org/10.3389/fpubh.2020.561924.
76. Zamberg I, Manzano S, Posfay-Barbe K, Windisch O, Agoritsas T, Schiffer E. A mobile health platform to disseminate validated institutional measurements during the COVID-19 outbreak: utilization-focused evaluation study. JMIR Public Health Surveill. 2020;6(2):e18668. https://doi.org/10.2196/18668.
77. Brownson RC, Eyler AA, Harris JK, Moore JB, Tabak RG. Getting the word out: new approaches for disseminating public health science. J Public Health Manag Pract JPHMP. 2018;24(2):102–11. https://doi.org/10.1097/PHH.0000000000000673.
78. Chan AKM, Nickson CP, Rudolph JW, Lee A, Joynt GM. Social media for rapid knowledge dissemination: early experience from the COVID-19 pandemic. Anaesthesia. 2020;75(12):1579–82. https://doi.org/10.1111/anae.15057.
79. Martin LJ, Turnquist A, Groot B, Huang SYM, Kok E, Thoma B, van Merriënboer JJG. Exploring the role of infographics for summarizing medical literature. Health Prof Educ. 2019;5(1):48–57. https://doi.org/10.1016/j.hpe.2018.03.005.
80. Anaya J. Biology preprints over time. San Francisco: ASAPbio; 2020. p. 1–5.
81. Brierley L. Lessons from the influx of preprints during the early COVID-19 pandemic. Lancet Planet Health. 2021;5(3):e115–7. https://doi.org/10.1016/s2542-5196(21)00011-5.
82. Yozwiak NL, Schaffner SF, Sabeti PC. Data sharing: make outbreak research open access. Nature. 2015;518(7540):477–9. https://doi.org/10.1038/518477a.
83. Horbach SPJM. Pandemic Publishing: Medical journals drastically speed up their publication process for Covid-19. bioRxiv. 2020;2020:045963. https://doi.org/10.1101/2020.04.18.045963.

84. Brock J. Rapid registered reports initiative aims to stop coronavirus researchers following false leads. Nat Index. 2020;14:1–8.
85. Talley NJ. SARS-CoV-2, the medical profession, ventilator beds, and mortality predictions: personal reflections of an Australian clinician. Med J Aust. 2020;212(7):302–3. https://doi.org/10.5694/mja2.50579.
86. Pellien J. & Abbas EP. The MIT Press and UC Berkeley launch rapid reviews: COVID-19. MIT News (2020). https://mitpress.mit.edu/blog/mit-press-and-uc-berkeley-launch-rapid-reviews-covid-19.
87. Irvine A. Fast science: vetting rapid research during the COVID-19 pandemic. Amsterdam: Elsevier; 2020.
88. Chan L, Kirsop B, Arunachalam S. Open access archiving: the fast track to building research capacity in developing countries. London: Open Access; 2008. p. 1–27.
89. Curioso WH, Carrasco-Escobar G. Collaboration in times of COVID-19: the urgent need for open-data sharing in Latin America. BMJ Health Care Inform. 2020;27(1):e100159. https://doi.org/10.1136/bmjhci-2020-100159.
90. Lancet. Transparency during global health emergencies. Lancet Digit Health. 2020;2(9):e441. https://doi.org/10.1016/S2589-7500(20)30198-9.
91. Smith ER, Flaherman VJ. Why you should share your data during a pandemic. BMJ Glob Health. 2021;6(3):e004940. https://doi.org/10.1136/bmjgh-2021-004940.
92. Gao F, Tao L, Huang Y, Shu Z. Management and data sharing of COVID-19 pandemic information. Biopreserv Biobank. 2020;18(6):570–80. https://doi.org/10.1089/bio.2020.0134.
93. Gardner L, Ratcliff J, Dong E, Katz A. A need for open public data standards and sharing in light of COVID-19. Lancet Infect Dis. 2020;21(4):e80. https://doi.org/10.1016/S1473-3099(20)30635-6.
94. Rios RS, Zheng KI, Zheng MH. Data sharing during COVID-19 pandemic: what to take away. Expert Rev Gastroenterol Hepatol. 2020;14(12):1125–30. https://doi.org/10.1080/17474124.2020.1815533.

# Chapter 30
# Anticipated Long-Term Neurobehavioral Outcomes Following COVID-19

**Erin K. Bailey, Joel E. Kamper, and Becky Gius**

Chapter objectives are as follows

1. Knowledge of medical and mental health factors which contribute to long-term cognitive symptomology in COVID-19 patients.
2. Identification of potential underlying causes of chronic cognitive, mental health, and physical complaints.
3. Familiarity with treatment directions for COVID-19 patients with chronic symptomology.

## Physiological Mechanisms of Long-Term Cognitive Change

Neuroinvasive properties of coronaviruses are well documented. Following entry, SARS-CoV-2 hijacks the host cells and uses the existing cell structures to promote viral replication. The result is a preferential excess of $O_2$ and metabolic resources

Portions of this chapter have been adapted from: *Bailey, E. K., Steward, K. A., VandenBussche Jantz, A. B., Kamper, J. E., Mahoney, E. J., and Duchnick, J. J. (2021). Neuropsychology of COVID-19: Anticipated cognitive and mental health outcomes. Neuropsychology, 35(4), 335.*

E. K. Bailey (✉) · J. E. Kamper
James A. Haley Veterans' Hospital, Tampa, FL, USA
e-mail: Erin.Bailey@va.gov; Joel.Kamper@va.gov

B. Gius
James A. Haley Veterans' Hospital, Tampa, FL, USA

University of South Florida, Tampa, FL, USA
e-mail: BkGius@usf.edu



S. Adibi et al. (eds.), *Frontiers of COVID-19*,
https://doi.org/10.1007/978-3-031-08045-6_30

supporting viral proliferation at the expense of uninfected cells, resulting in neuronal death [1]. Neuroimmune activation, as well as systemic and CNS inflammatory responses to SARS-CoV-2 infection triggers prolonged hyperactivation of the autoimmune cytokine network. The resulting dysregulated autoimmune response (cytokine storm) can cause metabolic derangements with possible subsequent organ failure, respiratory distress, blood coagulation abnormalities, and damage to endothelial cells in an attempt to return the body to homoeostasis [2]. Unfortunately, all these outcomes pose a risk for neurobehavioral change [3, 4]. While acute symptoms tend to remit with treatment of the underlying viral infection, protracted recovery and prolonged inflammatory responses beyond acute illness may place patients at risk for persisting neuropsychiatric symptoms or neurocognitive changes [5–7], despite eventual treatment and immune stabilization. Further, cognitive symptoms secondary to COVID-19 may not be directly due to the virus itself [8], but rather the outcome of downstream effects, as will be described in the sections below. In this section, we will discuss possible physiological mechanisms for prolonged neurocognitive outcomes that may be associated with COVID-19.

## *Hypoxia and Hypoxemia*

As primarily a respiratory disease, hypoxia (poor oxygenation at the tissue level) and hypoxemia (low blood oxygen levels) and both are manifestations of COVID-19 [9–11]. While acute hypoxic encephalopathy (HIE) typically follows the natural course of delirium (i.e., acute onset, with gradual resolution following resolution of the underlying medical cause), given the vital role of oxygen in cerebral functioning, severe or prolonged hypoperfusion can result in hypoxic–ischemic injury [12–14], coma [15, 16], and increased likelihood of residual cognitive impairments. Hypoxic brain injuries result from disruption of oxygen to critical brain areas. Due to its high metabolic demands, the hippocampus is typically involved, with dense anterograde amnesia being a classic sign of hypoxic injury [17, 18]. However, other gray matter regions including the thalamus, cerebellum, and areas of the cerebral cortex are also often involved [19]. Research has shown that while memory deficits remain a primary finding, changes in personality and behavior, visuospatial defects, and global cognitive impairments are also frequent findings [18, 20]. Watershed infarcts are also a common consequence of hypoxia. These often caused by prolonged hypoperfusion of the cerebral cortex at the terminal ends of the major arterial distributions, causing a characteristic "string of pearls" radiographic pattern [16, 21]. Watershed infarcts are associated with reduced working memory and visuospatial abilities [22].

Acute Respiratory Distress Syndrome (ARDS) is an often-fatal condition in which fluid collects within the air sacs of the lungs, causing extreme shortness of breath and severe hypoxemia [23]. Survivors of hypoxemia due to ARDS can also experience poor long-term outcomes [24]. In Hopkins et al.'s [25] longitudinal study following 55 individuals with ARDS, 100% of cases demonstrated cognitive impairments at the time of hospital discharge, including impaired memory, attention, and processing speed. When followed up a year later, many subjects saw mild improvements; however, 78% of these individuals continued to exhibit impairment in at least one of the aforementioned domains. Notably, $PaO_2$ (partial pressure of oxygen, a measurement of oxygen pressure in arterial blood) at baseline was significantly related to long-term outcomes on memory, attention, and processing speed tasks.

## *Stroke*

Cerebrovascular complications among COVID-19 are well-established [26, 27]. In addition to hypoxic-mediated ischemic change (described above), pro-inflammatory cytokine storms can alter blood coagulability by causing endothelial injury to blood vessels [26, 28]. The resulting prothrombic state raises risk of cardioembolic events and intracranial hemorrhage (ICH; [29]). As such, long-term cognitive complications from stroke syndromes and other cerebrovascular disease are broad in scope and nature. Injury to subcortical white matter can result in reduced processing speed, executive functioning, attention, and learning abilities [30]. However, large-vessel and/or focal insults may also produce circumscribed deficits in other areas of cognitive functioning—such as language, visuospatial processing, sensory/motor abilities, and memory [31]. Further, these patients may be more susceptible to post-stroke psychiatric changes, such as depression—a phenomenon attributed to biochemical changes as well as functional disability [32–34]. While severity of COVID-19 may play a role in increased risk for cerebrovascular disease, there is documentation of vascular dysfunction even among mild cases of COVID-19 [35, 36]. Ultimately, the full nature and extend of cardiovascular and cerebrovascular disease in COVID-19 is beyond the scope of this chapter. However, the increased risk of cerebrovascular compromise renders patients vulnerable to long-term cognitive and psychiatric change. See other chapters for detailed summaries of COVID-19-related vascular compromise.

## *Post-Intensive Care Syndrome*

Along with the increased survival rates of critical illness over the past several decades, it has been observed that many patients experience residual cognitive, physical, and psychiatric symptoms that can last for months, years, or reflect permanent changes [37–40]. Coined post-intensive care syndrome (PICS; [38]), this phenomenon encompasses new-onset or worsening cognitive, physical, or psychiatric symptoms following hospitalization for a critical illness may meet criteria for PICS, although the presence of multiple novel symptoms is more common, particularly in patients with pulmonary involvement [38, 41–43]. Pre-COVID-19 studies of mechanically ventilated patients suggest that up to 79% of patients had measurable cognitive changes at 3 months, and 71% had findings at 12 months postdischarge (with 36% of those having severe cognitive changes; [44]). A larger study of 821 ICU patients with history of respiratory failure or shock, found that 24% had global cognitive dysfunction >2 standard deviations below population means (~second percentile or lower) with only 6% having had cognitive impairments at baseline [40]. An even larger case-controlled observational study of 98,227 critically ill patients noted that 22% of ICU patients were cognitively impaired, with 2.5% of the total sample having new and persistent cognitive dysfunction at least 24 months postdischarge [45].

While many studies evaluating persistent post-ICU cognitive impairments have utilized brief screening tools, studies that have utilized more comprehensive examinations have demonstrated primary impairments in attention, memory, and executive functioning [40, 46, 47]. These data are consistent with the so-called subcortical pattern of cognitive impairment, which is commonly seen in patients with diffuse causes of cognitive dysfunction. Various mechanisms and predictors of PICS have been proposed, including hypoxia, metabolic or endocrine dysregulation, hypotension, use of sedatives, immobilization, sleep/wake disruptions, and intubation or ventilation [38]. Studies that have evaluated cognitive outcomes have identified the duration of delirium as a primary risk factor [44], as well as the number of ICU stays, hypotension, and hypoxemia [43, 45]. Interestingly, after controlling for other factors the duration of mechanical ventilation was not independently associated with PICS [44, 45].

## *Chronic Metabolic Dysfunction*

Emerging research also demonstrates that the lungs are not the only organ at risk of damage from COVID-19. Patients diagnosed with this virus are also at risk of experiencing acute liver and kidney dysfunction [48–50] which, in some cases, can have chronic effects. Elevated ammonia levels can increase cerebral edema, depress action potentials, and increase brain glutamate, all of which can disrupt normal brain metabolism. While patients with preexisting hepatic dysfunction may be more susceptible to severe cases of COVID-19 [51], data from prior coronavirus epidemics has demonstrated the ability of coronavirus to cause chronic liver and kidney injury [52] directly via ACE-2 receptors, as well as secondarily via inflammatory disorders and ischemia. In the short term, liver dysfunction can cause impairments in attention and concentration consistent with hepatic encephalopathy. Chronic hepatic disease is not only associated with these same decrements in attention, but also declines in motor praxis, calculations, visuospatial abilities, spatial scanning, processing speed, and some aspects of memory [53]. While, cognitive functions such as language, learning, abstraction, and general intelligence remain largely intact. Cognitive impairments associated with chronic kidney disease include decrements in immediate and long-term memory, executive functions, naming, visual scanning, and attention in the context of preserved verbal fluency [54, 55].

## *Neurodegenerative Risk*

Already vulnerable to deleterious cognitive, psychiatric, and medical outcomes [56, 57], COVID-19 patients with dementia may be at risk for acceleration of neurodegenerative processes. In this section, we nonexhaustively review three neurodegenerative conditions: Alzheimer's disease, degenerative demyelination, and Parkinson's disease in conjunction with emerging COVID-19 literature. Please see Figs. 30.1 and 30.2 as illustrated by Ferini-Strambi and Salsone [58] at the end of this section for an overview of main points in the associations between COVID-19 and the neurodegenerative conditions described below.

*Alzheimer's disease:* Viral invasion of the CNS by coronaviruses is hypothesized to occur through multiple mechanisms—both direct and indirect—including

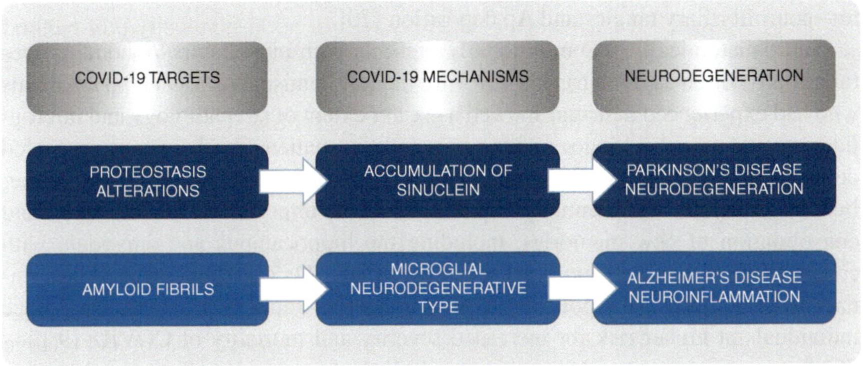


**Fig. 30.1** Schematic representation of main targets and pathogenetic mechanisms linking COVID-19 infection to Parkinson's disease and Alzheimer's disease neurodegeneration [58]

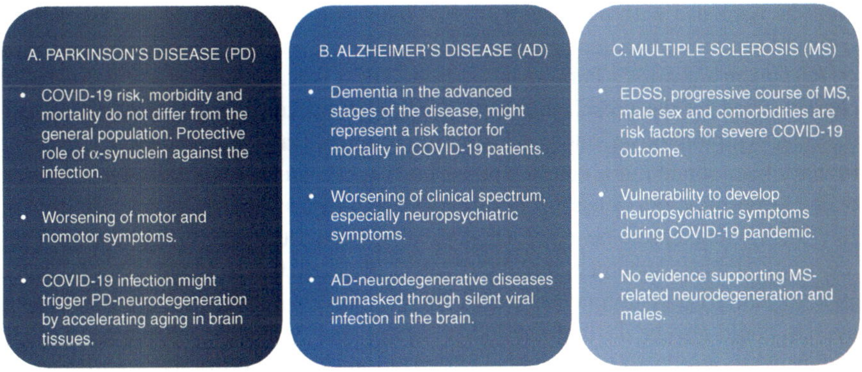


**Fig. 30.2** Key learning points on the interaction between COVID-19 infection and Parkinson's disease (**a**), Alzheimer's disease (**b**) and multiple sclerosis (**c**). [58]

infiltration of neuron and glial cells by binding to angiotensin-converting enzyme 2 (ACE2) receptors [59–61] through epithelium infiltration of the olfactory nerve [62] and damage of endothelial cells in blood vessels [63] resulting degeneration of the blood brain barrier. Neurotropism generates a neuroimmune response with activation of astrocytes and microglial cells resulting in the misfolding of proteins [64, 65] or myelin degeneration [66]. Microglial cells play a significant role in removing extracellular waste, regulating synaptic plasticity and neuronal activity, and supporting myelination, and regulating blood vessel permeability [67]. Alzheimer's disease (AD) is a neurodegenerative condition with two hallmark pathological underpinnings: neurofibrillary tangles, or accumulations of abnormally phosphorylated tau protein, and deposition of beta-amyloid (Aβ) plaques [68]. Although beyond the scope of this chapter, these pathologies have been linked to protein misfolding, accumulation of neuronal debris, and similar synaptic alterations or loss as seen in neuroimmune responses [5, 67, 69]. Myelin damage and death of oligodendrocytes is also seen in AD and has been theorized as a trigger of—or corollary to—neurofibrillary tangles and Aβ deposition [70].

Neuroanatomically, AD traditionally presents with hippocampal/medial temporal atrophy, often asymmetrically favoring the left hemisphere. COVID-19 patients who had experienced delirium showed a greater extent of tau pathology and microglial activation in the hippocampus, especially in patients with who experienced delirium earlier on in their hospital course [71]. Neurotropism via olfactory epithelium [62] may also differentially impact brain areas important to the formation and consolidation of new memories, including the hippocampus and amygdala with connect directly with olfactory nerve pathways [10, 72, 73]. While there is preliminary evidence that the ApoE ε4 allele, a genotype implicated in AD, may place individuals at higher risk for increased severity and mortality of COVID-19 [74–76], more research is needed in this area [77]. However, it is safe to conclude that AD may create circumstances in which patients are (1) more likely to contract COVID-19—such as nursing homes, (2) result in more severe COVID-19 symptoms due to premorbid health and cognitive vulnerability, and (3) predispose patients to a higher likelihood of delirium. Conversely, COVID-19 may result in a cascading immune response with neurotropism thus triggering, or exacerbating, AD pathology [78].

*Parkinson's disease:* Parkinson's disease (PD) is a neurodegenerative disorder characterized by the presence of extrapyramidal, parkinsonism symptoms, asymmetrical symptom onset, and good response to levodopa [79]. Coronavirus antibodies have been found in the cerebrospinal fluid of individuals with PD [80]. Anosmia, or impaired olfactory sense, is a commonly reported symptom in both PD and in COVID-19 and could be representative of a possible overlapping feature with respect to alpha-synuclein pathology [81, 82], although this is not necessarily indicative of definitive symbiotic or directional relationship between the two. Symptom overlap could also be attributed to other factors such as ICU-related complications and medication side effects during hospitalization [83]. PD is often accompanied by other well-established COVID-19 risk factors such as older age and premorbid health conditions (e.g., obesity, chronic obstructive pulmonary disease). Vitamin D deficiency is commonly reported in patients with Parkinson's disease [84] and has also been proposed as a potential risk factor for COVID-19 [85]. Lastly, individuals with Parkinson's disease may also be at greater risk for contracting COVID-19 due to socioenvironmental factors associated with their condition, such as residing in a nursing facility or receiving home-based medical care [83].

Infections have also been shown to exacerbate Parkinson's disease symptoms [86, 87]. Evidence from two studies with small sample sizes suggest that COVID-19 may result in worsening of motor symptoms [88, 89]. Another study found that new motor symptoms were reported by 18% of individuals with Parkinson's disease who endorsed confirmed or probable COVID-19 diagnosis, while 55% reported worsening of at least one motor symptom [90]. This study also described new or worsened nonmotor symptoms including mood (20% new; 51% worsening), self-reported cognitive changes (7.8% new; 41% worsening), and sleep disturbance (12% new; 59% worsening). Indirect sequalae of the COVID-19 pandemic may also play a role in symptom exacerbation. In one study, almost a quarter of individuals with PD reported new or worsened sleep disturbances, such as REM sleep behavior disorder or restless leg syndrome [91], during home confinement periods of the COVID-19 pandemic. New or worsened sleep disturbance was also associated with worsened motor features of PD and an increase in subjective mental health complaints, such as greater instances of hallucinations, anxiety, depression, and impulsive behavior compared to PD patients without sleep disturbance. Those reporting changes in sleep disturbance were also more likely to report longer duration of PD diagnosis and longer periods of home confinement.

*Demyelination:* Several case studies over the last few decades have found links between demyelinating disorders and human coronavirus [92, 93]. To this end, elucidating the relationship between demyelination and COVID-19 is necessary to better understand the risk of symptom exacerbation and associated cognitive changes in demyelinating disorders due to COVID-19. COVID-19 patients demonstrate greater microglial activation in the brain stem and myelin loss in the subcortical and deep white matter compared to controls [94]. In patients with preexisting autoimmune demyelinating diseases, COVID-19 infection may trigger worsened inflammatory responses that progress neurodegeneration. With regard to exacerbation of MS symptoms, approximately one-fifth of MS patients with COVID-19 reported recurrence of neurologic symptoms before or during COVID-19 symptom onset [95]. There is also evidence that COVID-19 can trigger other immune-mediated diseases such as Guillain–Barre syndrome [96]. Both inflammatory responses and immune-mediated organ damage have been identified as protentional mechanisms for exacerbation of demyelinating conditions among patient with viral infections [97, 98], including COVID-19 [99]. For this reason, current literature favors continuation of disease-modifying therapies for COVID-19 patients with demyelinating disorders [100].

## Psychiatric Conditions That Impact Cognition

To compliment identification of possible organic causes cognitive changes related to COVID-19 (described above), we will also offer a review of literature examining nonneurological factors which may promote protracted resolution of cognitive and physical complaints which would otherwise be expected to resolve or improve over time. The presence of persistent cognitive symptoms from COVID-19 may not be related to the disease itself, but to secondary health factors, preexisting conditions, or co-occurring psychiatric factors, or beliefs/expectations which perpetuate functional disability. Many individuals have experienced trauma associated with the pandemic such as personal illness, illness or death of a loved one, and loss of employment or housing, which may lead to increased psychiatric illness [101, 102]. At the individual level, financial difficulties and unemployment have also accompanied the COVID-19 pandemic, which are associated with depression and anxiety even under nonpandemic circumstances [103, 104]. At the community level, day-to-day social and occupational functioning have been altered for both those with and without infection light of government requirements and other sanctioned restrictions of social distancing and self-quarantine, which may reasonably result in feelings of social isolation and worry about one's own health as well as the safety and health of loved ones. To this end, it is imperative to elucidate the role psychiatric conditions may play in observed cognitive changes following COVID-19 infection [105, 106].

### *Depression*

Depression is characterized by feelings of sadness, anhedonia, changes in sleep or appetite, reduced energy, poor concentration, and thoughts of guilt [107]. Depression is not uncommon among those hospitalized for COVID-19, with greater symptom endorsement reported among those who were older, reported a family member also had COVID-19, or reported lower social support [108, 109]. In some, depressive symptoms persist postdischarge [110] and interferes with overall quality of life. Cognitive change associated with depression is well-established. Severity of depressive symptoms has been associated with decline in episodic memory, executive function, attention, and processing speed [111, 112].

*Sleep disturbance and lockdowns:* Sleep disturbance is a known contributor to day-to-day cognitive problems and depression. Sleep disruptions are associated with reduced attention, working memory, processing speed, and memory retrieval deficits on cognitive testing [113, 114]. During lockdown, studies show changes in sleep patterns compared to prelockdown sleep. These include a shift to later bedtimes and waking times, a reduction of nighttime sleep, and an increase in daytime napping [115]. Quality of sleep also declined in the study sample, with ~25% of participants reporting poor quality of sleep during lockdown. Depression and increased latency of sleep onset were associated with reduced quality of sleep after lockdown [115]. Geriatric populations in general are more prone to isolation, and thus be distinctively impacted by lockdown and social distancing [91].

*Bereavement/death of loved ones:* Grief, or bereavement, is defined as the change in thoughts, feelings, and behaviors associated with the death of a loved one [116] and is another potential source of depression during the COVID-19 pandemic. In approximately 9% of individuals experiencing grief, symptoms persist beyond the typical 6-month acute stage and become both persisting and functionally debilitating. The resulting complex grief disorder (also called *Complicated Grief* or *Persisting Grief Disorder*) further predisposes individuals to deleterious outcomes [117]. The COVID-19 pandemic places individuals at higher risk for of long-term grief symptoms due to several factors. These include an abrupt or unexpected loss, the loss of traditional death rituals—such as burial and saying goodbye—because of COVID-19 restrictions and lockdowns, and the total absence or alteration in physical social support due to social distancing and travel regulations [118]. Grief has also been linked to immunocompromise, further adding risk of cascading psychiatric and general health consequences [119]. Older adults with complex grief may show increased signs of slowed processing speed, reduced attention, and difficulties with verbal fluency [118]. However, this may be mediated by co-occurring depression and anxiety, thus able to be fully or partially treated with mental health interventions, such as antidepressant medications or psychotherapy techniques [120, 121].

## *Anxiety*

In addition to depressive symptoms, patients with COVID-19 also report symptoms of anxiety, including persistent worry that is difficult to control, physiological symptoms (e.g., increased heart rate, muscle tension), restlessness, fatigue, and poor sleep [107]. Pathological mechanisms of COVID-19 may help explain elevated anxiety among these patients, either via direct viral infection of the central nervous system [10, 122] or secondary to neuroinflammation [123, 124] Regarding the latter, immune response and systemic inflammation markers (e.g., lymphocyte, platelet, and neutrophil counts) have been found to be associated with both anxiety and depression symptoms 1 month postcharge for COVID-19 infection [125]. Nonmedical risk factors for anxiety include hospitalization, female gender, older age, and lower social support [108]. Lower oxygen saturation (a clinical marker for COVID-19 severity) was also associated with greater anxiety symptoms among those hospitalized for COVID-19. Acute anxiety is linked to impaired cognitive performance in domains of attention, executive function, language (i.e., word finding difficulties), and memory [126–128]. Chronic anxiety is also associated with cognitive symptoms. For example, anxiety and depression were associated with subjective cognitive complaints, including anomia and attention difficulties, among COVID-19 patients who completed a follow-up, 10–35 days postdischarge [129].

Given the potential for depression and anxiety symptoms to persist postdischarge, continued monitoring of psychiatric cognitive symptomology, as well as any clinically indicated psychotherapeutic treatment, will be an important component of follow up care for COVID-19 survivors.

## *Posttraumatic Stress Disorder*

Posttraumatic stress disorder (PTSD) is an emotional stress reaction to a traumatic event, typically (but not necessarily) in response to a threat to life or well-being of an individual or loved one [107]. Individual psychological factors associated with development and maintenance of PTSD symptoms can include emotional status at the time of the trauma (e.g., depression and anxiety), lack of perceived control over the outcome, and fear of permanent change after the traumatic event [130].

Microglial activation and autoimmune responses to a biologic or environmental trigger, such as COVID-19, are implicated in psychiatric disease [131, 132]. For example, pro-inflammatory responses, such as elevated levels of cytokines are documented in patients with PTSD [133]. To this end, pro-inflammatory responses may be one potential bio-mechanism linking PTSD symptomology to COVID-19 infection. Specifically, elevated cortisol levels and dysregulation of the hypothalamic–pituitary–adrenal axis (HPA) in response to psychophysiological shock [134] is implicated as a physiological underpinning of PTSD. This dysregulation results in downstream neuroendocrine and metabolic change which mediate immune functioning. As such, COVID-19-mediated autoimmune dysfunction may render these patients more susceptible to development of PTSD symptomology—independent of other psychological and situational risk factors.

*PTSD after critical illness:* Respiratory compromise while hospitalized is shown to correlate with subsequent psychiatric outcomes, including PTSD [135]. Specifically, the occurrence of dyspnea among patients with respiratory distress is associated with PTSD [136]. Dyspnea, also known as "air hunger," is a CNS-mediated increase in respiratory drive and can activate neural pathways associated with anxiety and psychological trauma [137]. Psychiatric outcomes following dyspnea can persist for years despite physical recovery [41]. As respiratory diseases, it is not unsurprising that PTSD is prevalent among individuals recovering from coronaviruses [8]. For example, a review on emotional distress following SARS survivors found that symptoms of PTSD were prevalent across all stages of the disease process, including in the years following recovery from infection [138]. Rates of psychiatric sequalae vary, although estimated to be up to a quarter to almost half of those hospitalized for COVID-19 [102]. However, during pandemics, both those *with and without* history of viral infection are at risk for developing psychiatric symptomology (including depression, anxiety, and PTSD) considering the individual and collective social impact of pandemic-related restrictions and illness. For example, community-level PTSD is not uncommon during pandemics, with prevalence rates during prior coronavirus pandemics upwards of 25% in study populations [139]. In addition to patients and their families, those at-risk for PTSD during the COVID-19 pandemic include front-line works, such as health-care professionals, or others with repeated exposure to viral risk [140–142].

*Cognitive change in PTSD:* Cognitive changes associated with PTSD are well-established, with individuals demonstrating decline in attention and working memory abilities relative to non-PTSD controls [143–145]. Secondary effects of PTSD, such as sleep disturbance, can also exacerbate both psychological and cognitive outcomes over time [146–149]. Specific sleep abnormalities in PTSD include insomnia, disturbed sleep–wake cycle [150], changes in sleep architecture [151, 152] and trauma-related nightmares [153]. The presence of sleep disturbance in PTSD has also been linked to elevated levels of pro-inflammatory cytokines [131], again suggestive of additional risk for cognitive decline in COVID-19 patients with PTSD-associated sleep disorders. PTSD is associated with reduced neural integrity and accelerating biomarkers of aging [154], as well as increased incidence of dementia in later life [155].

Although pathologically dissimilar, drawing parallels between chronic postconcussive symptoms (PCS) and emerging chronic cognitive and physical complaints seen in recovered "Long COVID-19" patients—especially those with mild infection [156]—may provide insight into mediating variables which can contribute to persistent symptoms, as well as possible treatment approaches. Common complaints which overlap in these two phenomena include reduced quality of life, fatigue, memory/attention difficulties, and sleep disturbance [157, 158]. In one study [159], over half of participants who initially presented to acute trauma ICU settings with concussion or skull fracture—in the absence of intracranial hemorrhage—had cognitive impairment at follow-up (12–24 months). Cognitive impairment was characterized by reduced performance on measures of delayed memory, processing speed, attention, and verbal fluency compared to nonconcussion/non-skull fractured trauma ICU controls. Overall performance on a cognitive screening measure was also significantly lower in the concussion/skull fracture group compared to controls. Nearly 40% of subjects reported posttraumatic symptoms and over half of the participants reported depressive symptoms. Changes in functional status at follow-up—namely, employment—was also reported across groups, although especially prominent in individuals with reduced cognitive functioning. This study describes persisting cognitive and psychiatric changes in patients with high illness severity yet no radiographic evidence of intracranial hemorrhage, as well as highlights the need for follow-up in populations which would normally not be identified as at-risk, given relatively milder acute pathology. In military populations, the presence of PTSD has been shown to mediate chronic cognitive complaints associated with mild concussive injuries [160]. In these studies, cognitive complaints included attention changes, memory disturbance, and slowed processing speed which lasted months to years after the initial traumatic event [161–163].

Although full review and comparison of this literature is beyond the scope of this chapter, interventions which have shown to aid in cognitive recovery of mTBI patients include: a biopsychosocial approach to symptoms management, gradually resumption of premorbid lifestyle include employment and other cognitively or emotionally demanding roles, education regarding stress management and sleep hygiene, reassurance of anticipated positive outcomes, and provision of support resources [164]. Trauma-Informed Psychotherapy is also an effective for treatment of anxiety and depression. It is based on the understanding that traumatic events and associated chronic stress may have long-term impacts on how the central nervous system and endocrine system responds to and regulates fear and stress [165, 166]. For this reason, trauma-informed psychotherapy may be an effective treatment approach to fully appreciate the widespread impacts of the COVID-19 pandemic on emotional and social functioning [167].

## Additional Clinical Considerations

Literature describing neuropsychiatric outcomes of prior pandemics as well as mental health considerations among similar neuropathological medical conditions illustrate correlated risks of neuropsychiatric symptomatology in individuals affected both directly and indirectly by COVID-19. Globally, it will be critical for healthcare providers of all disciplines to be aware of neuropsychiatric manifestations, correlates, and strategies to manage them in ways which address the biopsychosocial needs of identifiable populations [4, 168].

### *The Neuropsychological Evaluation*

As referenced above, while there is certainly concern for acute and chronic cognitive dysfunction due to SARS-CoV-2 both directly and indirectly. In this context, it is important to remember that signs are not symptoms, and reported cognitive symptoms are not always reflective of true neurocognitive impairment. To help elucidate etiology, we recommend referring such patients for a neuropsychological evaluation, which will be able to help differentiate organic cognitive disorders from cognitive symptoms due to secondary psychiatric factors. Such a distinction is helpful to avoid iatrogenic effects and help inform treatment. For example, psychoeducation regarding expected outcomes and recovery trajectories for patients with more mild disease can play a large role in resolving lingering symptoms and concerns. Preliminary research has shown that survivors of prior CoV epidemics experienced higher rates of PTSD, which may account for some (or all) of their persistent cognitive complaints [160]. As psychiatric conditions like PTSD can have adverse effects on cognition, educating patients with nonspecific memory complaints can help them to understand and treat modifiable causes of cognitive symptoms [169]. The multifaceted benefits of a neuropsychological evaluation include monitoring resolution of delirium, measuring acute and long-term nature and extent of cognitive decline, providing education regarding nature and etiology of symptoms less likely to be the direct result of viral infection, and provision of prognostic feedback to patients, families, and referring providers.

## *Patient, Caregiver, and Community Factors*

In the above sections, we describe factors which are known to impact both chronic cognitive and mental health functioning. Yet, in order to fully appreciate the breadth of possible long-term consequence, tertiary influences should be also be included in identification of vulnerable populations. Known social and financial inequities, as well as institutional discrimination, across health-care systems may be exponentially magnified in the setting of limited resources, isolation, and stigma. Further, individuals disadvantaged by these disparities may have elevated levels of baseline immune dysfunction [170]—which can predispose higher chances of contraction, or severity, of disease (Fig. 30.3). Issues like food insecurity and adoption of poor nutritional habits can have a cascading negative impact for those who are depressed, suffer from PTSD, or who—because of social distancing and lockdowns—have even less contact with health-care providers than in normal circumstances [172]. In a world with increased need for telehealth, options should be explored for patients with limited health literacy, access to Internet, and other technological devices [173].

Additionally, one need not have a personal history of COVID-19 infection to develop negative mental health outcomes and these interventions may be useful for both patients and caregivers, as well as general members of the community [170]. For example, Zhang and Ma [174] investigated the immediate impact of COVID-19 on mental health and quality of life among community-living Chinese individuals. Overall, 52.1% of participants felt horrified and apprehensive due to the pandemic. While the COVID-19 pandemic can arouse health-related fears, those from

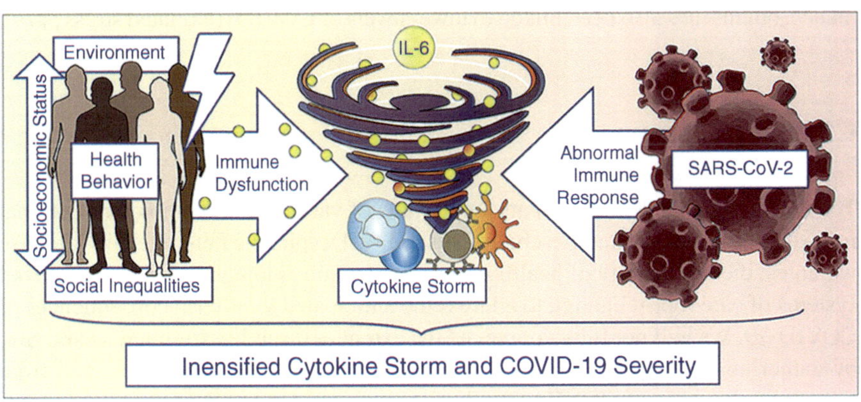


**Fig. 30.3** Accelerating the storm in vulnerable populations during COVID-19. Race/ethnicity, gender, and social determinants are important factors driving inflammation and immune cell dysfunction [171]

marginalized or stigmatized groups face compounded distress. Due to circumstances surrounding the origin and spread of COVID-19, entire cultural groups, communities, and geographic populations may become targets of stigmatization. The Asian community, particularly, has been the target of anger and fear during the COVID-19 pandemic [175]. Individuals from and within this group have been subjected to microaggressions and overtly hostile acts. Thus, they are at risk for poorer mental health outcomes and may face further barriers to care [8]. Similarly, family members of hospitalized patients may develop anxiety or panic responses given visitation restrictions and perceived limited access to information from both their loved one and medical teams. For patients, the cascading impact of loss of income or employment after COVID-19 may further trigger anxiety, as well as depression. Fiorillo and Gorwood [176] proposed that the mental health and psychosocial consequences of COVID-19 could be particularly serious for at least four groups of people: (a) those who have been directly or indirectly in contact with the virus; (b) those who are already vulnerable to biological or psychosocial stressors (e.g., people affected by mental health symptoms, those with unstable financial resources); (c) health professionals (due to higher levels of exposure); and (d) people who follow the news through numerous media channels. Social media exposure is particularly associated with an increased prevalence of anxiety and depression in community samples [177].

In addition to trauma-informed psychotherapy, another possible point of intervention for COVID-19 related stress during lockdowns is reinforcement of self-agency. In a Chinese study of over 3000 community members, those that reported feeling more control, self-confidence, and self-agency during lockdown had lower rates of depression and anxiety [178]. Thus, interventions aimed at cognitive and behavioral strategies which promote a sense of purpose and control may be effective in warding off psychiatric consequences of lockdowns or social distancing. Approaches which assist in developing emotional intelligence may be of particular benefit. Not only is higher emotional intelligence associated with better job performance, but this has also been linked to lower levels of COVID-19 related stress [179].

## Chapter Summary

The COVID-19 pandemic presents a multitude of variables which hold protentional for extended cognitive and psychiatric disability. Despite the heterogeneity of these variables, the equifinality of health-care burden requires integrated, and specialized systems of care robust enough to address the anticipated long-term consequences of COVID-19. We will not fully appreciate the extent of disability for many years. But, by gathering our knowledge of associated conditions, prior pandemics, and from known mechanisms of COVID-19-related injury, we can preemptively create standards of practice which match projected clinical needs. For example, knowing that acute factors such as ARDS, delirium, and metabolic encephalopathy increase risk for PICS as well as PTSD—especially in patients suffering from dyspnea, can lead to earlier detection, screening, and treatment for these and other syndromes. Prothrombotic states render patients at-risk for cerebrovascular and cardiovascular complications—especially in those with preexisting conditions. The neurologic burden of COVID-19 (from both direct neurotropic, and indirect inflammatory responses) may increase cognitive vulnerability to, or exacerbate, neurodegenerative disease [180]. Further, the indirect and social/societal impacts of COVID-19 (such as experiencing dyspnea or the death of a loved one), broad societal shifts (such as lockdowns and isolation), and other personal characteristics (such as the nature of one's employment, discrimination or other stigmas faced) pose additional risk for psychiatric illness such as PTSD, depression, and anxiety—irrespective of patient status and personal history of viral infection. As such, systems of care should not only seek to mitigate controllable factors related to long-term cognitive and mental health consequences for patients but also develop a broader range of individual and community interventions which target individual and societal change.

**Acknowledgements** All authors are thankful to their fellow collaborators. To the patients, families, health-care workers, community members, and researchers on the front lines of the COVID-19 pandemic, we extend our most heartful appreciation and support.

**Disclosure Statement** This material is the result of work supported by resources and the use of facilities at the James A. Haley Veterans' Hospital. The views, opinions, and/or findings contained here are those of the authors and may not represent the views of the Department of Veterans Affairs, Department of Defense, or other federal agency, policy, or decision unless designated by other official documentation.

## References

1. Song E, Zhang C, Israelow B, Lu-Culligan A, Prado AV, Skriabine S, Iwasaki A. Neuroinvasion of SARS-CoV-2 in human and mouse brain. J Exp Med. 2021;218(3):e20202135.
2. Fajgenbaum DC, June CH. Cytokine storm. N Engl J Med. 2020;383(23):2255–73.
3. Brown EG, Chahine LM, Goldman SM, Korell M, Mann E, Kinel DR, Tanner CM. The effect of the COVID-19 pandemic on people with Parkinson's disease. J Parkinsons Dis. 2020a;10(4):1365–77.
4. Yang J, Zheng Y, Gou X, Pu K, Chen Z, Guo Q, Zhou Y. Prevalence of comorbidities in the novel Wuhan coronavirus (COVID-19) infection: a systematic review and meta-analysis. Int J Infect Dis. 2020;10:1016.
5. Bisht K, Sharma K, Tremblay MÈ. Chronic stress as a risk factor for Alzheimer's disease: roles of microglia-mediated synaptic remodeling, inflammation, and oxidative stress. Neurobiol Stress. 2018;9:9–21.
6. Tay TL, Savage JC, Hui CW, Bisht K, Tremblay MÈ. Microglia across the lifespan: from origin to function in brain development, plasticity and cognition. J Physiol. 2017;595(6):1929–45.
7. Zhou H, Lu S, Chen J, Wei N, Wang D, Lyu H, Hu S. The landscape of cognitive function in recovered COVID-19 patients. J Psychiatr Res. 2020;129:98–102.
8. Bailey EK, Steward KA, VandenBussche Jantz AB, Kamper JE, Mahoney EJ, Duchnick JJ. Neuropsychology of COVID-19: anticipated cognitive and mental health outcomes. Neuropsychology. 2021;35(4):335.

9. Samuel J, Franklin C. Hypoxemia and hypoxia. In: Common surgical diseases. New York: Springer; 2008. p. 391–4.
10. Wu Y, Xiaolin X, Chen Z, Duan J, Hashimoto K, Yang L, Liu C, Yang C. Nervous system involvement after infection with COVID-19 and other coronaviruses. Brain Behav Immun. 2020;87:18–22.
11. Zhu N, Zhang D, Wang W, Li X, Yang B, Song J, Tan W. A novel coronavirus from patients with pneumonia in China, 2019. N Engl J Med. 2020;382(8):727–33.
12. Klok FA, Kruip MJHA, Van der Meer NJM, Arbous MS, Gommers DAMPJ, Kant KM, Kaptein FHJ, Paassen JV, Stals MAM, Huisman MV, Endeman H. Incidence of thrombotic complications in critically ill ICU patients with COVID-19. Thromb Res. 2020a;191:145–7.
13. Klok FA, Kruip MJHA, Van der Meer NJM, Arbous MS, Gommers DAMPJ, Kant KM, Endeman H. Confirmation of the high cumulative incidence of thrombotic complications in critically ill ICU patients with COVID-19: an updated analysis. Thromb Res. 2020b;191:148–50.
14. Nuzzo D, Cambula G, Bacile I, Rizzo M, Galia M, Mangiapane P, Scalisi L, et al. Long-term brain disorders in post Covid-19 neurological syndrome (PCNS) patient. Brain Sci. 2021;11(4):454.
15. Bernat JL. The natural history of chronic disorders of consciousness. Neurology. 2010;75(3):206–7.
16. Earnest MP, Parker WD. Metabolic encephalopathies and coma from medical causes. Management of the acutely ill neurological patient. New York: Churchill Livingstone; 1993. p. 1.
17. Di Paola M, Caltagirone C, Fadda L, Sabatini U, Serra L, Carlesimo GA. Hippocampal atrophy is the critical brain change in patients with hypoxic amnesia. Hippocampus. 2008;18(7):719–28.
18. Garcia-Molina A, Roig-Rovira T, Enseñat-Cantallops A, Sanchez-Carrion R, Pico-Azanza N, Bernabeu M, Tormos JM. Neuropsychological profile of persons with anoxic brain injury: differences regarding physiopathological mechanism. Brain Inj. 2006;20(11):1139–45.
19. Ramiro JI, Kumar A. Updates on management of anoxic brain injury after cardiac arrest. Mo Med. 2015;112(2):136–41.
20. Caine D, Watson JD. Neuropsychological and neuropathological sequelae of cerebral anoxia: a critical review. J Int Neuropsychol Soc. 2000;6(1):86–99.
21. Young GB, DeRubeis DA. Metabolic encephalopathies. In: Young GB, Ropper AH, Bolton CF, editors. Coma and impaired consciousness. New York: McGraw-Hill; 1998.
22. Kapasi A, Leurgans SE, James BD, Boyle PA, Arvanitakis Z, Nag S, Schneider JA. Watershed microinfarct pathology and cognition in older persons. Neurobiol Aging. 2018;70:10–7.
23. Acute Respiratory Distress Syndrome Definition Task Force, Ranieri VM, Rubenfeld GD, Thompson BT, Ferguson N, Caldwell E, Slutsky AS. Acute respiratory distress syndrome. JAMA. 2012;307(23):2526–33.
24. Wilcox ME, Herridge MS. Long-term outcomes in patients surviving acute respiratory distress syndrome. Semin Respir Crit Care Med. 2010;31(1):55–65.
25. Hopkins RO, Weaver LK, Pope D, Orme JF Jr, Bigler ED, Larson-Lohr V. Neuropsychological sequelae and impaired health status in survivors of severe acute respiratory distress syndrome. Am J Respir Crit Care Med. 1999;160(1):50–6.
26. Connors JM, Levy JH. COVID-19 and its implications for thrombosis and anticoagulation. Blood. 2020;135(23):2033–40.
27. Hernández-Fernández F, Sandoval Valencia H, Barbella-Aponte RA, Collado-Jiménez R, Ayo-Martín Ó, Barrena C, Segura T. Cerebrovascular disease in patients with COVID-19: neuroimaging, histological and clinical description. Brain. 2020;143(10):3089–103.
28. Marín-Medina DS, Orozco-Hernández JP, Martínez-Muñoz MA, Sánchez-Duque JA. Stroke as a complication of coronavirus disease 2019 (COVID-19). Le infezioni inmedicina. 2020;28:3.

29. Tan YK, Goh C, Leow AS, Tambyah PA, Ang A, Yap ES, Tan BY. COVID-19 and ischemic stroke: a systematic review and meta-summary of the literature. J Thromb Thrombolysis. 2020;50(3):587–95.
30. Jokinen H, Kalska H, Mäntylä R, Pohjasvaara T, Ylikoski R, Hietanen M, Erkinjuntti T. Cognitive profile of subcortical ischaemic vascular disease. J Neurol Neurosurg Psychiatry. 2006;77(1):28–33.
31. Sila C, Schoenberg MR. Cerebrovascular disease and stroke. In: The little black book of neuropsychology. Boston: Springer; 2011. p. 293–356.
32. Loubinoux I, Kronenberg G, Endres M, Schumann-Bard P, Freret T, Filipkowski RK, Popa-Wagner A. Post-stroke depression: mechanisms, translation and therapy. J Cell Mol Med. 2012;16(9):1961–9.
33. Paolucci S. Epidemiology and treatment of post-stroke depression. Neuropsychiatr Dis Treat. 2008;4(1):145.
34. Robinson RG, Jorge RE. Post-stroke depression: a review. Am J Psychiatry. 2016;173(3):221–31.
35. Crippa S, Kägi G, Graf L, Sauteur PM, Kohler P. Stroke in a young adult with mild COVID-19 suggesting endotheliitis. New Microb New Infect. 2020;38:100781.
36. Fara MG, Stein LK, Skliut M, Morgello S, Fifi JT, Dhamoon MS. Macrothrombosis and stroke in patients with mild Covid-19 infection. J Thromb Haemost. 2020;18(8):2031–3.
37. Griffiths J, Hatch RA, Bishop J, Morgan K, Jenkinson C, Cuthbertson BH, Brett SJ. An exploration of social and economic outcome and associated health-related quality of life after critical illness in general intensive care unit survivors: a 12-month follow-up study. Crit Care. 2013;17(3):1–12.
38. Needham DM, Davidson J, Cohen H, Hopkins RO, Weinert C, Wunsch H, Brady SL. Improving long-term outcomes after discharge from intensive care unit: report from a stakeholders' conference. Crit Care Med. 2012;40(2):502–9.
39. Needham DM, Dinglas VD, Morris PE, Jackson JC, Hough CL, Mendez-Tellez PA, Hopkins RO. Physical and cognitive performance of patients with acute lung injury 1 year after initial trophic versus full enteral feeding. EDEN trial follow-up. Am J Respir Crit Care Med. 2013;188(5):567–76.
40. Pandharipande PP, Girard TD, Jackson JC, Morandi A, Thompson JL, Pun BT, Ely EW. Long-term cognitive impairment after critical illness. N Engl J Med. 2013;369(14):1306–16.
41. Bienvenu OJ, Friedman LA, Colantuoni E, Dinglas VD, Sepulveda KA, Mendez-Tellez P, Needham DM. Psychiatric symptoms after acute respiratory distress syndrome: a 5-year longitudinal study. Intensive Care Med. 2018;44(1):38–47.
42. Marra A, Pandharipande PP, Girard TD, Patel MB, Hughes CG, Jackson JC, Brummel NE. Co-occurrence of post-intensive care syndrome problems among 406 survivors of critical illness. Crit Care Med. 2018;46(9):1393.
43. Mikkelsen ME, Christie JD, Lanken PN, Biester RC, Thompson BT, Bellamy SL, Angus DC. The ARDS Cognitive Outcomes Study (ACOS): long-term neuropsychological function in acute lung injury survivors. Am J Respir Crit Care Med. 2012;185(12):1307–15.
44. Girard TD, Jackson JC, Pandharipande PP, Pun BT, Thompson JL, Shintani AK, Ely EW. Delirium as a predictor of long-term cognitive impairment in survivors of critical illness. Crit Care Med. 2010;38(7):1513.
45. Sakusic A, Ognjen G, Singh T, O'Horo J, Jenkins G, Wilson G, Petersen R, Fryer J, Kashyap R, Rabinstein A. Risk factors for persistent cognitive impairment after critical illness, nested case control study. Crit Care Med. 2018;46(12):1977–84.
46. Jackson JC, Hart RP, Gordon SM, Shintani A, Truman B, May L, Ely EW. Six-month neuropsychological outcome of medical intensive care unit patients. Crit Care Med. 2003;31(4):1226–34.
47. Sukantarat KT, Burgess PW, Williamson RCN, Brett SJ. Prolonged cognitive dysfunction in survivors of critical illness. Anaesthesia. 2005;60(9):847–53.

48. Hirsch JS, Ng JH, Ross DW, Sharma P, Shah HH, Barnett RL, Northwell COVID-19 Research Consortium. Acute kidney injury in patients hospitalized with COVID-19. Kidney Int. 2020;98(1):209–18.
49. Portincasa P, Krawczyk M, Machill A, Lammert F, Di Ciaula A. Hepatic consequences of COVID-19 infection. Lapping or biting? Eur J Intern Med. 2020;77:18–24.
50. Sun J, Aghemo A, Forner A, Valenti L. COVID-19 and liver disease. Liver Int. 2020;40(6):1278–81.
51. Martinez MA, Franco S. Impact of COVID-19 in liver disease progression. Hepatol Commun. 2021;5(7):1138–50.
52. Tian D, Ye Q. Hepatic complications of COVID-19 and its treatment. J Med Virol. 2020;92(10):1818–24.
53. Harris MK, Elliott D, Schwendimann RN, Minagar A, Jaffe SL. Neurologic presentations of hepatic disease. Neurol Clin. 2010;28(1):89–105.
54. Kurella M, Chertow GM, Luan J, Yaffe K. Cognitive impairment in chronic kidney disease. J Am Geriatr Soc. 2004;52(11):1863–9.
55. Yaffe K, Ackerson L, Tamura MK, Le Blanc P, Kusek JW, Sehgal AR, Chronic Renal Insufficiency Cohort Investigators. Chronic kidney disease and cognitive function in older adults: findings from the chronic renal insufficiency cohort cognitive study. J Am Geriatr Soc. 2010a;58(2):338–45.
56. Brown E, Gray R, Monaco SL, O'Donoghue B, Nelson B, Thompson A, McGorry P. The potential impact of COVID-19 on psychosis: a rapid review of contemporary epidemic and pandemic research. Schizophr Res. 2020b;222:79–87.
57. Wang H, Li T, Barbarino P, Gauthier S, Brodaty H, Molinuevo JL, Weidner W. Dementia care during COVID-19. Lancet. 2020a;395(10231):1190–1.
58. Ferini-Strambi L, Salsone M. COVID-19 and neurological disorders: are neurodegenerative or neuroimmunological diseases more vulnerable? J Neurol. 2021;268(2):409–19.
59. Chen L, Wang G, Long X, Hou H, Wei J, Cao Y, Zhou J. Dynamics of blood viral load is strongly associated with clinical outcomes in coronavirus disease 2019 (COVID-19) patients: a prospective cohort study. J Mol Diagn. 2021;23(1):10–8.
60. Hoffmann, M., Kleine-Weber, H., Schroeder, S., Krüger, N., Herrler, T., Erichsen, S., . and Pöhlmann, S. (2020). SARS-CoV-2 cell entry depends on ACE2 and TMPRSS2 and is blocked by a clinically proven protease inhibitor. Cell, 181(2), 271–280.
61. Iadecola C, Anrather J, Kamel H. Effects of COVID-19 on the nervous system. Cell. 2020;183(1):16–27.e1.
62. Dubé M, Le Coupanec A, Wong AH, Rini JM, Desforges M, Talbot PJ. Axonal transport enables neuron-to-neuron propagation of human coronavirus OC43. J Virol. 2018;92(17):e00404–18.
63. Giordo R, Paliogiannis P, Mangoni AA, Pintus G. SARS-CoV-2 and endothelial cell interaction in COVID-19: molecular perspectives. Vasc Biol. 2021;3(1):R15–23.
64. Soto C. Unfolding the role of protein misfolding in neurodegenerative diseases. Nat Rev Neurosci. 2003;4(1):49–60.
65. Wan Q, Song D, Li H, He ML. Stress proteins: the biological functions in virus infection, present and challenges for target-based antiviral drug development. Signal Transduct Target Ther. 2020;5(1):1–40.
66. Reza-Zaldívar EE, Hernández-Sapiéns MA, Minjarez B, Gómez-Pinedo U, Márquez-Aguirre AL, Mateos-Díaz JC, Canales-Aguirre AA. Infection mechanism of SARS-COV-2 and its implication on the nervous system. Front Immunol. 2020;11:3738.
67. Tremblay ME, Madore C, Bordeleau M, Tian L, Verkhratsky A. Neuropathobiology of COVID-19: the role for glia. Front Cell Neurosci. 2020;14:363.
68. Wenk GL. Neuropathologic changes in Alzheimer's disease. J Clin Psychiatry. 2003;64:7–10.
69. Soto C, Estrada LD. Protein misfolding and neurodegeneration. Arch Neurol. 2008;65(2):184–9.
70. Papuć E, Rejdak K. The role of myelin damage in Alzheimer's disease pathology. Arch Med Sci. 2020;16(2):345.

71. Manca R, De Marco M, Ince PG, Venneri A. Heterogeneity in regional damage detected by neuroimaging and neuropathological studies in older adults with COVID-19: a cognitive-neuroscience systematic review to inform the long-term impact of the virus on neurocognitive trajectories. Front Aging Neurosci. 2021;13:646908.
72. Kerslake R, Hall M, Randeva HS, Spandidos DA, Chatha K, Kyrou I, Karteris E. Co-expression of peripheral olfactory receptors with SARS-CoV-2 infection mediators: potential implications beyond loss of smell as a COVID-19 symptom. Int J Mol Med. 2020;46(3):949–56.
73. Pantelis C, Jayaram M, Hannan AJ, Wesselingh R, Nithianantharajah J, Wannan CM, O'Brien TJ. Neurological, neuropsychiatric and neurodevelopmental complications of COVID-19. Aust N Z J Psychiatry. 2020;55(8):750–62.
74. Inal J. Biological factors linking ApoE ε4 variant and severe COVID-19. Curr Atheroscler Rep. 2020;22(11):1–2.
75. Kuo CL, Pilling LC, Atkins JL, Masoli JA, Delgado J, Kuchel GA, Melzer D. ApoE e4e4 genotype and mortality with COVID-19 in UK biobank. J Gerontol Ser A. 2020;75(9):1801–3.
76. Rodrigues JCG, Pinto P, Leitão LPC, Vinagre LWMS, Monte N, Fernandes MR, dos Santos SEB. Influence of APOE locus on poor prognosis of COVID-19. Heliyon. 2021;7(6):e07379.
77. Nikogosov DA, Shevlyakov AD, Baranova AV. Comment on "ApoE e4e4 genotype and mortality with COVID-19 in UK biobank" by Kuo et al. J Gerontol Ser A. 2020;75(11):2233–4.
78. Koenigsknecht-Talboo J, Landreth GE. Microglial phagocytosis induced by fibrillar β-amyloid and IgGs are differentially regulated by proinflammatory cytokines. J Neurosci. 2005;25(36):8240–9.
79. Dauer W, Przedborski S. Parkinson's disease: mechanisms and models. Neuron. 2003;39(6):889–909.
80. Fazzini E, Fleming J, Fahn S. Cerebrospinal fluid antibodies to coronavirus in patients with Parkinson's disease. Mov Disord. 1992;7(2):153–8.
81. Antonini A, Leta V, Teo J, Chaudhuri KR. Outcome of Parkinson's disease patients affected by COVID-19. Mov Disord. 2020;35(6):905–8.
82. Braak H, Rüb U, Gai WP, Del Tredici K. Idiopathic Parkinson's disease: possible routes by which vulnerable neuronal types may be subject to neuroinvasion by an unknown pathogen. J Neural Transm. 2003;110(5):517–36.
83. Fearon C, Fasano A. Parkinson's disease and the COVID-19 pandemic. J Parkinsons Dis. 2021;11(2):431–44.
84. Lv Z, Qi H, Wang L, Fan X, Han F, Wang H, Bi S. Vitamin D status and Parkinson's disease: a systematic review and meta-analysis. Neurol Sci. 2014;35(11):1723–30.
85. Ilie PC, Stefanescu S, Smith L. The role of vitamin D in the prevention of coronavirus disease 2019 infection and mortality. Aging Clin Exp Res. 2020;32(7):1195–8.
86. Brugger F, Erro R, Balint B, Kägi G, Barone P, Bhatia KP. Why is there motor deterioration in Parkinson's disease during systemic infections—a hypothetical view. NPJ Parkinsons Dis. 2015;1(1):1–5.
87. Zheng KS, Dorfman BJ, Christos PJ, Khadem NR, Henchcliffe C, Piboolnurak P, Nirenberg MJ. Clinical characteristics of exacerbations in Parkinson disease. Neurologist. 2012;18(3):120.
88. Cilia R, Bonvegna S, Straccia G, Andreasi NG, Elia AE, Romito LM, Eleopra R. Effects of COVID-19 on Parkinson's disease clinical features: a community-based case-control study. Mov Disord. 2020;35(8):1287–92.
89. Leta V, Rodríguez-Violante M, Abundes A, Rukavina K, Teo JT, Falup-Pecurariu C, Irincu L, Rota S, Bhidayasiri R, Storch A. Parkinson's disease and post-COVID-19 syndrome: the Parkinson's long-COVID spectrum. Mov Disord. 2021;36(6):1287.
90. Brown EE, Kumar S, Rajji TK, Pollock BG, Mulsant BH. Anticipating and mitigating the impact of the COVID-19 pandemic on Alzheimer's disease and related dementias. Am J Geriatr Psychiatry. 2020c;28(7):712–21.

91. Kumar N, Gupta R, Kumar H, Mehta S, Rajan R, Kumar D, Kandadai RM, Desai S, Wadia P, Basu P. Impact of home confinement during COVID-19 pandemic on Parkinson's disease. Parkinsonism Relat Disord. 2020;80:32.
92. Arbour N, Day R, Newcombe J, Talbot PJ. Neuroinvasion by human respiratory coronaviruses. J Virol. 2000;74(19):8913–21.
93. Nilsson A, Edner N, Albert J, Ternhag A. Fatal encephalitis associated with coronavirus OC43 in an immunocompromised child. Infect Dis. 2020;52(6):419–22.
94. Poloni TE, Medici V, Moretti M, Visonà SD, Cirrincione A, Carlos AF, Davin A, et al. COVID-19-related neuropathology and microglial activation in elderly with and without dementia. Brain Pathol. 2021;31:e12997.
95. Parrotta E, Kister I, Charvet L, Sammarco C, Saha V, Charlson RE, Howard J, Gutman JM, Gottesman M, Abou-Fayssal N. COVID-19 outcomes in MS: observational study of early experience from NYU multiple sclerosis comprehensive care center. Neurol Neuroimmunol Neuroinflamm. 2020;7(5):e835.
96. Bigaut K, Mallaret M, Baloglu S, Nemoz B, Morand P, Baicry F, Godon A, Voulleminot P, Kremer L, Chanson J-B. Guillain–Barré syndrome related to SARS-CoV-2 infection. Neurol Neuroimmunol Neuroinflamm. 2020;7(5):e785.
97. Berti R, Jacobson S. Role of viral infection in the aetiology of multiple sclerosis. CNS Drugs. 1999;12(1):1–7.
98. Cook S, Rohowsky-Kochan C, Bansil S, Dowling P. Evidence for multiple sclerosis as an infectious disease. Acta Neurol Scand. 1995;91(S161):34–42.
99. Boziki MK, Mentis AFA, Shumilina M, Makshakov G, Evdoshenko E, Grigoriadis N. COVID-19 immunopathology and the central nervous system: implication for multiple sclerosis and other autoimmune diseases with associated demyelination. Brain Sci. 2020;10(6):345.
100. Sharifian-Dorche M, Sahraian MA, Fadda G, Osherov M, Sharifian-Dorche A, Karaminia M, Giacomini PS. COVID-19 and disease-modifying therapies in patients with demyelinating diseases of the central nervous system: a systematic review. Mult Scler Relat Disord. 2021;50:102800.
101. Rogers JP, Chesney E, Oliver D, Pollak TA, McGuire P, Fusar-Poli P, David AS. Psychiatric and neuropsychiatric presentations associated with severe coronavirus infections: a systematic review and meta-analysis with comparison to the COVID-19 pandemic. Lancet Psychiatry. 2020;7(7):611–27.
102. Wang PR, Oyem PC, Viguera AC. Prevalence of psychiatric morbidity following discharge after COVID-19 hospitalization. Gen Hosp Psychiatry. 2020b;69:131–2.
103. Dijkstra-Kersten SM, Biesheuvel-Leliefeld KE, van der Wouden JC, Penninx BW, van Marwijk HW. Associations of financial strain and income with depressive and anxiety disorders. J Epidemiol Community Health. 2015;69(7):660–5.
104. Kessler RC, Turner JB, House JS. Effects of unemployment on health in a community survey: main, modifying, and mediating effects. J Soc Issues. 1988;44(4):69–85.
105. Jak AJ, Crocker LD, Aupperle RL, Clausen A, Bomyea J. Neurocognition in PTSD: treatment insights and implications. In: Behavioral neurobiology of PTSD. Cham: Springer; 2016. p. 93–116.
106. Keller J, Nitschke JB, Bhargava T, Deldin PJ, Gergen JA, Miller GA, Heller W. Neuropsychological differentiation of depression and anxiety. J Abnorm Psychol. 2000;109(1):3.
107. American Psychiatric Association. Diagnostic and statistical manual of mental disorders. 5th ed. Washington, DC: American Psychiatric Association; 2013. https://doi.org/10.1176/appi.books.9780890425596.
108. Kong X, Zheng K, Tang M, Kong F, Zhou J, Diao L, Wu S, Jiao P, Su T, Dong Y. Prevalence and factors associated with depression and anxiety of hospitalized patients with COVID-19. MedRxiv. 2020;2020:e0260819.

109. Zandifar A, Badrfam R, Yazdani S, Arzaghi SM, Rahimi F, Ghasemi S, Khamisabadi S, Khonsari NM, Qorbani M. Prevalence and severity of depression, anxiety, stress and perceived stress in hospitalized patients with COVID-19. J Diabetes Metab Disord. 2020;19(2):1431–8.
110. Garrigues E, Janvier P, Kherabi Y, Le Bot A, Hamon A, Gouze H, Nguyen Y, et al. Post-discharge persistent symptoms and health-related quality of life after hospitalization for COVID-19. J Infect. 2020;81(6):e4–6.
111. McDermott LM, Ebmeier KP. A meta-analysis of depression severity and cognitive function. J Affect Disord. 2009;119(1–3):1–8.
112. Rock P, Roiser J, Riedel W, Blackwell A. Cognitive impairment in depression: a systematic review and meta-analysis. Psychol Med. 2014;44(10):2029–40.
113. Alhola P, Polo-Kantola P. Sleep deprivation: impact on cognitive performance. Neuropsychiatr Dis Treat. 2007;3(5):553–67.
114. Killgore WD, Weber M. Sleep deprivation and cognitive performance. In: Sleep deprivation and disease. New York: Springer; 2014. p. 209–29.
115. Gupta R, Grover S, Basu A, Krishnan V, Tripathi A, Subramanyam A, Avasthi A. Changes in sleep pattern and sleep quality during COVID-19 lockdown. Indian J Psychiatry. 2020;62(4):370.
116. Bonanno GA, Kaltman S. The varieties of grief experience. Clin Psychol Rev. 2001;21(5):705–34.
117. Middleton W, Burnett P, Raphael B, Martinek N. The bereavement response: a cluster analysis. Br J Psychiatry. 1996;169(2):167–71.
118. Eisma MC, Boelen PA, Lenferink LI. Prolonged grief disorder following the coronavirus (COVID-19) pandemic. Psychiatry Res. 2020;288:113031.
119. Schleifer SJ, Keller SE, Camerino M, Thornton JC, Stein M. Suppression of lymphocyte stimulation following bereavement. JAMA. 1983;250(3):374–7.
120. Rozenzweig A, Prigerson H, Miller MD, Reynolds CF 3rd. Bereavement and late-life depression: grief and its complications in the elderly. Annu Rev Med. 1997;48(1):421–8.
121. Ward L, Mathias JL, Hitchings SE. Relationships between bereavement and cognitive functioning in older adults. Gerontology. 2007;53(6):362–72.
122. Mazza MG, Palladini M, De Lorenzo R, Magnaghi C, Poletti S, Furlan R, COVID-19 BioB Outpatient Clinic Study Group. Persistent psychopathology and neurocognitive impairment in COVID-19 survivors: effect of inflammatory biomarkers at three-month follow-up. Brain Behav Immun. 2021;94:138–47.
123. Dantzer R. Neuroimmune interactions: from the brain to the immune system and vice versa. Physiol Rev. 2018;98(1):477–504.
124. Netland J, Meyerholz DK, Moore S, Cassell M, Perlman S. Severe acute respiratory syndrome coronavirus infection causes neuronal death in the absence of encephalitis in mice transgenic for human ACE2. J Virol. 2008;82(15):7264–75.
125. Mazza MG, De Lorenzo R, Conte C, Poletti S, Vai B, Bollettini I, Melloni EMT, Furlan R, Ciceri F, Rovere-Querini P. Anxiety and depression in COVID-19 survivors: role of inflammatory and clinical predictors. Brain Behav Immun. 2020;89:594–600.
126. Clarke P, MacLeod C. The impact of anxiety on cognitive task performance. Secondary influences on neuropsychological test performance. Cambridge: Cambridge University Press; 2013. p. 93–116.
127. Robinson OJ, Vytal K, Cornwell BR, Grillon C. The impact of anxiety upon cognition: perspectives from human threat of shock studies. Front Hum Neurosci. 2013;7:203.
128. Schoen CB, Holtzer R. Differential relationships of somatic and cognitive anxiety with measures of processing speed in older adults. Aging Neuropsychol Cognit. 2017;24(5):481–95.
129. Almeria M, Cejudo JC, Sotoca J, Deus J, Krupinski J. Cognitive profile following COVID-19 infection: clinical predictors leading to neuropsychological impairment. Brain Behav Immun Health. 2020;9:100163.

130. Dunmore E, Clark DM, Ehlers A. Cognitive factors involved in the onset and maintenance of posttraumatic stress disorder (PTSD) after physical or sexual assault. Behav Res Ther. 1999;37(9):809–29.
131. Küffer A, Straus LD, Prather AA, Inslicht SS, Richards A, Shigenaga JK, O'Donovan A. Altered overnight levels of pro-inflammatory cytokines in men and women with posttraumatic stress disorder. Psychoneuroendocrinology. 2019;102:114–20.
132. Tay TL, Béchade C, D'Andrea I, St-Pierre MK, Henry MS, Roumier A, Tremblay ME. Microglia gone rogue: impacts on psychiatric disorders across the lifespan. Front Mol Neurosci. 2018;10:421.
133. Sutherland AG, Alexander DA, Hutchison JD. Disturbance of pro-inflammatory cytokines in post-traumatic psychopathology. Cytokine. 2003;24(5):219–25.
134. Hadad NA, Schwendt M, Knackstedt LA. Hypothalamic–pituitary–adrenal axis activity in post-traumatic stress disorder and cocaine use disorder. Stress. 2020;23(6):638–50.
135. Jiang YN, Zhou W, Zhao XH, Hong X, Wei J. Post-traumatic stress disorder in convalescent patients of severe acute respiratory syndrome:(1) H-MRS study. Zhonghua Yi Xue Za Zhi. 2013;93(5):366–9.
136. Worsham CM, Banzett RB, Schwartzstein R. Dyspnea, acute respiratory failure, psychological trauma, and post-ICU mental health: a caution and a call for research. Chest. 2020a;159(2):749–56.
137. Worsham CM, Banzett RB, Schwartzstein RM. Air hunger and psychological trauma in ventilated patients with COVID-19. An urgent problem. Ann Am Thorac Soc. 2020b;17(8):926–7.
138. Gardner PJ, Moallef P. Psychological impact on SARS survivors: critical review of the English language literature. Can Psychol. 2015;56(1):123.
139. Mak IWC, Chu CM, Pan PC, Yiu MGC, Chan VL. Long-term psychiatric morbidities among SARS survivors. Gen Hosp Psychiatry. 2009;31(4):318–26.
140. Carmassi C, Foghi C, Dell'Oste V, Cordone A, Bertelloni CA, Bui E, Dell'Osso L. PTSD symptoms in healthcare workers facing the three coronavirus outbreaks: what can we expect after the COVID-19 pandemic. Psychiatry Res. 2020;292:113312.
141. Johnson SU, Ebrahimi OV, Hoffart A. PTSD symptoms among health workers and public service providers during the COVID-19 outbreak. PLoS One. 2020;15(10):e0241032.
142. Marvaldi M, Mallet J, Dubertret C, Moro MR, Guessoum SB. Anxiety, depression, trauma-related, and sleep disorders among healthcare workers during the COVID-19 pandemic: a systematic review and meta-analysis. Neurosci Biobehav Rev. 2021;126:252–64.
143. Brandes D, Ben-Schachar G, Gilboa A, Bonne O, Freedman S, Shalev AY. PTSD symptoms and cognitive performance in recent trauma survivors. Psychiatry Res. 2002;110(3):231–8.
144. Gilbertson MW, Gurvits TV, Lasko NB, Pitman RK. Neuropsychological assessment of Vietnam combat veterans with and without PTSD. Ann N Y Acad Sci. 1997;821:476–9.
145. Vasterling JJ, Brailey K, Constans JI, Sutker PB. Attention and memory dysfunction in post-traumatic stress disorder. Neuropsychology. 1998;12(1):125–33.
146. Borders A, Rothman DJ, McAndrew LM. Sleep problems may mediate associations between rumination and PTSD and depressive symptoms among OIF/OEF veterans. Psychol Trauma Theory Res Pract Policy. 2015;7(1):76.
147. Martindale SL, Morissette SB, Rowland JA, Dolan SL. Sleep quality affects cognitive functioning in returning combat veterans beyond combat exposure, PTSD, and mild TBI history. Neuropsychology. 2017;31(1):93.
148. Verfaellie M, Lee LO, Lafleche G, Spiro A. Self-reported sleep disturbance mediates the relationship between PTSD and cognitive outcome in blast-exposed OEF/OIF veterans. J Head Trauma Rehabil. 2016;31(5):309.
149. Wright KM, Britt TW, Bliese PD, Adler AB, Picchioni D, Moore D. Insomnia as predictor versus outcome of PTSD and depression among Iraq combat veterans. J Clin Psychol. 2011;67(12):1240–58.

150. Mellman TA, Nolan B, Hebding J, Kulick-Bell R, Dominguez R. A polysomnographic comparison of veterans with combat-related PTSD, depressed men, and non-ill controls. Sleep. 1997;20(1):46–51.
151. Kobayashi I, Boarts JM, Delahanty DL. Polysomnographically measured sleep abnormalities in PTSD: a meta-analytic review. Psychophysiology. 2007;44(4):660–9.
152. Otte C, Lenoci M, Metzler T, Yehuda R, Marmar CR, Neylan TC. Hypothalamic–pituitary–adrenal axis activity and sleep in posttraumatic stress disorder. Neuropsychopharmacology. 2005;30(6):1173–80.
153. Neylan TC, Marmar CR, Metzler TJ, Weiss DS, Zatzick DF, Delucchi KL, Wu RM, Schoenfeld FB. Sleep disturbances in the Vietnam generation: findings from a nationally representative sample of male Vietnam veterans. Am J Psychiatry. 1998;155(7):929–33.
154. Wolf EJ, Logue MW, Hayes JP, Sadeh N, Schichman SA, Stone A, Miller MW. Accelerated DNA methylation age: associations with PTSD and neural integrity. Psychoneuroendocrinology. 2016;63:155–62.
155. Yaffe K, Vittinghoff E, Lindquist K, Barnes D, Covinsky KE, Neylan T, Kluse M, Marmar C. Posttraumatic stress disorder and risk of dementia among US veterans. Arch Gen Psychiatry. 2010b;67(6):608–13.
156. Hellmuth, J., Barnett, T. A., Asken, B. M., Kelly, J. D., Torres, L., Stephens, M. L., . and Peluso, M. J. (2021). Persistent COVID-19-associated neurocognitive symptoms in non-hospitalized patients. J Neurovirol, 27(1), 191–195.
157. Bryant RA, Harvey AG. Postconcussive symptoms and posttraumatic stress disorder after mild traumatic brain injury. J Nerv Ment Dis. 1999;187(5):302–5.
158. Taquet M, Luciano S, Geddes JR, Harrison PJ. Bidirectional associations between COVID-19 and psychiatric disorder: retrospective cohort studies of 62,354 COVID-19 cases in the USA. Lancet Psychiatry. 2021;8(2):130–40.
159. Jackson JC, Obremskey W, Bauer R, Greevy R, Cotton BA, Anderson V, Ely EW. Long-term cognitive, emotional, and functional outcomes in trauma intensive care unit survivors without intracranial hemorrhage. J Trauma Acute Care Surg. 2007;62(1):80–8.
160. Kaseda ET, Levine AJ. Post-traumatic stress disorder: a differential diagnostic consideration for COVID-19 survivors. Clin Neuropsychol. 2020;34(7–8):1498–514.
161. Campbell TA, Nelson LA, Lumpkin R, Yoash-Gantz RE, Pickett TC, McCormick CL. Neuropsychological measures of processing speed and executive functioning in combat veterans with PTSD, TBI, and comorbid TBI/PTSD. Psychiatr Ann. 2009;39(8):796–803.
162. Jurick SM, Crocker LD, Sanderson-Cimino M, Keller AV, Trenova LS, Boyd BL, Twamley EW, Rodgers CS, Schiehser DM, Aupperle RL. Contributions to executive dysfunction in operation enduring freedom/operation Iraqi freedom veterans with posttraumatic stress disorder and history of mild traumatic brain injury. J Head Trauma Rehabil. 2018;33(2):E41–52.
163. Nelson LA, Yoash-Gantz RE, Pickett TC, Campbell TA. Relationship between processing speed and executive functioning performance among OEF/OIF veterans: implications for postdeployment rehabilitation. J Head Trauma Rehabil. 2009;24(1):32–40.
164. Marshall S, Bayley M, McCullagh S, Velikonja D, Berrigan L. Clinical practice guidelines for mild traumatic brain injury and persistent symptoms. Can Fam Physician. 2012;58(3):257–67.
165. Hamberger LK, Barry C, Franco Z. Implementing trauma-informed care in primary medical settings: evidence-based rationale and approaches. J Aggress Maltreat Trauma. 2019;28(4):425–44.
166. Raja S, Hasnain M, Hoersch M, Gove-Yin S, Rajagopalan C. Trauma informed care in medicine. Fam Community Health. 2015;38(3):216–26.
167. Tomaz T, Castro-Vale I. Trauma-informed care in primary health settings—which is even more needed in times of COVID-19. Healthcare (Basel). 2020;8(3):340.
168. Stuart K, Faghy MA, Bidmead E, Browning R, Roberts C, Grimwood S, Winn-Reed T. A biopsychosocial framework for recovery from COVID-19. Int J Sociol Soc Policy. 2020;40:1021–39.

169. Bryant RA, Moulds M, Guthrie R, Nixon RD. Treating acute stress disorder following mild traumatic brain injury. Am J Psychiatry. 2003;160(3):585–7.
170. Zhang J, Lu H, Zeng H, Zhang S, Du Q, Jiang T, Du B. The differential psychological distress of populations affected by the COVID-19 pandemic. Brain Behav Immun. 2020;87:49.
171. Baumer Y, Farmer N, Premeaux TA, Wallen GR, Powell-Wiley TM. Health disparities in COVID-19: addressing the role of social determinants of health in immune system dysfunction to turn the tide. Front Public Health. 2020;8:589.
172. Ripon RK, El-Sabban F, Sikder T, Hossain S, Mim SS, Ahmed HU, Mehta N. Psychological and nutritional effects on a COVID-19-quarantined population in Bangladesh. J Hum Behav Soc Environ. 2021;31(1–4):271–82.
173. Feeney MP, Xu Y, Surface M, Shah H, Vanegas-Arroyave N, Chan AK, Alcalay RN. The impact of COVID-19 and social distancing on people with Parkinson's disease: a survey study. NPJ Parkinsons Dis. 2021;7(1):1–10.
174. Zhang Y, Ma ZF. Impact of the COVID-19 pandemic on mental health and quality of life among local residents in Liaoning Province, China: a cross-sectional study. Int J Environ Res Public Health. 2020;17(7):2381.
175. Choi S. "People look at me like I AM the virus": fear, stigma, and discrimination during the COVID-19 pandemic. Qual Soc Work. 2021;20(1–2):233–9.
176. Fiorillo A, Gorwood P. The consequences of the COVID-19 pandemic on mental health and implications for clinical practice. Eur Psychiatry. 2020;63(1):e32.
177. Gao J, Zheng P, Jia Y, Chen H, Mao Y, Chen S, Dai J. Mental health problems and social media exposure during COVID-19 outbreak. PLoS One. 2020;15(4):e0231924.
178. Gan Y, Ma J, Wu J, Chen Y, Zhu H, Hall BJ. Immediate and delayed psychological effects of province-wide lockdown and personal quarantine during the COVID-19 outbreak in China. Psychol Med. 2020;52(7):1321–32.
179. Sadovyy M, Sánchez-Gómez M, Bresó E. COVID-19: how the stress generated by the pandemic may affect work performance through the moderating role of emotional intelligence. Personal Individ Differ. 2021;180:110986.
180. Ciaccio M, Lo Sasso B, Scazzone C, Gambino CM, Ciaccio AM, Bivona G, Agnello L. COVID-19 and Alzheimer's disease. Brain Sci. 2021;11(3):305.

# Chapter 31
# The Road Ahead (Editors)

**Sasan Adibi, Paul Griffin, Melvin Sanicas, Maryam Rashidi, and Francesco Lanfranchi**

In 2015, Bill Gates at TED talked about how the world avoided a global outbreak of Ebola, thanks to thousands of selfless health-care workers and some good luck but the world needs to be ready for the next one [1]. In 2019, the medical historian and journalist Mark Honigsbaum concluded his book *The Pandemic Century* [2] by saying: "The only thing that is certain is that there will be new plagues and new pandemics. It is not a question of if, but when", and so it happened.

On 31 December 2019, the World Health Organization (WHO) was informed of cases of pneumonia of unknown cause in Wuhan City, China. This novel coronavirus was identified as the cause by Chinese authorities on 7 January 2020 and was temporarily named 2019-nCoV, considered a public health emergency of international concern on 30 January 2020, and declared a pandemic on March 11, 2020 after more than 118,000 cases reported in 114 countries, and 4291 deaths recorded,

S. Adibi (✉)
School of Information Technology, Deakin University, Melbourne, VIC, Australia
e-mail: sasan.adibi@deakin.edu.au

P. Griffin (✉)
School of Medicine, University of Queensland, Brisbane, QLD, Australia
e-mail: paul.griffin@uq.edu.au

M. Sanicas (✉)
Clinical - Vaccines, Clover Biopharmaceuticals, Zürich, Switzerland
e-mail: melvin.sanicas@cloverbiopharma.com

M. Rashidi (✉)
Inflammation Division, Walter and Eliza Hall Institute of Medical Research, Melbourne, VIC, Australia
e-mail: rashidi@wehi.edu.au

F. Lanfranchi (✉)
Department of Health Sciences (DISSAL), University of Genoa, Genoa, Italy
e-mail: flanfranchi@hotmail.com


S. Adibi et al. (eds.), *Frontiers of COVID-19*,
https://doi.org/10.1007/978-3-031-08045-6_31

**Table 31.1** Known vs. unknown matrix for COVID-19

| | | |
|---|---|---|
| Known | Things about COVID-19 we are aware of and understand | Things about COVID-19 we are aware of but do not understand |
| Unknown | Things about COVID-19 we understand but are not aware of | Things about COVID-19 we are neither aware of nor understand |
| | Knowns | Unknowns |

mostly in China. This was an event that has never been witnessed by almost everyone in the world apart from those who lived through the 1918 influenza pandemic that killed an estimated 50 million people. This once-in-a-lifetime global public health event was met by an unprecedented cooperation and collaboration by the medical, scientific, and public health community and after more than 2 years we already know a lot about the novel coronavirus disease (COVID-19).

We tried to categorize our knowledge about COVID-19 in terms of the known vs. unknown matrix which has been used since the Greek era and in several areas of knowledge (Table 31.1).

About this new disease we have accumulated a vast amount of medical and scientific data in the known known category. Because we are still amid the pandemic and knowledge about the severe acute respiratory syndrome coronavirus 2 (SARS-CoV-2) is evolving rapidly, some of the information and recommendations can still change.

## The Known Knowns

### *Prevention*

Infection prevention is the key. According to the last update of the WHO advice for the public [3], the main measures to be adopted included vaccine administration, physical distance maintenance, mask wearing, frequent cleaning of hands, and self-isolation in case of onset of suspicious symptoms.

### *Risk Stratification*

The virus affects people differently. Though COVID-19 is a respiratory virus, it does not limit itself to damaging the lungs. It can infect the cells that line blood vessels and affect a range of other important organs, such as the heart, brain, kidneys, liver, pancreas, and spleen. The effect has been found even in young, low-risk people.

**Table 31.2** SARS-CoV-2 diagnostic tests

| | PCR test | Antigen test | Antibody test |
|---|---|---|---|
| Specimen | Respiratory tract specimens | Respiratory tract specimens | Blood |
| Purpose | Diagnosis of active infection | Diagnosis of active infection | Diagnosis of past infection |
| Method | In most cases, a nasopharyngeal or nasal swab is taken and tested; oral swabs and saliva are also acceptable. Most commonly, the swab needs to be sent to a lab for testing | In most cases, a nasopharyngeal or nasal swab is taken and tested. Most often the test can be run while you wait | In most cases, a blood sample is taken and is sent to a lab for testing |
| Turnaround time | As early as 12–24 h after sample collection | As early as 30 min after sample collection | 2–3 days, longer in some cases |
| Limitations | It gives you a result for the point and time when the specimen was collected and cannot predict if you will remain negative<br>In some people, the virus can be found by PCR in the nose and throat for several weeks, even longer than their infectious period (the time they are contagious to other people)<br>The test requires certain kinds of swabs and reagents that may be in short supply | Best results are achieved with those who are symptomatic, and it will not help determine who had an infection in the past<br>Lower sensitivity than PCR tests, so there may be false-negative results<br>In persons with known exposure, negative tests must be treated as a preliminary result and confirmed with PCR testing | If used too close to the beginning of an infection, this may result in a negative test which is why it must not be used to detect active COVID-19 infection<br>Some antibody tests have low sensitivity and specificity and thus may not produce reliable results<br>Some antibody tests may cross-react with other coronaviruses that are not SARS-CoV-2, leading to false-positive test results |

## *Diagnosis*

A quick and accurate diagnosis is crucial for both infected patients and their contacts. To date, different tests were approved (Table 31.2). Cheap and reliable techniques could be helpful for screening procedures in specific situations requiring a strict monitoring such as in settings with a high risk of exposure.

## *Treatments*

Several approved therapeutics demonstrated a specific efficacy in COVID-19 symptoms treatment and prevention [4, 5]. More molecules are under evaluation in clinical trials [6] and regulators around the world have allowed additional treatments to be used on an emergency-use basis.

In general, in most cases of COVID-19, there is clearly no need for antiviral therapy and most patients can be managed by taking medicine to reduce fever and supportive care. The more severe cases require hospitalization, with treatment that might include IV antivirals such as Veklury™ (remdesivir, nucleotide prodrug of an adenosine analog), corticosteroids (such as dexamethasone), supplemental oxygen, assisted ventilation, and other supportive measures.

Antiviral pills such as Paxlovid™ (nirmatrelvir, 3C-like protease inhibitor) [7] or Lagevrio™ (molnupiravir or MK-4482/EIDD-2801) [8] may be prescribed by a doctor if a patient is eligible, according to the Food and Drug Administration (FDA). Both molecules have shown varying levels of effectiveness in treating mild to moderate COVID-19 for those most at risk. Paxlovid consists of nirmatrelvir, which inhibits a SARS-CoV-2 protein to stop the virus from replicating, and ritonavir, which slows down nirmatrelvir's breakdown to help it remain in the body for a longer period at higher concentrations. In the EPIC-HR trial [9], nirmatrelvir significantly reduced the proportion of people with COVID-19 related hospitalization or death from any cause by 88% compared to placebo in patients treated within 5 days of symptom onset. Molnupiravir is a medication that works by introducing errors into the SARS-CoV-2 virus's genetic code, which prevents the virus from further replicating. In the MOVe-OUT trial [10], Molnupiravir reduces hospitalization or death by 30%. Both antivirals are not authorized for use for longer than five consecutive days. These new oral antivirals have the potential to reshape the trajectory

**Table 31.3** March 2022 updated worldwide authorized/approved vaccines (RAPS COVID-19 vaccine tracker; https://www.raps.org/news-and-articles/news-articles/2020/3/covid-19-vaccine-tracker)

| Name | Vaccine type | Primary developers | Country |
|---|---|---|---|
| Comirnaty (BNT162b2) | mRNA-based vaccine | Pfizer, BioNTech; Fosun Pharma | Multinational |
| Spikevax (mRNA-1273) | mRNA-based vaccine | Moderna, BARDA, NIAID | USA |
| COVID-19 Vaccine AstraZeneca (AZD1222); also known as Vaxzevria and Covishield | Adenovirus vaccine | BARDA, OWS | UK |
| Sputnik V | Recombinant adenovirus vaccine (rAd26 and rAd5) | Gamaleya Research Institute, Acellena Contract Drug Research and Development | Russia |
| Sputnik Light | Recombinant adenovirus vaccine (rAd26) | Gamaleya Research Institute, Acellena Contract Drug Research and Development | Russia |
| COVID-19 Vaccine Janssen (JNJ-78436735; Ad26.COV2.S) | Nonreplicating viral vector | Janssen Vaccines (Johnson & Johnson) | The Netherlands USA |

**Table 31.3** (continued)

| Name | Vaccine type | Primary developers | Country |
|---|---|---|---|
| CoronaVac | Inactivated vaccine (formalin with alum adjuvant) | Sinovac | China |
| BBIBP-CorV/ NVSI-06-07 | Inactivated vaccine | Beijing Institute of Biological Products; China National Pharmaceutical Group (Sinopharm) | China |
| EpiVacCorona | Peptide vaccine | Federal Budgetary Research Institution State Research Center of Virology and Biotechnology | Russia |
| Convidicea (PakVac, Ad5-nCoV) | Recombinant vaccine (adenovirus type 5 vector) | CanSino Biologics | China |
| Covaxin (BBV152) | Inactivated vaccine | Bharat Biotech, ICMR; Ocugen; ViroVax | India |
| WIBP-CorV | Inactivated vaccine | Wuhan Institute of Biological Products; China National Pharmaceutical Group (Sinopharm) | China |
| CoviVac | Inactivated vaccine | Chumakov Federal Scientific Center for Research and Development of Immune and Biological Products | Russia |
| ZF2001 (ZIFIVAX) | Recombinant vaccine | Anhui Zhifei Longcom Biopharmaceutical, Institute of Microbiology of the Chinese Academy of Sciences | China Uzbekistan |
| QazVac (QazCovid-in) | Inactivated vaccine | Research Institute for Biological Safety Problems | Kazakhstan |
| Unnamed vaccine | Inactivated vaccine | Minhai Biotechnology Co.; Kangtai Biological Products Co. Ltd | China |
| COVIran Barekat | Inactivated vaccine | Shifa Pharmed Industrial Group | Iran |
| Unnamed vaccine | Inactivated vaccine | Chinese Academy of Medical Sciences, Institute of Medical Biology | China |
| Abdala (CIGB 66) | Protein subunit vaccine | Center for Genetic Engineering and Biotechnology | Cuba |
| Soberana 02/Soberana Plus | Conjugate vaccine | Finlay Institute of Vaccines; Pasteur Institute | Cuba Iran |
| MVC-COV1901 | Protein subunit vaccine | Medigen Vaccine Biologics Corp.; Dynavax | Taiwan |
| ZyCoV-D | DNA vaccine (plasmid) | Zydus Cadila | India |

(continued)

**Table 31.3** (continued)

| Name | Vaccine type | Primary developers | Country |
|---|---|---|---|
| Spikogen (COVAX-19) | Monovalent recombinant protein vaccine | Vaxine Pty Ltd.; CinnaGen | Iran |
| FAKHRAVAC (MIVAC) | Inactivated vaccine | The Stem Cell Technology Research Center; Organization of Defensive Innovation and Research | Iran |
| Nuvaxovid (Covovax in India; previously NVX-CoV2373) | Recombinant nanoparticle vaccine | Novavax; CEPI, Serum Institute of India | USA |
| Turkovac (ERUCOV-VAC) | Inactivated vaccine | Health Institutes of Turkey | Turkey |
| Corbevax | Adjuvanted protein subunit vaccine | Biological E, Baylor College of Medicine, Dynavax, CEPI | India USA |
| Covifenz (CoVLP) | Plant-based adjuvant vaccine | Medicago; GSK; Dynavax | Canada |
| VLA2001 | Inactivated vaccine | Valneva;UK National Institute for Health Research; Dynavax | USA |
| Noora | Recombinant protein vaccine | Baqiyatallah University of Medical Sciences | Iran |

of the pandemic going forward especially for those at high risk of severe COVID. At the time of writing, Paxlovid™ and Lagevrio™ are not available worldwide.

### *Vaccines*

Several safe and effective COVID-19 vaccines have been authorized or approved for use around the world (Table 31.3). Updated information about approved and candidates vaccines are provided by different institutions, including the WHO [11] and the Regulatory Affairs Professional Society [12].

## The Known Unknowns

### *New Drugs*

To find effective and easily available treatments for COVID-19 is one of the most active field of research. There are over 6000 ongoing and completed COVID-19 studies listed on the World Health Organization's International Clinical Trials

**Table 31.4** ClinicalTrials.gov vaccine and drug studies

| Selected search of ClinicalTrials.gov | Studies | Vaccine studies | Drug studies | Mapped drug names |
|---|---|---|---|---|
| COVID-19 studies | 7605 | 685 | 2030 | 655 |

**Table 31.5** Current and previous COVID-19 variants of concern (VOC), variants of interest (VOI), and variants under monitoring (VUM) according to the WHO (March 2022)

| Who label | Pango lineage | GISAID clade | Nextstrain clade | Earliest documented samples | Date of designation | Type |
|---|---|---|---|---|---|---|
| Delta | B.1.617.2 | G/478K.V1 | 21A<br>21I<br>21J | 2020, Oct<br>India | 11th May, 2021 | Current VOC |
| Omicron | B.1.1.529 | GR/484A | 21K | 2021, Nov<br>Multiple countries | 26th Nov, 2021 | Current VOC |
| Alpha | B.1.1.7 | GRY | 20I (V1) | 2020, Sep<br>UK | VOC: 18th Dec, 2020<br>Previous VOC: 9th Mar, 2022 | Previous VOC |
| Beta | B.1.351 | GH/501Y.V2 | 20H (V2) | 2020, May<br>South Africa | VOC: 18th Dec, 2020<br>Previous VOC: 9th Mar, 2022 | Previous VOC |
| Gamma | P.1 | GR/501Y.V3 | 20J (V3) | 2020, Nov<br>Brazil | VOC: 11th Jan, 2021<br>Previous VOC: 9th Mar, 2022 | Previous VOC |
| Epsilon | B.1.427<br>B.1.429 | GH/452R.V1 | 21C | 2020, Mar<br>US | VOI: 5th Mar, 2021<br>Previous VOI: 6th Jul, 2021 | Previous VOI |
| Zeta | P.2 | GR/484K.V2 | 20B/S.484K | 2020, Apr<br>Brazil | VOI: 17th Mar, 2021<br>Previous VOI: 6th Jul, 2021 | Previous VOI |
| Eta | B.1.525 | G/484K.V3 | 21D | 2020, Dec<br>Multiple countries | VOI: 17th Mar, 2021<br>Previous VOI: 20th Sep, 2021 | Previous VOI |
| Theta | P.3 | GR/1092K.V1 | 21E | 2021, Jan<br>Philippines | VOI: 24th Mar, 2021<br>Previous VOI: 6th Jul, 2021 | Previous VOI |
| Iota | B.1.526 | GH/253G.V1 | 21F | 2020, Nov<br>US | VOI: 24th Mar, 2021<br>Previous VOI: 20th Sep, 2021 | Previous VOI |

(continued)

**Table 31.5** (continued)

| Who label | Pango lineage | GISAID clade | Nextstrain clade | Earliest documented samples | Date of designation | Type |
|---|---|---|---|---|---|---|
| Kappa | B.1.617.1 | G/452R.V3 | 21B | 2020, Oct India | VOI: 4th Apr, 2021 Previous VOI: 20th Sep, 2021 | Previous VOI |
| Lambda | C.37 | GR/452Q. V1 | 21G | 2020, Dec Peru | VOI: 14th Jun, 2021 Previous VOI: 9th Mar, 2022 | Previous VOI |
| Mu | B.1.621 | GH | 21H | 2021, Jan Colombia | VOI: 30th Aug, 2021 Previous VOI: 9th Mar, 2022 | Previous VOI |
| – | B.1.640 | GH/490R | – | 2021, Sep Multiple countries | 22nd Nov, 2021 | VUM |
| – | XD | – | – | 2022, Jan France | 9th Mar, 2022 | VUM |

Registry Platform. A continuously updated list of ongoing trial can be found at ClinicalTrials.gov [6]. Table 31.4 shows the number of registered COVID-19 studies that are either vaccine related or have at least one drug intervention.

## *Variants*

SARS-CoV-2 variants (Table 31.5) represent a major challenge in a continuous development. Among the two current variants of concern (VOC), the Delta variant seems to be linked with a higher risk of pneumonia with respect with the wild-type virus [13]. Moreover, the prolonged viral shedding could be a determinant of an increased transmissibility of this variant [13, 14]. On the other hand, our knowledges about the second circulating VOC, Omicron, and further studies are necessary to a better comprehension of this new variant. However, it seems to be associated with a higher transmissibility but even with a milder clinical presentation [15, 16].

## *Long COVID*

Long COVID syndrome represent the topics of greater concern, not just for the present but even for the future. The pathogenesis of postacute sequelae of COVID-19 (PASC) is still unclear, and to identify the molecular mechanisms underlying this condition is critical. To date, it is clear that PASC are frequent and multifaceted [17–20], involving both somatic and neuropsychiatric symptoms (Figs. 31.1 and

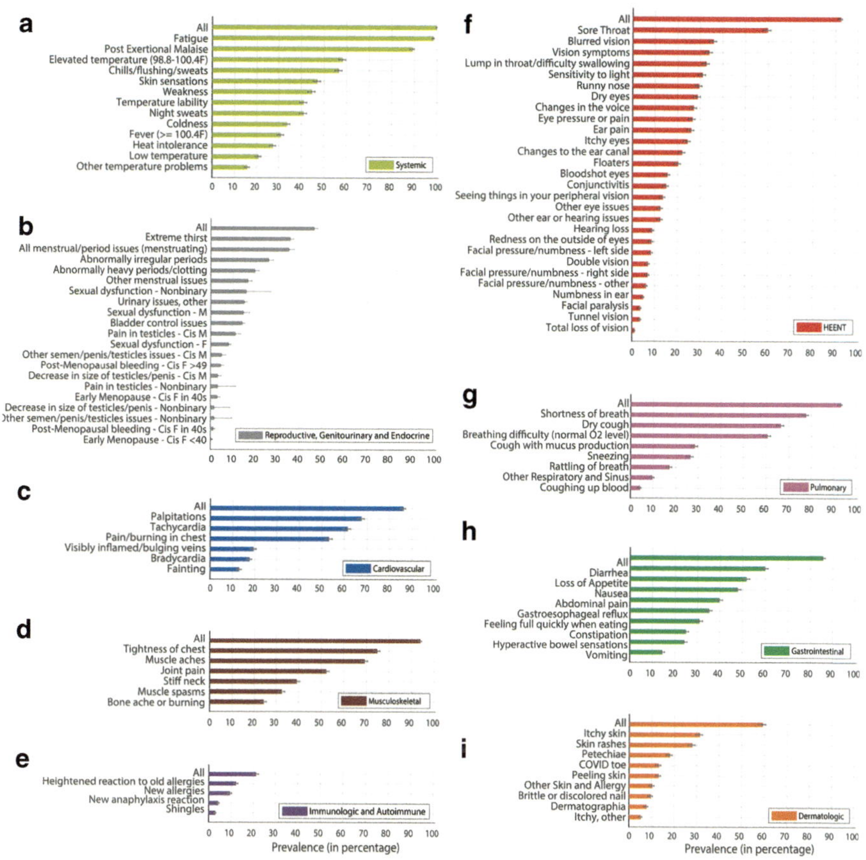


**Fig. 31.1** Symptom prevalence estimates (non-neuropsychiatric symptoms). Bars represent the percentage of respondents who experienced each symptom at any point in their illness. Symptoms are categorized by the affected organ systems (systemic, panel **a**; reproductive, genitourinary and endocrine, panel **b**; cardiovascular, panel **c**; musculoskeletal, panel **d**; immunologic and autoimmune, panel **e**; head, eyes, ears, nose, and throat (HEENT), panel **f**; pulmonary, panel **g**; gastrointestinal, panel **h**; dermatologic, panel **i**). When all rows in a given panel use the same denominator, the first row, labeled "All," indicates the percentage of respondents who experienced any symptoms in that category. Error bars are bootstrap 95% confidence intervals. In panel **b**, sexual dysfunction is broken up into male (sexual dysfunction—M) and female (sexual dysfunction—F). "Cis M" refers to cisgender males, "Cis F" refers to cisgender females, and cisgender females are further broken down by age group: "Cis F < 4000 indicates cisgender females age 39 or younger, "Cis F in 40s" indicates cisgender females age 40–49, and "Cis F > 4900 indicates cisgender females age 50 or older. (Figure and caption modified from Davis et al. [18] and licensed under Creative Common License CC BY 4.0, http://creativecommons.org/licenses/by/4.0/)

31.2, respectively). Systematic in vivo imaging studies as well as postmortem autoptic examinations are the only way to obtain deeper knowledges of these manifestations and their mechanisms.

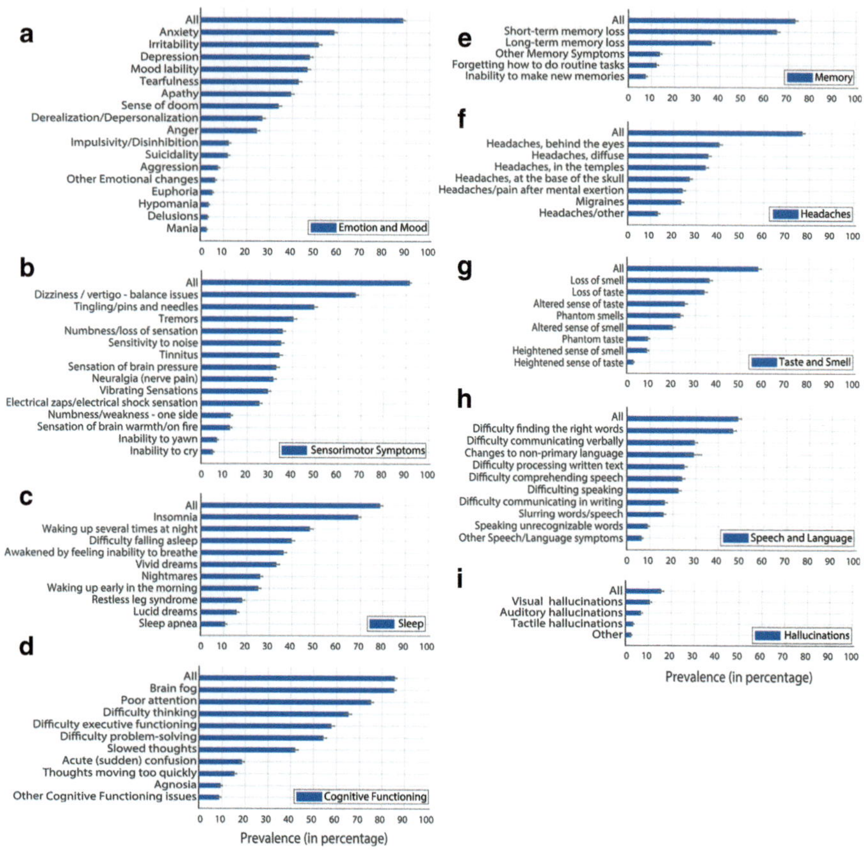


**Fig. 31.2** Symptom prevalence estimates for neuropsychiatric symptoms, divided into nine subcategories (emotion and mood, panel **a**; sensorimotor symptoms, panel **b**; sleep, panel **c**; cognitive functioning, panel **d**; memory, panel **e**; headaches, panel **f**; taste and smell, panel **g**; speech and language, panel **h**; hallucinations, panel **i**). Each bar represents the percentage of respondents who experienced that symptom. Error bars are bootstrap 95% confidence intervals. (Figure and caption modified from Davis et al. [18] and licensed under Creative Common License CC BY 4.0, http://creativecommons.org/licenses/by/4.0/)

## *Main Topics of Concern*

Two years since the pandemic started, science has delivered more than we could have imagined prepandemic. We now have all the tools we need but the world needs to work together to ensure that everyone, everywhere has access to these life-saving tools. While working on equity, we need to continue research on the following research topics: (1) vaccines to develop a pancoronavirus or variantproof vaccines; thermostable formulations that do not need ultracold chain; oral or nasal vaccines; (2) drugs and therapeutics: more antiviral options that are cheap and widely available; monoclonal antibody therapies that are delivered though IM route instead of

IV; (3) diagnostic tests: scientific validation of existing tests to be able to accurately identify new variants, and quicker tests that can be mass produced and used even in low- and middle-income countries; (4) mechanism of and treatment for long-term effects of COVID-19.

## The Unknown Knowns

What about the next global pandemic? Will it be another coronavirus? Will it be a relative of SARS-CoV-2? What is COVID-19 impact on the environment? How will the virus develop resistance to antiviral drug? Three quarters of emerging infectious diseases originate in wildlife [21]. HIV, West Nile encephalitis, SARS-CoV-1, MERS-CoV, Lujo, Lassa, Nipah, Dandenong, Ebola, Marburg, dengue, monkey-pox, Zika, influenza, and SARS-CoV-2 all came from animals. For SARS-CoV-2, we understand that, but we are not aware of when or where this animal-to-human jump happened.

## The Unknown Unknowns

There are things that we are neither aware of nor understand. As the medical and scientific world continue to study COVID-19, some of these situations may move to become unknown known or known unknown. In the past 2 years, we have become better at treating COVID-19 and mortality rates have come down, but there is only one exit strategy: prevention through vaccination and other interventions that change the fundamentals of infection, transmission and illness. The ways in which different Countries will work together on COVID-19 in the next coming years will define how and when this pandemic will end.

## References

1. TED. 2015. https://www.ted.com/talks/bill_gates_the_next_outbreak_we_re_not_ready?.
2. Honigsbaum M. The pandemic century: a history of global contagion from the Spanish flu to Covid-19. Cambridge: Penguin; 2020.
3. WHO. 2021. https://www.who.int/emergencies/diseases/novel-coronavirus-2019/advice-for-public#:~:text=Avoid%20crowds%20and%20close%20contact,when%20you%20cough%20or%20sneeze.
4. WHO. 2022a. https://www.who.int/publications/i/item/WHO-2019-nCoV-therapeutics-2022.2.
5. WHO. 2022b. https://www.who.int/publications/i/item/WHO-2019-nCoV-prophylaxes-2021-1.
6. ClinicalTrials.gov. 2022. https://clinicaltrials.gov/ct2/results?cond=COVID-19.

7. FDA. 2022a. https://www.fda.gov/news-events/press-announcements/coronavirus-covid-19-update-fda-authorizes-first-oral-antiviral-treatment-covid-19.
8. FDA. 2022b. https://www.fda.gov/news-events/press-announcements/coronavirus-covid-19-update-fda-authorizes-additional-oral-antiviral-treatment-covid-19-certain.
9. Hammond J, Leister-Tebbe H, Gardner A, Abreu P, Bao W, Wisemandle W, Baniecki M, Hendrick VM, Damle B, Simón-Campos A, Pypstra R, Rusnak JM, EPIC-HR Investigators. Oral nirmatrelvir for high-risk, nonhospitalized adults with Covid-19. N Engl J Med. 2022;386(15):1397–408. https://doi.org/10.1056/NEJMoa2118542.
10. Jayk Bernal A, Gomes da Silva MM, Musungaie DB, Kovalchuk E, Gonzalez A, Delos Reyes V, Martín-Quirós A, Caraco Y, Williams-Diaz A, Brown ML, Du J, Pedley A, Assaid C, Strizki J, Grobler JA, Shamsuddin HH, Tipping R, Wan H, Paschke A, Butterton JR, MOVe-OUT Study Group. Molnupiravir for oral treatment of Covid-19 in nonhospitalized patients. N Engl J Med. 2022;386(6):509–20. https://doi.org/10.1056/NEJMoa2116044.
11. WHO. 2022c. https://www.who.int/publications/m/item/draft-landscape-of-covid-19-candidate-vaccines.
12. RAPS. 2022. https://www.raps.org/news-and-articles/news-articles/2020/3/covid-19-vaccine-tracker.
13. Ong S, Chiew CJ, Ang LW, Mak TM, Cui L, Toh M, Lim YD, Lee PH, Lee TH, Chia PY, Maurer-Stroh S, Lin R, Leo YS, Lee VJ, Lye DC, Young BE. Clinical and virological features of SARS-CoV-2 variants of concern: a retrospective cohort study comparing B.1.1.7 (alpha), B.1.315 (beta), and B.1.617.2 (delta). Clin Infect Dis. 2021;2020:ciab721. https://doi.org/10.1093/cid/ciab721.
14. Park S, Lim SY, Kim JY, Park H, Lim JS, Bae S, Kim J, Jung J, Kim MJ, Chong YP, Choi SH, Lee SO, Kim YS, Park MS, Kim SH. Clinical and virological characteristics of SARS-CoV-2 B.1.617.2 (delta) variant: a prospective cohort study. Clin Infect Dis. 2022;2022:ciac239. https://doi.org/10.1093/cid/ciac239.
15. Meo SA, Meo AS, Al-Jassir FF, Klonoff DC. Omicron SARS-CoV-2 new variant: global prevalence and biological and clinical characteristics. Eur Rev Med Pharmacol Sci. 2021;25(24):8012–8. https://doi.org/10.26355/eurrev_202112_27652.
16. Modes ME, Directo MP, Melgar M, Johnson LR, Yang H, Chaudhary P, Bartolini S, Kho N, Noble PW, Isonaka S, Chen P. Clinical characteristics and outcomes among adults hospitalized with laboratory-confirmed SARS-CoV-2 infection during periods of B.1.617.2 (delta) and B.1.1.529 (omicron) variant predominance—One Hospital, California, July 15–September 23, 2021, and December 21, 2021–January 27, 2022. MMWR Morb Mortal Wkly Rep. 2022;71(6):217–23. https://doi.org/10.15585/mmwr.mm7106e2.
17. Anaya JM, Rojas M, Salinas ML, Rodríguez Y, Roa G, Lozano M, Rodríguez-Jiménez M, Montoya N, Zapata E, Post-COVID Study Group, Monsalve DM, Acosta-Ampudia Y, Ramírez-Santana C. Post-COVID syndrome. A case series and comprehensive review. Autoimmun Rev. 2021;20(11):102947. https://doi.org/10.1016/j.autrev.2021.102947.
18. Davis HE, Assaf GS, McCorkell L, Wei H, Low RJ, Re'em Y, Redfield S, Austin JP, Akrami A. Characterizing long COVID in an international cohort: 7 months of symptoms and their impact. EClinicalMedicine. 2021;38:101019. https://doi.org/10.1016/j.eclinm.2021.101019.
19. Groff D, Sun A, Ssentongo AE, Ba DM, Parsons N, Poudel GR, Lekoubou A, Oh JS, Ericson JE, Ssentongo P, Chinchilli VM. Short-term and long-term rates of postacute sequelae of SARS-CoV-2 infection: a systematic review. JAMA Netw Open. 2021;4(10):e2128568. https://doi.org/10.1001/jamanetworkopen.2021.28568.
20. Lopez-Leon S, Wegman-Ostrosky T, Perelman C, Sepulveda R, Rebolledo PA, Cuapio A, Villapol S. More than 50 long-term effects of COVID-19: a systematic review and meta-analysis. Sci Rep. 2021;11(1):16144. https://doi.org/10.1038/s41598-021-95565-8.
21. CDC. 2021. https://www.cdc.gov/onehealth/basics/zoonotic-diseases.html.

# Index




S. Adibi et al. (eds.), *Frontiers of COVID-19*,
https://doi.org/10.1007/978-3-031-08045-6

## C

**Q**



**R**

## S

GPSR Compliance

*The European Union's (EU) General Product Safety Regulation (GPSR) is a set of rules that requires consumer products to be safe and our obligations to ensure this.*

*If you have any concerns about our products, you can contact us on ProductSafety@springernature.com*

In case Publisher is established outside the EU, the EU authorized representative is:

Springer Nature Customer Service Center GmbH
Europaplatz 3
69115 Heidelberg, Germany

**Batch number: 10732064**

Printed by Printforce, the Netherlands